Blindness, Visual
Impairment, Deaf-Blindness:
Annotated Listing of the
Literature, 1953–75

Blindness, Visual Impairment, Deaf-Blindness

Annotated Listing of the Literature, 1953–75

Compiled by
Mary K. Bauman

Ahmed ElShami, Index Consultant

Carol A. Kropf, Editor

Carla deHaas, Coordinator

Temple University Press
Philadelphia

Temple University Press, Philadelphia 19122
© 1976 by Temple University. All rights reserved
Published 1976
Developed under a grant to Temple University from Nevil Trust Funds,
    Philadelphia, Pennsylvania
A Bicentennial Activity
Printed in the United States of America

International Standard Book Number: 0-87722-067-0
Library of Congress Catalog Card Number: 76-14724

Preface

The first significant attempt to list nonmedical literature related to visual impairment was made by Helga Lende in her *Books about the Blind*, published by the American Foundation for the Blind in 1953. This book, which includes a number of listings in foreign languages as well as most of the professional literature printed in the English language, is still a classic in the field and should be consulted by the student interested in material published prior to 1953. Almost none of this material is included in the present publication.

A second listing of literature about blindness was made in the form of a dictionary card catalogue by Isabella S. Diamond under a grant from the Department of Health, Education, and Welfare to the American Association of Workers for the Blind. Unfortunately, problems inherent in the card catalogue itself and a seriously limited distribution of the catalogue resulted in great frustration for scholars and practitioners who needed easy access to the growing literature in the field of blindness. The supporting grant was discontinued in mid-1972, so that even the rare library or agency which possesses a Dictionary Card Catalogue has no way of keeping it up to date except by its own individual efforts.

To fill this gap, and in response to a strongly expressed need in the Philadelphia area for a reference library on blindness and deafness, the Nevil Trust Funds have provided a grant to Temple University. The Nevil Reference Library and Resource Center for Sensory Disabilities, providing access to many of the documents here described, is housed in the Paley Library on the campus of Temple University in Philadelphia.

This book is the second product of the grant of the Nevil Trust Funds to Temple University. An advisory committee representing professionals and consumers was appointed by the presidents of the Association for Education of the Visually Handicapped and the American Association of Workers for the Blind. After much consideration, this committee recommended that the card catalogue be replaced by a single publication more complete yet more compact, more readily housed in the student's library, and easily accessible through author and content indexes. This volume grew out of that recommendation.

Beginning with 1976, the relevant literature will be listed and annotated in semiannual issues of a periodical of similar name, made possible by a grant from the Rauch Foundation. This book and the periodical match in form and index. The periodical is intended to represent a constant updating of this book.

Thus it is hoped that through the Nevil Reference Library at Temple University, through Lende's *Books about the Blind*, through this publication, and through the continuing periodical, the student, the research worker, the professional in the field, and the layman can find easy access to the printed information about the nonmedical aspects of blindness and visual impairment.

For much larger, older, and more complete library collections, the scholar is referred to the two famous American libraries in the field of blindness: The M. C. Migel Memorial Library of the American Foundation for the Blind in New York City, and the Library of Perkins School for the Blind, including the Samuel P. Hayes Memorial Library, in Watertown, Massachusetts.

Acknowledgments

It seems impossible that a year ago the thought of producing this book had not yet taken shape. Within a span of nine months, the small staff of Nevil Interagency Referral Service has researched and annotated the documents listed here, organized them within broad groupings, learned from a kind but firm master teacher, Ahmed ElShami, how to index the material, and produced the finished manuscript. How monumental our task was, we could not appreciate at its inception since our best advice was that the number of documents available for listing was far smaller than it proved to be.

The work could not have been accomplished without the cooperation and support of many people. Those whose names appear on the title page were the key figures, among whom I would especially like to thank Carol Kropf, whose devotion to the task has gone far beyond the call of duty. Other NIRS staff who have made great contributions are Evelyn Paslawski and William Bauman.

For sound advice, representing professionals and consumers, we owe a debt of gratitude to the two men who were presidents of American Association of Workers for the Blind during this period, Robert H. Whitstock and Harold G. Roberts, and to the president of Association for Education of the Visually Handicapped, Ferne R. Roberts. They selected and appointed our Advisory Committee, which developed the guidelines for this publication: Bruce Blasch, Michael Coyle, Eleanor Dym, Vahram Kashmanian, Michael Monbeck, Ralph Peabody, Judy Sharko, Elaine Siegel, and Etheldra Templeton.

The cooperation of representatives of Temple University has smoothed the path toward publication so that we feel most warmly toward them. Our special thank you goes to Dr. Nettie Bartel, Dr. Edward P. Adkins, and Dr. Millard Gladfelter, who facilitated the entire contact with Temple University.

Above all, we are grateful to Louis Rives, chairman of the Nevil Advisory Committee, whose awareness of the needs in the field of blindness made him supportive to this project and whose advice at its inception was invaluable.

Mary K. Bauman
March 26, 1976

Contents

How to Use This Book

Scope

This book is intended to serve individuals who have some serious concern about blindness, visual impairment, or related topics. Such individuals are not necessarily professional workers, but they want information in greater depth than can be found in the typical newspaper article or popular journal. Consequently, newspapers and popular journals have not been reviewed to identify documents for listing in this book even though excellent material on our subject does occasionally appear in these media.

Since medical literature is well indexed through *Index Medicus* and since, in most cases, it appeals to a different readership, it has not been included.

With the exception of a mere handful of books which are regarded as foundations of the literature on blindness, all documents listed were published between 1953 and 1975.

Documents published prior to 1953 are listed in *Books about the Blind* by Helga Lende (American Foundation for the Blind, 1953). The scholar seeking older material should consult *Books about the Blind*.

Since there is always some lag between the publication of a document and its listing in professional abstracts or indexes, some material published in 1975 may not have been known to us when this volume went to press. That literature will be annotated and indexed in the periodical *Blindness, Visual Impairment, Deaf-Blindness: Semiannual Listing of Current Literature*, of which the first volume will appear in 1976.

Although fully recognizing the great professional contributions made by the associations of and for the blind, visually handicapped, and deaf-blind, and by agencies serving the field, it has not seemed appropriate to include in this listing articles chiefly concerned about the business, meetings, special projects, personnel, or financial reports of those associations and agencies. Such information can be readily found in their reports and publications, usually available directly from their central offices. Under Associations and Agencies will be found a list of the names and addresses of the larger associations and agencies serving the English-speaking countries.

Because of their restricted and specialized nature, most dissertations have been excluded from this listing. The student interested in such material is referred to *Dissertation Abstracts International,* available in most large libraries.

Other esoteric materials, such as papers delivered at meetings, masters' theses, and special reports, few of which are listed in this publication, may appear on bibliographies serving very specific interests. A number of these bibliographies are listed in this book, and the student seeking in-depth coverage is strongly urged to consult them.

We regret that considerations of time and space forbade listing by author and title every paper presented in conference reports but, to the extent that they were available to us, many conference reports have been listed as single units. The student is referred to such conference reports as very likely to include excellent papers on current topics.

In selecting the documents to be listed, an effort was made to include all material of evident professional value. However, the compiler has probably made the human error of omitting some documents either through oversight or because she believed their content was more currently available in some later publication. We apologize to those who may seek a favorite article and not find it listed here.

Listing and annotation are for record and reference only and do not constitute an endorsement or evaluation of any document.

Arrangement

The contents of this book have been arranged in four sections: Annotated Listing (chapters 1–35), Associations and Agencies, Author Index, Analytical Subject Index.

Annotated Listing

Division of the annotated listing into major content sections (chapters 1–35) is intended especially for the novice in the field of blindness who is seeking a general overview of the literature available. The Contents will guide the reader to the broad interest areas with which he is most concerned. Since no document is listed more than once, and since many documents might with logic be placed under several of the chapter headings, the decision upon placement of a specific document is admittedly colored by the experience of the compiler.

Following each chapter heading, documents appear alphabetically by author and, for any particular author, by chronology of publication.

Documents are numbered in the order of their appearance in the book, and it is document numbers only which appear in the Author and Analytical Subject Indexes.

A quick way to get a rough picture of what is available in your area of interest is to skim the contents of the chapter or chapters which appear most relevant to your concern. This will provide an estimate of the amount of literature produced between 1953 and 1975 on your topic of interest and perhaps disclose a few titles which seem particularly promising reading.

Associations and Agencies

Rather more than has traditionally been true for other disability groups, blind people and professionals serving blind people have tended to band together in associations. Those with national scope in this country, Canada, and Great Britain are listed in this part.

Visually impaired and deaf-blind people are served by a very large number of agencies and schools, many on a local level, many at the state level, and a few providing nationwide service. The older and larger agencies which serve on a nationwide basis in United States, Canada, and Great Britain are included.

Letters to any or all of these associations and agencies will provide the inquirer with a wealth of information about them and, if reviewed longitudinally, would provide raw data for a rather complete history of work with the blind and deaf-blind.

Author Index

If you know the names of writers who have addressed their work to your particular concern, turn to the Author Index. Following each name are the numbers of the documents authored or coauthored by that person.

Analytical Subject Index

This index offers an analysis of the contents of the documents shown in the annotated listing. Some documents have been indexed under four or five different subject headings.

The Analytical Subject Index is arranged by subject headings in alphabetical order; subheadings are arranged alphabetically under the subject headings. Following each heading are the numbers of the documents in the chapters that refer to that subject. The subject headings are in capital letters, with subheadings in capital and lower-case letters. Documents listed under general headings, i.e., preceding the subheads, have been so listed because they include more than one of the subheads; therefore, all general heading documents should be considered in order to get thorough coverage of the area.

Abbreviations and Symbols

AFB	American Foundation for the Blind
app.	publication contains appendix or appendices
Bib.	publication contains a bibliography
Comp(s).	Compiler(s)
Ed(s).	Editor(s)
illus.	publication includes illustrations—diagrams, drawings, photographs, etc.
Mimeo.	publication is mimeographed
n.d.	no publication date given
n.p.	no place of publication given
O & M	orientation and mobility
Proj. Dir.	Project Director
Ref.	publication contains a number of references
rev. ed.	revised edition
$S(s)$	subject(s)
Trans.	Translator
VA	Veterans Administration
wpm	words per minute
–	following first three digits of calendar year, indicates uncertainty of year of publication, but presumes publication in decade indicated
?	following date, indicates presumption, but not certainty, that year indicated is year of publication

Blindness, Visual Impairment, Deaf-Blindness: Annotated Listing of the Literature, 1953–75

1. General and Historical: The Broad Field

1. **American Assoc. of Workers for the Blind.** *Blindness 1964.* Washington, D.C.: Author, 1964, 175 pp.

   Annual publication covering: Government-sponsored research, Mary E. Switzer & C. Warren Bledsoe; welfare, Wilbur J. Cohen; aging, Douglas C. MacFarland; definition of blindness, Richard E. Hoover; mobility, Martha J. Ball; world organization, M. Robert Barnett; AAWB history, Norman M. Yoder.

2. ———. *Blindness 1965.* Washington, D.C.: Author, 1965, 188 pp.

   Annual publication covering: Randolph-Sheppard Act, Jennings Randolph; World Council for the Welfare of the Blind, Berthold Lowenfeld; rehabilitation centers, C. Warren Bledsoe, Russell C. Williams, H. Kenneth Fitzgerald, & J. Albert Asenjo; treatment of blindness, David Paton; performance tests of intelligence, Mary K. Bauman & Susan C. Mullen; blindness statistics, John Wilson; library services, Robert S. Bray; government-sponsored research, Mary E. Switzer & C. Warren Bledsoe; personnel training, Margaret Ryan; and reprint of an address by Samuel Gridley Howe.

3. ———. *Blindness 1966.* Washington, D.C.: Author, 1966, 235 pp.

   Annual publication covering: Law, Louis J. Rives; deaf-blind, Peter J. Salmon & Herbert Rusalem; Canada, E. A. Baker & Marjorie Campbell; education and rehabilitation, Salvatore G. DiMichael; Israel, Berthold Lowenfeld; placement, George A. Magers; Randolph-Sheppard Act, Joseph F. Clunk; funding, George G. Mallinson; sensory aids, Howard Freiberger; library services, Robert S. Bray; government-sponsored research, Mary E. Switzer & C. Warren Bledsoe; and a reprint from Diderot.

4. ———. *Blindness 1967.* Washington, D.C.: Author, 1967, 199 pp.

   Annual publication covering: Agency philosophy, George Werntz; compressed speech, Emerson Foulke; the arts, Mary E. Switzer; eye institute, Thomas D. Duane; international program, Joseph M. LaRocca; anthology, C. Warren Bledsoe; multiply handicapped, Lawrence Goodman; teacher training, Georgie Lee Abel; government-sponsored research, Mary E. Switzer & C. Warren Bledsoe; and reprints from Maurice de la Sizeranne and Valentin Hauy.

5. ———. *Blindness 1968.* Washington, D.C.: Author, 1968, 183 pp.

   Annual publication covering: Canada, Paul C. O'Neill; SRS philosophy and function, Mary E. Switzer; statistics, Theodore D. Woolsey & Ronald

Wilson; architecture, F. Cuthbert Salmon & Christine F. Salmon; aural reading, Robert S. Bray & Edward S. Steffen; psychiatry, H. Robert Blank; Valley Forge story, Richard E. Hoover; public relations, Robert H. Whitstock; eye bank, R. Townley Paton; workshops, Henry C. Seward; Shotwell awardees, C. Warren Bledsoe; government-sponsored research, Mary E. Switzer & C. Warren Bledsoe; and reprint from Robert B. Irwin.

6. ———. *Blindness 1969.* Washington, D.C.: Author, 1969, 207 pp.

Annual publication covering: Counseling, Clayton A. Morgan; interprofessional communication, W. Alfred McCauley; diabetic blindness, Arnall Patz; Royal National Institute, John C. Colligan; state agencies, George A. Magers; South America, Richard Kinney; mobility, C. Warren Bledsoe; historians, James J. Barnes; Hawaii, Elizabeth H. Morrison; government-sponsored research, Mary E. Switzer & C. Warren Bledsoe; reprints from Edward E. Allen.

7. ———. *Blindness 1970.* Washington, D.C.: Author, 1970, 245 pp.

Annual publication covering: National Eye Institute, Carl Kupfer; causes of blindness, Roy O. Scholz; rubella, Powrie V. Doctor; South Vietnam, Rodney J. Kossick; mobility, John D. Malamazian; war-blinded, Baynard Kendrick; optometry, Sterling B. Brickley; optical aids, Ruth Heron; communication aids, Charles E. Hallenbeck; an interview and government-sponsored research, Mary E. Switzer & C. Warren Bledsoe; and reprints from the past.

8. ———. *Blindness 1971.* Washington, D.C.: Author, 1971, 242 pp.

Annual publication covering: Poetry, Richard Kinney & Robert J. Smithdas; mobility, Donald Blasch & Ruth Kaarlela; residential schools, C. Warren Bledsoe; counseling, G. D. Carnes; advice about college, Betty Bird and students; counseling, Clayton A. Morgan; financial aid, George A. Magers & Stanton C. Craigie; emotionally disturbed, Mary K. Bauman; retarded, Joanne M. Davidoff; volunteer transcribers, Mary S. Bradley; international grants, Martin E. McCavitt; government-sponsored research; and reprint from the past.

9. ———. *Blindness 1972.* Washington, D.C.: Author, 1972, 223 pp.

Annual publication covering: AAIB, Francis M. Andrews & C. Warren Bledsoe; musicians, George G. Mallinson & Jacqueline V. Mallinson; mobile medical service, Paul C. O'Neill; mobility, Richard L. Welsh; library services, Charles Gallozzi; activation of mobility program, Daniel N. Head; psychological testing, Mary K. Bauman; typewriter and education, Donald J. Wonderling; and government-sponsored research.

10. ———. *Blindness 1973.* Washington, D.C.: Author, 1973, 124 pp.

Annual publication covering: Library services, Frank K. Cylke; mobility, William R. Wiener & Everett Hill; service delivery, Joseph Kohn; diabetes, Arnall Patz; the server and the served, W. Payton Kolb; Perkins brailler, Edward J. Waterhouse; reprints from the past; and government-sponsored research.

11. ———. *Blindness 1974–75.* Washington, D.C.: Author, 1975, 141 pp.

Annual publication including: Nature of blindness, Berthold Lowenfeld; lawyers, Peter Putnam; deaf-blind, Frank Lasky, also Peter J. Salmon; genetic counseling, H. E. Cross; papers on low vision services by Loyal

E. Apple, Randall T. Jose, Pat Carpenter, Clare M. Hood, Eleanor E. Faye, Beth Phillips, Roy J. Ward, & J. J. Hennessy; and a reprint on rehabilitation codes.

12. ———. *Contemporary papers, Volume I.* Washington, D.C.: Author, 1966, 23 pp.

Papers on the following topics: Value of vision as a sense, Richard E. Hoover; nursing the blind, C. Warren Bledsoe & Russell C. Williams; services from voluntary sector, Isabella S. Diamond; social isolation, Douglas C. MacFarland.

13. ———. *Contemporary papers, Volume VI: A group of discussion papers.* Washington, D.C.: Author, 1970, 38 pp.

Papers on varied topics by Joseph Kohn, Gerard J. DeAngelis, Constance Gant, William Cornwell, & Kenneth Z. Altshuler.

14. American Foundation for the Blind. *Blindness at home and abroad.* New York: Author, 1956, 16 pp.

Rather general descriptions of incidence and causes of blindness, education, rehabilitation, and services in U.S. with brief comparisons abroad.

15. ———. *Proceedings of the West Coast Regional Conference on Research Related to Blind and Severely Visually Impaired Children.* New York: Author, 1965, 156 pp.

Includes papers on demography and causes of blindness, educational research, and orientation and mobility research.

16. ———. *Who is the visually handicapped child?* New York: Author, 1969, 12 pp.

Nature and incidence and types of educational programs.

17. ———. *Index of publications issued by International Research Information Service through Summer 1970.* New York: Author, 1970, 38 pp.

Outlines proceedings of several conferences on the visually handicapped between 1964 and 1968. Indexing by definitions, psychological and attitudinal studies and surveys, mobility, communications, sensory studies, and medical studies.

18. Anderson, Paul H. *Statistics on blindness in the Model Reporting Area, 1968.* Washington, D.C.: Govt. Printing Office, 1971, 66 pp., 65¢.

Presents statistics on blindness in the Model Reporting Area (MRA) for Blindness Statistics, a voluntary association of 16 states which maintain registers of blind persons.

19. Attleweed, George, et al., Eds. *Sensory disabilities study group report.* Calif. Conference on Rehabilitation, October 8–10, 1974. n.p., n.d., v + 100 pp.

Discusses sensory disabilities presentation demonstrating that deaf and blind can plan and work together. Topics include: Sensory aids, higher education, legislation, needs of multiply handicapped. Ten papers.

20. Barraga, Natalie C. International Conference of Educators of Blind Youth—1972. *Education of the Visually Handicapped,* Oct. 1972, Vol. 4, No. 3, pp. 91–93.

Briefly summarized are the conference proceedings and resolutions. Provides paper titles but not the papers themselves.

21. Best, Harry. *Blindness and the blind in the United States.* New York: Macmillan, 1934, 714 pp.
One of the early classics in the field.

22. Bledsoe, C. Warren. The "typhlo-" words. *New Outlook for the Blind,* Mar. 1969, Vol. 63, No. 3, pp. 89–93.
Presents with sense of humor some of the vocabulary problems of the field of blindness, with special attention to "typhlology."

23. ————. Gearing to meet the challenge of the decade. *New Outlook for the Blind,* Apr. 1971, Vol. 65, No. 4, pp. 105–7, 116.
An inspirational talk for workers with the blind.

24. ————. The state of blindness; its counselors of state; and its citizens. *Rehabilitation Record,* Mar.–Apr. 1972, Vol. 13, No. 2, pp. 11–13. Also in *New Beacon,* Aug. 1972.
Excerpt from keynote address to Mid-Atlantic Regional Conference of the American Assoc. of Workers for the Blind, Sept. 1970.

25. Bonner, Ruth E., & Lovett, Mary E. *The visually limited child.* New York: MSS Educational Publishing, 1970, 74 pp., $2.50.
Recounts historical background of blindness, milestones in treatment, and important personages in the education of the blind. Discusses structure of the eye and visual defects. Also has a general discussion of the organization and administration of special educational facilities for the visually handicapped. Glossary.

26. Bourgeault, Stanley E. Blindness—a label. *Education of the Visually Handicapped,* Mar. 1974, Vol. 6, No. 1, pp. 1–6.
Examines cultural patterns, issues, and trends associated with proposed changes in the labeling and classification of blind people.

27. ————, **Ed.** *Glossary of professional terms.* Malaysia: American Foundation for Overseas Blind, 1969, 56 pp.
A short glossary compiled to facilitate interchange of information and understanding of reports and other professional literature.

28. Bowley, Agatha H., & Gardner, Leslie. *The handicapped child: Educational and psychological guidance for the organically handicapped.* 3rd ed. Baltimore: Williams & Wilkins, 1972, 203 pp., $8.25.
Each chapter on a type of handicap considers incidence, causes, and lists relevant organizations, literature, and references.

29. Carroll, Thomas J. Tin cups and free rides. *New Outlook for the Blind,* June 1954, Vol. 48, No. 6, pp. 192–94.
Free transportation emphasizes the concept of blind persons as afflicted and dependent, separate from the rest of society.

30. ————. Developing public understanding about the blind. *New Outlook for the Blind,* Oct. 1954, Vol. 48, No. 8, pp. 259–66.
Developing public understanding is impossible until workers in the field develop their own understanding and full acceptance of blind people. Often, the staff needs therapy, not just admonitions. Publicity must conform to helping the blind person take his place in the community and the words used in publicity must be chosen carefully.

31. ————. The philosophy of the rights of the individual. *New Outlook for the Blind,* Jan. 1956, Vol. 50, No. 1, pp. 3–7.

Relates to workshops specifically and the social philosophy on which they are based, their purpose, and whom they should serve. Depends on whether a training shop or a terminal shop. Workers have right to organize, be trained, and placed outside the shop—the right to rehabilitation.

32. ————. On integration. *New Outlook for the Blind*, Dec. 1959, Vol. 53, No. 10, pp. 371–73.

Rather general and philosophical discussion of the meaning and importance of integration in our society.

33. ————. *Blindness: What it is, what it does, and how to live with it.* Boston: Little, Brown, 1961, 382 pp.

A rehabilitation guide for the blinded and those working with them. Discusses loss of basic skills, psychological security, and occupation, and how to restore or substitute for these losses. Considers congenitally blind, multiply handicapped, and partially sighted, and discusses organized work for the blind.

34. **Charen, Thelma G.** Blind and blindness: An etymological note. *American Journal of Ophthalmology*, 1953, Vol. 36, pp. 839–40.

Derivation of words referring to blindness in various languages stem from words meaning darkness.

35. **Committee on Statistics of the Blind.** Revision of the standard classification of the causes of blindness. *New Outlook for the Blind*, Nov. 1957, Vol. 51, No. 9, pp. 421–24.

Short report of the committee activity and the actual classification by site and type of affection, and by etiology.

36. **Cutsforth, Thomas D.** *The blind in school and society.* New York: AFB, 1951, 269 pp.

Reissued manual presented as a pioneer work in the study of the mental and emotional problems of the blind, laying the foundations for a social psychology of the blind. Chapters discuss the preschool blind child, inadequate social and motor development, verbalisms, the fantasy life of the blind, and speech defects.

37. ————. Are we truly part of the community? *New Outlook for the Blind*, Apr. 1961, Vol. 55, No. 4, pp. 121–25.

A blind M.D.-psychologist feels that blind persons are better off participating in existing activities with sighted people than forming their own exclusive groups.

38. ————. Are we truly part of the community? *American Foundation for the Blind Research Bulletin 12*, Jan. 1966, pp. 69–75.

Takes position that blind people should be concerned with the problems of all people, the improvement of the total community. Until they stop concentrating on the problems of blindness, they will not be part of the community.

39. **Dickinson, Raymond M.** The humanitarian spirit in work for the blind. *New Outlook for the Blind*, Nov. 1953, Vol. 47, No. 9, pp. 264–70.

The humanitarian spirit is a necessary component of, and in fact the primary reason for, work for the blind, why it is in danger of being lost, and what can be done about this.

40. DiMichael, Salvatore G. The value of research in the field of blindness. *New Outlook for the Blind*, Jan. 1965, Vol. 59, No. 1, pp. 21–23.

Whereas 10 or more years ago the small amount of research done was privately financed, government now recognizes the value of research by providing significant sums of public money for it. Calls for an organized, total-group involvement in the support and effective use of research.

41. Evensen, Richard H. Factors in integration. *New Outlook for the Blind*, Mar. 1957, Vol. 51, No. 3, pp. 120–22.

Three groups must work together for true integration: The public, blind persons, and workers with the blind.

42. Farrell, Gabriel. *The story of blindness.* Cambridge, Mass.: Harvard Univ. Press, 1956, 270 pp.

Historical development, changing attitudes, and present statement of awareness and treatment of blindness.

43. Ferree, John W. The blind population: 1967–1977. *New Outlook for the Blind*, Nov. 1967, Vol. 61, No. 9, pp. 290–95, 308. Reprinted from *Sight-Saving Review*, Fall 1967.

How predictions of incidence of blindness are made, factors which might result in changes, and projections of incidence figures for 1977.

44. Fitzsimmons, Ellen. *It's about time visual impairments came out into the open.* Madison: Univ. of Wis., Center for Studies in Vocational & Technical Educ., 1975, 18 pp., illus.

Discusses definitions of blindness and visual impairment, considering causes and effects of each. Also discusses special problems, benefits, classroom aids, and employment opportunities. Bib.

45. Flemming, Arthur S. Welfare activities on the defensive. *New Outlook for the Blind*, Sept. 1962, Vol. 56, No. 7, pp. 240–42.

Discusses residence laws, unemployment, welfare achievements, and social work in relationship to a rehabilitative service.

46. Fonda, Gerald. Definition and classification of blindness with respect to ability to use residual vision. *New Outlook for the Blind*, May 1961, Vol. 55, No. 5, pp. 169–72.

Proposes detailed standards for judging blindness. Says overall intelligence and other factors must be considered, as well as visual acuity.

47. Fraser, G. R., & Friedmann, A. I. *The causes of blindness in childhood.* Baltimore: Johns Hopkins Press, 1967, 245 pp., illus., $12.

Report of results of a clinical and genetic study of 776 children with severe visual handicaps. In each case the cause of blindness was diagnosed as exactly as possible. Resulting data was subjected to statistical analysis in an attempt to define the roles and relative importance of heredity and environment in childhood blindness.

48. French, Richard S. *From Homer to Helen Keller: A social and educational study of the blind.* New York: AFB, 1932, 298 pp.

One of the early histories of the field.

49. Fried, Joseph J. Problems, care, and rehabilitation of blind and almost blind. *New York State Journal of Medicine*, 1968, Vol. 68, No. 20, pp. 2690–96.

Reviews recent statistics concerning age and race of the blind, and causes of blindness. Also discusses organizations for care and rehabilitation of the blind, schools for them, and aids which are available.

50. Froelich, Walter. That the sightless may see. *World Health*, Aug.–Sept. 1972, pp. 12–17.

Causes of blindness. What WHO is doing about it. Discussions of various devices that can help sightless, Optacon, Braille-emboss, folding cane, etc.

51. Genensky, Samuel M. *A functional classification system of the visually impaired to replace the legal definition of blindness.* Santa Monica, Calif.: Rand Corp., 1970, 26 pp.

Basis of a proposed new system is the capacity of the visually impaired to perform normal tasks. Author makes recommendations which he believes would clarify impairments, improve public understanding of the capabilities and needs of the visually handicapped, improve the quality and quantity of services and increase educational and economic opportunities.

52. George, Nolene H., & McPhee, William M. The isolation of the rural blind adults in Utah. *American Foundation for the Blind Research Bulletin 7*, Dec. 1964, pp. 63–70.

A study of the social characteristics, mobility, activities, and interests of 291 blind adults in Utah.

53. Gill, J. M., Comp. *International register of research on blindness and visual impairment.* Coventry, England: Warwick Research Unit f/t Blind, 1975, £5. (Also in braille.)

Covers research in natural, behavioral and technological sciences bearing on problems arising from sensory impairment, and especially visual impairment.

54. Gill, J. M., & Tobin, M. J., Comps. *European register of research on visual impairment.* Birmingham, England: Birmingham Univ. Research Center f/t Education of the Visually Handicapped, 1974, 27 pp.

This register of research currently underway contains a scan-column index of approximately 60 research topics and an alphabetical list of 204 research workers including postal addresses and a brief description of the current research project of each. Examples of projects: Evaluation of closed-circuit television aids, spatial organization in blindness, development of program to teach blind children to read embossed maps.

55. Goldberg, Maxwell H., & Swinton, John R., Eds. *Blindness research: The expanding frontiers: A liberal studies perspective.* University Park: Pa. State Univ. Press, 1969, 544 pp., $12.50.

Papers presented at a national conference on research on blindness including the following areas: Parent-child relationships, old age, childhood and adolescence, motivation, education. Also discusses stress and reaction to loss, counseling, the agency and the person, placement and occupation, multiply handicapped blind.

56. Goldstein, Harris K. Guidelines for obtaining funds for training, services, and research. *New Outlook for the Blind*, Nov. 1968, Vol. 62, No. 9, pp. 270–76.

Procedures for obtaining grants are often misunderstood. Describes these procedures in some detail: Selecting an appropriate source of fund-ing, content of the application, screening of applications by the grantor with the possibility of different kinds of approval.

57. Goldstein, Hyman. So that all may see. *New Outlook for the Blind,* Nov. 1964, Vol. 58, No. 9, pp. 280–84.

Discussion of difficulties in obtaining statistics relating to the blind. Information on reporting program and other work of the Biometrics Branch of the National Institute of Neurological Diseases and Blindness.

58. ———. Role of blindness statistics in prevention and control. *New Outlook for the Blind,* Sept. 1966, Vol. 60, No. 7, pp. 205–9.

Lack of comparability of international data on incidence of blindness might be improved by a concise record form allowing delineation of ocular conditions leading to blindness. Statistical discussion of geriatric and younger blind indicates importance of prevention for latter.

59. ———. *The demography and causes of blindness.* New York: AFB, June 1968, 103 pp.

Outlines difficulties of collecting and comparing statistics on incidence, prevalence, and causes of blindness. Thirty-three tables of blindness statistics are included.

60. Goldstein, Hyman, & Josephson, E. The social demography of vision impairment in the United States. *Public Health Reviews,* Jan.–Mar. 1975, Vol. 4, No. 1, pp. 5–38.

Describes major social and health characteristics based primarily on 16-state register and sample examinations and interviews. Problems in defining and measuring prevalence of vision impairment also discussed.

61. Gowman, Alan G. *The war blind in American social structure.* New York: AFB, 1957, xv + 237 pp.

A sociopsychological analysis of the behavior patterns of the war-blinded. Bib.

62. Graham, Earl C., & Mullen, Marjorie M., Comps. *Rehabilitation Literature 1950–1955,* New York: McGraw-Hill, 1956, 621 pp.

Includes 21 pages of references on blindness with comprehensive annotations.

63. Graham, Milton D. Toward a functional definition of blindness. *New Outlook for the Blind,* Oct. 1959, Vol. 53, No. 8, pp. 285–88.

Varying definitions of blindness result in widely varied estimates of the incidence of blindness and make sound planning for services difficult.

64. ———. *Social research on blindness: Present status and future potentials.* New York: AFB, 1960, 177 pp.

Analyzes characteristics of the literature of social research on blindness, providing statistical evidence of areas of research activity and the kinds of literature resulting from the activity. Lists specific research projects in some detail. Provides lengthy reference lists, many annotated.

65. ———, Ed. *Science and blindness: Retrospective and prospective.* New York: AFB, 1972, 212 pp., $3.75.

Selected readings. Among the areas covered are demography of blindness, psychosocial research, education, evaluation, professional preparation of the visually impaired, the blindness delivery system, nonvisual information processing, orientation, reading, and cognition.

66. Graham, Milton D., & Clark, Leslie L. Trends of the research and development process on the sensorily impaired: Europe and U.S.A. 1966. *American Foundation for the Blind Research Bulletin 14*, Mar. 1967, pp. 1–30.

A state-of-the-art report about trends of research and development on sensory impairment and the behavioral effects of such impairment. Concludes that European view of rehabilitation is much broader than simply returning the individual to employment. Ref.

67. ———. Trends of the research and development process on the sensorily impaired—Part one. *New Outlook for the Blind*, Nov. 1968. Vol. 62, No. 9, pp. 265–69. 1st of 2-part article adapted from longer one in *Research Bulletin 14*.

Describes research and development process as having 6 steps: Posing problem, evolution of experimental design, seeking financial support, presenting reports, trial with controlled evaluation, and delineation of techniques affecting practice.

68. ———. Trends of the research and development process on the sensorily impaired—Part two. *New Outlook for the Blind*, Dec. 1968, Vol. 62, No. 10, pp. 301–6. 2nd of 2-part article (Part one, Nov. 1968) adapted from longer one in *Research Bulletin 14*.

Dissemination of professional knowledge is essential but difficult. Best accomplished by personal visits among researchers, but conferences and written reports are good and include the practitioner. Training should precede evaluation of a device and application precede evaluation of of research findings.

69. Graham, Milton D.; Robinson, Robert L.; Lowrey, Austin; et al. *851 blinded veterans: A success story.* New York: AFB, 1968, 338 pp., $4.25.

Reports very detailed follow-up data, including general characteristics of the sample, family and health data, and activities. Appropriate comparisons are made with other groups. Concludes that "blindness is not an insurmountable barrier to a productive and rewarding life."

70. Gruber, Kathern F. Work with the blind: A pilot program? *New Outlook for the Blind*, Jan. 1960, Vol. 54, No. 1, pp. 18–22.

Author cites the dramatic emotional impact made upon the public by words and causes associated with blindness, stating that this situation can be exploited constructively. Review advances spurred by needs of the blind, lagging areas, personnel standards.

71. Handel, Alexander F. Principles and standards in service for the blind. *New Outlook for the Blind*, Oct. 1954, Vol. 48, No. 8, pp. 281–85.

Briefly reviews the history of concern about service standards in American Assoc. of Workers for the Blind. There is a public demand for standards and cooperation is necessary among agencies. Procedures for development of standards are suggested.

72. ———. A view of things to come: Community services for the blind, 1980. *New Outlook for the Blind*, Jan. 1960, Vol. 54, No. 1, pp. 1–11.

Following examples of progress in past 20 years, sets goals for services in 1980, including funding, vocational rehabilitation, research, and organizations of the blind. Predictions based on 3 assumptions and perspectives.

73. Hardy, Richard E., & Cull, John G. *Social and rehabilitation services* *for the blind.* Springfield, Ill.: Charles C Thomas, 1972, 403 pp., $15.75.

With many chapters by individual authors, reviews history and philosophy of work for the blind, special projects and programs. Part II discusses blindness and its impact with emphasis on attitudes and psychological factors. Part III discusses the rehabilitation process, including psychological and counseling services, occupational information and placement procedures. Part IV reviews social and educational services.

74. ————, Eds. *Mental retardation and physical disability.* Springfield, Ill.: Charles C Thomas, 1974, 250 pp., $9.75.

Intended chiefly for social workers, includes material on the visually handicapped child's attitudes, retardation in blind children, and effect of diabetes on orientation and mobility.

75. Hatfield, Elizabeth M. Causes of blindness in school children. *Sight-Saving Review,* Winter 1963, Vol. 33, No. 4, pp. 218–33.

Report of study of 7,757 legally blind children in residential and public day schools in 1958–59. Analysis of trends showed: Prevalence rate of blindness increased 81% 1951–52 (RLF); blindness due to injuries and diseases declining; blindness due to prenatal factors and unknown causes remains high.

76. ————. Estimates of blindness in the United States. *Sight-Saving Review,* Summer 1973, Vol. 43, No. 2, pp. 69–80.

Presentation of revised prevalence rates and new case rates for blindness in the entire U.S. and in each individual state.

77. ————. Why are they blind? *Sight-Saving Review,* Spring 1975, Vol. 45, No. 1, pp. 3–22.

Latest in a series of studies undertaken by the National Society for the Prevention of Blindness for children enrolled in residential schools for the blind and public schools during 1968–69. The studies have provided valuable information on the most important problems to be dealt with in preventing blindness in this age group.

78. ————, Comp. *Estimated statistics on blindness and vision problems.* New York: National Society for the Prevention of Blindness, 1966, illus.

Estimates and some trend data are presented on the following subjects: Population growth (1940–60), and prevalence of legal blindness, new cases of legal blindness, age distribution of legally blind persons, causes of legal blindness, changing patterns in causes of legal blindness, cases of glaucoma, school children needing eye care, partially seeing school children, and eye injuries to school children. Ref., glossary.

79. Held, Marian. The challenge of change—Are you prepared? *New Outlook for the Blind,* Oct. 1963, Vol. 57, No. 8, pp. 302–7.

Discusses developments over the past 30 years, specific areas for further development including psychological testing, low vision lens clinic, vending stands, transcribing-typing, the field of music and piano tuning. Cites need to design programs with flexibility.

80. Hoover, Richard E. A new look at the definition of blindness. *Optometric Weekly,* 1958, Vol. 49, pp. 1227–32.

Discussion of 1955 AMA statement on the "appraisal of loss of visual acuity."

81. **Hurlin, Ralph G.** Estimated prevalence of blindness in the United States. *New Outlook for the Blind*, Sept. 1953, Vol. 47, No. 7, pp. 189–96.

Defines blindness and gives method for estimating prevalence in each state. Table of estimates by state as of July 1952. Reviews N.C. Census of Blind Persons.

82. **Jernigan, Kenneth.** Blindness: Handicap or characteristic? *New Outlook for the Blind*, Sept. 1965, Vol. 59, No. 7, pp. 244–49.

Argues that blindness is not a handicap, that its handicapping effects actually come from social attitudes. Decisions should be made by the blind person himself.

83. **Jones, John W.** Problems in defining and classifying blindness. *New Outlook for the Blind*, Apr. 1962, Vol. 56, No. 4, pp. 115–21.

Discusses old idea that use of remaining vision by visually impaired caused further loss. Discusses seeking new guidelines based on mode of reading and visual acuity and refining selection and dismissal processes for special classes. Suggests need for realistic definitions and guidelines for educational classification of the visually handicapped.

84. **Josephson, Eric.** Screening for visual impairment. *American Foundation for the Blind Research Bulletin 14*, Mar. 1967, pp. 139–50. Reprinted from *Public Health Reports*, Jan. 1965.

Compares results of telephone and face-to-face interviews about presence of visual impairment. Concludes that telephone interviews are equally dependable to determine crude rates of visual impairment but must be supplemented by a sample of nontelephone households because of important demographic differences between telephone and nontelephone populations.

85. **Kahn, Harold A., & Moorhead, Helen B.** *Statistics on blindness in the Model Reporting Area 1969–1970.* Washington, D.C.: Dept. of Health, Education & Welfare, Public Health Service, National Institute of Health, 1973, 149 pp., $2.10.

Presents statistics in 16 states in 30 tables including cause of blindness and demographic information.

86. **Kans. State Dept. of Education.** *A study of the visually impaired young people of Kansas and a review of educational services.* Topeka: State Dept. of Social & Rehabilitation Services, 1974, 74 pp.

Reports study of 708 Kansans up to 21 years of age. Includes descriptions of legal provisions, residential and home care, rationale for residential care, sample questionnaire, and brief discussion of normalization principle.

87. **Knudson, A. B. C.** The blinded veteran in the United States. *New Outlook for the Blind*, May 1955, Vol. 49, No. 5, pp. 176–78.

Rather general discussion of procedures and accomplishments in the rehabilitation of blinded veterans with some comparison with what has been done in England.

88. **Kozier, Ada.** Human welfare in the next half century. *New Outlook for the Blind*, June 1964, Vol. 58, No. 6, pp. 181–82.

Development of social welfare services in general. Role of specialized agencies for the blind.

89. Langdon, J. N. Services for blind children and young persons. *New Beacon*, June 1971, Vol. 55, No. 650, pp. 142–48.

Study of case histories and interviews with parents of visually handicapped children and with mature teenagers and young adults yields information about services available to them in England. Suggests ophthalmological referral to appropriate local agency for nonmedical counseling. Table on attitudes of young adults' feelings on social and occupational activities in which they participate.

90. Lende, Helga. *What of the blind? A survey of the development and scope of present-day work with the blind.* New York: AFB, 1938, 214 pp. Vol. II, 1941, 206 pp.

A collection of papers by experts in various fields of work with the blind.

91. ———. *Books about the blind: An annotated bibliographical guide to literature relating to the blind.* New York: AFB, 1953, 357 pp.

Lists literature related to blindness through 1952, chiefly in the English language but some foreign.

92. Lewis, Carol. Alice meets a blind hatter. *New Beacon*, June 1975, Vol. 59, No. 698, pp. 147–50.

Amusing but thought-provoking commentary on terminology and integration/segregation in blindness.

93. Library of Congress, Congressional Research Service. *Key facts on the handicapped.* Washington, D.C.: Author, 1975, 32 pp.

Includes a statistical overview of the total handicapped population as well as separate sections on 4 disability groups (blind is 1) for which detailed recent statistics are available.

94. Lindqvist, B., & Trowald, N., Eds. *European conference on educational research for the visually handicapped.* Stockholm: Swedish Assoc. for the Blind, 1972, 91 pp.

Proceedings of Oct. 1971 international conference in Stockholm review research activities among British, German, Soviet, and Swedish visual impairment research centers.

95. Liska, James S. What does it mean to be "legally blind"? *New Outlook for the Blind*, Jan. 1973, Vol. 67, No. 1, pp. 19–20.

A short article from the Australian magazine *Faithfully Theirs* which defines the term "legally blind."

96. Love, Harold D. *Exceptional children in a modern society.* 2nd ed. Dubuque: Kendall/Hunt, 1967, 184 pp.

Attempt to cover the entire spectrum of exceptionalities in children aims at both graduate and undergraduate students. Includes sections dealing with the classifications, history, types, education, future possibilities of, parental attitudes toward, and special education plans for the visually handicapped.

97. Lowenfeld, Berthold. The role and status of the blind person—A historical review. *New Outlook for the Blind*, Feb. 1964, Vol. 58, No. 2, pp. 36–40.

Comprehensive discussion of noteworthy developments in blindness in past 40 years. Includes changes in social legislation, growth of organization and vocational rehabilitation for the blind, adoption of braille grade 2, advent of the talking book, growth in mobility training and use of low vision aids, work with deaf-blind, elimination of homes for blind, raising professional standards, changes in education.

98. ————. 100 years ago: The Vienna Congress of Teachers of the Blind. *New Outlook for the Blind,* Oct. 1973, Vol. 67, No. 8, pp. 337–45.

The First European Congress of Teachers of the Blind, held in Vienna, Austria, in 1873, is described. Its origin and originator, its discussion topics, and its historical importance are discussed.

99. ————. *The changing status of the blind: From separation to integration.* Springfield, Ill.: Charles C Thomas, 1975, xiv + 336 pp., $23.50.

A history of blindness, of the status of blind people from earliest history to the present, and of the social, economic, and legislative forces which have contributed to moving blind people from a condition of separation and rejection to one of moderate acceptance in the socioeconomic fabric of the U.S. Ref.

100. McPhee, William M., & Magleby, F. LeGrand. *Activities and problems of the rural blind in Utah.* Salt Lake City: Univ. of Utah Press, 1963, 45 pp.

One hundred legally blind Ss living in rural Utah were interviewed to determine: (1) Their characteristics, (2) their psychological attitudes, (3) their degree of vision, (4) how they occupied their leisure time, and (5) to make comparisons between rural blind in Utah and the blind in the AFB survey of Mass., Oreg., Minn., and N.C.

101. Morris, June E., & Nolan, Carson Y., Comps. *Bibliography of research on the visually handicapped. 1953–1971.* Louisville, Ky.: American Printing House for the Blind, 1972, 109 pp.

Covers approximately 1,300 entries published between 1953 and 1971. Only those references containing reports of empirical research on the visually handicapped are included, excluding medical research on the eye and blindness. Includes journal articles and bulletins, theses, books, and foreign publications.

102. Morrison, Elizabeth H. Characteristics of blind persons living in Hawaii. *New Outlook for the Blind,* Feb. 1964, Vol. 58, No. 2, pp. 58–60.

Vital statistics relating to characteristics of blind persons in Hawaii based on state-wide study.

103. National Center for Health Statistics. *Eye examination findings among children, United States.* Washington, D.C.: Public Health Service, HEW, 1972, 55 pp., 50¢.

The Health Examination Survey of 1963–65 reports on the prevalence of abnormal eye conditions, history of eye problems, heterophoria, test results, as well as interrelationship between eye examination and vision test results among children aged 6 to 11 years.

104. ————. Binocular visual acuity of children: Demographic and socioeconomic characteristics, United States. *Vital and Health Statistics,* Feb. 1972, Series 11, No. 112, iv + 33 pp.

Results of Health Examination Survey of 1963–65 for a probability sample of 7,317 children 6–11 years of age, presented by age, sex, race, region, size of place of residence, rate of population change in size of place 1950–60, family income, education of parents, and grade in school.

105. ————. Eye examination findings among children, United States. *Vital and Health Statistics*, June 1972, Series 11, No. 115, iv + 47 pp.

Report is subtitled "Eye examination findings, phoria test results, visual acuity, color deficiency, the history of eye trouble, and their relationship among children 6–11 years of age." Data analyzed is from the Health Examination Survey of 1963–65.

106. **National Committee for Research on Ophthalmology and Blindness.** *Proceedings of the symposium on research in blindness and severe visual impairment.* New York: Author, May 1964, 118 pp.

In Oct. 1963 specialists reported findings of studies then underway and outlined research possibilities in their agencies. Definition of blindness questioned, data sources discussed.

107. **National Institute of Neurological Diseases and Blindness.** Report of workshop on classification of causes of blindness. *American Foundation for the Blind Research Bulletin 3*, Aug. 1963, pp. 200–208.

Ophthalmologists and coders from 6 Model Reporting Area states and 3 other states discussed the difficulties in getting consistent reporting and coding of the causes of blindness. Some guidelines were developed.

108. **Nolan, Carson Y., & Morris, June E., Comps.** *Bibliography of research on the visually handicapped 1953–1967.* Louisville, Ky.: American Printing House, 1967, 59 pp.

This supplement to Lende's 1953 bibliography on research on the visually handicapped cites only articles reporting research in which empirical data were collected.

109. **Organization for Social and Technical Innovation.** *Blindness and services to the blind in the United States.* Cambridge, Mass.: OSTI Press, 1971, 212 pp.

Results of study of characteristics and problems of the blindness system in the U.S. Appended are 6 papers discussing allocation of resources to various constituencies of the blind population, rehabilitation issues, new sources for manpower in the field, the role of technology in relation to visual impairment, psychosocial problems of the blind, and the ophthalmologist's role in rehabilitation.

110. **Perkins School for the Blind.** General bibliography on blindness. Watertown, Mass.: Author, n.d., 6 pp. Mimeo.

A selected bibliography including documents available from Perkins. Also provides list of other publishers.

111. **Pollock, Franklyn J.** Survey of 200 blind veterans as to age, visual acuity and etiology. *Eye, Ear, Nose and Throat Monthly*, Feb. 1972, Vol. 51, No. 2, pp. 58–60.

Survey based on statistics compiled at the VA Outpatient Clinic in Los Angeles. The men were examined prior to rehabilitation.

112. **Riviere, Maya.** Rehabilitation codes: Code for impairment of visual function. *American Foundation for the Blind Research Bulletin 8*, Jan. 1965, pp. 45–69, app.

Presents a detailed coding system for all ages and types of visual impairment, usable by all services and agencies. Provides for classification of personal history, health history, impairment-etiology code, evaluation-service code, and cumulative record.

113. Roberts, Jean, & Duyan, Kenneth R. *Visual acuity of children.* Washington, D.C.: Govt. Printing Office, Feb. 1970, 42 pp., 45¢.

Reports findings from the Health Examination Survey (1963–65) on uncorrected monocular and binocular visual acuity levels.

114. Roberts, Jean, & Slaby, David. *Visual acuity of youths 12–17 years, United States.* Rockville, Md.: National Health Statistics, May 1973, 50 pp., 75¢.

Presents findings of national survey of 7,514 noninstitutionalized youth analyzed with respect to age, sex, race, geographic region, size of place of residence, and annual family income.

115. Robinson, Robert L. Blinded veterans today. *New Outlook for the Blind,* Oct. 1967, Vol. 61, No. 8, pp. 241–45.

Summarizes the major findings in the 1964 study published as *851 Blinded Veterans—A Success Story.* As result of these findings, VA is changing a number of policies as part of generally improved social and health services.

116. ———. *Blinded veterans of the Vietnam era.* AFB, 1973, 33 pp., $2.

Little in the way of hard facts about this group of veterans is known. This book pulls together what is known in order that information that can provide a basis for further research and the establishment of appropriate services is easily available.

117. Rusalem, Herbert. A hard look at research on blindness. *New Outlook for the Blind,* Apr. 1961, Vol. 55, No. 4, pp. 115–20.

Author feels more research needed. Disputes many excuses put forward for not doing more research. Thinks that results are seldom practically applied but that research is increasing and outlook is bright.

118. Salmon, Peter J. The role of the private agency in 1990. *New Outlook for the Blind,* Jan. 1963, Vol. 57, No. 1, pp. 15–21.

Discusses functions worth preserving and hurdles for voluntary agencies.

119. ———. The role of the specialized agency in the rehabilitation of blind persons. *Journal of Rehabilitation,* July–Aug. 1970, Vol. 36, No. 4, pp. 11–13.

General discussion of role based on tradition, definitions, and special aspects of hearing and touch.

120. Sausser, Doris P. Community resources—and volunteers. *New Outlook for the Blind,* Feb. 1963, Vol. 57, No. 2, pp. 56–61.

Discusses wide availability of, and how to use community resources effectively.

121. Schloss, Irvin P.; Hoover, Richard E.; Braley, A.E., et al. Implications of altering the definition of blindness. *American Foundation for the Blind Research Bulletin 3,* Aug. 1963, pp. 111–33.

The various authors present the implications of altering definition of blindness from following points of view: Legislative, service needs, medico-legal, education, practical and functional considerations.

122. Scholl, Geraldine T. The visually handicapped and the Great Society.

International Journal for the Education of the Blind, May 1966, Vol. 15, No. 4, pp. 102–6.

To make the Great Society meaningful for the visually handicapped many improvements are needed in medical, educational, and social services. Author indicates how some of these are either planned or being initiated.

123. **Schon, Donald A.** The blindness system. *New Outlook for the Blind*, June 1970, Vol. 64, No. 6, pp. 169–80.

Defines the system as the network of all visually handicapped persons, agencies and groups which serve them, all training and research that affects this group, and all laws and policies concerning services to them. Describes the problems of the system and suggests areas of improvement.

124. **Schottland, Charles I.** Striving for excellence in community services for the blind. *New Outlook for the Blind*, Jan. 1966, Vol. 60, No. 1, pp. 7–11.

Discusses need for standardization, accreditation groups, elements of accreditation, relevancy to government programs.

125. **Scott, Robert A.** *The making of blind men.* New York: Russell Sage Foundation, 1969, 145 pp., $6.

Based on sociological study concerned with the processes by which persons with serious or total loss of vision learn to play the role of a blind person, argues that agencies contribute to dependence.

126. **Scott, Robert A., & Bassoff, Bruce.** Organizational processes in social welfare programs: A case study. *American Foundation for the Blind Research Bulletin 16*, May 1968, pp. 1–16.

Reports a sociological analysis of workshops for the blind as typical of social welfare programs in America.

127. **The Seeing Eye.** *If blindness occurs.* Morristown, N.J.: Author, 196—, 20 pp., illus.

Intended for the guidance of family, friends, hospital personnel, and others concerned with the care of newly blinded persons. Covers orientation, walking, personal appearance, eating, social contacts, and other daily living situations.

128. **Shaw, John A.** Visually handicapped or blind? *New Beacon*, Feb. 1975, Vol. 59, No. 694, pp. 35–37.

Discusses various interpretations of the terms "blind" and "visually handicapped," suggesting ways to define and clarify their use.

129. **Social and Rehabilitation Service.** *Social services for persons who are blind.* Washington, D.C.: Dept. of Health, Education & Welfare, 1975, 44 pp., free.

An introduction to blindness, special problems of the population and services available to them, written for the social service worker.

130. **Sorieri, Antonio A.** Shifts in the partnership of public and voluntary agencies serving families and children. *New Outlook for the Blind*, Sept. 1963, Vol. 57, No. 7, pp. 250–56.

Discusses history of the partnership, and federal legislative amendments of 1962 because of their effect on public agencies which are now under mandate.

131. Sundquist, Perry. *Aid to the blind in California: Fifty years of program development 1919–1969.* Los Angeles: Calif. Council of the Blind, 1969, 55 pp.

Reports on the history and present status of Calif.'s progressive public assistance programs for the blind. Includes determination of degree of blindness, causes, social characteristics, program administration, and caseload and grant trends.

132. Switzer, Mary E. The contribution of the handicapped to the world economy. *New Outlook for the Blind,* Dec. 1960, Vol. 54, No. 10, pp. 356–60.

Concept that rehabilitation contributes to the productivity of the individual and the world. Broad discussion of rehabilitation on an international scale.

133. ———. "Hope is the anchor of life": The changing role of government in provision of services for rehabilitation of the disabled. *New Outlook for the Blind,* Jan. 1965, Vol. 59, No. 1, pp. 8–12.

"The role of government is one of leadership in initiating services and supporting them in such a manner that there is really equal opportunity for all to obtain them." Historical review of legislation but with emphasis on the importance of the participation of the disabled person.

134. Tisdall, William J. The visually impaired. In G. O. Johnson, & H. D. Blank, Eds., *Exceptional Children Research Review,* Washington, D.C.: Council for Exceptional Children, 1968, pp. 110–34.

135. Townsend, M. Roberta. A trend toward integration. *New Outlook for the Blind,* Jan. 1959, Vol. 53, No. 1, pp. 20–24.

A somewhat philosophical and value-oriented discussion of integration. Concludes that the measure for integration vs. special services is what serves the blind individual well.

136. U.S. Dept. of Health, Education & Welfare. Selected impairments by etiology and activity limitation, United States, July 1959–June 1961. *American Foundation for the Blind Research Bulletin 2,* Dec. 1962, pp. 1–11. Reprinted from Health Statistics Series 5–35, July 1962.

Twelve tables and 2 figures present statistical data reporting prevalence, rate per 1,000 population, etiology of visual and hearing impairments for age groups. Degree of activity limitation reported on visual impairments.

137. ———. *Statistics for 1966 on blindness in the Model Reporting Area.* Washington, D.C.: Author, 1966, v + 63 pp.

With very brief explanation, presents in complex tables the above data.

138. ———. *District of Columbia directory of services for handicapping conditions.* Washington, D.C.: Author, 1968, 223 pp.

Services for persons living in Washington, D.C., with handicaps due to mental, physical, sensory, or special health conditions are described.

139. U.S. Rehabilitation Services Admin. *Services to the blind: A community concern; A report from prime study group III of the Institute on Rehabilitation Services.* Washington, D.C.: Author, 1973?, 110 pp.

140. Upshaw, McAllister. Services to the blind in historical perspective. *New Outlook for the Blind,* Oct. 1959, Vol. 53, No. 8, pp. 281–85.

Rather philosophical review of attitudes toward blindness and blind people over the years, and of the blind person's temptation to use some of these attitudes to exploit society.

141. ——. Statesmanship in social welfare. *New Outlook for the Blind,* Sept. 1963, Vol. 57, No. 7, pp. 241–49.

Part 1: Basis of authorizing service, interpretation of need, community interests, statesmanship vs. lobby. Part 2: Employment, including requests for preferential treatment, unity of philosophy and purpose. Lists 40 philosophical bases, compared through juxtaposition, for planning and offering services.

142. Veterans Administration. *War-blinded veterans in a postwar setting.* Washington, D.C.: Govt. Printing Office, 1958, xiv + 260 pp.

Interviews with 1949 blinded veterans. Data tabulated and interpreted.

143. ——. *Report on visual impairment services teams, July 1, 1971– June 30, 1972.* Washington, D.C.: Author, 1972, vi + 148 pp.

This is subtitled "An analysis of VA outpatient services given to and characteristic of severely visually impaired and blinded veterans."

144. Waterhouse, Edward J. *History of the Howe Press of Perkins School for the Blind.* Watertown, Mass.: Howe Press, 1975, 32 pp., illus.

Traces history from establishment when the school opened. Howe Press is essentially an organization dealing with braille, writing devices as well as books.

145. West, Doral N. Integration: For whom? How? *New Outlook for the Blind,* June 1957, Vol. 51, No. 6, pp. 253–55.

Criticizes much of the current discussion about integrating "the blind" into "society" as vague generalization which poorly serves the individual blind person and his special needs.

146. Wiehn, Virginia. *Bibliography of the blind.* Lansing, Mich.: State Dept. of Education, Sept. 1966, 13 pp.

Annotated bibliography listing books and other publications dealing with the blind at the State Library of the Michigan Dept. of Education. Categories include: Education of the visually handicapped, books for parents of visually handicapped children, bibliographies for educators of the visually handicapped, teaching manuals, publications on aids and materials for the visually handicapped.

147. Wilson, John. The blind in a changing world—New trends seen. *New Outlook for the Blind,* Apr. 1965, Vol. 59, No. 4, pp. 138–40.

Reviews blindness statistics around the world and gives projections for the future with reasons for those projections.

148. Wood, Maxine. *Blindness . . . Ability not disability.* New York: Public Affairs Committee, 1968, 32 pp.

Estimates number of blind people. Gives definitions of legal and functional blindness. Delineates rehabilitation services. Presents special provisions of Social Security and income tax laws. Lists 9 organizations for the blind.

149. World Council for the Welfare of the Blind. *Proceedings of the World Assembly of the World Council for the Welfare of the Blind (New Delhi, India, Oct. 8–17, 1969).* Paris: 1970, 363 pp., $2.

Includes papers on communication in an age of science, preparing the blind to live in an age of science, employment, social services, medical research on blindness, recreation, technical aids, and the roles of the United Nations, UNICEF, ILO, UNESCO, and WHO.

150. World Veterans Federation. *European Seminar on the Rehabilitation of the Blind.* Paris: Author, 1965, 194 pp.

Results of a seminar in which representatives from 18 European countries, the U.S. and Canada presented discussions on the rehabilitation programs of their respective countries.

151. Zahl, Paul A., Ed. *Blindness: Modern approaches to the unseen environment.* New York: Hafner, 1962, 589 pp. (Reprint ed. with new bib.)

Chapters by various contributors on: History and welfare, education and psychology, vocational considerations, the military blinded, various time-tested aids and new technical developments, and ophthalmological factors.

152. Zelditch, Morris. Social change and its impact on the services we render. *New Outlook for the Blind*, Dec. 1962, Vol. 56, No. 10, pp. 347–52.

Presents broad review of technological and sociological change: Automation, population change, change in family structure. Discusses these changes in terms of their relevance to health and welfare agencies in the community, and raises 3 questions of economic relevance for agency consideration.

153. Ziemer, Gregor. This hoax must be routed. *New Outlook for the Blind*, May 1957, Vol. 51, No. 5, pp. 202–4.

Cigar bands and empty match books do not get guide dogs or other aids for blind people.

2. Organizations, Agencies, Volunteers, Public Relations, and Selected Services

154. Allen, Alfred. The code of ethics—An appraisal. *New Outlook for the Blind*, Nov. 1955, Vol. 49, No. 9, pp. 317–20.

Describes and argues the need for the AAWB Seal of Good Practice and its supporting code of ethics.

155. American Foundation for the Blind. *The changing American scene as it relates to health, education and welfare services for visually handicapped: An institute for executives and board members of agencies serving visually handicapped persons in Region I.* New York: Author, 1967, 37 pp.

Considers social welfare programming and practice. Summarizes implications for administrative practice and executive responsibility.

156. ———. *Directory of agencies serving the visually handicapped in the United States, 18th ed.* New York: Author, 1973, 381 pp., $10.

Lists several hundred agencies, institutions, organizations, included on the basis of incorporation as nonprofit, services of at least 1 full-time paid executive and a board of directors, or establishment through local, state, or federal legislation.

157. ———. *Directory of agencies serving the visually handicapped in the U.S., 19th ed.* New York: Author, 1975, 398 pp., $10.

A state-by-state listing of all governmental and voluntary services for the blind plus a category-by-category listing of national services. Listings include name, address, telephone number, chief executive, and description of services.

158. American Printing House for the Blind. *American Printing House for the Blind, Inc.: Its history, purposes, and policies.* Louisville, Ky.: Author, 1966, 15 pp.

A history of the development and growth of APH includes controversy resulting in the final choice standard English braille grade 2 as the standard type for the English-speaking world. Published are braille books, talking books, large-type books, tangible materials, braille music, and literature for adult blind. Research in the education of blind children is conducted.

159. American Printing House for the Blind, Inc. *International Journal for the Education of the Blind*, Dec. 1964, Vol. 14, No. 2, pp. 33–41.

Gives history, purposes and policies of APH with particular attention to administrative procedures and requirements under federal legislation. However, APH is an entity in its own right with services to all blind people, at once a private and a federal agency.

160. Bartoo, Margaret A., & Schwind, Bernard. Alaska's rural home helper program. *New Outlook for the Blind*, June 1972, Vol. 66, No. 6, pp. 167–68.

Report of how the Homemaker Service of the Dept. of Health and Social Services enabled an elderly couple, 1 of whom had a visual handicap, to remain self-sufficient in a remote Eskimo village.

161. Berkowitz, Sidney J. Public subsidy of private programs. *New Outlook for the Blind*, June 1963, Vol. 57, No. 6, pp. 206–8.

Five serious drawbacks to public subsidy of private programs. There is reason to believe that partial or major dependence on public subsidy seriously distorts the program of any private agency or institution and interferes with its vigorous pursuit of independent ideas.

162. Black, Winifred. Volunteers: A community resource. *New Outlook for the Blind*, Dec. 1961, Vol. 55, No. 10, pp. 325–28.

General treatise on volunteerism: Volunteer as a community resource, how and why to use volunteers.

163. Blake, Ruth, et al. *Visually handicapped: An approach to program development.* Indianapolis, Ind.: West Central Joint Services for Handicapped, 1972, 30 pp.

Includes guidelines on physical facilities, low vision aids, curriculum, materials, and equipment. Presents a description of a partially sighted child. Includes a bib., lists of national organizations, and a glossary of terms relating to the eye.

164. Brieland, Donald M. Suggestions for a coordinated research program. *International Journal for the Education of the Blind*, June 1952, Vol. 1, No. 4, pp. 80–81.

Presents suggestions to assist in the development of a coordinated research program designed to assist those who work with the visually handicapped, and involve them in cooperation with researchers.

165. Brown, Charles E. Defining and measuring agency services to improve their effectiveness. *New Outlook for the Blind*, June 1974, Vol. 68, No. 6, pp. 241–46.

Discussion of the United Way of America Services Identification System as a tool for program definition and measurement and how Seattle's Community Services for the Blind uses it.

166. Bureau of Labor Statistics. *Salaries for selected occupations in services for the blind. January 1966.* Washington, D.C.: Dept. of Labor, 1966, 39 pp. Bulletin No. 1500.

Chiefly in the form of statistical tables, reports results of a mail survey with breakdowns by agency, sex, region, etc.

167. ———. Salaries for selected occupations in services for the blind, Jan. 1966. *New Outlook for the Blind*, Apr. 1967, Vol. 61, No. 4, pp. 120–28.

Detailed results of salary study done by Div. of Occupational Pay of the Bureau of Labor Statistics, with extensive tables and interpretation.

168. Burnside, Freda F. Social work: Three views. Welfare problems and community services. *New Outlook for the Blind*, May 1957, Vol. 51, No. 5, pp. 184–88.

Tells how and why community agencies, and especially volunteers, are an important force in social welfare.

169. Butts, Sarah A. *Social services for persons who are blind: A guide for staff in departments of public social services.* Washington, D.C.: Social & Rehabilitation Service, 1975, 44 pp., free.

Types of and eligibility requirements for financial aid, medical, remedial, vocational, and rehabilitation care and services available to the blind from the government. Separate sections on the child, the young adult, and the elderly.

170. Cleary, Helen. You and the agency: Client-centered or agency-centered. *New Outlook for the Blind*, Apr. 1968, Vol. 62, No. 4, pp. 105–10.

In a project to facilitate integrated service to blind clients by agencies not specific to the blind, attitudes and problems were identified. By a series of penetrating questions the author challenges agencies to more client-centered service.

171. Cohen, Wilbur J. The role of the service agency. *New Outlook for the Blind*, Nov. 1961, Vol. 55, No. 9, pp. 275–80.

Review of present programs and those proposed for the future, to be sponsored by the federal government, that would affect those with vision problems.

172. Cohn, Theodore. A board takes a look at its executive. *New Outlook for the Blind*, Apr. 1960, Vol. 54, No. 4, pp. 133–35.

Describes the reasons for, limitations in, and results of examining the executive. Cites the Family Service Assoc. of America booklet *Guide and Outline for Evaluation of the Agency Executive* as helpful.

173. Coleman, Thomas J. Community relations: Public information and education. *New Outlook for the Blind*, May 1966, Vol. 60, No. 5, pp. 146–49.

Discusses communication relevant to public relations and education, particularly in relationship to public health and welfare agencies: Results of inadequate communication; utilization, enumeration of 5 problems; benefits from successful programs.

174. Colwell, Nancy. "Put yourself in Solomon's shoes." *International Journal for the Education of the Blind*, Mar. 1958, Vol. 7, No. 3, pp. 69–74.

How to develop a PR program for a school or agency, examples of good public relations material, and the benefits it can bring.

175. Cowell, Eugene I. Some PR methods in a metropolitan agency. *New Outlook for the Blind*, Mar. 1962, Vol. 56, No. 3, pp. 89–91.

Discusses what makes news, radio and TV channels, and measuring responses.

176. Crawford, Fred L. *A manual of practices and procedures in the establishment and operation of a professional counseling and placement service.* New York: N.Y. Assoc. for the Blind, 1965, 40 pp.

Manual designed to facilitate establishment of programs to assist the blind in securing suitable positions in professional, administrative, and related occupations.

177. Davis, Finis E. 99 years of service to blind children. *New Outlook* *for the Blind,* Mar. 1957, Vol. 51, No. 3, pp. 109–16. Also, *International Journal for the Education of the Blind,* Mar. 1957, Vol. 6, No. 3, pp. 49–55.

History and current status of American Printing House for the Blind.

178. Davison, Owen R. The accountability of nonprofit institutions in a free society. *New Outlook for the Blind,* Nov. 1973, Vol. 67, No. 9, pp. 389–95.

Since nonprofit institutions are public institutions, they are accountable to the public. The internal monitoring and evaluation necessary in accountability improve services. Reviews role of COMSTAC Report and NAC.

179. Daygee, John L. Public assistance for the blind. *New Outlook for the Blind,* May 1959, Vol. 53, No. 5, pp. 170–76.

Warm and human discussion of some of the legal and casework problems related to public assistance.

180. DeAngelis, Gerard J. The seminar series: A strategy for acquainting professional workers with the problems of the blind. *New Outlook for the Blind,* Apr. 1969, Vol. 63, No. 4, pp. 97–102.

A 10-week series of seminars for professional workers was formed to develop services and community influences to minimize the causes and effects of blindness and to minimize some of the negative attitudes toward blindness. Success of this series led to development of new programs and additional seminars.

181. Dickinson, Frances. An effective public relations project. *New Outlook for the Blind,* Apr. 1954, Vol. 48, No. 4, pp. 95–99.

A utility company and the N. J. State Commission for the Blind use a cooking class for blind individuals as a PR project.

182. *The directory for exceptional children: A listing of educational and training facilities,* 7th ed. Boston: Porter Sargent, 1972.

Federal and state agencies listed. State maps showing location of facilities. Listings for Canada also.

183. Donnelly, Eleanor, & Hill, John G. Functional budgeting: A description of the system now in use at the Association for the Blind of Rochester and Monroe County, Inc. *New Outlook for the Blind,* Mar. 1964, Vol. 58, No. 3, pp. 65–68.

Details of a budgetary system that enabled this agency for the blind to cut costs and streamline services.

184. Dumpson, James R. A time of change—A challenge to administrators. *New Outlook for the Blind,* Jan. 1968, Vol. 62, No. 1, pp. 25–29.

Acceptance and implementation of the concept of the welfare state changes government's relationship to people and affects delivery of service. Lists 5 implications of these changing concepts for voluntary agencies.

185. Dye, Arthur M. Racial segregation in agencies for the blind. *New Outlook for the Blind,* Dec. 1963, Vol. 57, No. 10, pp. 393–95.

Agencies for blind persons can eliminate discrimination through administrative action and board decisions.

186. Eastman, E. Elaine. The establishment of state-wide volunteer services in Oregon. *New Outlook for the Blind,* Apr. 1970, Vol. 64, No. 4, pp. 97–103.

Organization and administration of a state-wide volunteer group discussed. Describes needs for volunteer workers, services they can provide, methods of providing independence for the blind, tailoring each program to the specific community, and the coordination necessary in each program.

187. Fitzgerald, H. Kenneth. Program planning and development within the social agency. *New Outlook for the Blind*, Oct. 1962, Vol. 56, No. 8, pp. 271–78.

Cites lack of literature on program planning. Suggests such planning is part of administration and lists 8 steps in administration process. Discusses relevance to agency objectives and standards, technical purposes. Bib.

188. ———. Volunteer work with the handicapped. *New Outlook for the Blind*, Jan. 1963, Vol. 57, No. 1, pp. 4–9.

Discusses the effects of a disability, shock and depression, team work, and specialized training.

189. ———. A brief overview of services to blind persons. *New Outlook for the Blind*, Sept. 1964, Vol. 58, No. 7, pp. 213–14.

Review of present services, of progress made and changes ahead.

190. Fitzgerald, H. Kenneth, & Handel, Alexander F. Accreditation—Some background and observations. *New Outlook for the Blind*, June 1964, Vol. 58, No. 6, pp. 177–80.

Discussion of accreditation in general. Role of AAWB and AAIB in setting standards for workers with the blind that may lead to an accreditation system in work for the blind.

191. Flury, Ablett H. Accreditation is plus. *New Outlook for the Blind*, Mar. 1966, Vol. 60, No. 3, pp. 93–95.

Relates development of accrediting process used for secondary schools, hoping similarities will be helpful to development of proposed accreditation program for agencies, etc., serving the blind.

192. Forer, Lois G. The obligations of board members. *New Outlook for the Blind*, Nov. 1963, Vol. 57, No. 9, pp. 343–47.

Discusses board member as trustee, annual budget, duty to consult experts, legal restrictions on fund raising, charitable funds, the obsolete agency, merger or consolidation, and public accountability.

193. Fowler, Herbert S. Public relations—The administrator's indispensable. *New Outlook for the Blind*, Sept. 1966, Vol. 60, No. 7, pp. 222–25.

The PR man should be a key staff advisor on PR and public information policy as it relates to all agency operations. Methods of involvement with the community, citizen visitation program, and production of PR materials discussed.

194. Friedensohn, Oscar. A symposium on accreditation. *New Outlook for the Blind*, Dec. 1967, Vol. 61, No. 10, pp. 313–22.

With introduction by Friedensohn, presents abstracts of papers: A state agency point of view, Joseph Kohn; large private agency point of view, Wesley D. Sprague; agency planning and program development, Helen M. Worden & Marcella C. Goldberg.

195. Froistad, Wilmer. Development and use of community resources. *New Outlook for the Blind*, Sept. 1961, Vol. 55, No. 7, pp. 237–42.

Realistic overview of community resources and suggestions as to how these can best be used. Focus is especially on blind and on type of worker necessary to deliver optimum services.

196. General Accounting Office. *Charges made by the National Federation of the Blind against the National Accreditation Council for agencies serving the blind and visually handicapped.* Washington, D.C.: Author, Sept. 1974, 106 pp.

Finds no cause to revoke NAC's status. Describes NAC.

197. Gluck, Samuel. Blindness plus—An approach tailored to individual need. *New Outlook for the Blind*, May 1965, Vol. 59, No. 5, pp. 163–67.

With illustrative case reports, describes the services of Jewish Guild for the Blind, New York City.

198. Graham, Milton D. "What good are statistics?" *New Outlook for the Blind*, Sept. 1965, Vol. 59, No. 7, pp. 229–32.

Shows some of the many ways in which statistics can be effectively used in operational programs. Statistics are a tool; research suggests answers, statistics define the data, but it is up to management to use both with imagination and wisdom.

199. Greenhalgh, Robert. Services for the visually handicapped. *New Beacon*, June 1973, Vol. 57, No. 674, pp. 146–48.

Discusses criticism of services provided by social services depts., major developments and reorganization undertaken to deal with the problems and provide firm foundation for establishment of effective comprehensive specialist service.

200. Hayes, Harry E. The county board—arm of the state agency. *New Outlook for the Blind*, Mar. 1955, Vol. 49, No. 3, pp. 77–86.

Describes the Kans. program with its state-county team with increased county responsibility. Ultimate objective is total assimilation of the individual blind person into community life.

201. Heeren, Ethel. Means and ends in direct services to blind people. *New Outlook for the Blind*, Oct. 1955, Vol. 49, No. 8, pp. 275–81.

Detailed description, with many examples, of the effect upon an agency of having as its purpose assisting blind people, in every possible way, to develop and use their own abilities.

202. Held, Marian. The private agency program in the critical years ahead. *New Outlook for the Blind*, Dec. 1958, Vol. 52, No. 10, pp. 376–81.

Presents broad general discussion of questionable need for professional personnel, using early programs eclectically to build better programs, integrated vs. segregated recreation, camping, agency philosophies, future problems.

203. Hollem, Adele P. Some implications for supervision of the paraprofessional in home services for the visually handicapped. *New Outlook for the Blind*, Feb. 1975, Vol. 69, No. 2, pp. 73–76, 87.

Interagency cooperation and coordination of efforts are necessary to provide complete and high quality services to the visually handicapped person. Gives examples with case histories.

204. Hughes, Norma E. Partnership of the blind with the agency for the blind—on behalf of the blind. *New Outlook for the Blind*, Oct. 1957, Vol. 51, No. 8, pp. 344–50.

A brief history of the Canadian Council of the Blind and more extended discussion of its functions and relationships with the Canadian National Institute for the Blind.

205. Hush, Howard. What is an agency executive? *New Outlook for the Blind*, Apr. 1960, Vol. 54, No. 4, pp. 131–33.

Prefacing his discussion by stating that social workers are often seen as "peddlers of gloom," the author proceeds to 5 job satisfactions of an agency executive.

206. Jahoda, Milton A. Implications of BLS survey for standard of service. *New Outlook for the Blind*, Oct. 1956, Vol. 50, No. 8, pp. 306–8.

In light of the results of a Bureau of Labor Standards survey, recommends 8 ways to improve agency services.

207. Johnson, J. Arthur. Utilization of standards and accreditation. *New Outlook for the Blind*, May 1970, Vol. 64, No. 5, pp. 148–53.

Discussion of initial development and formation of standards, resulting improvement of staffing policies, and the need for positive utilization of accreditation requirements.

208. Johnson, J. Arthur, & Dishart, Martin. Letting the client judge. *New Outlook for the Blind*, Mar. 1958, Vol. 52, No. 3, pp. 75–77.

Discusses services of the Columbia Lighthouse for the Blind and how the Lighthouse subjected itself to an evaluation by the most qualified of judges—the clients, in terms of how they personally benefitted from the program. New skills assessed.

209. Johnson, Suzanne. Sources of agency referrals. *New Outlook for the Blind*, Feb. 1971, Vol. 65, No. 2, pp. 49–50.

Raises question of how to encourage more persons to seek assistance from agencies for the blind. Stresses need for public education about services, especially for physicians, nursing homes, hospitals, and professional persons in other social agencies.

210. Jones, Charles P. Symposium—Self-image: A guide to adjustment. The private agency's role. *New Outlook for the Blind*, Mar. 1961, Vol. 55, No. 3, p. 102.

Briefly discusses the role of a private agency in a community in dealing with the visually handicapped.

211. Kahlert, Janet M. Medical aspects of aid to the blind. *New Outlook for the Blind*, May 1962, Vol. 56, No. 5, pp. 159–65.

Discusses organizational relationships between the agency and the ophthalmologist, determination of blindness, administrative relationships with the medical director or ophthalmologist.

212. Kanninen, Tovio P., et al. *Salaries for selected occupations in service for the blind.* New York: AFB, 1966, 43 pp.

Nationwide survey of agencies with full-time workers spending over 50% of their time serving blind clients provided authoritative salary data to assist salary planning by local organizations.

213. Klein, Earl T. Staff competency—key to effective service. *New Outlook for the Blind*, Dec. 1955, Vol. 49, No. 10, pp. 351–55.

The Vocational Amendments of 1954 provided funds for staff within the Federal-State Employment Service to work with the handicapped. This is good, but more careful selection of interviewers, training, and interchange with vocational rehabilitation counselors is necessary.

214. Koestler, Frances A. Five days at Vinton: The birth of the American Foundation for the Blind—Part one. *New Outlook for the Blind*, Oct. 1971, Vol. 65, No. 8, pp. 241–260.

An excerpt from a book being written on the history of work with the blind, article focuses on the role of American Foundation for the Blind, beginning with its creation at the 1921 convention of the American Association of Workers for the Blind in Vinton, Iowa.

215. ———, Ed. *The COMSTAC report: Standards for strengthened services.* New York: Commission on Standards and Accreditation of Services for the Blind, 1966, 393 pp.

After fairly detailed history of the commission, its policies and principles, outlines standards for: Agency function and structure, financial accounting and service reporting, personnel administration and volunteer service, physical facilities, public relations and fund-raising, education, library services, orientation and mobility services, rehabilitation centers, sheltered workshops, social services, and vocational services.

216. Kohn, Joseph. The future of services by state agencies for the blind. *New Outlook for the Blind*, Nov. 1970, Vol. 64, No. 9, pp. 301–305.

Describes trends in the services by state agencies. Also discusses the misconception that programs designed for general handicapping conditions can also serve the blind.

217. ———. Volunteers in a state agency for the blind. *Rehabilitation Record*, Jan.–Feb. 1973, Vol. 14, No. 1, pp. 17–20.

Describes the major activities of the more than 2,000 volunteers who work with the N. J. Commission for the Blind and Visually Impaired each year.

218. Koocher, Robin C. *What does the social worker do anyway?* Boston: Boston Center for Blind Children, 1974, 9 pp., 60¢.

Describes the function of social workers at the Boston Center, emphasizing information dissemination and work with parents.

219. Lacy, Bernard. AFOB's fifty years of service around the globe. *New Outlook for the Blind*, Nov. 1965, Vol. 59, No. 9, pp. 325–29.

Fifty years of accomplishment of the American Foundation for Overseas Blind are described, including the countries and services involved.

220. Little, Regina. Coordinating the services of caseworker and volunteer. *New Outlook for the Blind*, Oct. 1963, Vol. 57, No. 8, pp. 312–16.

Discusses the work of a volunteer, the rehabilitation counselor and casework. Tries to show how a better understanding of respective roles can improve services and how a misunderstanding and misuse of functions can destroy client's chance to use the help available.

221. Lowenfeld, Berthold. Review of a major study: Services to blind children in the State of New York. *New Outlook for the Blind*, Jan. 1960, Vol. 54, No. 1, pp. 11–18.

Reviews Cruickshank's & Trippe's *Service to Blind Children*, a study to determine scope and status to blind persons under age of 21 years. Reports study's most important observations and recommendations. Criticizes organization of data/tables and questions significance in many cases. Reports on lacks in study.

222. MacDonald, Anne L. National Committee's special recording services show growth. *New Outlook for the Blind*, May 1953, Vol. 47, No. 5, pp. 130–33.

Describes the National Committee for Recording for the Blind, its brief history, how it functions, and general characteristics of blind persons served.

223. Magill, Arthur N. Partnership of the blind with the agency for the blind—on behalf of the agency. *New Outlook for the Blind*, Oct. 1957, Vol. 51, No. 8, pp. 339–43.

How the Canadian National Institute for the Blind was developed in response to the needs of blind people while the Canadian Council of the Blind interprets those needs. Major decisions are made through a joint national committee of leaders of both organizations.

224. Mallas, Aris A., Jr. *An evaluation of the organization of state programs to serve the blind . . . . and a suggested evaluation sequence.* Austin, Tex.: Management Services Assoc., 1975, 58 pp. + app., $6. 1st of 2 volumes.

Review ways in which state services for the blind have been changing and suggests procedures to evaluate that change and its results for blind people.

225. Mallinson, George G., & Blasch, Donald. *Planning services for the blind for the decade of the 70's: Final report.* Kalamazoo: W. Mich. Univ., 1973, 149 pp., app.

Reports a conference on the state of the art in 4 major areas: Services to the older blind, vocational training and job placement, clerical and secretarial occupations, and development of hardware.

226. Maloney, Elizabeth. Social casework approach to the visually handicapped client. *New Outlook for the Blind*, Apr. 1956, Vol. 50, No. 4, pp. 129–31. Also in *Field of Vision*, Winter 1955.

Work with blind clients must be built on 4 fundamental principles of casework: Self-determination, particularization, acceptance, and relationship. Adjustment to blindness requires time, and referrals for other services must be made at just the right moment. The social worker's acceptance helps the client to reestablish his place in the community.

227. ———. Social work function in an agency for the blind. *New Outlook for the Blind*, Mar. 1959, Vol. 53, No. 3, pp. 91–94.

Describes the major areas of service and varied roles of the social service department of a private agency.

228. ———. Examining the adequacy of programming for blind children. *New Outlook for the Blind*, Feb. 1965, Vol. 59, No. 2, pp. 54–57.

Analysis of 60 case records of children at the Industrial Home for the Blind, Brooklyn, leads to 6 recommendations for improved service.

229. Manning, Seaton W. Cultural and value factors affecting the Negro's use of agency services. *New Outlook for the Blind*, Feb. 1961, Vol. 55, No. 2, pp. 49–60.

Fairly extensive review of factors affecting Negroes in our society. Examination of common stereotypes about them. Discussion of Negroes' attitudes toward social agencies and special questions that arise when working with them.

230. Martin, C. Lewis, & Travis, John T. *Exceptional children: A special ministry.* Valley Forge, Pa.: Judson Press, 1968, 63 pp., $1.25.

Addressed to clergy and laymen, provides information on the inclusion in church activities of children who are hard of hearing, deaf, blind, physically, multiply, or emotionally handicapped.

231. Mayo, Leonard W. Rehabilitation and social work. *New Outlook for the Blind,* Nov. 1957, Vol. 51, No. 9, pp. 397–401.

Differentiates between rehabilitation and social work but shows their mutually supporting roles.

232. Monbeck, Michael E. The on-site review: NAC at IHB. *New Outlook for the Blind,* Apr. 1972, Vol. 66, No. 4, pp. 109–14, illus.

Article intended to clarify one of the steps of NAC accreditation—on-site review—through a description of part of the first day of the 3-day review at the Industrial Home for the Blind, N.Y.

233. Morris, Alfred. Integration and the disabled. *New Beacon,* Aug. 1974, Vol. 58, No. 688, pp. 197–201.

Printed from an address by the Minister of the Disabled to the RNIB, discusses relevant legislation, philosophy of integration, and cooperation between the government and the Institute.

234. Mungovan, John F. Aid to the blind: A tool of rehabilitation. *New Outlook for the Blind,* Nov. 1960, Vol. 54, No. 9, pp. 313–20.

Following a history of aid to the blind in Mass., presents organizational and administrative guidelines for a new plan.

235. ———. A social work training unit in an agency for the blind. *New Outlook for the Blind,* Feb. 1962, Vol. 56, No. 2, pp. 43–45.

Discusses student orientation, history, effects of the unit on the agency, and client reaction.

236. National Accreditation Council. *Self-study and evaluation guide.* New York: AFB, 1968, 348 pp.

Presents standards developed for agencies over a 3-year period and includes a manual of procedures for agency self-study, agency function and structure, orientation and mobility services, social and vocational services, and an evaluation summary and report.

237. ———. NAC assesses the impact of accreditation. *New Outlook for the Blind,* Jan. 1973, Vol. 67, No. 1, p. 6.

Report of survey on improving services for blind Americans. Survey covered 32 agencies which submitted comprehensive self-study reports to NAC before Dec. 31, 1971. In summation, the need was pointed out for short- and long-term followup by agencies and greater involvement and input from blind people themselves.

238. National Rehabilitation Association. *State agency exchange: Services to the blind and the deaf.* Washington, D.C.: State Agency Exchange, Interagency Project, May 1972, 97 pp.

Summarizes responses to questionnaires sent to vocational rehabilitation agencies in each state. Unmet needs and relevant recommendations reported.

239. New, Anne L., Ed. Strengthening services for the blind and visually handicapped through the application of standards: Final report. New York: National Accreditation Council, 1975, v + 67 pp. Mimeo.

Report of a project begun in 1967 concludes that standards have brought identifiable improvements in agency management and operations.

240. O'Neill, Kitty. IHB adds volunteer visitor service. *New Outlook for the Blind,* Dec. 1953, Vol. 47, No. 10, pp. 296–300.

Planning and organization required to initiate a volunteer visitor service which would also provide guides, readers, chore services in homes and hospitals. Clients, as well as volunteers, must be prepared for this relationship.

241. O'Neill, Paul C. The power to change the world. *New Outlook for the Blind,* Oct. 1958, Vol. 52, No. 8, pp. 303–7.

Describes a PR program to change negative public attitudes, recruit volunteers, and raise funds.

242. Ortof, Murray E. Identification of varied needs of blind persons. *New Outlook for the Blind,* Oct. 1964, Vol. 58, No. 8, pp. 253–56.

Discussion of how blind can be treated as a less segregated group and integrated into society. Adjustments need to be made in agencies to prepare clients for today's rapidly changing society.

243. Platt, Philip S., & Reiser, Neil. The interdependence of an agency's program and its financial support. *New Outlook for the Blind,* June 1958, Vol. 52, No. 6, pp. 203–9.

General discussion of fund-raising problems and solutions.

244. Plunkett, Margaret L. National survey of personnel standards and personnel practices in services for the blind, 1955. *New Outlook for the Blind,* Nov. 1957, Vol. 51, No. 9, pp. 418–20.

Analyzes results of questionnaires to 400 voluntary and public agencies serving the blind. Data include age and sex of workers, education, occupations, wages, agency services, and fringe benefits.

245. Rabinoff, George W. Social work: Three views. What can a community expect of social workers? *New Outlook for the Blind,* May 1957, Vol. 51, No. 5, pp. 188–96.

Three elements which produced the social worker are: Industrialization, interdependence, and concept of the dignity of man. Social work must adapt old values to the demands of today's new world.

246. Register, Joe S. Management by objectives: A tool for management. *New Outlook for the Blind,* June 1974, Vol. 68, No. 6, pp. 247–51.

This approach to management involves specific techniques for identifying goals and establishing a process for achieving them. The training of staff who are to work within such a program includes the development of a training manual and sessions to teach the necessary skills. Examples are given.

247. Risley, Burt L. Toward more effective services: Cooperation and coordination as the imperative for relevance. *Education of the Visually Handicapped,* Oct. 1971, Vol. 3, No. 3, pp. 73–79.

Discusses the inadequacy of services to blind children and youth resulting from poor service coverage, inefficient approach to services, and insufficient practical results.

248. Rives, Louis H., Jr. Basic philosophy of the Office of Vocational Rehabilitation. *New Outlook for the Blind,* Nov. 1959, Vol. 53, No. 9, pp. 322–25.

The OVR goal is to provide "services for the disabled which will help them to help themselves to their fullest potentialities. . . ."

249. **Roberts, Harold G.** The role of a national voluntary agency in meeting the challenge of the 1970's. *New Outlook for the Blind*, Apr. 1971, Vol. 65, No. 4, pp. 108–11.

Briefly reviews current status of voluntary agencies and indicates several new challenges. Suggests ways in which AFB hopes to meet these.

250. **Rougagnac, Jeri.** Are you public relations wise? *International Journal for the Education of the Blind*, Dec. 1958, Vol. 8, No. 2, pp. 63–64.

Defines 6 problems related to PR and suggests solutions.

251. **Science for the Blind.** *Science for the Blind.* Bala-Cynwyd, Pa.: Author, 1967, 70 pp.

Report details past (since 1955) and planned growth of this nonprofit organization. Current and future projects and equipment are detailed.

252. **Scott, Robert A.** The selection of clients by social welfare agencies: The case of the blind. *Social Problems*, 1967, Vol. 14, No. 3, pp. 248–57.

Contends that social welfare programs for the blind are often more responsive to community pressures and the organizational needs of agencies through which services are offered than they are to the needs of blind persons.

253. **Seider, Violet M.** Community organization in the direct-service agency. *New Outlook for the Blind*, Sept. 1963, Vol. 57, No. 7, pp. 256–63.

Discusses organizational interaction, mobilization of community support, change of community resources. Also discusses 4 basic steps of the community organization process which offer a rational approach to planned change.

254. **Shapiro, Robert, & Saul, Shura.** Effective use of volunteers in group work and recreation programs. *New Outlook for the Blind*, Dec. 1959, Vol. 53, No. 10, pp. 361–66.

Discusses importance and ways in which volunteer is of value. Describes recruitment and orientation of volunteers, development of attitudes and relationships, and use of workshops for these purposes.

255. **Sherman, Allan W.** Some basic guideposts in public relations and fund raising. *New Outlook for the Blind*, Oct. 1958, Vol. 52, No. 8, pp. 293–97.

PR guidelines with suggestions for application, discussion of benefits.

256. **Smith, Patricia S.** Press relations: One tool in a community relations program. *New Outlook for the Blind*, May 1967, Vol. 61, No. 5, pp. 146–50.

Guidelines for relating to the press in an agency public relations program, including a list of agency events which might make good publicity.

257. **Sperry, A. W.** Social work with the blind in the Veterans Administration. *New Outlook for the Blind*, Jan. 1966, Vol. 60, No. 1, pp. 16–19.

Outlines significant points in VA's work with blind veterans since 1944, emphasizing areas in which social work has made major contributions.

258. **Spitzer, Carlton E.** The administrator's function in a rehab public information program. *New Outlook for the Blind*, Nov. 1966, Vol. 60, No. 9, pp. 283–85.

Discusses the unfortunate administrative tendency to downgrade importance of public information in obtaining results; the need for personal administrative concern about public information and attitudes (especially relevant to vocational rehabilitation agencies).

259. Sprague, Wesley D. Determining objectives of agencies. *New Outlook for the Blind*, Sept. 1966, Vol. 60, No. 7, pp. 216–17.

Author notes that agency programs, rather than being formulated on clients' demonstrated needs, force clients to conform to the program. Discusses why this is so, why this is unfortunate, and what can be done to change the situation.

260. Storey, Frederick G. The case of the white convertible: Accreditation system for agencies will help prevent community scandals. *New Outlook for the Blind*, Jan. 1966, Vol. 60, No. 1, pp. 11–13.

Discusses the work of AFB's COMSTAC and gives examples of why such a commission is necessary.

261. Tekawa, Toshi. Volunteers: A boon or a nuisance? *Education of the Visually Handicapped*, Oct. 1971, Vol. 3, No. 3, pp. 95–96.

Discusses motivations, acceptance procedure, attendance consistency, orientation, and functions of volunteers in programs for the blind.

262. tenBroek, Jacobus. Within the grace of God. *New Outlook for the Blind*, Oct. 1956, Vol. 50, No. 8, pp. 328–35.

Explains the animosity between agencies and Federation for the Blind, showing that it is the result of attitudes of agency heads.

263. tenBroek, Jacobus, & Matson, Floyd W. *Hope deferred: Public welfare and the blind.* Berkeley: Univ. of Calif. Press, 1959, 272 pp.

The experience of the blind under the welfare system is used to examine and assess the maturity and consequences of our social philosophies and human values. "Public assistance must be directed toward opportunity as well as security. . . . rehabilitation, employment, and self support, as well as to relief."

264. Tobin, Michael J. The Research Centre for the Education of the Visually Handicapped, University of Birmingham, England. *New Outlook for the Blind*, Mar. 1975, Vol. 69, No. 3, pp. 97–102.

Gives the origins and broad aims of the Centre and brief descriptions of some of their major projects. Also describes the way in which classroom teachers are actively involved in the planning of the projects.

265. Townsend, M. Roberta. The world is too big a client. *New Outlook for the Blind*, June 1958, Vol. 52, No. 6, pp. 210–15.

Discusses the problems in a world teeming with opportunities while bristling with confusing contradictions. Declares agencies for the blind must band together as a needed and democratic medium through which the blind individual may be helped to move from position of dependency to that of participating citizenship.

266. Upshaw, McAllister. Development of program support. *New Outlook for the Blind*, Dec. 1964, Vol. 58, No. 10, pp. 316–22.

Example of a prototype report used in mobilizing support for a program to train blind children in use of special techniques, aids, and appliances.

267. Urrows, H. H. Effect of fund raising on public opinion and education. *New Outlook for the Blind*, Oct. 1958, Vol. 52, No. 8, pp. 298–302.

Author doubts effectiveness of single projects such as brochures, designed to raise money and educate simultaneously. Reflects a number of doubt about effectiveness of various media.

268. ———. Shoals and storms ahead? Funding trends. *New Outlook for the Blind*, Nov. 1973, Vol. 67, No. 9, pp. 396–406.

Discusses fund-raising trends which affect agencies, including patterns of federal funding and private philanthropy, financial reporting, state laws, volunteer and professional fund raisers, cost, training, and tax considerations.

269. Van Vranken, Inez. Recruitment of service volunteers. *New Outlook for the Blind*, June 1959, Vol. 53, No. 6, pp. 206–8.

Five important factors in recruitment of service volunteers are: Public attitudes, agency attitudes, agency functions, need for volunteers, and available budget. An informal, personal approach is necessary.

270. Va. Commission for the Visually Handicapped. *New approaches to the delivery of total services for blind people: A final report.* Richmond: Author, 1971, 55 pp., app.

Results of project conducted to develop innovative methods of locating visually handicapped persons in 2 selected geographical areas of Va., and to establish a Service Determination Unit to expedite delivery of services to persons referred.

271. Wagner, Robert. "Right to organize," greeting card mailings major themes of Federation New Orleans meeting. *New Outlook for the Blind*, Sept. 1957, Vol. 51, No. 7, pp. 316–23.

Reports the meeting of the National Federation of the Blind, New Orleans, 1957.

272. Werntz, George. Principles of accreditation. *New Outlook for the Blind*, Jan. 1959, Vol. 53, No. 1, pp. 24–28.

Paper based on a meeting of executive heads of national agencies for the blind at the 1958 convention of the AAWB. Describes purpose and procedure of accrediting process.

273. Wolf, Benjamin. Some guideposts for public education at the grass roots. *New Outlook for the Blind*, Feb. 1964, Vol. 58, No. 2, pp. 40–43.

Objectives in public education about blindness are to stimulate authentic attitudes about blind people and to spur community action to provide opportunities for blind people. Gives guidelines for a program of public education for agencies serving the blind.

274. ———. Voluntary agencies: A new look. *New Outlook for the Blind*, Nov. 1973, Vol. 67, No. 9, pp. 385–88.

Because of the changing role of federal and state governments, services of private agencies must be reexamined and updated to insure that all necessary services are provided. Services must be tailored to meet the needs of each individual. Includes discussion of the increased responsibility of agencies serving the blind and the use of volunteers in conjunction with professional staff.

275. Yoder, Norman M. Program developments from the state's viewpoint. *New Outlook for the Blind*, Mar. 1959, Vol. 53, No. 3, pp. 88–91.

State agencies should (1) coordinate staff skills and services, (2) decentralize to bring service to the community level, and (3) improve services through developing new ideas, demonstration projects, and research.

276. Ziemer, Gregor. Public Relations Workshop. *New Outlook for the Blind*, Apr. 1958, Vol. 52, No. 4, pp. 143–45.

Discusses problems of PR in work for the blind.

277. ———. 5,000 years of bad advertising is enough! *New Outlook for the Blind*, Oct. 1958, Vol. 52, No. 8, pp. 287–92.

Encourages social welfare agencies to explore public relations techniques and employ PR experts. Discusses, briefly, the need to do so, contact with mass media, relevant AFB projects, requirements for an effective PR program.

278. ———. Public relations is what we make it. *New Outlook for the Blind*, Mar. 1962, Vol. 56, No. 3, pp. 85–88.

Discusses public relations, its purpose relative to work with the blind, and obstacles to effective PR activity in areas related to blindness.

3.   Legislation

279. Alexander Graham Bell Assoc. for the Deaf. Legislation progress, 1967: ESEA provisions for the handicapped. *Volta Review*, Apr. 1968, Vol. 70, No. 4, pp. 247–49.

Summarized then current changes in Titles I, III, VI of the National Elementary and Secondary School Act. Resumes, including services and amount of expenditure, are given for many provisions.

280. Alford, Albert L. The Education Amendments of 1974. *American Education*, Jan.–Feb. 1975, pp. 6–11.

Highlights the most important provisions of the Amendments (Public Law 93–380) on a title-by-title basis.

281. Barnett, M. Robert, Ed. Hearings on minimum wage for blind workers: A report. *New Outlook for the Blind*, Oct. 1960, Vol. 54, No. 8, pp. 275–79.

Discusses and reprints excerpts of testimony heard by the Subcommittee on Labor Standards of the House Committee on Education and Labor, in May 1960, on the H.R. 9801 bill. Testimony from Jacobus tenBroek (pro) and Irvin P. Schloss (con) and Peter J. Salmon (con).

282. Committee on Labor and Public Welfare, U.S. Congress. *Handicapped workers legislation, 1970.* Washington, D.C.: Govt. Printing Office, 1970, 155 pp.

Congressional testimony presented on S.2461 Randolph-Sheppard Act to amend and improve it, and on S.3425 Wagner-O'Day Act to extend the provisions to nonblind severely handicapped individuals. Testimony topics included retirement and fringe benefits, job opportunities, needed safety standards, hourly wages.

283. Corder, W. Owens, & Walker, Don L. The effects of Public Law 89–10, Title VI, on programs for visually impaired children. *Education of the Visually Handicapped*, May 1969, Vol. 1, No. 2, pp. 52–57.

Questionnaire was sent to 50 state directors of special education to ascertain the effects of Title VI funds on programs for visually impaired children. Future needs are to expand services and to improve the programs which are now in effect.

284. Cummings, Francis J. Association policy and aid to the blind. *New Outlook for the Blind*, Sept. 1956, Vol. 50, No. 7, pp. 268–70.

Statement of position regarding Social Security Act and reasons for that position.

285. Davis, Finis E. Expanded provisions under the federal act "To Promote the Education of the Blind." *International Journal for the Education of the Blind*, Dec. 1956, Vol. 6, No. 2, pp. 29–30.

Comments on new legislation related to the American Printing House for the Blind and how its products and services are made available to schools.

286. Erisman, Charles M. Benefits and the blind—Rights and requirements under the Social Security Disability Insurance. *New Outlook for the Blind*, Oct. 1962, Vol. 56, No. 8, pp. 267–70.

Discusses OASDI program provisions, definitions of disability (including those specific to blindness), eligibility requirements, disability determinations, and trial work period.

287. Farrell, Gabriel. Today's legislative picture in historical perspective. *New Outlook for the Blind*, Nov. 1958, Vol. 52, No. 9, pp. 325–29.

With examples from A.D. 3 to present, reviews attitudes toward blindness, vocational potential of blind, and legislated assistance to blind, with predictions for the future.

288. Froistad, Wilbur M. Does receiving blind persons' allowances make good citizens? *New Outlook for the Blind*, Feb. 1962, Vol. 56, No. 2, pp. 46–51.

Discusses whether financial assistance should be a policy of government as a means of preserving dignity of all citizens. Also discusses previous history of this assistance, a progress report of a study completed in Feb. 1960, and the present picture.

289. Godfrey, Joseph. Insurance benefits and the disability freeze. *New Outlook for the Blind*, Apr. 1958, Vol. 52, No. 4, pp. 123–27.

Discusses disability freeze, disability insurance benefits at age 50, and general eligibility. Defines disability for the disability "freeze" and for disability insurance benefits. Also discusses substantial gainful activity, temporary disability, remediability, vocational rehabilitation, offset and determination of disability by state agency.

290. Gruber, Kathern F. Education program liberalized by Congress. *New Outlook for the Blind*, Sept. 1956, Vol. 50, No. 7, pp. 245–53.

Details of new legislation providing books and materials for the education of blind children.

291. Handel, Alexander F. Social services and blindness. *New Outlook for the Blind*, Oct. 1963, Vol. 57, No. 8, pp. 295–301.

Discusses income maintenance, services for blind children, aging persons, rehabilitation services for the handicapped in their own homes.

292. Hess, Arthur E. How Social Security affects blind people. *New Outlook for the Blind*, Nov. 1959, Vol. 53, No. 9, pp. 325–27.

Detailed discussion and description of benefits available to the handicapped.

293. Lansdale, Robert T. The role of a voluntary agency in a welfare state. *New Outlook for the Blind*, Sept. 1962, Vol. 56, No. 7, pp. 233–39.

Discusses public welfare prior to the Social Security Act, the Social Security Act, the new emphasis in public assistance, state services, and the responsibility of metropolitan communities, as related to the role of the voluntary agencies.

294. Laski, Frank. Post secondary education and handicapped students, some legal considerations. In George Attleweed, et al., Eds., *Sensory disabilities study group report.* Calif. Conference on Rehabilitation, Oct. 8–10, 1974. n.p., n.d., pp. 23–44.

A review of relevant legal decisions is presented. Court actions on education for the handicapped; state constitutions and statutes; federal laws; as well as the topic of "equal protection of the law" are covered.

295. Lende, Helga. Survey of state legislation in 1953. *New Outlook for the Blind,* Jan. 1954, Vol. 48, No. 1, pp. 9–15.

Legislation for this year related to: Education, financial aid, residence requirements, agencies, vocational opportunities, state use laws, tax exemptions, and guide dogs.

296. ————. A survey of state legislation in 1955. *New Outlook for the Blind,* Feb. 1956, Vol. 50, No. 2, pp. 35–41.

Covers state legislation re education, financial aid, vocational rehabilitation and other agencies for the blind, fund raising, state use of blind-made products, mandatory reporting, libraries, and guide dogs.

297. ————. A survey of state legislation in 1957. *New Outlook for the Blind,* Jan. 1958, Vol. 52, No. 1, pp. 1–7.

Discusses measures indicating intended improvement in service or administrative structure relevant to the blind such as education, financial aid, vocational opportunities, agencies' fund raising, mandatory reporting of blindness, libraries, guide dogs, tax exemptions, and election laws.

298. ————. A survey of state legislation in 1959. *New Outlook for the Blind,* Feb. 1960, Vol. 54, No. 2, pp. 49–54.

Presents information on legislation relevant to many areas of service to the blind including education, financial aid, agencies, library service, tax exemption.

299. ————. A survey of state legislation in 1961. *New Outlook for the Blind,* Feb. 1962, Vol. 56, No. 2, pp. 58–62.

Discusses education of the young blind, financial aid, agencies serving blind persons, vocational opportunities, State Use laws, blind-made products, library services, travel, election laws, eye banks, tax exemption, fishing and hunting licenses, right to organize.

300. Lister, Charles. Confidentiality and the law. *New Outlook for the Blind,* Feb. 1973, Vol. 67, No. 2, pp. 50, 52.

Excerpted from *Privacy in the schools: Controlling the maintenance and usage of students' public school records,* an unpublished study by the author completed under a grant from the Russell Sage Foundation. Covers individual vs. public interests, record-keeping policies, decisions of the Supreme Court, change of rhetoric, and the leading case of Van Allen v. McCleary.

301. MacFarland, Douglas C. Challenges and opportunities under the Randolph-Sheppard Act. *New Outlook for the Blind,* Nov. 1967, Vol. 61, No. 9, pp. 279–82, 303.

On a national basis, discusses broad needs in the vending stand program, especially for maintenance and appropriate replacement of equipment, training operators, and techniques to meet competition. Describes proposed amendments to the Randolph-Sheppard Act and why desirable.

302. **Mallas, Aris A., Jr.** *The legal analysis of the organization of state programs to serve the blind.* Austin, Tex.: Management Services Assoc., 1975, 171 pp. + app., $6.

Examines, state by state, the statutes concerning the creation, organization, duties, and funding of the agency for the blind.

303. **President's Committee on Employment of the Handicapped.** *Wagner-O'Day Act program: How to join it.* Washington, D.C.: Author, 1974, 11 pp., free.

Summarizes background and content of the Act (1938) and the additional provisions of Public Law 92–28 (1971) which established the Committee for Purchase of Products and Services of the Blind and Other Severely Handicapped.

304. **PRO, National Federation of the Blind.** *Educational provisions for the visually handicapped: Comments on the "Vernon Report." Jointly submitted to the Secretary of State for Education and Science by the National Federation of the Blind of the United Kingdom and the Assoc. of Blind and Partially Sighted Teachers and Students.* Leeds, England: Univ. of Leeds, 1973, 64 pp., app., £1.

A response to the Report of the Committee of Enquiry into the Education of the Handicapped (issued Nov. 1972.) Part 1 indicates report's strengths and weaknesses and offers proposals. Part 2 comments in detail on report's recommendations, especially in the area of integration. Part 3 summarizes principal conclusions and recommendations.

305. **Risley, Burt L., & Hoehne, Charles W.** The vocational rehabilitation act related to the blind. *Journal of Rehabilitation*, Sept.–Oct. 1970, Vol. 36, No. 5, pp. 26–31.

Traces the history of the state-federal vocational rehabilitation program and federal legislation as they have affected the lives of the blind. Includes examination of the Vocational Rehabilitation Act, the Randolph-Sheppard Act, and the Wagner-O'Day Act, as well as the later amendments to the Vocational Rehabilitation Act.

306. **Rives, Louis H., Jr.** Plans and progress of the OVR Division of Services to the Blind. *New Outlook for the Blind*, Dec. 1958, Vol. 52, No. 10, pp. 382–85.

Discusses the 1954 Vocational Rehabilitation Act and some resultant grants, and objectives of the DSB-OVR. Discusses the 3 major functions of DSB: Provision of leadership; technical consultation; personnel training.

307. **Robinson, Leonard A.** *Light at the tunnel end.* Silver Spring, Md.: Foundation for the Handicapped and Elderly, 1975, 190 pp., app., illus., $6. (Forward by Senator Jennings Randolph.)

Somewhat autobiographical, tells history of the vending stand program and Randolph-Sheppard Act.

308. **Ross, Sterling L.** Beyond education for the handicapped: Overcoming barriers of access to employment, transportation, and buildings. In George Attleweed, et al., Eds., *Sensory disabilities study group report.* Calif. Conference on Rehabilitation, Oct. 8–10, 1974. n.p., n.d., pp. 61–74.

Summarizes the recent legal efforts in Calif. to make employment, public transportation, and buildings as accessible to handicapped individuals as they are to nonhandicapped.

309. Salmon, Peter J. IHB statement on interpretation. *New Outlook for the Blind*, Nov. 1956, Vol. 50, No. 9, pp. 360–62.

In relation to the 1956 Amendment to the Social Security Act, Title II, expresses anxiety that very limiting interpretations are possible. However, properly interpreted, the amendment can strengthen rehabilitation.

310. ———. Legislation—past and present. *New Outlook for the Blind*, Jan. 1958, Vol. 52, No. 1, pp. 28–30.

Discusses essentials of favorable legislation in the past and predicts future success based on that experience.

311. Schloss, Irvin P. Blinded veterans oppose S. 2411. *New Outlook for the Blind*, Oct. 1957, Vol. 51, No. 8, pp. 370–72.

Report of the Twelfth Annual Convention of the Blinded Veterans Association with emphasis upon the reasons for opposition to the above legislation.

312. ———. Unmet needs in services to blind persons. *New Outlook for the Blind*, Sept. 1966, Vol. 60, No. 7, pp. 210–15.

Presents statistical information on the U.S. blind population. Discusses such areas as prevention, education, rehabilitation, income maintenance, reading material, and special problems, such as deaf-blindness, all in terms of relevant legislation.

313. ———. Legislation for the aging. *New Outlook for the Blind*, Feb. 1971, Vol. 65, No. 2, pp. 51–55.

Discusses problems of the aged in receiving adequate income, health care, rehabilitation services, and housing, and the existing federal laws designed to meet these needs. Amendments to the Vocational Rehabilitation Act are proposed.

314. Schottland, Charles I. Gains in social legislation for the blind. *New Outlook for the Blind*, June 1955, Vol. 49, No. 6, pp. 215–21.

Reviews benefits to the blind in legislation related to social security, vocational rehabilitation, public assistance, public health services, etc.

315. ———. 1956 amendment to Title II of the Social Security Act: Summary of disability insurance benefits. *New Outlook for the Blind*, Nov. 1956, Vol. 50, No. 9, pp. 358–60.

Details how the new amendment to the Social Security Act should affect disability benefits.

316. Segal, Arthur. Report of the conference of blind vendors. *Braille Monitor*, June 1975, pp. 239–47.

Summarizes 2-day workshop held in Philadelphia Mar. 1975 to inform vendors of ramifications of Randolph-Sheppard Act Amendments of 1974 (Public Law 93–516).

317. Selis, Sara N. Modernizing assistance for the blind. *New Outlook for the Blind*, May 1956, Vol. 50, No. 5, pp. 181–84.

Modern social policy is reevaluating the aims of financial assistance and liberalizing the definition of blindness as shown in the legislation.

318. Sherberg, Albert N. Reporting blindness. *New Outlook for the Blind*, June 1957, Vol. 51, No. 6, pp. 248–49.

Conn.'s 1955 law requiring that physicians and optometrists report all blind persons to the Board of Education of the Blind and procedures to implement that law.

319. Social Security for the blind. *Performance*, Oct. 1972, Vol. 23, No. 4, pp. 1–4.

Report on the development of the Social Security Administration's program to train and place blind persons as telephone service representatives answering questions relating to Social Security and, in some cases, initiating action.

320. Taylor, William, Jr. Practical and legal operation and effects of white cane laws. *New Outlook for the Blind*, Nov. 1961, Vol. 55, No. 9, pp. 281–84.

A lawyer discusses the white cane and its legal ramifications. Prompted by the article in May 1961 *Outlook* pointing out weak points in law.

321. tenBroek, Jacobus. The Eighty-third Congress and the blind. *New Outlook for the Blind*, Jan. 1955, Vol. 49, No. 1, pp. 16–20.

From the point of view of the blind consumer, an analysis of the effects upon the blind of the new vocational rehabilitation law, the new vending stand act, and the expanded and altered program of social security.

322. U.S. Dept. of Health, Education & Welfare. *Introducing Supplemental Security Income.* Washington, D.C.: Social Security Admin., 1974, 16 pp.

Explains supplemental income for aged, blind, etc., eligibility, and optional/mandatory state supplementation. Gives 6 brief examples.

323. Watson, Charles W., Comp. *Laws and regulations relating to education and health services for exceptional children in California.* Sacramento: State Dept. of Education, 1966, 163 pp.

Discussion of laws and regulations up to July 1966. Provisions pertain to the physically, aurally, visually, educationally, and mentally handicapped as well as to the mentally gifted.

324. Wickenden, Elizabeth. The challenge of a changing social policy. *New Outlook for the Blind*, May 1957, Vol. 51, No. 5, pp. 177–83.

After briefly discussing the place of the blind in other societies, uses the initiation of Old Age and Survivors Insurance to spark consideration of relevant public policy in U.S.

4. Prevention and Vision Screening

325. American Optometric Assoc. *Vision care and the nation's children.* St. Louis, Mo.: Author, 1968, 46 pp.

Considers aspects of vision and vision care such as extent and types of defects of American children, importance and extent of vision care in children and adults. Charts present data on vision problems of children, analysis of optometric needs in 1970, etc. Preschool vision screening tests.

326. Ames, A. C., & Swift, P. N. Lead poisoning in blind children. *British Medical Journal*, 1968, Vol. 3, No. 5611, pp. 152–53.

Many visually handicapped children have the habit of discrimination and identification by use of the mouth, lips, and tongue. This practice can cause lead poisoning.

327. Aubuchon, Marie T. Vision screening for preschoolers. *Optometric Weekly*, June 28, 1973, Vol. 64, No. 26, pp. 630–32.

Stresses need for mandatory screening and lists 10 signs displayed by children with poor vision.

328. Bacharach, John A., et al. Vision testing by parents of 3½-year-old children. *Public Health Reports*, May 1970, Vol. 85, No. 5, pp. 426–32.

Screening kit for visual problems, especially amblyopia, developed and mailed to parents of 1,040 3½-year-old children. Of 579 responses, 94% indicated that the child had never had an eye examination. Results indicated parents could screen effectively and 52% of the children could be reached inexpensively.

329. Bader, Dennis. Visual defects in children. *Phoenix Journal*, Mar. 1974, Vol. 7, No. 1, pp. 3–6.

Describes visual tasks demanded by classroom activities. Checklist to help teachers identify children having difficulty in each task area is provided.

330. Bettman, Jerome W., & Weisenheimer, Frederic S. A regional eye screening program for senior citizens. *Sight-Saving Review*, Spring 1975, Vol. 45, No. 1, pp. 23–29.

A report on the planning, operation, standards of procedure, and funding of a series of screening centers in northern Calif.

331. Bishop, Virginia E. *School vision screening: Policies, procedures, practices.* Chester, Pa.: Chester School District, 1967, 46 pp.

Study provides supportive data to reinforce request for revision of Pa.'s school vision screening standards in order to properly identify visually limited children. Surveys screening policies of 35 states, discusses problems of screening practices. Includes copies of questionnaires.

332. Boyce, Virginia S. The home eye test program. *Sight-Saving Review.* Spring 1973, Vol. 43, No. 1, pp. 43–48.

Main objectives are location of preschool children with previously undiagnosed eye conditions, education of parents and health care professionals about importance of early detection and treatment.

333. Burian, Hermann M. Treatment of functional amblyopia. *Sight-Saving Review*, 1971, Vol. 41, No. 2, pp. 69–81.

Considers neurologic base of amblyopia, defines clinical features of the disease, and stresses prevention with aid of an ophthalmologist.

334. Carter, Kent D., & Carter, Constance A. Itinerant low vision services. *New Outlook for the Blind*, June 1975, Vol. 69, No. 6, pp. 225–60, 265.

Low-vision service in the student's own environment through a professional team approach in N.H.

335. Davis, Alice H.; McConnell, Corinne R.; Michelotti, Anna S.; et al. Pre-school vision screening conducted through joint efforts of Armstrong-Indiana branch association for the blind and special education staff Indiana County Public Schools, Indiana, Pennsylvania. Indiana: Indiana Co. Public Schools, 1970, 14 pp. Mimeo.

A report on the preschool screening program in the Indiana Co. school system.

336. Dickman, Irving R. *What can we do about limited vision?* New York: Public Affairs Committee, 1973, 28 pp., 35¢.

Discusses prevention, detection, and rehabilitation of visual limitations in children and adults. Recommended changes include more limited-vision clinics, more trained personnel, increased research on limited vision, and programs to inform patients and doctors of available facilities.

337. Dvorine, Israel. What you should know about sight: III. Symptoms of abnormal function of the visual process. *Education*, 1958, Vol. 79, pp. 240–46.

Author analyzes symptoms of visual disorders.

338. Gibbons, Helen, & McCaslin, Murray F. Prevention of blindness—The contribution of medical, social and statistical research. *International Journal for the Education of the Blind*, May 1962, Vol. 11, No. 4, pp. 116–20.

Shows how research, resulting in both prevention and correction of blindness, has changed the statistics on incidence of blindness.

339. Gibbons, Robert D. Beware the home eye test for preschoolers. *Reading Teacher*, Mar. 1974, Vol. 27, No. 6, pp. 566–71.

Focuses on inadequacies of the test developed by National Society for the Prevention of Blindness. States research indicates over 50% of children with visual problems can pass this test.

340. Ginzberg, Eli. Preventive health: No easy answers. *Sight-Saving Review*, Winter 1973–74, Vol. 43, No. 4, pp. 187–93.

Discussion of general preventive care and the fact that it is not always practiced. Implications for blindness prevention discussed.

341. Grier, Timothy L. Visual acuity development and evaluation in the preschool child. *Optometric Weekly*, Apr. 19, 1973, Vol. 64, No. 16, pp. 370–73.

Reviews literature on optometric evaluation of the child from birth to 5 years of age, with the aid of graphs and a comparison of several screening tests.

342. Haase, Kenneth W., & Bryant, E. Earl. Development of a scale designed to measure functional distance vision loss using an interview technique. *American Foundation for the Blind Research Bulletin 28*, Oct. 1974, pp. 81–89.

Results of a survey by National Center for Health Statistics in cooperation with AFB and National Society for the Prevention of Blindness. A short series of questions shows some potential for identifying persons with limited vision although comparison with acuity measures yields a positive but relatively weak statistical association.

343. Hanson, Howard H. Vision screening of the aged. *New Outlook for the Blind*, Sept. 1971, Vol. 65, No. 7, pp. 213–15.

Describes a project to screen the vision of 2,578 elderly persons in S. Dak. nursing homes. Thirty-two percent were in need of services from an agency serving the blind or an optometrist. 13% were legally blind.

344. Harley, Randall K. Children with visual disabilities. In L. M. Dunn, Ed., *Exceptional children in the schools: Special education in transition.* 2nd ed. New York: Holt, Reinhart, Winston, 1973, xiii + 610 pp.

Discusses the child's eye, common defects, and the screening and identification of vision problems. Behavioral characteristics, social and personal adjustment problems, and special educational procedures for the visually disabled child are detailed. Ref.

345. Harley, Randall, & Spollen, John. A study of the reliability and validity of the Visual Efficiency Scale with low vision children. *Education of the Visually Handicapped*, Dec. 1973, Vol. 5, No. 4, pp. 110–14.

This revision of the Visual Discrimination Test was administered to 78 children between the ages of 6 and 14 years with visual acuities of 6/200 or less. Evaluation results indicated Scale had content validity and acceptable internal consistency. Notes item analysis.

346. ———. A study of the reliability and validity of the Visual Efficiency Scale with first grade children. *Education of the Visually Handicapped*, Oct. 1974, Vol. 6, No. 3, pp. 88–93.

Study found that Scale has content validity and acceptable internal consistency. A large number of test items do not discriminate between high and low scorers. Results agree with previous studies.

347. Harley, Randall; Spollen, John; & Long, Susan. A study of the reliability and validity of the Visual Efficiency Scale with preschool children. *Education of the Visually Handicapped*, May 1973, Vol. 5, No. 2, pp. 38–42.

Content validity and internal consistency shown. Some items questionable.

348. Havener, William. What you can do to help prevent blindness. *Nursing Care*, Mar. 1974, Vol. 7, No. 3, pp. 29–31.

Seven danger signals that precede blindness. When eyes should be checked. First-aid hints.

349. Henkind, Paul, & Saurez, Michael F. An urban mobile eye clinic. *Sight-Saving Review*, Spring 1974, Vol. 44, No. 1, pp. 23–30.

A report of 2 years experience in Bronx, N.Y., in bringing eye care to communities and individuals that previously had not had such services.

350. Hunt, Joseph. Why prevent blindness? *New Outlook for the Blind*, Feb. 1962, Vol. 56, No. 2, pp. 52–56.

Discusses blindness prevention, research, needs including the need for ophthalmic personnel, and individual and community responsibility.

351. James, George. Intensifying preventive programs. *Sight-Saving Review*, Fall 1971, Vol. 41, No. 3, pp. 121–27.

Text of paper presented at 1971 Annual Conference of National Society for the Prevention of Blindness in New York City. Data cited to emphasize stated research needs in prevention of blindness.

352. Kripke, Sidney S., et al. Vision screening of preschool children in mobile clinics in Iowa. *Public Health Reports*, Jan. 1970, Vol. 85, No. 1, pp. 41–44.

Description of 2 years of a vision screening program for children aged 4–6. Improvements noted in follow-up examinations found in second year because of modifications in referral system. Suggestions made for early identification so that preventive measures can be undertaken.

353. Kuehn, Patricia M. Tonometry training for nurses in Vermont. *Sight-Saving Review*, Spring 1975, Vol. 45, No. 1, pp. 35–40.

Report of 121 registered nurses having been instructed by a registered nurse in Schiøtz tonometry techniques, and having experienced supervised practice in nurse-run community screening clinics.

354. Kugel, Robert B. Vision screening of preschool children. *Pediatrics*, Dec. 1972, Vol. 50, No. 6, pp. 966–67.

Describes proposed program and lists conditions said to be detectable by screening.

355. Lead poisoning can cause blindness. *Sight-Saving Review*, 1971, Vol. 41, No. 2, pp. 65–68.

Cites statistics on the problem of lead poisoning in children, particularly as it involves visual problems. Physiology of lead poisoning and the eye reviewed.

356. Leopold, Irving H. POB programming and diabetes. *Sight-Saving Review*, Spring 1975, Vol. 45, No. 1, pp. 31–33.

An editorial discussing whether or not excellent control of diabetes makes any difference.

357. Lin-Fu, Jane S. *Vision screening of children.* Washington, D.C.: Govt. Printing Office, 1971, 24 pp., 25¢.

Discusses the importance of vision screening and the prevalence and types of vision problems, including a discussion of special problems in screening of preschool children and some tests of visual acuity which can be used with preschool children.

358. Lippmann, Otto. Vision of young children. *Archives of Ophthalmology*, June 1969, Vol. 81, No. 6, pp. 763–75.

Vision testing must be appropriate to age of child. British Stycar test recommended. Need for early testing stressed.

359. Marshall, G. H. Detecting visual dysfunction. *Journal of Special Education*, Sept. 1969, Vol. 58, No. 3, pp. 21–22.

Role of teacher in detecting visual difficulties emphasized with attention given to testing limitations, understanding of visual development, specific danger signals, and the need for comprehensive testing.

360. Michaelson, I. C., & Berman, Elaine R., Eds. *Causes and prevention of blindness: Proceedings of the Jerusalem Seminar on the Prevention of Blindness, August 25–27, 1971.* New York: Academic Press, 1972, 656 pp., $11.

Proceedings of seminar in which about 450 participants from 45 countries delivered 150 papers and spoke in numerous panel discussions. There were presentations in the areas of public health ophthalmology, clinical problems in developing and developed countries, and basic laboratory research.

361. Moore, Thomas R. Challenges. *Sight-Saving Review,* Fall 1975, Vol. 45, No. 3, pp. 101–4.

Discusses need by National Society for the Prevention of Blindness for volunteers and funds. Briefly touches on differences between U.S. and Russia PoB programs.

362. Patz, Arnall, & Hoover, Richard E. *Protection of vision in children.* Springfield, Ill.: Charles C Thomas, 1969, 172 pp., $10.

Methods for prevention, early detection, and management of visual defects presented along with guidelines for professionals interested in screening programs. Special concerns include roles of health personnel, genetic counseling, the child with severe vision impairment, and the school child with a reading problem. Glossary.

363. Petersen, Robert A. Vision screening and the detection of amblyopia in children. *Sight-Saving Review,* Summer-Fall 1974, Vol. 44, No. 2, pp. 85–88.

Information on importance and methods of testing vision in children long before school age; detailed description of 3 kinds of amblyopia.

364. Press, Edward, & Austin, Caroline. Screening of preschool children for amblyopia: Administration of tests by parents. *Journal of the American Medical Association,* May 1968, Vol. 204, No. 9, pp. 767–70.

Description of a simplified method of screening vision of 3- and 4-year-old children by parents. Results of trials by pediatricians who gave the screening card to parents and the correlation with later confirmation by ophthalmologists provided.

365. Roberts, Jean. *Vision test validation study for the health examination survey among youths 12–17 years.* Washington, D.C.: Govt. Printing Office, 1973, 43 pp., 65¢.

The study was designed to discover the degree of correspondence between survey test results and clinical examination by an ophthalmologist in determining the incidence of myopia and lateral heterophoria.

366. Sherman, Allan W. Glaucoma detection programs. *New Outlook for the Blind,* June 1960, Vol. 54, No. 6, pp. 210–15.

Discusses the needed organization, augmentation of detection programs, program goals, standards, values. Makes a plea for tonometric testing to become part of routine physical exams. Suggests several approaches to implementation and use of detection programs.

367. Velasquez, Osvaldo. A prevention of blindness program for underdeveloped nations. *Sight-Saving Review*, Winter 1973–74, Vol. 43, No. 4, pp. 217–21.

Study done for the Ministry of Public Health in Ecuador. Discusses importance of a program, purpose, objectives, a working plan, assistance to rural hospitals without ophthalmology services, dispensing of glasses, and aids as well as organization of a PoB society.

368. Williams, Mary T. Community screening for glaucoma and diabetes. *Sight-Saving Review*, Summer–Fall 1974, Vol. 44, No. 2, pp. 79–83.

Detailed description of operation, procedures of testing, follow-up, costs, etc., of screening sponsored by Sight Conservation Research Center in Santa Clara Co., Calif.

369. Winkley, William M. The geographically deprived. *New Outlook for the Blind*, Jan. 1971, Vol. 65, No. 1, pp. 21–24.

Notes the difficulties in providing eye care and other services in remote and sparsely populated areas. Method used in doing eye examinations in a traveling clinic-like operation is detailed.

5. Countries Other than the United States

370. **Alavi, S. Hassan.** The blind in Iran—A report. *New Outlook for the Blind*, June 1966, Vol. 60, No. 6, pp. 198–99.

Brief overview of advances in ophthalmological practice, establishment of the Reza Pahlavi School for the Blind, general arrangements for the education of the blind in Iran.

371. **American Foundation for Overseas Blind.** *The Third Asian Conference on Work for the Blind.* New York: Author, 1969, 354 pp.

Record of reports presented at the conference by each of the invited delegations on development of services for the blind in their respective countries. Attention was focused on three major areas: Education, rehabilitation, and coordination of services.

372. **Arnstein, Eliezer.** Testing and guiding the blind. Jerusalem: Hadassah Vocational Guidance Dept., 1956, 16 pp. Mimeo.

Detailed study of 35 blind adults, 20–51 years old, who were new immigrants living in a transition camp.

373. **Ashcroft, Samuel C.** Assignment Philippines. *International Journal for the Education of the Blind*, Oct. 1960, Vol. 10, No. 1, pp. 8–11.

A 10-week assignment of consultation in the Philippines provided opportunity to study their education of the blind. Findings and recommendations are reported.

374. **Bell, Donald, Ed.** *An experiment in education: The history of Worcester College for the blind, 1866–1966.* New York: Humanities Press, 1968, 80 pp.

Development of an English elementary and secondary school for blind boys is examined from its inception in 1866. Also mentioned are recent developments in education of the visually handicapped there.

375. **Bellini, Mario P.** Education of blind children in Italy. *International Journal for the Education of the Blind*, June 1953, Vol. 2, No. 4, p. 184.

Gives overview of the types of education and placement available for the blind in Italy since 1923.

376. **Bisbee, Margaret K.** Blindness in Kenya. *Rehabilitation Teacher*, June 1972, Vol. 4, No. 6, pp. 25–31.

Discusses medical and social aspects of blindness and stresses the need for more education on eye diseases, prevention of eye diseases, and personal hygiene. Describes 2 pilot projects which involve an equipped Land Rover to provide diagnostic services.

377. ————. The Nippon Lighthouse for the Blind, Osaka, Japan. *Rehabilitation Teacher*, May 1973, Vol. 5, No. 5, pp. 33–38.

Describes a visit which included a tour of the braille printing plant, the library, the rehabilitation facilities. Discusses observed aspects of volunteerism, housekeeping, and mobility procedures.

378. **Blank, H. Robert.** Rehabilitation in Israel. *New Outlook for the Blind*, Mar. 1962, Vol. 56, No. 3, pp. 92–95.

Discusses the obstacles to vocational rehabilitation of the blind, and notes that accomplishments of the American-Israeli Lighthouse have demonstrated not only that a large percentage of the blind can be rehabilitated socially, educationally, and vocationally, but also that this can be done with people having relatively poor initial prognoses.

379. **Boulter, Eric T.** World-wide services to blind people. *New Outlook for the Blind*, Jan. 1965, Vol. 59, No. 1, pp. 4–7.

Services have changed largely because attitudes toward blindness have changed greatly. Details the changes in service under the headings: Preschool blind child, education of blind children, adjustment and rehabilitation, and employment.

380. **Bourgeault, Stanley E.** *Integrated education for blind children.* Kuala Lumpur, Malaysia: American Foundation for Overseas Blind, 1970, 59 pp.

Describes integrated education for blind children in Asia with specific suggestions for educators.

381. **Brunner, P.** The Shelter for the Blind in Lausanne, Switzerland. *International Journal for the Education of the Blind*, Oct. 1952, Vol. 2, No. 1, pp. 123–24.

Describes the Shelter as distinctive, because it is a complete establishment offering instruction, lodging, employment, treatment. Gives overview of program for normal blind children, mentioning their integration with sighted at secondary levels, and travel training goals.

382. **Childs, J.** Training for independence and leisure. *Teacher of the Blind*, Summer 1974, Vol. 62, No. 4, pp. 116–28.

Results of questionnaire survey of 9 schools for the partially sighted and 8 schools for the blind in England. Most significant finding was that 50% felt not sufficiently prepared for life after school, and 33% referred to lack of social contacts as the main reason for this. Of those in employment, 50% had difficulties in seeking jobs. Some further education was pursued by 67%. Of 77% who lived in their family homes, only 2 shared in running the home despite school training in home management.

383. **Cruz, Gloria V.** Observations on work for the blind in the Philippines. *New Outlook for the Blind*, Mar. 1959, Vol. 53, No. 3, pp. 94–97.

Describes the early problems and gradual development of education and rehabilitation for the blind of the Philippines.

384. **Culbertson, Edwin J.** The blind in the Philippines. *International Journal for the Education of the Blind*, June 1954, Vol. 3, No. 4, pp. 268–70.

Describes postwar setbacks in education: Destruction of buildings, books, equipment, and loss of teachers. Explanation of gradual reconstruction of blind education under extreme difficulties. Details of problems and attempts to cope with them.

385. Cypihot, Jean. The Louis Braille Institute. *International Journal for the Education of the Blind*, Mar. 1955, Vol. 4, No. 3, pp. 53–54.

Often detailed description of comprehensive education program for boys 12–21 years of age, stresses economic and social independence.

386. Dajani, S. T. The blind in the Hashimite Kingdom of Jordan. *International Journal for the Education of the Blind*, June 1952, Vol. 1, No. 4, pp. 104–5.

Author believes criteria of civilization depends on standard of social services. Education and work for blind in Jordan backward. Author believes can and will be improved but funds needed. Tribute to UNESCO. Hope of handling problems of blind on international scale.

387. Danish National Institute of Social Research. The physically handicapped in Denmark. *American Foundation for the Blind Research Bulletin 15*, Jan. 1968, pp. 103–46.

As a model for a national study of all forms of physical impairment, this is a collation of the English summaries to four volumes of a study in Denmark. Statistical data, graphs.

388. Dassanaike, Kingsley C. Education of the blind in the U.S.S.R. *International Journal for the Education of the Blind*, Oct. 1960, Vol. 10, No. 1, pp. 5–8.

Education of the blind follows the national pattern with four schools under the Ministry of Education in each republic of the U.S.S.R. A Russian school and services to the adult blind are described.

389. Davis, Patricia A. Education of the visually impaired in the Soviet Union. *Education of the Visually Handicapped*, Dec. 1973, Vol. 5, No. 4, pp. 120–24.

Describes program and curriculum in special separate residential schools for the visually handicapped in the Soviet Union, and relates this to regular program followed in other Soviet schools. Discusses teacher training, subjects included in programs, and relevant, characteristically Soviet, research.

390. ———. The adult blind in the Soviet Union. *Education of the Visually Handicapped*, May 1975, Vol. 7, No. 2, pp. 60–62.

Discussion/description of the All-Russia Society of the Blind (Vserossijskoe Obščestivo Slepyx), vocational training, higher education, and social benefits.

391. *The Education of the Visually Handicapped: Report of the Committee of Enquiry appointed by the Secretary of State for Education and Science in October, 1968.* London: Her Majesty's Stationery Office, 1972, viii + 154 pp., £1.

The study was undertaken "to consider the organization of education services for the blind and the partially sighted and to make recommendations." Report covers organization of schools, teacher training, curriculum, teaching aids, etc., for the visually handicapped in England and Wales.

392. Enc, Mitat. Bright horizons of hope in Turkey. *International Journal for the Education of the Blind*, June 1952, Vol. 1, No. 4, pp. 96–97.

Briefly reviews Turkey's history of development of education for the blind. Improvement is only recent. Necessary teaching materials very short. Credit to help from other countries. Much more needed.

393. Engbere, Eugenie, et al. *Rehabilitation and care of the handicapped.* Copenhagen: International Relations Div. Ministries of Labour and Social Affairs, 1967, 84 pp.

An overview of services to help the handicapped is given in light of the characteristics of social development in Denmark.

394. Fine, Shirley R. *Blind and partially sighted children.* London: Her Majesty's Stationery Office, 1968, 43 pp.

Report of survey of 817 blind and partially sighted children between 1962 and 1965 in England and Wales. Reports on following topics: Clinical diagnosis, etiology, visual acuity and visual fields, schools previously attended, use of visual aids, mobility, intelligence, additional handicaps, mannerisms, and attitudes of children, parents, and teachers.

395. Folley, Mary. Seebohm and after. *New Beacon,* Apr. 1974, Vol. 58, No. 684, p. 92.

A volunteer worker for the blind describes beginning the work, her apprehensions, her work.

396. Franks, Frank L. An approach for initiating educational programs for the blind in Asia: The Philippine Program, Phase One. *New Outlook for the Blind,* June 1966, Vol. 60, No. 6, pp. 191–97.

Discussion includes: Need for diversiphased approach, implementation process, teacher education program, preschool services, integration into regular classes, special classes, goals. Suggests countries or school systems starting to establish programs will find diversiphased approach has most possibilities and is most economical.

397. Freudenberger, Herbert J. Some observations on work for the blind in Israel. *New Outlook for the Blind,* Jan. 1961, Vol. 55, No. 1, pp. 21–24.

Author visited most schools and agencies working with the blind in Israel. He mentions specific problems pertaining to the immigrant population and how they are handled. Thinks there is possibility of new ideas in a new land.

398. Friedman, Ruth. Inside Russia today: Preparing the blind to lead useful lives. *New Outlook for the Blind,* Nov. 1962, Vol. 56, No. 9, pp. 326–31. Reprinted from *Journal of Rehabilitation,* Jan.–Feb. 1962.

Describes many aspects of education, vocational training, and socialization of the blind in the U.S.S.R.

399. ⸺. Looking at blind education and welfare in Europe and the Near East. *New Outlook for the Blind,* Sept. 1964, Vol. 58, No. 7, pp. 211–13.

Report of the author's basic philosophy about blindness and how it was agreed with or disagreed with in programs used in other countries.

400. Fyson, Marjory. Lahore revisited. *New Beacon,* Oct. 1973, Vol. 57, No. 678, pp. 258–60.

Article, by founder and principal of Lahore's "Sunrise" School for blind children, conveys ambience of work for the blind in Pakistan.

401. Gaster, S. M. G. The Nur Ayin School for the Blind. *International*

Journal for the Education of the Blind, Dec. 1961, Vol. 11, No. 2, pp. 40–41.

Gives history and present status of this school in Iran.

402. Gaukroger, Betty. Teacher training in India. *International Journal for the Education of the Blind*, Oct. 1961, Vol. 11, No. 1, pp. 18–19.

Reports on the first teacher training program in India in which there were 9 trainees, 4 of them blind.

403. Getliff, E. H. The College of Teachers of the Blind. *International Journal for the Education of the Blind*, May 1961, Vol. 10, No. 4, pp. 97–102.

History and present activities of this British institution.

404. Gissler, Tore. Work for adult blind in Sweden. *International Journal for the Education of the Blind*, Feb. 1952, Vol. 1, No. 3, pp. 66–68.

Detailed description of Swedish governmental arrangements for handicapped, especially blind, with various types of pensions and help for training and education.

405. Gray, P. G., & Todd, Jean E. *Mobility and reading habits of the blind: An inquiry made for the Ministry of Health, covering the registered blind of England and Wales in 1965*. London: Her Majesty's Stationery Office, 1968, 119 pp., illus.

A random sample of registered blind people in England and Wales was interviewed in 1965 regarding mobility, orientation, and reading. A copy of the questionnaire is provided.

406. Grosvenor, Theodore. Refractive state, intelligence test scores, and academic ability. *American Journal of Optometry and Archives of American Academy of Optometry*, May 1970, Vol. 47, No. 5, pp. 355–61.

In an experiment with 707 European and Maori intermediate school children, it was found that myopes had higher mean scores than hypermetropes on both the Otis Self-Administered Test and the Raven Progressive Matrices Test.

407. Groth, Hilde. *An evaluation of the pre-industrial selection and training program for blind workers in Malaysia*. Kuala Lumpur, Malaysia: American Foundation for Overseas Blind, 1970, 25 pp., app., illus.

Study of skills needed by the blind to compete within framework of current industrial development in Malaysia. A series of separate investigations show need for modification of current program and long-range plan for development of an industrial training program.

408. Gwaltney, John L. *The thrice shy: Cultural accomodation* [sic] *to blindness and other disasters in a Mexican Community*. New York: Columbia Univ. Press, 1970, xii + 219 pp., illus., $6.95.

Anthropological field study of a Mexican village, deals with cultural accommodation to a particular form of blindness native to region.

409. Harley, Randall K. The development of a program for education of blind children in Ceylon. *Peabody Journal of Education*, July 1971, Vol. 48, No. 4, pp. 314–20.

Development traced from 1912 to today. Considers a three-year project begun in 1967 by AFB which identified visually handicapped children, embossed braille books, and trained teachers.

410. Holmes, Christine M. Helen Keller House. *International Journal for the Education of the Blind*, Mar. 1962, Vol. 11, No. 3, pp. 82–83.

History and present status of a vocational training center for blind girls in Jordan.

411. Holowinsky, Ivan Z. Special education in Eastern Europe: Serious sensory defects. *Journal of Special Education*, Feb. 1973, Vol. 7, No. 3, pp. 329–31.

Reviews special education related research on aurally or visually handicapped in Eastern Europe, U.S.S.R. Areas reviewed include tactile adaptations, occupational opportunities, mental development.

412. House, Roger. *A proposal for the development of a computerized system for Swedish braille: Interim report number 17.* Stockholm: Research Group for Quantitative Linguistics, 1970, 12 pp.

Proposes a computerized production system for Swedish braille. Describes characteristics and development of a new abbreviation scheme, plans for computer translation of Swedish text, and the production system and its development.

413. International Conference of Educators of Blind Youth. *The second quinquennial conference, Oslo, Norway, Aug. 2–10, 1957.* Watertown, Mass.: Author, 1957, 200 pp.

Summaries of educational facilities in 34 countries and papers on special services such as guidance, vocational and extracurricular activities.

414. ———. *Third quinquennial conference proceedings. Aug. 6–18, 1962.* Watertown, Mass.: Author, 1962, 196 pp.

Papers on education of the blind in many countries but especially in Asia, Africa, and Latin America, and on methods and materials and problems of special groups, such as deaf-blind.

415. ———. *Fifth Quinquennial Conference, Madrid, Spain, 1972.* Madrid: Author, 1972, 381 pp.

Papers and abstracts of papers grouped as follows: Reports from research centers, the new math, programmed learning, open education programs, education for life in the community, occupational training and placement, embossed diagrams and maps, and partially sighted.

416. Jackson, Stephen. *Special education in England and Wales.* New York: Oxford Univ. Press, 1966, 147 pp.

Includes outline and discussion of visually impaired children and those with other handicaps. Cites references for suggested reading and lists 27 films about handicapped children.

417. Jackson, W. Rehabilitation in Uganda: "The blind are indeed emerging in emergent Africa." *New Outlook for the Blind*, May 1963, Vol. 57, No. 5, pp. 170–74.

Discusses the country, finding the blind, the center, training, the future, requests for land.

418. Jaekle, Robert C. Orientation and mobility in Asia: The hazards. *New Outlook for the Blind*, Sept. 1975, Vol. 69, No. 7, pp. 295–99.

Greater flexibility in basic cane techniques needed in Asia. Orientation and mobility skills must be adapted to true needs of blind traveler.

419. Jain, I. S. A report on blindness in two rural blocks in northwestern India. *American Foundation for the Blind Research Bulletin 27*, Apr. 1974, pp. 45–86, app.

Detailed statistical and interpretive report of the incidence and characteristics of blindness in a remote section of India, including results of a house-to-house survey.

420. Jarvis, John E. A world review of work for the blind. *New Outlook for the Blind*, Sept. 1955, Vol. 49, No. 7, pp. 251–61.

Describes work with the blind in many countries, contribution of the British Empire Society for the Blind, developments in Latin America, influence of U.N., and the World Council and its committees.

421. Jensen, Ole, & Truelsen, Hans Tage. People with sensory handicaps (English summary from *Maend Med Synshandicap*). *American Foundation for the Blind Research Bulletin 28*, Oct. 1974, pp. 225–31.

Discussion of visually handicapped individuals in Denmark. Includes educational opportunities, relationships with sighted society, role of the visually handicapped man, and attitude of the individual to his handicap.

422. Jensen, Svend. Computerized braille production in Denmark. *American Foundation for the Blind Research Bulletin 28*, Oct. 1974, p. 223.

Brief note. Names equipment used.

423. Jones, Gideon. A look at programs for the blind child with additional handicaps in England. *Education of the Visually Handicapped*, Mar. 1974, Vol. 6, No. 1, pp. 14–18.

Includes discussion of residential facilities for children 7–14 and older, education/training based on fostering independence and use of verbal communication, staff responsibility, diagnostic teaching, vocational orientation. Attributes program success to traditional British education patterns appropriate for multiply handicapped children.

424. Jorgensen, Ernest. A Danish view of allowances to the blind without means test. *New Outlook for the Blind*, May 1953, Vol. 47, No. 5, pp. 126–29.

Arguments for such allowances and the history of efforts to obtain them in Denmark.

425. Jussawala, K. N. K. Blind children and their rehabilitation. *Indian Journal of Social Work*, 1953, Vol. 13, pp. 257–69.

Attention is focused on India's national needs for its 2,000,000 blind. Ways and means of organizing programs of prevention, treatment, education, training, and employment are discussed.

426. Kasemsri, M. R. Sermsri. Problems of the care and education of the blind in Thailand. *International Journal for the Education of the Blind*, Feb. 1953, Vol. 2, No. 2, pp. 144–47.

Presents a short history of work for the blind in Thailand, and the history of development, goals, curriculum, procedures, problems of the School for the Blind there, and mentions plans for a vocational center.

427. Katz, Alfred H. Poland's self-help rehabilitation program. *New Outlook for the Blind*, June 1965, Vol. 59, No. 6, pp. 216–18.

General account of rehabilitation in Poland with some brief mention of the blind.

428. Kavalgikar, Ramchandra Rav. Education and employment of blind and deaf-mute children. *Indian Journal of Social Work,* 1953, Vol. 14, pp. 160–67.

Services for education and welfare of blind and deaf in India are surveyed and compared with U.S. statistics. Need for vast improvement is noted.

429. Keizer, R. Rehabilitation of the adult blind in the Netherlands. *New Outlook for the Blind,* June 1958, Vol. 52, No. 6, pp. 225–29.

Discusses origin and organization, methods, developments, overcoming limitations, cooperating organizations, and results.

430. Keller, Helen. My work in the Near East. *New Outlook for the Blind,* June 1953, Vol. 47, No. 6, pp. 151–71.

Detailed description of her trip through Egypt, Lebanon, Syria, Jordan, Palestine, and Israel, and services for blind people in those countries.

431. ———. My experiences in Latin America. *New Outlook for the Blind,* May 1954, Vol. 48, No. 5, pp. 129–48.

Detailed account of her trip and observations in Brazil, Chile, Peru, Panama, and Mexico.

432. ———. My tour around the globe. *New Outlook for the Blind,* Oct. 1956, Vol. 50, No. 8, pp. 310–25.

Observations on services to the blind in India, Indonesia, the Philippines, and Japan.

433. Kenmore, Jeanne R. Establishing special education programs in developing countries. *New Outlook for the Blind,* Oct. 1970, Vol. 64, No. 8, pp. 270–74.

Participation of the country's government, quality of foreign technical assistance consultants, and consideration of local conditions are stressed as important factors for success. Examples show influence of initial patterns in establishing future standards. Various outside sources of aid are discussed.

434. Klinkhart, Emily J. Some observations on work for the blind in the U.S.S.R. *New Outlook for the Blind,* Dec. 1958, Vol. 52, No. 10, pp. 386–89.

The author notes some interesting items such as type of work at the Institute for Defectology, existence of schools for the totally blind and separate schools for the partially sighted, procedures at the Leningrad School, sophisticated levels of work for blind children in a less-than-sheltered atmosphere, and role of the All-Union Society for the Blind in placement activities.

435. Knox, Barbara. Modern approaches to financial assistance to the blind. *New Outlook for the Blind,* Mar. 1965, Vol. 59, No. 3, pp. 86–89.

Briefly reviews assistance in a number of countries and suggests the broader security, education, and employment which would be ideal.

436. Kohler, Lennart. Health of preschool children in Sweden. *Sight-Saving Review,* Summer 1975, Vol. 45, No. 2, pp. 59–67.

Background and description of pilot study of the health of 4-year-olds—purpose, items covered by program, personnel, methods, and results. Ninety-seven percent of the children with eye disorders were detected with the visual screening part of the program. Over-referral was found in 16.5% and significant eye disorders in 43%.

437. Kulicheva, N. *Organization of recreation for the blind in the U.S.S.R.* Moscow: All-Russia Society for the Blind, 1972, 41 pp.

Description of recreation under the auspices of the Society. Mentions such areas as drama, music, sports, art. Contains photographs illustrating activities.

438. Langerhans, Clara. A continent awakes: South America's developing program for the blind. *New Outlook for the Blind*, Mar. 1957, Vol. 51, No. 3, pp. 98–107.

Incidence of blindness in various South American countries and growth of services in the preceding 5 years, especially the part played by the Center for the Training of Teachers in Special Education. Braille literature and tangible teaching equipment are much needed.

439. Miller, Andrew S. Educating the blind in Kalimpong. *New Outlook for the Blind*, Dec. 1968, Vol. 62, No. 10, pp. 323–24.

With 6 teachers, a residential school in India serves 50 students offering a program similar to the public schools. Describes typical day.

440. Mulholland, Mary E. The Royal National Institute for the Blind 1868–1968. *New Outlook for the Blind*, June 1968, Vol. 62, No. 6, pp. 169–72.

With pictures, recounts the history of this British institution.

441. Neleson, Leonard. A non-institutional program for the education of blind children in Israel. *New Outlook for the Blind*, Dec. 1957, Vol. 51, No. 10, pp. 457–65.

A plan for education of blind children in the normal community schools of Israel with discussion of proposed staff, program coordination, and implications.

442. ———. The current status of work with the blind in Israel. *New Outlook for the Blind*, Apr. 1961, Vol. 55, No. 4, pp. 129–32.

Largely a supplement to and critique of Freudenberger's article (*Outlook*, Jan. 1961). Present author gives what he thinks is more fair and up-to-date state of work with the blind in Israel.

443. Ogiyama, Jiro. The Braille Mainichi—Pioneer in Japan. *New Outlook for the Blind*, Feb. 1956, Vol. 50, No. 2, pp. 62–64. Reprinted from the *Matilda Ziegler Magazine for the Blind.*

This newspaper for the blind has been published by a newspaper company for 34 years; it has also published books in braille, and sponsors or supports various enterprises for the schools for the blind of Japan.

444. Rau, P. N. Venkata. The handicapped. *International Journal for the Education of the Blind*, June 1953, Vol. 2, No. 4, pp. 179–82.

Suggests that "handicapped" is too general a term and that, in India, legislation specific to blindness and deafness would be desirable.

445. Republic of China, Ministry of Education. *Special education programs in the Republic of China.* Taiwan: Dept. of Social Education, Ministry of Education, 1971, 14 pp.

Describes Taiwan's present state and future outlook for education of 4 special groups, 1 being the blind. Since only 350 of 2,000 visually handicapped children are in residential schools, an integrated program is recommended. Specific preparation of special education teachers is recent but expanding.

446. Robson, Howard. Some aspects of welfare services for blind persons in Japan. *New Outlook for the Blind*, Apr. 1973, Vol. 67, No. 4, pp. 175–80.

With the exception of rehabilitation, the entire spectrum of services for blind and visually handicapped persons in Japan—library services, the weekly newspaper, government benefits, the employment situation, provisions for education—is discussed. Article concludes that in general the services are adequate but that improvement could be noted in areas of vocational training and gainful employment.

447. Roose, Herman. Observations of a Hollander on work for the blind in America. *New Outlook for the Blind*, Apr. 1953, Vol. 47, No. 4, pp. 101–14.

Rather detailed comparison of all aspects of education and work for the blind in this country with those in Holland.

448. Royal National Institute for the Blind. Blindness in England. *New Outlook for the Blind*, Apr. 1972, Vol. 66, No. 4, pp. 120–21. Excerpted from *New Beacon*, Oct. 1971.

Statistics relating to the blind and partially sighted for the year 1970. Gives some comparisons with previous year's figures.

449. Said, Mohyi-Eldin; Goldstein, Hyman; Korra, Ahmad; et al. Blindness prevalence rates in Egypt. *HSMHA Health Reports*, Feb. 1972, Vol. 87, No. 2, pp. 177–84.

Prevalence of blindness among persons residing around Alexandria. Comparison of rates between a randomly selected population and a self-selected population sample.

450. ———. Blindness prevalence rates in Egypt. *Health Services Reports*, Jan. 1973, Vol. 88, No. 1, pp. 89–96.

Article based on data from the U.S. Govt.-sponsored Blindness Register Demonstration Project in Egypt. The diagnostic classification is comparable to that used by the Model Reporting Area for Blindness Statistics in the U.S.

451. Salisbury, Geoffrey E. Assignment in Africa. *International Journal for the Education of the Blind*, Mar. 1960, Vol. 9, No. 3, pp. 63–66.

Describes numbers of blind and public attitudes toward the blind in Africa. Schools and training centers for adults have been recently established, and this paper reports their progress.

452. Schiff, Yehuda. A pioneer experiment in training blind persons in Israel. *New Outlook for the Blind*, Apr. 1963, Vol. 57, No. 4, pp. 134–35.

Discusses Israel's lack of resources to implement a program for research and demonstration, and application to the U.S. Dept. of Health, Education & Welfare. It was recognized that a research program could be of importance in countries which have a textile industry and also a need to find employment for blind persons.

453. Snider, Harold. Crossing the Atlantic does make a difference. *New Beacon*, Aug. 1974, Vol. 58, No. 688, pp. 203–7.

Compares British blind welfare system with the system in the U.S. Based on personal observations.

454. Solntseva, Lujdmila. The upbringing of blind children in the Soviet Union. *New Outlook for the Blind,* Feb. 1969, Vol. 63, No. 2, pp. 42–44. Adapted from Soviet journal, *Special School,* Vol. 114, No. 2.

Guidelines for upbringing of Soviet blind preschool child within the family, including orientation, self-care, healthy attitudes, learning the arts, etc.

455. Sorsby, Arnold. *The incidence and causes of blindness in England and Wales 1963–68; With an appendix on services available for incipient blindness.* London: Her Majesty's Stationery Office, 1972, ix + 72 pp.

456. Spurgeon, E. Education of the blind in India. *Teacher of the Blind,* Winter 1974–75, Vol. 63, No. 2, pp. 46–48.

Description of the blind population and their schooling in India.

457. Taylor, Wallace W. The education of the blind in Western Europe. *International Journal for the Education of the Blind,* Dec. 1959, Vol. 9, No. 2, pp. 25–31.

After a short historical introduction, discusses the identification and incidence of blind children in various countries of Western Europe, various kinds of educational provisions, and some of the problems including shortage of special teachers.

458. Taylor, Wallace W., & Taylor, Isabelle W. *Special education of physically handicapped children in Western Europe.* New York: International Society f/t Welfare of Cripples, 1960, 497 pp.

Includes an account of education of the blind in 21 countries. Lists definitions of disabilities, incidence and prevalence of disabilities, services for children, and the organization and administration of services for each country. Ref.

459. Thatcher, Margaret. After Vernon. *New Beacon,* Aug. 1973, Vol. 57, No. 676, pp. 202–6.

Discusses the Royal National Institute and other organizations for the blind, their relationship to relevant depts. of the government, criticism by the Vernon Committee of services to the blind.

460. Tobin, Michael J. Report on overseas research. *Teacher of the Blind,* Apr. & July 1971, Vol. 59, Nos. 3 & 4, pp. 117–26, 154–70.

The "overseas research" of the title is mostly that done in the U.S., although Russia, Japan, Sweden, and other countries are included. Bib.

461. Townsend, Alex H. Middle East seminar for instructors of blind children and youth. *New Outlook for the Blind,* Feb. 1966, Vol. 60, No. 2, pp. 59–60.

Notes pressures for change on traditional Islamic concept of the blind. Presents seminar curriculum.

462. Townsend, M. Roberta. A U.N. mission to Guatemala. *New Outlook for the Blind,* Apr. 1953, Vol. 47, No. 4, pp. 97–100.

After rather lengthy comments on the history of the country, describes services to the blind and the development of a program to improve those services.

463. Trutneva, K. *Prevention of blindness in the U.S.S.R.* Moscow: All-Russia Society for the Blind, 1972, 25 pp.

Contrasts conditions prior to 1917 with those in 1971. Mentioned among achievements are a state standard on protective glasses, methods of locating foreign bodies in the eye, treatment of the eye, new methods of surgery.

464. Uzelac, Stevo. Life and work of the blind in Yugoslavia. *New Outlook for the Blind*, June 1964, Vol. 58, No. 6, pp. 188–89.

Detailed description of education and other special services provided for the blind in Yugoslavia.

465. Watson, L. S. The assessment and placement of the blind worker in industry. *American Foundation for the Blind Research Bulletin 24*, Mar. 1972, pp. 113–41.

Detailed description of a complex assessment program for potential blind workers in South Africa.

466. Westaway, D. L. Alternatives to the blindness system in Australia. *New Outlook for the Blind*, Feb. 1973, Vol. 67, No. 2, pp. 66–71.

Suggests that integration into regular community services would provide better service and eliminate the present complex of agencies. Makes specific suggestions.

467. ———. What if it happened to you? *Guide Dog Magazine*, Sept. 1974, Vol. 9, No. 3, pp. 10–11.

Discusses mobility training, counseling, mobility aids available from Australia's National Guide Dog and Mobility Training Center. Describes research and expansion efforts and eligibility criteria.

468. Wexler, Abraham. Education and welfare of the blind in Japan. *New Outlook for the Blind*, May 1966, Vol. 60, No. 5, pp. 159–63.

Discusses establishment, plans, activities of the Nippon Lighthouse; elementary, secondary, and higher education; research on blind welfare; employment. Figures on blind population, graduates, and employees given.

469. Wilson, John. Blindness in Africa. *New Outlook for the Blind*, Oct. 1955, Vol. 49, No. 8, pp. 291–93.

Describes the huge problems presented by blindness, its prevention and treatment, in Africa. Local schools, rooted in African village economy, seem the most promising answer.

470. ———. Blind children in rural communities. *New Outlook for the Blind*, Oct. 1957, Vol. 51, No. 8, pp. 351–56.

Broad discussion of the needs of blind children in rural settings all over the world but especially in developing countries. Realistic education and training are much needed.

471. ———. Past and present. *New Beacon*, Aug. 1975, Vol. 59, No. 700, pp. 197–99.

Brief history of work with the blind in the United Kingdom and especially of the Royal National Institute for the Blind.

472. Yazina, A. *General principles of organization of production.* Moscow: All-Russia Society for the Blind, 1972, 23 pp.

Describes the development of employment opportunities for the blind and the current states of production by the blind in the U.S.S.R.

473. Zacho, Zlata. Are the blind always cheerful? *New Beacon*, Nov. 1975, Vol. 59, No. 703, pp. 283–85.

Account of a PR program in Denmark.

474. Zemtsova, M. *Education of the blind and people with weak sight in the U.S.S.R.* Moscow: All-Russia Society for the Blind, 1972, 15 pp.

475. Zimin, Boris. Employment and vocational training of the blind in the U.S.S.R. *New Outlook for the Blind*, Dec. 1962, Vol. 56, No. 10, pp. 363–66.

Describes "special enterprises" employing from 50% to 75% blind workers who are preferably involved in industrial processing, pressing, and fitting. Enumerates blind-made products and tools used in woodworking and metal industries. Discusses special safety measures, the "special enterprises" rationale, vocational training procedures, leisure activities.

476. ———. *Raising the welfare of the blind in the U.S.S.R.* Moscow: All-Russia Society for the Blind, 1972, 21 pp.

Describes activities and plans of the All-Russia Society for the Blind.

477. ———. *To live and work.* Moscow: All-Russia Society for the Blind, 1972, 79 pp.

Describes the history and functions of the Society which was founded in 1925 to improve the physical, educational, and employment conditions of the blind.

6. Parents and Younger Children

478. Adelson, Edna, & Fraiberg, Selma. Gross motor development in infants blind from birth. *Child Development,* Mar. 1974, Vol. 45, No. 1, pp. 114–26.

Report on a longitudinal study of 10 infants observed from birth to 2 years at the Univ. of Mich. Medical Center's Child Development Project.

479. Allegheny County Schools (Pa.). *A demonstration project on developing independence in preschool visually handicapped children.* Washington, D.C.: Office of Education, 1969, 62 pp.

Seven children participated in a 6-week program for developing independence in movement in space, self-help skills, effective use of residual vision, socialization, and body image. Parent education meetings were held and caseworkers provided counseling. Self-help and other skills did improve.

480. Allegheny Intermediate Unit No. 3, Exceptional Children's Program, Pittsburgh, Pa. *A plan for itinerant educational consultant services for preschool visually handicapped children.* Harrisburg: State Dept. of Education, 1972, 79 pp.

Describes 2-year program: Procedures of identification, referral, interviewing, and instruction; use of paraprofessionals, mobility specialists, and student teachers; development of a toy library with entries catalogued according to age levels and developmental goals. Six case studies.

481. American Association of Instructors of the Blind. *AAIB National Conference on Pre-School Services for Visually Handicapped Children and Their Families (St. Louis, Mo., March 28–30, 1965).* St. Louis: Author, 1965, 102 pp., $2.

Topics of 11 papers include defining blind children, role of pediatrician in identification of infants with visual defects, eye diseases, counseling with parents, emotional development of preschool children, and use of community resources.

482. American Foundation for the Blind. *Is your child blind?* New York: Author, 1970, 8 pp., free.

Pamphlet shows parents of blind children how these children develop and grow, and how parents can help them to achieve their maximum potential.

483. ———. *Proceedings of the National Seminar on Services to Young Children with Visual Impairment.* Author, 1970, 78 pp., $2.

This publication deals with the need for changes in services caused by the increase in the number of multiply handicapped young blind children. Subjects covered include cognitive development, perception, and the family of the blind child.

484. Axline, Virginia M. That the blind may see. *New Outlook for the Blind*, Feb. 1955, Vol. 49, No. 2, pp. 45–48. Reprinted from *Teachers College Record*, 1954.

Discusses attitudes of parents and others in the environment of a blind child and how these affect the child's concept of himself.

485. ———. Understanding and accepting the child who is blind. *New Outlook for the Blind*, Apr. 1955, Vol. 49, No. 4, pp. 132–35. Reprinted from *Childhood Education*, 1954.

Attitudes of parents upon discovering that the child is blind and attitudes of others around the child help to determine the child's life.

486. Bakalis, Michael J., & Calovini, Gloria. *Toys for early development of the young blind child.* Springfield, Ill.: State Office of Supt. of Public Instruction, 1971, 16 pp., illus.

Suggests toys which tend to encourage development of certain skills. Lists types of toys, purposes, ways to use, and manufacturers.

487. Barraga, Natalie, et al. *Aids for teaching basic concepts of sensory development.* Louisville, Ky.: American Printing House for the Blind, 1973, 157 pp.

Presents instructions for use and construction of approximately 58 instructional materials to aid young visually handicapped children in developing basic sensory concepts, numerical concepts, and manual dexterity.

488. Barry, H., Jr., & Marshall, Frances E. Maladjustment and maternal rejection in retrolental fibroplasia. *Mental Hygiene*, 1953, Vol. 37, pp. 570–80.

Study of 17 children with RLF and a control group of 13 children blind due to other causes. Conclusion was that maternal rejection is associated with poor school adjustment of RLF children.

489. Barry, M. Adelaide. How to play with your partially sighted preschool child: Suggestions for early sensory and educational activities. *New Outlook for the Blind*, Dec. 1973, Vol. 67, No. 10, pp. 457–65, 467.

An explanation of a visual stimulation program for a partially sighted child is explained in detail from infancy through 2 years of age. Concludes with overall guidelines which should be considered in a program of visual stimulation.

490. Barsch, Ray H. *The parent of the handicapped child: The study of child-rearing practices. American lecture series.* Springfield, Ill.: Charles C Thomas, 1968, 445 pp., app.

Report of 3-year study of parents of blind and other handicapped children includes data collection process, demography of 5 populations, information on identification and early infancy, communication, toilet training, rest, restrictions, demands, allowances, sex, attitudes, schooling, religion. Gives handicapped ranking scale, summary, critique, proposals, parent questionnaires.

491. Basic concepts of blind children. *New Outlook for the Blind*, Dec. 1965, Vol. 59, No. 10, pp. 341–43.

A committee of teachers reviews the development of basic concepts in blind children, especially concepts upon which orientation and mobility must build. Practical suggestions are made for parents and teachers for useful experiences from when child is in the crib to elementary school.

492. Bell, Donald, Ed. Hints for blind mothers, *New Beacon*, Mar. 1970, Vol. 54, No. 635, pp. 58–63.

Written by a blind mother, provides advice on child care.

493. Benson, Jo, & Ross, Linda. Teaching parents to teach their children. *TEACHING Exceptional Children*, Fall 1972, Vol. 5, No. 1, pp. 32–35, illus.

Report of a parent volunteer project in which some of the 13 trainable mentally retarded children were visually impaired as well. Parents became more interested and involved in their children's educational development.

494. Benton, Arthur L. Language learning: Perceptual bases. *Proceedings of the Annual Reading Institute*, Mar. 1968, Vol. 7, pp. 23–31.

Considers the nature, functions, and early development of language, including in children with visual deficiencies.

495. Bledsoe, C. Warren. For parents looking ahead to future mobility needs of their blind children. *International Journal for the Education of the Blind*, Oct. 1963, Vol. 13, No. 1, pp. 13–16.

With attention to the history, gives reasons for training for independent mobility.

496. Blos, Joan W. Traditional nursery rhymes and games: Language learning experiences for preschool blind children. *New Outlook for the Blind*, June 1974, Vol. 68, No. 6, pp. 268–75.

Suggestions for a definite, but informal, sequence of language-related activities, using songs, rhymes, records, and stories.

497. ———. Rhymes, songs, records, and stories: Language learning experiences for preschool blind children. *New Outlook for the Blind*, Sept. 1974, Vol. 68, No. 7, pp. 300–307.

Sources of tales and songs are suggested, as are hints for presenting them and adapting them to real-life situations. The use of recorded materials is explored.

498. Bornstein, Susan. *Why severely impaired infants and their families need help: The earlier—the better.* Boston: Boston Center for Blind Children, 1974, 25 pp., app., $1.20.

Describes home teaching program for children whose visual handicaps are often accompanied by severe developmental disorders. App. includes record forms, bib., and lists of materials and equipment.

499. Bowley, Agatha H., & Gardner, Leslie. *The young handicapped child: Educational guidance for the young cerebral palsied, deaf, blind, & autistic child.* London: E. & S. Livingstone, 1969, 167 pp.

The different classes of handicaps, the size of the problem, the causes, and the principles and methods of psychological and education care concerning children with partial and total blindness, cerebral palsy, deafness, or autism are discussed.

500. Branson, Helen K. The blind mother. *American Journal of Nursing.* Mar. 1975, Vol. 75, No. 3, pp. 414–16.

Information for the obstetrical nurse about blindness and instructing a blind mother in the best care for her baby.

501. Branson, Helen K., & Branson, Ralph. The blind child and his special problems. *New Outlook for the Blind,* Apr. 1956, Vol. 50, No. 4, pp. 122–28.

Two blind counselors offer information and advice to parents of blind children. "The sightless child needs to be treated as an individual capable of living his own life."

502. Brown, Charles E.; Briller, Stanley; & Richards, Susan S. A new program for young blind children: A cornerstone for future service. *New Outlook for the Blind,* Sept. 1967, Vol. 61, No. 7, pp. 210–17.

Needs of the child must be met effectively all through his developmental growth. These needs and effective approaches to these needs are discussed in detail.

503. Brown, Jean D. Storytelling and the blind child. *New Outlook for the Blind,* Dec. 1972, Vol. 66, No. 10, pp. 356–60.

A discussion of storytelling as a tool for aiding a child's mental development. Suggestions for making storytelling meaningful to blind children. Lists some stories enjoyed by blind children.

504. Bryan, Dorothy. *Guide for parents of pre-school visually handicapped children.* Springfield, Ill.: State Office of Supt. of Public Instruction, 1972, 66 pp.

A guide booklet offering attitudinal and early training experience necessary for the child's development into a happy, well-rounded adult. Descriptive listings of national and Ill. state agencies serving visually handicapped persons.

505. Burgess, Caroline B. Counseling parents of children with handicaps. *New Outlook for the Blind,* Jan. 1955, Vol. 49, No. 1, pp. 1–5.

It is extremely important that the counselor understand the depth of the parent's emotion and that the help be practical. The goal is not just giving answers but counseling together. "It is deliberation together which is the essence of counseling."

506. Burlingham, Dorothy. Some notes on the development of the blind. *Psychoanalytic Study of the Child,* 1961, Vol. 16, pp. 121–45.

Observations on a nursery group of blind children and their mothers.

507. Burnham, Rose K. Blind parents and their children. *Dialogue,* Spring 1972, Vol. 11, No. 1, pp. 7–10.

Reports on interviews with 2 mothers of grown children, the parents of 2 young children, and the sighted daughter of blind parents.

508. Cargill, Joanna. Our set of circumstances. *New Outlook for the Blind,* June 1971, Vol. 65, No. 6, pp. 174–80.

The very normal story of the birth and development of a blind child of blind parents.

509. Carolan, Robert H. Sensory stimulation and the blind infant. *New Outlook for the Blind,* Mar. 1973, Vol. 67, No. 3, pp. 119–26.

A blind infant needs a rich environment of sensory stimulation; parents can be helped in a variety of ways to provide this. The concept of an infant curriculum, as developed by Barsch, is suggested as a particularly useful means of insuring that appropriate kinds and amounts of sensory stimulation are provided at each developmental stage.

510. Carr, Lela B. Pre-school blind children and their parents. *Children,* May-June 1955, Vol. 2, No. 3, pp. 83–88.

Explanation of a counseling service, the case worker's job, and use of nursery schools. Also notes institutes for parents.

511. Cauffman, Josef G. The way he should go. *International Journal for the Education of the Blind,* Mar. 1956, Vol. 5, No. 3, pp. 64–65.

Discusses increase in blindness and increase in parents and agencies looking for final and new answers to blindness. Considers recognition of handicap, acceptance, education.

512. Caulfield, Thomas E. Guides to improving parental attitudes. *New Outlook for the Blind,* Apr. 1959, Vol. 53, No. 4, pp. 128–31.

Speaks directly to parents about their attitudes and emotions. Recommends self-appraisal and provides a few suggestions for handling the child.

513. Cegelka, Walter J. *Readings in counseling parents of exceptional children.* New York: Selected Academic Readings, 1965, 134 pp.

Mentions parent-teacher conferences, psychotherapy for parents, group counseling, therapy and consultation among counseling methods for parents of handicapped children.

514. Chase, Joan B. *Retrolental fibroplasia and autistic symptomatology: An investigation into some relationships among neonatal, environmental, developmental and affective variables in blind prematures.* New York: AFB, 1972, 215 pp., $4.

Data were collected through parent interviews, professional ratings, and medical and psychological case histories of 263 children and adults. App. gives parent questionnaires, counselor's checklist, data tables.

515. ———. A retrospective study of retrolental fibroplasia. *New Outlook for the Blind,* Feb. 1974, Vol. 68, No. 2, pp. 61–71.

The relationship between RLF and severe affect disturbances was investigated. Data on 263 *S*s was studied. Of some 11 variables, autistic symptomatology was found to be correlated only with high birth weight (rather than low as expected), long gestation or extreme prematurity, and parental intellectuality. A multifactor theory of etiology is suggested. Ref.

516. ———. Developmental assessment of handicapped infants and young children: With special attention to the visually impaired. *New Outlook for the Blind,* Oct. 1975, Vol. 69, No. 8, pp. 341–49, 364.

Early objective developmental assessments are necessary to effectively plan for services for young handicapped children. Lists some widely used measures. Case history given. Ref.

517. Clark, Leslie L.; Freedman, D. G.; & Dumas, Georges. The expression of emotion by the blind. *New Outlook for the Blind,* May 1967, Vol. 61, No. 5, pp. 155–63, & June 1967, Vol. 61, No. 6, pp. 194–204.

Following introduction by Clark, Freedman reviews the literature on smiling by all infants and reports a study of smiling in four congenitally blind infants. Dumas discusses mimicry as a voluntary imitation of spontaneous expressions and summarizes his rather informal experiments in mimicry with blind persons.

518. Clay, Frances. Social work and the blind child. *New Outlook for the Blind*, Dec. 1961, Vol. 55, No. 10, pp. 321–25.

Overview of role of social worker in dealing with family that has a visually handicapped child. Long-range nature of relationship is emphasized.

519. Cohen, Jerome; Alfano, Joseph E.; Boshes, Louis D.; et al. Clinical evaluation of school-age children with retrolental fibroplasia. *American Foundation for the Blind Research Bulletin 7*, Dec. 1964, pp. 71–96, illus.

A longitudinal interdisciplinary study of 43 children with RLF from a total research group of 66 blind children previously described by Norris, et al. Interrelated ophthalmologic findings, birth characteristics, X-rays, electroencephalograms, and other pediatric disorders.

520. Cohen, Pauline C. The impact of the handicapped child on the family. *New Outlook for the Blind*, Jan. 1964, Vol. 58, No. 1, pp. 11–15.

Dealing with stages of grief, anger, necessity of adjusting adaptive patterns, and effect of reality on total family are discussed from point of view of caseworker.

521. Connelly, Winnifred. *Visually handicapped children—Birth to three years.* Ann Arbor: Mich. Univ. Medical Center, Dec. 1969, 10 pp.

Early development discussed. Mother's role stressed with attention to providing love and an environment for learning, manipulative and motor activities, and nutrition.

522. Coon, Nelson. French views on the education of the pre-school blind child. *International Journal for the Education of the Blind*, June 1953, Vol. 2, No. 4, pp. 178–79.

Presents comments on a Paris conference in 1889 on topics such as parent education and living skills. Lists 17 suggestions to parents of blind children.

523. Council for Exceptional Children. *Exceptional children conference papers: Curriculum, methods, and materials in early childhood education programs.* Arlington, Va.: Author, 1969, 175 pp.

Papers presented at Dec. 1969 conference in New Orleans on early childhood education include the following topics: Stimulation and cognitive development, curriculum development, sequencing instructional activities, nursery school observation, assessing cognitive development, preschool programs for cerebral palsied children, a service for parents of the visually impaired, techniques in speech therapy.

524. Coyne, Peggy H.; Peterson, Linda W.; & Peterson, Robert F. The development of spoon-feeding behavior in a blind child. *International Journal for the Education of the Blind*, Dec. 1968, Vol. 18, No. 4, pp. 108–12.

A blind child, age 3, who had not developed independent spoon-feeding skills, was the subject of a study of reinforcement procedures. Results are reported with aid of graphs.

525. Cratty, Bryant J. *Some implications of movement.* Seattle: Special Child Publications, 1970, 248 pp., $4.65.

Deals with movement experiences and how they may be used bene-
ficially by children with mild or severe sensory-motor deficiencies. Positive
suggestions made for improvement through movement; relations between
movement, intelligence, and perception explored. Final section elaborates
upon the use of motor activities in education of exceptional children concentrating on mentally retarded and blind.

526. ―――. *Movement and spatial awareness in blind children and youth.*
Springfield, Ill.: Charles C Thomas, 1971, 240 pp., $12.

Clinical observations and research evidence presented to aid children
to move and deal with space more effectively.

527. **Cratty, Bryant J.; Peterson, Carl; Harris, Janet; et al.** The development of perceptual-motor abilities in blind children and adolescents. *New
Outlook for the Blind,* Apr. 1968, Vol. 62, No. 4, pp. 111–17.

On the basis of reported experiments and experience, 3 improvements
are needed in education of blind children: Thorough tactile training, body
image training, and early mobility education.

528. **Curtis, John, et al., Eds.** *The guidance of exceptional children: A book
of readings.* 2nd ed. New York: David McKay, 1972, xi + 465 pp., $4.95.

A collection of reprinted articles and speeches. Chap. 6 (pp. 307–36) is
is on "The blind child."

529. **Cutsforth, Margery.** The pre-school blind child at home. *Exceptional
Children,* 1957, Vol. 24, pp. 58–65.

Discusses need for parental awareness and understanding of the pre-
school-age blind child's needs.

530. **DiCaprio, Nicholas S.** Factors affecting the child's evaluation of the
visually handicapped parent. *New Outlook for the Blind,* June 1971, Vol.
65, No. 6, pp. 181–86.

Reviews potential problems of child-rearing in a family where at least
1 parent is blind, including discipline, parental competition, difficulties
outside the home, explaining the handicap to the child, and the child
helping the parent.

531. **Dickinson, Raymond M.** *Questions asked by parents of visually handicapped children.* Springfield, Ill.: Dept. of Children & Family Services,
1968, 22 pp.

Offers information on a wide range of problem solutions. Walking, posture, exercise, play, eating, developing other senses and space concepts,
discipline, and sex education are covered.

532. **Duncan, James A.** "Buddies incorporated"—Companion dogs for blind
children: An observation of the dog training section of the animal hus-
bandry program at the New York Institute for the Education of the
Blind. *International Journal for the Education of the Blind,* May 1956,
Vol. 5, No. 4, pp. 80–86.

Details how to teach visually handicapped children the training and
care of dogs as pets or, later, for show ring. Possible fringe benefits are
development of responsibility, elimination of blindisms, integrated competition, self-confidence, and experience leading to vocational placement.

533. Eisenstadt, Arthur A. Psychological problems of the parents of a blind child. *International Journal for the Education of the Blind,* Oct. 1955, Vol. 5, No. 1, pp. 20–23.

Most handicapped children have emotional and psychological problems; parents do also. Stages of reactions of parents: Shock and grief, bewilderment and helplessness, fears, tension. Recommendations.

534. Eissler, Ruth S., et al., Eds. *The psychoanalytic study of the child. Volume XVI.* New York: International Univ. Press, 1961, 563 pp.

Discusses psychosexual development of the blind including psychological process operating during pregnancy and the earliest mother-child relationship; processes involved in symbol formation derived from the relationship between perception and reality testing; and the equilibrium between libido and aggression producing either structural synthesis or fragmentation.

535. Ellis, Jean M. The role of the preschool counselor. *New Outlook for the Blind,* Jan. 1957, Vol. 51, No. 1, pp. 25–30.

Partially through case histories, describes the educational, supportive, public relations, and intermediary roles of the preschool counselor in Massachusetts Div. of the Blind.

536. Fine, M. Ruth. Psychological considerations of the child with a progressive terminal condition in a residential setting. *New Outlook for the Blind,* Mar. 1975, Vol. 69, No. 3, pp. 121–30.

Areas of concern include parental and sibling attitudes and ways of coping with the fact that the child is dying, as well as the roles of teachers, houseparents, and other professionals.

537. Fitzgerald, H. Kenneth. Family life education and work with the blind. *New Outlook for the Blind,* Feb. 1962, Vol. 56, No. 2, pp. 39–42.

Discusses dissatisfaction with historical approach to dealing with blindness and cites numerous forward trends. Discusses parents' role in education of the blind child, and need for and possible structure of family education programs.

538. Fox, Julia V. Improving tactile discrimination of the blind. *American Journal of Occupational Therapy,* 1965, Vol. 19, No. 1, pp. 5–7.

Report of a study of effect of olfactory stimulation on scores of 10 blind children undergoing a test of tactual discrimination. Results indicated that cutaneous and olfactory stimulation may be useful in developing tactile discrimination in the blind child.

539. Fraiberg, Selma. Separation crisis in two blind children. *Psychoanalytic Study of the Child,* 1971, Vol. 26, pp. 355–71.

Describes the factors which aggravate the separation crisis for the blind child and his mother. Age 14 and 17 months.

540. Fraiberg, Selma; Siegel, Barry L.; & Gibson, Ralph. The role of sound in the search behavior of a blind infant. *Psychoanalytic Study of the Child,* 1966, Vol. 21, pp. 327–57.

The absence of vision at birth is seen to retard: (1) search for the source of sounds, (2) reaching for tactile objects in response to auditory cues, (3) establishment of coordination of hearing and prehension, and (4) ego development.

541. Freedman, D. G. Smiling in blind infants and the issue of innate vs. acquired. *Journal of Child Psychology and Psychiatry*, 1964, Vol. 5, Nos. 3–4, pp. 171–84.

A review of the literature and observations of 4 congenitally blind infants indicated smiling is an innate response. However, it is at first fleeting and reflex-like and its development into a social response is facilitated by vision.

542. Freedman, David A. Congenital and perinatal sensory deprivation: Some studies in early development. *American Journal of Psychiatry*, May 1971, Vol. 127, No. 11, pp. 1539–45.

Evidence is presented that the high incidence of autistic disturbances in the congenitally blind is due to coenesthetic deprivation.

543. Froyd, Helen E. Counseling families of severely visually handicapped children. *New Outlook for the Blind*, June 1973, Vol. 67, No. 6, pp. 251–57.

Discussion of the value of professional counseling to families of visually handicapped children from the family's first awareness of the impairment through each of the stages of the child's development. While many agencies now begin family counseling with preschool youngsters, there is still a void of service in the birth to age 3 period.

544. Gaines, Rosslyn. Experiencing the perceptually-deprived child. *Journal of Learning Disabilities*, Nov. 1969, Vol. 2, No. 11, pp. 559–65.

Suggests that the perceptually-blind child can experience his world more fully with intensive parental assistance. Perceptually-deprived means reduced perceptual intake due to blindness, deafness, neurological disorder, or retardation. Discussion of parental roles and psychological, social, and cultural difficulties involved. Solutions proposed.

545. Garrison, Karl C., & Force, Dewey G., Jr. *The psychology of exceptional children.* New York: Ronald Press, 1965, 571 pp.

Discusses the definition, characteristics, identification, socioemotional adjustment, economic needs and provisions of visually handicapped as well as other exceptional children. Annotates 10 references, lists films, film sources.

546. Gesell, Arnold. Development of the infant with retrolental fibroplastic blindness. *Field of Vision*, Dec. 15, 1953, Vol. 5, No. 1.

Notes factors to be considered in the development of an infant with RLF with illustrative case history. However, permanently serious retardation is not necessarily produced. Some guidance suggestions for parents.

547. Gillman, Arthur E. Handicap and cognition: Visual deprivation and the rate of motor development in infants. *New Outlook for the Blind*, Sept. 1973, Vol. 67, No. 7, pp. 309–14.

With review of literature and report of pilot study with 74 Ss, concludes delays in development are not due to blindness per se. Urges full understanding of the growth and development of the nonhandicapped child as a basis for work with all children.

548. Gillman, Arthur E., & Goddard, Dorothy R. The 20-year outcome of blind children two years old and younger: A preliminary survey. *New Outlook for the Blind*, Jan. 1974, Vol. 68, No. 1, pp. 1–7.

A study of 77 blind children, conducted through a survey of case records, including changes in visual acuity, additional handicaps, social status, and psychological test scores. Twenty-five percent were still active with the agency, 20% were institutionalized; 15% had attended college.

549. Grossman, Rose T. The preschool blind child. *Seer*, Mar. 1970, Vol. 41, No. 1, pp. 3–9.

Primarily for parents, presents simple suggestions and activities for the young blind child.

550. Groves, Doris, & Griffith, Carolynn. *Guiding the development of the young visually handicapped: A selected list of activities.* Columbus, Ohio: State School for the Blind, 1969, 43 pp.

Contains suggestions to help the child develop and prepare for the activities of a formal school program. Outline of activities for children 6 mos.–10 yrs. stresses auditory awareness, locomotion and preorientation, and body image. Eating skills and toilet training discussed separately. App. includes suggestions for books, toys, records, and games.

551. Hall, George C. *Parents' role.* Boston: Boston Center for Blind Children, 1974, 4 pp., 50¢.

A psychologist discusses Center's efforts to help parents adjust to the demands of their multiply handicapped, visually impaired children, and the programs found to be helpful in that attempt.

552. Hallam, Kris. Mother and teacher seeks acceptance for handicapped. *Braille Monitor*, Apr. 1975, pp. 159–61.

Apparently based on an interview with a teacher who is a mother of a blind child, relates experiences with that child.

553. Hallenbeck, Jane. Two essential factors in the development of young blind children. *New Outlook for the Blind*, Nov. 1954, Vol. 48, No. 9, pp. 308–15.

A close positive relationship with some person is important to development and adjustment. The degree of closeness must be greater the less vision the child has. A description of the degree and age of onset of blindness should precede any evaluation of the child.

554. Halliday, Carol. *The visually impaired child: Growth, learning, development—Infancy to school age.* Washington, D.C.: Office of Education, HEW, 1970, 85 pp.

Handbook delineates visual impairment and discusses child growth with references to the visually handicapped. Considers development of self-care skills, physical, social/personal, intellectual, and emotional development and contrasts these to the normal child.

555. Hatfield, Elizabeth M. Blindness in infants and young children. *Sight-Saving Review*, Summer 1972, Vol. 42, No. 2, pp. 69–89.

Report on a study undertaken in 1967 by the National Society for the Prevention of Blindness. Records of 3,115 children (legally blind or partially seeing) born in the years 1959 through 1966 provided the basic data for the study.

556. Held, Marian. New York Association faces challenge of the preschool child. *New Outlook for the Blind*, Dec. 1954, Vol. 48, No. 10, pp. 365–68.

Describes needs of preschool blind children and program of the Lighthouse, which consists of nursery school, home counseling, parent-teacher meetings, and country holidays. Discusses funding and transportation problems.

557. ———. Better community planning for the preschool blind child. *New Outlook for the Blind*, Oct. 1955, Vol. 49, No. 8, pp. 295–99.

Describes the nursery school program at the Lighthouse, New York City.

558. Henderson, Lois T. *The opening doors—My child's first eight years without sight.* New York: John Day, 1954, 242 pp.

Useful to parents, houseparents, educators, and social workers, this is a mother's frank account of the first 8 years of her blind child's development.

559. Hirst, C. C., & Machael, E. *Developmental activities for children in special education.* Springfield, Ill.: Charles C Thomas, 1972, 272 pp., $15.75.

Gives some attention to blind children.

560. Hoffman, Barbara Ann. Observations and work with preschool blind children. *International Journal for the Education of the Blind*, Mar. 1959, Vol. 8, No. 3, pp. 93–97.

Criteria for the readiness of the child to profit by nursery experience suggest that the normal blind child is ready at about age 3. Describes 2 nursery school groups, 1 normal blind and the other blind with social and emotional problems, and how both are handled.

561. Hollis, John H., Ed. *Developmental deficiencies: Volume 2.* New York: U.S.S. Information Corp., 1973, 398 pp., app., $15.

This 2nd in a series of textbooks integrating papers of historical interest with recent research presents 33 readings on developmental deficiencies in exceptional children. Includes 6 papers specifically on visual disabilities. Early identification and treatment of developmentally deficient children is generally stressed.

562. Huffman, Mildred B. Symposium—Self-image: A guide to adjustment. A call for recreation. *New Outlook for the Blind*, Mar. 1961, Vol. 55, No. 3, pp. 86–89.

Stresses that a developing child who is blind needs much the same things as any developing child. This is especially true when it comes to active play with other children.

563. Huffman, Mildred B., & DiPietro, Diana. Creating motivation through meaningful reading. *International Journal for the Education of the Blind*, Dec. 1962, Vol. 12, No. 2, pp. 33–39.

Meaningful reading creates motivation to read; therefore reading material must be chosen from the point of view of the child, his abilities and interests, and his real experiences. With the young and/or retarded child in mind, suggests ways to reach the child's interest.

564. Hull, Wilma A., & McCarthy, Daniel G. Supplementary program for preschool visually handicapped children: Utilization of vision/increased readiness. *Education of the Visually Handicapped*, Dec. 1973, Vol. 5, No. 4, pp. 97–104.

Describes visual efficiency and reading readiness training program of ancillary nature, program's staff and schedule. Curriculum content outlined. Reviews group profile of 24 partially sighted preschool children involved. Reports positive reactions, possible followup.

565. Hulza, Wilfred C. III. Denial and infantilization: Two pitfalls in the choice of setting. *New Outlook for the Blind*, Sept. 1958, Vol. 52, No. 7, pp. 257–60.

Last of 3 articles on early childhood. Discusses problems in determining which children need segregated, and which need integrated, classes. Complicating factors of attitudes of denial or infantilization in the parents or teachers.

566. Ill. State Office of the Supt. of Public Instruction. *Toys for early development of the young blind child: A guide for parents.* Springfield: Author, 1971, 18 pp.

Booklet lists various useful toys for the child in his early development and cognitive growth.

567. ———. *Preschool learning activities for the visually impaired child: A guide for parents.* Springfield: Author, 1972, 102 pp.

Lists games and activities to develop independence by means of tactual, aural, physical, self-care, social, visual, and mobility training. Includes glossary of helpful terms and lists of Ill. agencies serving the visually impaired.

568. Imamura, Sadako. *Mother and blind child.* New York: 1965, 78 pp., $1.50.

Behavior observation protocols were made of blind and sighted children aged 3–6 and their mothers. Despite some varying patterns in mother-child behavior for the blind and the sighted, the degree of self-reliance in the children could be predicted with greater certainty on the basis of their mother's compliant behavior than on the basis of whether they were blind or not.

569. Ind. Univ. (Pa.). *Visually handicapped children: A guide for parents.* Harrisburg: Pa. Dept. of Education, 1970, 10 pp.

Intended to answer basic questions of parents about the child at home and his future education. Gives preschool home activities to strengthen the child's potential, information on kinds of education available in Pa., and a list of reading materials for parents.

570. Jackson, Claire L. The blind child in the nursery school. *New Outlook for the Blind*, Feb. 1955, Vol. 49, No. 2, pp. 39–45.

With special reference to 2 Calif. programs of parent counseling and integrated nursery school, suggests that important factors in success are teachers' attitudes, the teacher's perception of the blind child's viewpoint, ample provision of sensory experience, and clear objectives.

571. Johnson, G. Orville, & Blank, Harriett D., Eds. *Exceptional children research review.* Washington, D.C.: Council for Exceptional Children, 1968, 343 pp., $6.75 (paper $4.75).

Research reviews for 8 areas of exceptionality include 20 on the visually impaired presented by William J. Tisdall and 18 on administration by James C. Chalfant and Robert A. Henderson.

572. Jones, John W. *The visually handicapped child at home and school.* Washington, D.C.: Govt. Printing Office, 1963, 55 pp.

Discussion of the child at home includes: Parent counseling program, levels of expectation, enriching and supplementing school experiences, and the older child. At school includes: Vision screening, identification, what the school should know about the child, trial placement, basic instructional needs. Also discusses sources of materials and aids.

573. Kaarlela, Ruth. The role of the family in developing independence in the blind child. *New Outlook for the Blind*, Sept. 1959, Vol. 53, No. 7, pp. 245–48.

In relation to the above, discusses selection of educational setting, socialization, mechanics of daily living, and beginnings of vocational objective. Suggests ways in which agencies can help.

574. Kakalik, James S., et al. *Improving services to handicapped children; with emphasis on hearing and vision impairments.* Santa Monica, Calif.: Rand Corp., 1974, 338 pp.

The second of 2 reports providing a comprehensive, cross-agency evaluation of federal and state programs, this report examines current policies and suggests alternative future policies for improved delivery of services. Presents extensive background information and recommendations for federal, state, and local-government-level changes in each of 8 major service areas. Also examines information gained through interviews of 77 families with hearing and visually handicapped children.

575. Kapela, Edith L. Junior high readiness and the blind child. *New Outlook for the Blind*, Jan. 1971, Vol. 65, No. 1, pp. 12–17.

Discusses general aims of education in preparing children for junior high school and the response to the needs of blind children. Attitudes, orientation and mobility skills, academic readiness, personality traits, listening skills, and social fulfillment are all considered.

576. Kaplan, Bert L., & Kaplan, Theadora. Developmental psychology and the visually handicapped. *Clinical Social Work Journal*, 1974, Vol. 2, No. 2, pp. 113–19.

Presents 4 brief case histories describing the behavior of each blind patient and interpreting it in light of M. Mahler's separation-individuation concept.

577. Kenyon, Eunice L. *Diagnostic study for the day preschool at the Boston Center for Blind Children.* Boston: Boston Center for Blind Children, 1974, 24 pp., $1.50.

Describes Center setting and diagnostic procedures for multiply and visually handicapped children from 3 to 12 years old functioning at the preschool level, and the function of diagnosis. Explains prestudy procedures. Notes roles of individual staff members in diagnosis.

578. Kerby, C. E. Blindness in pre-school children. *Sight-Saving Review*, 1954, Vol. 24, pp. 15–30.

Comparative data indicates an increase of about 50% in the number of preschool blind in U.S. between 1943 and 1950 due chiefly to increase in incidence of retrolental fibroplasia. However, a decrease in blindness due to other causes also occurred.

579. ———. Causes of blindness in children of school age. *Sight-Saving Review*, Spring 1958, Vol. 28, pp. 10–21.

An update of the 1954 report listed above.

580. Kirk, Samuel A., & Bateman, Barbara D. *Ten years of research at the Institute for Research on Exceptional Children.* Urbana: Institute for Research on Exceptional Children, Univ. of Ill., 1964, 52 pp.

Reviews research on prevalence studies, diagnostic instruments, children with sensory disabilities and their families, and programmed instruction.

581. Klein, George S. Blindness and isolation. *Psychoanalytic Study of the Child,* 1962, Vol. 17, pp. 82–93.

Case history of a blind twin girl is discussed in terms of the relation between sensory deficit and stimulus deprivation, and the implications of both handicaps for affect, cognitive development, and ego development in general.

582. Krause, Arlington C. Effect of retrolental fibroplasia in children. *Archives of Ophthalmology,* Apr. 1955, Vol. 53, pp. 522–29.

583. Kurzhals, Ina W. Creating with materials can be of value for young blind children. *International Journal for the Education of the Blind,* Mar. 1961, Vol. 10, No. 3, pp. 75–79.

Values of mental and emotional growth are found in work with materials in the kindergarten of Utah School for the Blind. A long list of projects is provided and some of the projects are described in detail.

584. ———. What is "readiness" for the blind child? *International Journal for the Education of the Blind,* Oct. 1968, Vol. 18, No. 3, pp. 90–93.

Describes 4 kinds of readiness: Physical, mental, social-emotional, and psychological. Lists activities which can help with development of these.

585. ———. Personality adjustment for the blind child in the classroom. *New Outlook for the Blind,* May 1970, Vol. 64, No. 5, pp. 129–34.

Personality development of blind child described including significance of parental attitudes, limitations of the impairment, development of self-image, and influence of the environment. Specific teaching techniques and desirable characteristics of the teacher and classroom setting presented.

586. Kvaraceus, William C., & Hayes, E. Nelson. *If your child is handicapped.* Boston: Porter Sargent, 1969, 413 pp., $7.95.

Intended for parents of handicapped children and the specialists who work with them. Highly personal accounts by parents of the experiences of having a handicapped child.

587. Lairy, Gabrielle-Catherine. Problems in the adjustment of the visually impaired child. *New Outlook for the Blind,* Feb. 1969, Vol. 63, No. 2, pp. 33–41. Translated and adapted from May 1967 *Les Annals d'occulistique.*

Very complete description of the psychosocial and educational variables affecting partially sighted children from birth through early school years. Corrective measures to meet the problems are suggested.

588. Lairy, Gabrielle-Catherine, & Harrison-Covello, A. The blind child and his parents: Congenital visual defect and the repercussion of family attitudes on the early development of the child. *American Foundation for the Blind Research Bulletin 25,* Jan. 1973, pp. 1–24.

Stresses the mother's role in providing a positive early educational environment. Reviews literature presenting common developmental patterns found in blind children in the areas of sensorimotor, motor, cognitive, and language skills.

589. Langley, Elizabeth. Symposium—Self-image: A guide to adjustment. Self-image: The formative years. *New Outlook for the Blind,* Mar. 1961, Vol. 55, No. 3, pp. 80–81.

Suggestions for handling a child in his younger years to promote mastery of physical and social skills. Suggestions also covering the first few school years.

590. Leach, Fay W. Educational materials for early childhood education. In *Selected papers: Methods and materials in the education of the visually handicapped.* Philadelphia: Association for Education of the Visually Handicapped, 1972, pp. 51–53.

Stresses importance of knowing the child and the goals before selecting educational materials. Lists 16 questions to be considered in the selection and encourages originating materials for the specific child.

591. LeZak, Raymond J., & Starbuck, Harold B. Identification of children with speech disorders in a residential school for the blind. *International Journal for the Education of the Blind,* Oct. 1964, Vol. 14, No. 1, pp. 8–12.

A speech survey with 173 blind students showed that almost 50% had various types and degrees of speech disorders. A formal program of speech therapy is recommended. Ref.

592. Love, Harold D. *Parental attitudes toward exceptional children.* Springfield, Ill.: Charles C Thomas, 1970, ix + 167 pp., $9.50.

Designed to help educators, physicians, psychologists, and others who counsel parents of exceptional children. Chap. 8 (pp. 127–46) concerns parental attitudes toward the deaf child and the blind child.

593. Lowenfeld, Berthold. The pre-school blind child and his needs. *Exceptional Children,* 1953, Vol. 20, pp. 50–55.

Indicates increase in number of pre-school age blind children and emphasizes need for parental acceptance and cooperation.

594. ———. If he is blind. *International Journal for the Education of the Blind,* Oct. 1954, Vol. 4, No. 1, pp. 1–6.

Emphasizes that the blind child is first a child like other children. Discusses attitudes toward blindness, parents' reactions, adaptations in equipment, skills, necessity of creative activity, physical education, recreation, concrete experiences, independence, close contact with families and communities, and how schools for the blind can help in all areas.

595. ———. Psychological problems of children with impaired vision. In William M. Cruickshank, Ed., *Psychology of exceptional children and youth.* New York: Prentice-Hall, 1955, pp. 214–83.

Independence and opportunity for development are stressed in a well-rounded discussion of the development of the visually handicapped child.

596. ———. Emotional growth. *International Journal for the Education of the Blind,* Oct. 1955, Vol. 5, No. 1, pp. 1–8. Chap. from *Our blind children: Growing and learning with them.*

Offers insight into problems of emotional nature frequently connected with blindness and parents' reactions; reactions of others and effects on child.

597. ————. The blind child as an integral part of the family and community. *New Outlook for the Blind*, Apr. 1965, Vol. 59, No. 4, pp. 117–21.

Discusses how the blind child can be part of the family and guidance needed by parents to accomplish this, challenges to schools and recreation. Suggests relevant vocational services and research.

598. ————. *Our blind children: Growing and learning with them.* Springfield, Ill.: Charles C Thomas, 1956, 205 pp. (2nd ed., 1964, 240 pp.; 3rd ed., 1971, xv + 244 pp., $8.50).

Designed especially for parents, describes child's growth stages, preschool, kindergarten, and school age, attitudes of parents, special methods of teaching, and some questions frequently asked by parents. (3rd ed. updates 2nd throughout and contains an added chapter re the multiply handicapped blind child.)

599. ————. Psychological considerations. In Berthold Lowenfeld, Ed., *The visually handicapped child in school.* New York: John Day, 1973, pp. 27–60.

Analyzes the effects of various factors in the visual impairment of a particular child and describes the special methods of early training through which the child's program can be individualized. Stresses concrete experiences, unifying experiences, and learning by doing.

600. Lowenfeld, Viktor. *Creative and mental growth*, 3rd ed. New York: Macmillan, 1957, 541 pp.

Although oriented toward art professionals, contains much information and advice which can be used effectively by parents. Chap. 8 deals with creative activity and handicapped children.

601. Magary, James F., & Eichorn, John R. *The exceptional child: A book of readings.* New York: Holt, Rinehart, Winston, 1966, 561 pp.

Selected readings by 78 authors give information on exceptional children including the visually handicapped.

602. Magdsick, Winifred. Meeting the needs of blind children. In *An institute for houseparents of visually handicapped children: Proceedings.* New York: AFB, 1957, pp. 9–12.

Reviews basic needs of all children and how these may be shown in the visually handicapped child. Suggests ways to meet behavioral expressions of need.

603. Michaels, Winifred M. Cooperative pre-school program. *International Journal for the Education of the Blind*, Dec. 1954, Vol. 4, No. 2, pp. 36–37.

New program combining schools and agencies in New York City for teaching and training children from 3 to 6 years of age. Social, medical, and psychological services to both children and parents. Further details on this and other services to older blind.

604. Middlewood, Esther L. A child—though blind. *New Outlook for the Blind*, Mar. 1954, Vol. 48, No. 3, pp. 61–65.

First of all a child, the blind child needs love, security, and opportunities for growth experiences, just as other children do. Recognition is important to feeling accepted, and basic drives must be received by the family as natural.

605. Miguel, Mary, & Cecilia, Mary. Helping the preschool blind child. *New Outlook for the Blind*, June 1964, Vol. 58, No. 6, pp. 170–72.

Description of need for a nursery school for blind children, and techniques used there.

606. Mikell, Robert F. *Normal growth and development of children with visual handicaps.* New York: AFB, 1953, 14 pp. Reprinted in *New Outlook for the Blind*, Apr. 1953.

Addressed specifically to parents of preschool blind children. Discusses child's needs, training, parental attitudes, and specific suggestions for developing desired behavior.

607. Miner, L. E. A study of the incidence of speech deviations among visually handicapped children. *New Outlook for the Blind*, Jan. 1963, Vol. 57, No. 1, pp. 10–14.

Discusses procedure, analysis of data, summary, and implications for further research.

608. ———. Speech improvement for visually handicapped children. *New Outlook for the Blind*, May 1963, Vol. 57, No. 5, pp. 160–63.

Discusses program justification, 9 general objectives, 9 items in the classroom teacher's role, program procedure, and introduction to the "alphabet of sounds."

609. Minturn, Emma H. The preschool blind child and his mother. *International Journal for the Education of the Blind*, Dec. 1960, Vol. 10, No. 2, pp. 57–59.

Reviews some of the ways in which early advice to parents of RLF children sometimes went wrong, producing poor results. But the professionals have learned from this and, with early referral, could provide better advice today. Pleads for use of this knowledge with parents of multiply handicapped blind children.

610. Mitchell, Ruth & Henderson, Freda. Prepare for school living. *International Journal for the Education of the Blind*, Mar. 1956, Vol. 5, No. 3, pp. 55–57.

Discusses ways in which parents can help their blind children prepare for attendance in a residential school. Offers some practical suggestions on activities for preschool blind children.

611. Monroe, Edith H. Team work approach in Ohio services for the preschool blind child. *New Outlook for the Blind*, Oct. 1954, Vol. 48, No. 8, pp. 274–77.

Describes committee to develop plans for full utilization of Ohio's resources for pre-school blind children.

612. Moor, Pauline M. Meeting the needs of the preschool blind child and his parents. *Education*, 1954, Vol. 74, pp. 382–89.

Discussion of specific needs of the child and of a variety of ways in which the parents may be assisted in providing for those needs.

613. ———. Meeting the needs of young blind children. In *An institute for houseparents of visually handicapped children: Proceedings.* New York: AFB, 1957, pp. 13–15.

Reviews interplay of physical facts about the young blind child and his parents' attitudes.

614. ———. *A blind child, too, can go to nursery school.* New York: AFB, 1962, 15 pp.

Discusses preschool blind children who have attended nursery schools with sighted children. Cites benefits as well as topics of concern.

615. ———. Comprehensive care services for the young child who is visually impaired. *New Outlook for the Blind,* May 1975, Vol. 69, No. 5, pp. 193–200.

Discusses comprehensive care as a concept and describes a theoretical model program. Covers 2 pilot projects that show how existing resources can be used in developing a program.

616. Moore, Charlotte. Jean questions blindness. *New Outlook for the Blind,* Jan. 1954, Vol. 48, No. 1, pp. 15–16.

Brief and charming account of a young child's first questions about her blindness.

617. Murray, Virginia. Report. In *An institute for houseparents of visually handicapped children: Proceedings.* New York: AFB, 1957, pp. 16–17.

Reports briefly on 6 young blind children and the backgrounds from which they come. Shows how these backgrounds have influenced the children.

618. ———. Parental attitudes affect growth and development of the young blind child. *New Outlook for the Blind,* Jan. 1958, Vol. 52, No. 1, pp. 8–10.

Sympathetic discussion of the important relationships between parents and child.

619. ———. Play and playthings for blind children. *International Journal for the Education of the Blind,* Oct. 1965, Vol. 15, No. 1, pp. 17–20.

Toys are the tools of play, and for each stage in the child's development there are toys which encourage new skills and increase understanding. Many are listed and their special values described.

620. ———. *Hints for parents of preschool visually handicapped children.* Lincoln: Nebr. State Dept. of Education, 1970, 29 pp.

Suggestions for parents of blind children, birth to kindergarten age, regarding development of skills, learning the environment, and developing normal social and emotional characteristics.

621. Napoli, P. J., & Harris, W. W. Finger painting for the blind. *Journal of Psychology,* 1948, Vol. 25, pp. 185–96.

Finger painting provides a psychotherapeutic outlet for the emotional strain under which many blind people live.

622. Nelson, Mary S., & Stevens, Godfrey D. Preschool services for visually handicapped children. *Exceptional Children,* 1953, Vol. 19, pp. 211–13.

Describes cooperation of Cincinnati Board of Education and association for the blind in nursery school (in which half the children are sighted), home counseling and parent activity programs, and the problems disclosed.

623. Norris, Miriam. What affects blind children's development? *New Out-*

look for the Blind, Sept. 1956, Vol. 50, No. 7, pp. 258–67. Reprinted from *Children*, July–Aug. 1956.

Brief report of Study of the Development of Preschool Blind Children, at Univ. of Chicago Clinics. Gives principles and objectives of study, methods, and summary of findings. Opportunities for child's freedom and initiative, and counseling service to parents and nursery schools are important.

624. ————. The blind child in the sighted nursery group. *New Outlook for the Blind*, Dec. 1956, Vol. 50, No. 10, pp. 375–79.

Developmental needs are the same for blind and sighted children, but skilled counseling is required for parents and nursery school teachers.

625. Norris, Miriam; Spaulding, Patricia J.; & Brodie, Fern H. *Blindness in children*. Chicago: Univ. of Chicago Press, 1957, 173 pp.

Reports a 5-year study of the development of nearly 300 preschool children. Concludes that blind children can develop into independent, freely functioning individuals who compare favorably with sighted children.

626. O'Brien, Rosemary. Early childhood services for visually impaired children: A model program. *New Outlook for the Blind*, May 1975, Vol. 69, No. 5, pp. 201–6.

A program, including educational services for the children and counseling and training for the parents, in a public school system.

627. Office of Child Development, HEW. *The preschool child who is blind*. Washington, D.C.: Govt. Printing Office, 1968, 27 pp., 20¢.

Information and guidelines for parents. Provide many and varied experiences; suggestions are made about playmates, learning by doing, and use of other senses.

628. Pa. Dept. of Education, Bureau of Special Education. *Visually handicapped children: A guide for parents*. Harrisburg: Author, 1970, 10 pp.

Brochure delineates those preschool activities which will strengthen the visually handicapped child's potential for formal school experience and provides general information on the kinds of special education available for a Pa. child who is visually handicapped. List of reading materials for parents and helpful organizations provided.

629. Park, Gloria G. *A plan for itinerant educational consultant services for preschool visually handicapped children*. Washington, D.C.: Bureau of Elementary and Secondary Education, 1971, 77 pp.

Report of a demonstration project with objective of preventing social and sensory deprivation and of developing personal independence.

630. Parten, Carroll B. Encouragement of sensory motor development in the preschool blind. *Exceptional Children*, Summer 1971, Vol. 37, No. 10, pp. 739–41.

Specific activities to develop child's self and body awareness, socially desirable behaviors and mobility.

631. Pittman, Yvette H. An exploratory study of the eating problems of blind children. *New Outlook for the Blind*, Oct. 1964, Vol. 58, No. 8, pp. 264–67.

Author points out lack of instructive materials available to help in teaching table skills to blind children. Details program designed to help teach these skills. Schools must provide more information for parents, take on job themselves or at least be partners in teaching table manners.

632. Pringle, M. L. K. The emotional and social adjustment of blind children. *Educational Research*, 1964, Vol. 6, No. 2, pp. 129–38.

Reviews literature published over preceding 34 years and groups it under 6 headings: General descriptive accounts, rehabilitation and therapy, case studies, explorations of suitable testing techniques, comparative studies of various kinds, and investigations of relationship between parental attitudes or those of society and adjustment of blind child.

633. Rawls, Horace D. Social factors in disability. *New Outlook for the Blind*, June 1957, Vol. 51, No. 6, pp. 231–36.

Against a background of sociology and anthropology, states that the feelings of a blind child about himself are largely determined by the attitudes of the people around him.

634. Rawls, Rachel F. Parental reactions and attitudes toward the blind child. *New Outlook for the Blind*, Mar. 1957, Vol. 51, No. 3, pp. 92–97.

Possible reactions of parents to having a blind child and how these reactions are affected by ignorance, religious views, anxiety, attitudes of relatives, and attitudes of physicians. Lists sources of help for parents.

635. Reger, Roger, Ed. *Preschool programming of children with disabilities.* Springfield, Ill.: Charles C Thomas, 1970, 123 pp.

Intended for those interested in special educational programming, the book contains a chapter on visually handicapped children.

636. Reid, Eleanor S. Helping parents of handicapped children. *New Outlook for the Blind*, Apr. 1959, Vol. 53, No. 4, pp. 123–28.

Describes some of the ways in which parents react to having a handicapped child and suggests how the professional may help them.

637. Richards, Susan S., & Briller, Stanley. Learning from experience: A revisit to the children's corner. *New Outlook for the Blind*, Mar. 1971, Vol. 65, No. 3, pp. 73–78.

Early childhood development program consists of group and individual parent counseling, child development, and home training. Describes how 3 years of experience have modified the program. Emphasizes intensive and varied use of volunteers.

638. Ritchie, Amy G. Nursery education helps blind children. *International Journal for the Education of the Blind*, Oct. 1957, Vol. 7, No. 1, pp. 17–21.

With the stories of a number of children as illustrations, tells about a nursery school for handicapped children, how it is organized, what it accomplishes, and how it does it.

639. Roberts, Alvin H. Child care information for blind parents. *Rehabilitation Teacher*, June 1973, Vol. 5, No. 6, pp. 3–13.

Intended for blind parents, the article gives information on feeding, bathing, diapering, sickness, and general management of the infant and young child.

640. Rowe, Emma D. *Speech problems of blind children: A survey of the North California area.* New York: AFB, 1958, 39 pp.

Report of survey to determine the percentage of significant speech defects in the speech of blind children with the hypothesis that blind children with normal experiences will have normal speech. 148 visually handicapped children in grades 1–6 participated. Hypothesis supported.

641. Rubin, Judith A. Mother-child art sessions II. Education in the community. *American Journal of Art Therapy*, Apr. 1974, Vol. 13, No. 3, pp. 219–27.

Describes sessions in 3 different settings with multiply handicapped blind and partially sighted children and their mothers. Analyzes reactions of mothers and children. Part 1 of this article is "Mother-child art sessions I. Treatment in the clinic."

642. Sandler, Anne-Marie. Aspects of passivity and ego development in the blind infant. In Ruth S. Eissler; Anna Freud; Heinz Hartmann; et al., Eds., *The psychoanalytic study of the child: XVIII.* New York: International Univ., 1963, pp. 343–60.

Concludes that children blind from birth show a degree of fixation to the very earliest phase of development, in which the passive experiencing of bodily gratification is dominant.

643. Sanford, Marvin. A program for the enhancement of motor skills in visually impaired children. *Florida School Herald*, Feb. 1975, Vol. 74, No. 6, pp. 1–2.

Workshop for public school teachers to help overcome their reluctance to have visually impaired children in their classes. Curriculum deals with the younger blind child and his physical development and covers body image, concept development, daily sensorimotor training activities, and movement-exploration of body parts.

644. Saul, Sidney R. Serving the blind child in the neighborhood community center: A professional challenge. *Journal of Jewish Communal Service*, 1959, Vol. 35, pp. 285–92.

The Guild for the Jewish Blind provided a program through which an integrated summer day camp evolved and proved effective for both blind and sighted children.

645. Schleifer, Maxwell J. Case history: "My brother, he's blind." *Exceptional Parent*, Mar.–Apr. 1973, Vol. 3, No. 1, pp. 31–34.

Family dynamics of a family with a blind son from the viewpoints of the other family members and the counselor.

646. Schulz, Paul J. A group approach to working with families of the blind. *New Outlook for the Blind*, Mar. 1968, Vol. 62, No. 3, pp. 82–86.

In a series of meetings, material was presented on a practical level to help family members understand and cope with problems of blindness in areas of physical adaptation and emotional adjustment. Describes several kinds of leadership for the meetings with panel structure evoking the greatest audience response.

647. Scott, Eileen. The preschool blind child and his parents. *International Journal for the Education of the Blind*, Oct. 1956, Vol. 6, No. 1, pp. 5–10.

Describes the possible reactions of parents to having a blind child, the family's need for casework and information, and 6 possible sources of anxiety in the parents. Describes a Canadian program for working with these parents and children.

648. ———. The blind child in the sighted nursery school. *New Outlook for the Blind,* Nov. 1957, Vol. 51, No. 9, pp. 406–10.

Important factors in the blind child's integration are selection of supervisors and how he is introduced into the group.

649. Shuey, Rebekah. II. The non-segregated setting: Positive values and problems. *New Outlook for the Blind,* Sept. 1958, Vol. 52, No. 7, pp. 254–57.

Second of 3 articles on early childhood. Describes a college laboratory school for 3–6-year-olds in which 2 blind children were enrolled. Describes their progress and policies for admission.

650. Shumway, H. Smith. The highway of the future. *Rehabilitation Teacher,* Nov. 1974, Vol. 6, No. 11, pp. 3–8.

The director of visually handicapped services in Wyo. discusses that state's consultant system, including such aspects as encouraging visually handicapped children to attend preschool nurseries, consultants' visits, provision of educational aids, benefits of integration for sighted students.

651. Sibert, Katie N. The "legally blind" child with useful residual vision. *International Journal for the Education of the Blind,* Dec. 1966, Vol. 16, No. 2, pp. 33–44.

A very detailed report with copies of forms used to determine usable vision and plan school placement. Typical individual needs are listed. A chart showing the placement and results for 40 children represents case history summaries.

652. Spache, George D., & Bing, Louis B. *Children's vision and school success.* St. Louis, Mo.: American Optometric Assoc., 1971, 33 pp.

Intended to assist discussion leaders in presenting information about the visual problems of children to educational groups or parents' groups, this manual includes nontechnical discussion of the vision process, educationally relevant visual abilities, the teacher's role relevant to visual difficulties, suggestions on adjustment. App. includes charts and glossary. For use with 33 slides and various charts.

653. Spencer, Marietta B. (Photographs by Frank Agar, Jr., & Carol Safer.) *Blind children in family and community.* Minneapolis: Univ. of Minn. Press, 1960, 138 pp.

Addressed to parents and professional workers, through pictures and brief, clear explanations shows how to start blind children on their way to becoming useful, independent adults.

654. Steinzor, Luciana V. Siblings of visually handicapped children. *New Outlook for the Blind,* Feb. 1967, Vol. 61, No. 2, pp. 48–52.

Exploratory study of 16 siblings' attitudes toward visually handicapped children in the family. Analysis of interviews shows siblings usually considered their blind brother or sister a special member of the family, in need of care and kindness, but capable of participation.

655. Strehl, Carl. What fundamental problems exist in the care and treatment of the blind, especially of blind youth. *International Journal for the Education of the Blind*, Mar. 1954, Vol. 3, No. 3, pp. 238–39.

General information on how a person can be helped to overcome disadvantages of blindness. Educational, vocational, and social aspects of life discussed.

656. Swartz, Edward M. Blindness in the toybox. *Sight-Saving Review*, Summer 1973, Vol. 43, No. 2, pp. 95–101.

Text of a paper presented at the National Conference of the National Society for the Prevention of Blindness, Apr. 1973.

657. Sykes, Kim C. Camp Challenge: Program for parents and their preschool children with visual handicaps. *New Outlook for the Blind*, Oct. 1974, Vol. 68, No. 8, pp. 344–47.

Recruitment, programming, and evaluation are discussed as well as the informal aspects of the camp. Scheduling allows parents to attend lectures while trainee teachers work with the children.

658. Tait, Perla. A descriptive analysis of the play of young blind children. *Education of the Visually Handicapped*, Mar. 1972, Vol. 4, No. 1, pp. 12–15. Also in *American Foundation for the Blind Research Bulletin 24*, Mar. 1972.

Play of 29 children (4–9 yrs.) compared to play of peer group. Blind children had difficulty understanding the spatial relationship of the party-room used and of the play materials.

659. ———. The effect of circumstantial rejection on infant behavior. *New Outlook for the Blind*, May 1972, Vol. 66, No. 5, pp. 139–51.

Discussion of blindisms as "acts which substitute for, or interfere with, the drive to explore the environment." Author contends that adequate mastery of the environment can only be accomplished if there is a secure mother-infant relationship. Suggests that a depth analysis of mothering patterns may provide a specific plan of action for raising a blind child. Ref.

660. ———. The implications of play as it relates to the emotional development of the blind child. *Education of the Visually Handicapped*, May 1972, Vol. 4, No. 2, pp. 52–54.

Discusses relationship between play and the blind child's emotional development. Advocates blind children be encouraged to develop spontaneous play behavior.

661. ———. Behavior of young blind children in a controlled play session. *Perceptual and Motor Skills*, June 1972, Vol. 34, No. 3, pp. 963–69.

In 29 blind and 29 seeing 4–9 year olds, 3 types of play were identified: Manipulative, dramatic, and other. Residential-nonresidential status and degree of blindness had no effect. Blind *S*s engaged in more manipulative play.

662. ———. Play and the intellectual development of blind children. *New Outlook for the Blind*, Dec. 1972, Vol. 66, No. 10, pp. 361–69.

Begins by defining "play" as "exploratory behavior." The lack of ability to engage in spontaneous play by blind children limits intellectual development, cognizance of reality, language and abstract functioning, the articulation of experience, and the ability to abstract. It is the responsibility of those working with blind children to teach them "to engage actively, creatively, and independently in spontaneous play activities." Ref.

663. ———. Method for quantitative analysis of dramatic play. *Perceptual and Motor Skills*, Oct. 1974, Vol. 39, No. 2, pp. 1012–14.

In developing her method for quantitative analysis, the author worked with data she had gathered for a previously published study concerning the play behavior of blind children.

664. Taylor, Billie M. *Blind Pre-school: A manual for parents and educators.* Colorado Springs, Colo.: Industrial Printers, 1974, 49 pp., $3.95.

Revised edition of a manual concerning general development and suggested activities for young blind children.

665. Taylor, Ian G. *The neurological mechanisms of hearing and speech in children.* Manchester, England: Manchester Univ. Press, 1964.

A 5-year longitudinal study of 78 children (min. age 11 mos.) referred to Dept. of Deaf Education at Univ. of Manchester is described. All children presented problems related to sound or linguistic development or both. Test methods and case histories are presented. Visually handicapped children included. Bib.

666. Telson, Sara. Parent counseling. *New Outlook for the Blind*, Apr. 1965, Vol. 59, No. 4, pp. 127–29.

Describes some typical problems of parents of blind children especially in the areas of attitudes and values, and how the counselor may meet these.

667. Toomer, Joan, & Brown, M. S. Colborne. Learning through play. *New Outlook for the Blind*, Jan. 1965, Vol. 59, No. 1, pp. 24–26. Reprinted from *New Beacon*, Mar. 1964.

Suggests toys and objects with which the child can play with illustrations and instructions for parents.

668. Turner, Hester. A mother joins the teacher in interpreting the blind child. *New Outlook for the Blind*, Dec. 1957, Vol. 51, No. 10, pp. 473–74.

Seven specific suggestions to teachers of young blind children in regular classes.

669. Ulrich, Sharon (with Anna W. M. Wolf). *Elizabeth.* Ann Arbor: Univ. of Mich. Press, 1972, 122 pp., $4.95.

A mother's account of the early growth, affective development, and cognitive learning of a blind child.

670. Vogel, Mary. Creating a toy for a blind child. *New Outlook for the Blind*, Oct. 1968, Vol. 62, No. 8, p. 253.

Important considerations in a toy for a blind child are size and weight, textural interest, changing exterior shape by insertion of moveable parts, and sound.

671. Wanger, Arlene E. Dinner in darkness. *Exceptional Parent*, Mar.–Apr. 1975, Vol. 5, No. 2, pp. 25–27.

Mother recounts her frustrations and resultant comprehension of the difficulties experienced by her youngster as result of blindfolded dinner.

672. Ware, Mary A., & Schwab, Lois O. The blind mother providing care for an infant. *New Outlook for the Blind*, June 1971, Vol. 65, No. 6, pp. 169–74.

By individual interviews, 10 blind mothers indicated the responsibilities carried in care for their infants and toddlers and how they carried those responsibilities without vision.

673. Warnick, Lillian. The effect upon a family of a child with a handicap. *New Outlook for the Blind,* Dec. 1969, Vol. 63, No. 10, pp. 299–304.

Main areas of concern are family reaction to early identification, periods of stress for the family, and parental counseling.

674. Weinberg, Bernd. Stuttering among blind and partially sighted children. *Journal of Speech and Hearing Disorders,* 1964, Vol. 29, No. 3, pp. 322–26.

Stuttering in blind children is within the range of incidence in the general population.

675. Weiner, Florence. *Help for the handicapped child.* New York: McGraw-Hill, 1973, xv + 221 pp., $7.95.

Describes resources throughout the U.S. on the community, state, and national levels. Has 12-page section on "blindness and partial sightedness."

676. Wessell, Margery H. A language development program for a blind language-disordered pre-school girl: A case report. *Journal of Speech and Hearing Disorders,* Aug. 1969, Vol. 34, No. 3, pp. 267–74.

Case report describes diagnostic examinations and a therapy program for a 3.9-year-old congenitally blind girl.

677. Wheeler, Jane G. A practical knowledge of color for the congenitally blind. *New Outlook for the Blind,* Oct. 1969, Vol. 63, No. 8, pp. 225–31.

Through discussion of the general properties of color and specifically the primary, secondary, and basic colors, followed by symbols or stereotypes of the meanings of the various colors, tries to convey for congenitally blind some sense of what colors are.

678. Whitcraft, Carol. *Gross motor engrams: An important spatial learning modality for preschool visually handicapped children.* Washington, D.C.: Bureau of Education for the Handicapped, 1971, 13 pp.

For visually handicapped children, the concept of motoric engrams is seen as an essential learning modality for motor orientation and spatial perception. Delineates four motor generalizations significant in the education of blind children: Balance and posture, contact, locomotion, and receipt and propulsion.

679. Williams, Cyril E. Behavior disorders in handicapped children. *Developmental Medicine and Child Neurology,* 1968, Vol. 10, No. 6, pp. 736–40.

Stresses need for studies to assess mechanisms contributing to faulty child-parent interaction in blind and autistic children; gives examples of common maladjustments.

680. Wills, Doris M. Problems of play and mastery in the blind child. *British Journal of Medical Psychology,* 1968, Vol. 41, No. 3, pp. 213–22.

Traces early development of blind child to suggest reasons for the observation that young blind children often withdraw from age-adequate play and revert to simple activities.

681. ———. Vulnerable periods in the early development of blind children. *Psychoanalytic Study of the Child,* 1970, Vol. 25, pp. 461–80.

682. Wolman, Marianne J. Interpreting the needs of the "special child" to the parents and children of the "normal" group. *New Outlook for the Blind*, Oct. 1954, Vol. 48, No. 8, pp. 267–69.

Discusses possible attitudes of parents, other children, and teachers when blind children become part of regular classes.

683. Zadnik, Donna. Social and medical aspects of the battered child with vision impairment. *New Outlook for the Blind*, June 1973, Vol. 67, No. 6, pp. 241–50.

Discussion of visual loss due to child abuse. Explanation of phenomena of child abuse with listings of medical conditions (including eye disorders) related to abuse. Role of agency or school in dealing with suspected cases. Includes discussion of working with parents and instigation of legal intervention.

684. Zahran, Hamed A. A study of personality differences between blind and sighted children. *British Journal of Educational Psychology*, 1965, Vol. 35, No. 3, pp. 329–38.

Matched groups of blind and sighted children were studied using 2 measures of intelligence and a variety of personality measures.

685. Zimmerman, Ruth E. *A classroom program.* Boston: Boston Center for Blind Children, 1974, 24 pp., app., $1.50.

Describes operations at Center's day preschool for visually impaired, multi-handicapped children 3–8 years old. Includes identification of stages of evaluation and planning and discussion of staff roles. Sample lists educational goals, educational evaluation procedure, the schedule, and lists of toys, records, books, etc.

7. Adolescents

686. Abel, Georgie Lee. The blind adolescent and his needs. *Exceptional Children*, Feb. 1961, pp. 309–34.

Discussion of basic needs of the blind adolescent in relation to needs of all people and to needs of the sighted adolescent. Relevant research mentioned.

687. ———. Symposium—Self-image: A guide to adjustment. Adolescence: Foothold on the future. *New Outlook for the Blind*, Mar. 1961, Vol. 55, No. 3, pp. 103–6.

Discusses problems of adolescence in general and more particularly how blindness adds to the adjustment difficulties. Points out most important areas of concern and where more work needs to be done.

688. Apple, Marianne M. Kinesic training for the blind: A program. *Education of the Visually Handicapped*, May 1972, Vol. 4, No. 2, pp. 55–60.

Seven congenitally blind adolescents participated in a 6-week nonverbal communication skills program which sought to acquaint the *S* with facial expressions and gestures common to daily sighted life and to teach appropriate use of the expressions and gestures.

689. Boldt, Werner. The development of scientific thinking in blind children and adolescents: Results of empirical research regarding the teaching of science in schools for the blind. *Education of the Visually Handicapped*, Mar. 1969, Vol. 1, No. 1, pp. 5–8.

How blind students develop scientific thinking in comparison to sighted students. Implications for teaching of science.

690. Canadian National Institute for the Blind. *Conference of blind youth: Selfhelp through collective action, Toronto, May 23–25, 1975.* [n.p.]: Author, 1975, 19 pp.

Results of a conference attended by 100 young blind people to discuss common problems of the blind and seek information and solutions.

691. Chandler, Margaret. Now I have a sister. *International Journal for the Education of the Blind*, Oct. 1959, Vol. 9, No. 1, pp. 11–13.

Describes the beneficial effects, social and motivational, of pairing older and younger girls and/or partially seeing and blind girls as "sisters."

692. Church, Ada. The happy teen-age girl. *International Journal for the Education of the Blind*, Mar. 1957, Vol. 6, No. 3, pp. 65–66.

A housemother argues for structure and discipline in the child's life. The happy girl has been imbued with good attitudes toward life, has learned to think of others, has learned to give and take, and practices the Golden Rule.

693. Cowen, Emory L.; Underberg, Rita P.; Verrillo, Ronald T.; et al. *Adjustment to visual disability in adolescence.* New York: AFB, 1961, 239 pp., $4 (paperback, $3).

Study collected data concerning adjustment, parental attitudes and parental understanding of visually handicapped and sighted adolescents. Results showed no difference in adjustment among larger groups of visually handicapped over sighted controls.

694. Cunliffe, W. "Hethersett," assessment centre for blind adolescents, Reigate, Surrey, England. *International Journal for the Education of the Blind,* May 1958, Vol. 7, No. 4, pp. 117–21.

History and physical plant of this center, which is neither school nor workshop. Provides prevocational and vocational experiences and acts as a pathway to independence.

695. Davidson, Terry M. The vocational development and success of visually impaired adolescents. *New Outlook for the Blind,* Sept. 1975, Vol. 69, No. 7, pp. 314–16, 319.

Based on Career Development Survey feels there is indication that visually impaired adolescents may not be as vocationally immature as they are often portrayed. However, does feel that improvements need to be made in career education and that negative attitudes toward the visually impaired need to be combated.

696. Eaglestein, A. Solomon. The social acceptance of blind high school students in an integrated school. *New Outlook for the Blind,* Dec. 1975, Vol. 69, No. 10, pp. 447–51.

Results of study (9 Ss) in Israel. Blind students' school marks were average, and they were well integrated into social framework of their classes. Some negatives.

697. Greenberg, Herbert M.; Allison, Louise; Fewell, Mildred; et al. The personality of junior high and high school students attending a residential school for the blind. *Journal of Educational Psychology,* 1957, Vol. 48, pp. 406–10.

103 students attending grades 6–12 were tested. They exhibited neurotic tendencies, low self-sufficiency, submissiveness, lack of self-confidence, lack of healthy sociability, authoritarianism, and discontent with the school.

698. Hatlen, Philip H.; Le Duc, Paula; & Canter, Patricia. The Blind Adolescent Life Skills Center. *New Outlook for the Blind,* Mar. 1975, Vol. 69, No. 3, pp. 109–15.

The Center provides individual and group instruction in mobility, living skills, communication, recreation, and social relations not in a traditional classroom but by providing real experiences.

699. Johanson, Daniel E., & Gilson, Charles. Teenagers evaluate mobility training. *New Outlook for the Blind,* Sept. 1967, Vol. 61, No. 7, pp. 227–31, 237.

Blind students undergoing mobility instruction were brought together to discuss their experiences and problems.

700. Karpen, Mary Lou, & Lipke, Lee Ann. Sex education as part of an agency's four-week summer workshop for visually impaired young people. *New Outlook for the Blind*, June 1974, Vol. 68, No. 6, pp. 260–67. Also in *Sex education for the visually handicapped in schools and agencies . . . Selected papers.* New York: AFB, 1975, pp. 35–42, $3.

Program developed by agency, parents, and resource persons. Teaching was student oriented and included group discussion, group activities, problem-solving, and demonstrations.

701. Karterud, Halvdan. The social needs of blind youth in a seeing world. *New Outlook for the Blind*, Jan. 1953, Vol. 47, No. 1, pp. 24–26.

Rather general discussion of how blind youth can acquire the social knowledge, acceptable manners, etc., to integrate in the seeing world.

702. Kramer, Rosanne. Personality and attitudes of blind teen-agers learning cane travel. *American Foundation for the Blind Research Bulletin 2*, Dec. 1962, pp. 57–71.

Discusses interaction between mobility aid and user. Reviews studies of blind child's ability to perform on tests and notes factors in child's mental outlook on handicap. Bib.

703. Lowenfeld, Berthold. The blind adolescent in a seeing world. *New Outlook for the Blind*, Oct. 1959, Vol. 53, No. 8, pp. 289–95. Also in *Exceptional Children*, Oct. 1959.

Describes the stages of adolescence and why progress through these stages is especially difficult for blind youth. Relates problems to sex curiosity, dating, mobility, and concern for the future.

704. Manaster, Al, & Kucharis, Sue. Experimental methods in a group counseling program with blind children. *New Outlook for the Blind*, Jan. 1972, Vol. 66, No. 1, pp. 15–19, 25. Reprinted from pamphlet of same title pub. by American Society Group, Psychotherapy & Psychodrama, Mar. 1968.

Description of experimental techniques and methods used in a group counseling situation with 7 blind adolescents.

705. Mayadas, Nazneen S. Role expectations and performance of blind children: Practice and implications. *Education of the Visually Handicapped*, May 1972, Vol. 4, No. 2, pp. 45–52.

Results and implications of a study that investigated the role perception and performance of 56 blind adolescents when compared with 4 categories of expectations: Significant other expectations (parents, houseparents, teachers, and counselors), blind child's perception of significant other expectations, blind child's self-expectations, and expectations of persons unfamiliar with blindness.

706. Meighan, Thomas. *An investigation of the self concept of blind and visually handicapped adolescents.* New York: AFB, 1971, vi + 43 pp., $2.50.

This brief monograph studies the relationship between self-concepts and academic achievement in language.

707. Miller, William H. Manifest anxiety in visually impaired adolescents. *Education of the Visually Handicapped*, Oct. 1970, Vol. 2, No. 3, pp. 91–95.

Hardy's Anxiety Scale for the Blind administered to students to examine relative levels of manifest anxiety between students in graded and special classes and between blind and partially sighted students. Results showed no differences; however, 11th and 12th graders had a higher anxiety level than other students.

708. Schleifer, Maxwell J. What's wrong with this town? *Exceptional Parent*, May–June 1974, Vol. 4, No. 3, pp. 31–35.

Adjustment problems of an adolescent blind boy and his family after moving to a new town are told by each parent, the boy, and his counselor.

709. Seelye, Wilma S., & Thomas, John E. A pattern to promote habilitation of blind youth. *International Journal for the Education of the Blind*, Dec. 1966, Vol. 16, No. 2, pp. 48–52.

A private agency and a residential school cooperate to provide a summer program to day school students, to improve their independence, living skills, relationships with others, and general physical and mental development. Details of program content and management are provided.

710. Splaver, Sarah. *Your handicap—don't let it handicap you.* New York: Julian Messner, 1967, illus., $3.95.

Addressed to young people with handicaps, gives practical advice and stresses need for positive thinking. Visual disabilities included.

711. Underberg, Rita P.; Verillo, Ronald T.; & Benham, Frank G.; et al. Factors relating to adjustment to visual disability in adolescence. *New Outlook for the Blind*, Sept. 1961, Vol. 55, No. 7, pp. 253–59.

Study reported in considerable detail comparing visually handicapped adolescents, both those living at home and those in residential schools, with sighted adolescents on various adjustment measures.

712. Wurster, Marion V. Now there's an idea. *New Outlook for the Blind*, Mar. 1965, Vol. 59, No. 3, p. 105.

Tells some of the ways in which youthful volunteers, usually Scouts, have helped agencies and associations for the blind.

8.   Education: General and Historical

713. Abel, Georgie Lee. New frontiers in the education of the young blind child. *New Outlook for the Blind*, Mar. 1955, Vol. 49, No. 3, pp. 87–97.

The increasing number of young blind children due to RLF and the positive reactions of most of their parents are forcing education to initiate new educational patterns in public and residential schools. Discusses many of these changes.

714. ———. *Concerning the education of blind children.* New York: AFB, 1959, 107 pp.

Includes discussions of the needs and resources of the preschool child, role of the residential school and public schools in education of blind children, the itinerant teaching program, and resource room. Additional papers on clay modeling, community resources, and problems and trends in the education of the blind.

715. Ala. State Dept. of Education. *Specific guidelines for teaching exceptional children.* Montgomery: Author, 1966, 164 pp.

Includes 9 pages dealing with teaching the visually handicapped, including a definition of resource programs.

716. Alaska State Dept. of Education. *Guidelines of programs of special education in Alaska.* Juneau: Author, 1966, 32 pp.

Six areas of exceptionality served by public schools are presented, including blind and partially sighted. Provides definition, criteria for placement, a section on evaluation, procedures for establishing programs, list of equipment, and relevant forms.

717. American Assoc. of Instructors of the Blind. *Proceedings of the Biennial Convention of the American Association of Instructors of the Blind, Inc. (46th, Miami Beach, Florida, June 28–July 2, 1962).* St. Louis, Mo.: Author, 1962, 146 pp., $2.

Topics covered include mobility, educational research, self-concept in blind children, and physical fitness.

718. ———. *Biennial convention of the American Association of Instructors of the Blind, Inc. (47th, Perkins School for the Blind, Watertown, Massachusetts, June 21–25, 1964).* St. Louis, Mo.: Author, 1964, 199 pp., $2.

Proceedings including address on directions in special education, panel discussions on research on technical devices, workshop summaries, description of demonstration project by deaf-blind pupils, and Association's business reports.

719. ———. *Biennial Conference of the American Association of Instructors of the Blind (48th, Salt Lake City, June 26–30, 1966).* Washington, D.C.: Author, 1966, 119 pp., $2.

Papers covered include research on: Teaching of reading and improving reading skills; independent living skills and orientation, mobility and travel; the child with limited but useful vision; the multihandicapped child; and listening, technical devices, and teaching methods.

720. Andrews, Francis M. Centennial address—Maryland School for the Blind.. *International Journal for the Education of the Blind,* Sept. 1953, Vol. 3, No. 1, pp. 196–97.

Discusses history and development of school, challenges for future, residential school vs. public school. Mention of doubly handicapped children.

721. ———. Is education for blind youth meeting the challenge of the changing times? *New Outlook for the Blind,* Dec. 1963, Vol. 57, No. 10, pp. 396–98.

Questions present adequacy and future directions.

722. Ariz. State Univ. *Mission: Possible.* Tempe, Ariz.: Author, 1969, 114 pp.

Discusses various exceptionalities, including visual impairment; gives bibliography, teaching methods, and sources of materials for each.

723. Ark. State Dept. of Education. *Guidebook for classes in special education.* Little Rock: Author, 1969, 62 pp.

Statements concerning the philosophy of special education, role of the state dept., and the steps in setting up special education programs. Gives program standards for various exceptionalities including the visually handicapped.

724. Ashcroft, Samuel C. The blind and partially seeing. *Review of Educational Research,* 1959, Vol. 29, No. 5, pp. 519–28.

Selective review of literature since 1953 written about the visually handicapped. Notes major trends such as the rise and fall in the incidence of retrolental fibroplasia, integrated education, and broader provision and application of improved optical aids. Bib.

725. ———. A new era in education and a paradox in research for the visually limited. *Exceptional Children,* 1963, Vol. 29, No. 8, pp. 371–76.

Review of recent research activity reveals a predominating interest in the area of test performance, adaptation or construction. Does not seem to be aimed toward discovery of needed educational modifications.

726. Assoc. for Education of the Visually Handicapped. *Selected papers: Fiftieth Biennial Conference. "A look at the child."* Philadelphia: Author, 1970, 232 pp., $3.

Presents 26 papers and 4 reports given at the Association's 1970 national conference. Paper topics include education and facilities for multiply handicapped deaf-blind children, mobility for young blind children, computer service, emotional disturbance and sensory deprivation, sexual and social adjustment, sensory aids, vision and hearing screening, guidance counselors and vocational success.

727. ———. *Selected papers: Fifty-second biennial conference. Equal educational opportunity for all the visually handicapped.* Philadelphia: Author, 1974, 106 pp., $3.

A selection of papers given at the Association's 1974 national conference.

728. ———. *Proceedings and selected papers of the First Biennial Conference of the Southeastern Region of AEVH, June 15–18, 1975, Atlanta, Georgia.* Philadelphia: Author, 1975, 70 pp.

Proceedings of conference concerned with "alternatives for educating the visually handicapped."

729. Barsch, Ray H. Concepts in programming for handicapped children. *New Outlook for the Blind,* Dec. 1963, Vol. 57, No. 10, pp. 379–84.

Discusses intake policy, developmental service, staff personnel, grouping of children, parent involvement.

730. Beaird, James H., et al. *Education of Oreg.'s sensory impaired youth.* Washington, D.C.: Bureau of Elementary and Secondary Education, 1972, 87 pp.

Reviews educational needs of deaf and blind children and reports on results of a 4-month study of Oreg.'s educational facilities and programs.

731. Best, John P. A comparison of the essential program components of residential schools for the blind. El Paso, Tex.: N.M. State Univ., 1963, 131 pp., app. Dissertation.

Study compares residential school program preferences of ex-students, houseparents, teachers, and administrators. Further comparisons were made between various groups of college, noncollege, independent, and nonindependent ex-students. Two instruments developed to conduct this study are included.

732. ———. The need for the residential school. *New Outlook for the Blind,* Apr. 1963, Vol. 57, No. 4, pp. 127–30.

States position of forward-looking residential school in rapidly changing field of special education. Discusses many areas of curriculum and services and general goals of the residential school.

733. Bishop, Virginia E. *Teaching the visually limited child.* Springfield, Ill.: Charles C Thomas, 1971, 214 pp., $9.50.

Written specifically for the beginning teacher of children with visual problems. Includes discussion of curriculum adaptations, listening skills, academic subject adaptations, typing and the communication process, and an outline of special classroom environments and materials. Detailed resource list includes: Educational games, teaching devices, equipment and tangible apparatus, resource books, resource organizations. Bib., glossary.

734. Board of Education of the City of New York. *Educating visually handicapped pupils.* New York: Author, 1967, 97 pp., app.

Explanation of current practices upgrading the educational program for visually handicapped pupils attending public schools with emphasis on integration of these pupils into the total curriculum of the regular school program.

735. Bodahl, Eleanor. *Guidelines for the referral of children who are sus-*

pected or known to be exceptional. Boise, Idaho: State Dept. of Education, 1966, 30 pp.

This booklet includes a definition, incidence figures, and characteristics of the blind and partially sighted.

736. Bommarito, James W. Visually handicapped children: A meaningful overview for school personnel. *Scientia Paedagogica Experimentalis,* 1968, Vol. 5, No. 2, pp. 160–86.

Areas discussed are: (1) definition, description, and incidence; (2) real limitations; (3) social and emotional characteristics; (4) potential difficulties; (5) educational considerations; and (6) psychological testing. Ref.

737. Bourgeault, Stanley E. The new look in special education. *New Outlook for the Blind,* Sept. 1961, Vol. 55, No. 7, pp. 246–51. Reprinted from *Minnesota Medicine,* Aug. 1960.

Presents some of the strengths and weaknesses of the various educational programs for the visually impaired child at various stages of development. Some historical perspective.

738. Browing, Philip L., et al. *Impact 3: The Title VI Program in the State of Oregon, June–August 1969.* Salem: Oreg. State Board of Education, 1969, 115 pp.

An overview of the summer 1969 activities which consisted of 24 projects designed for various exceptional populations including the visually handicapped. Detailed background and evaluation information on each project.

739. Buell, Charles. A survey of residential school policies of educating blind high school pupils. *International Journal for the Education of the Blind,* June 1953, Vol. 2, No. 4, pp. 174–77.

The author examines trends, in residential schools, of sending all or some of their high school students to public schools for all or part of their courses, and the reasons determining this policy. Gives lists of administrators' reasons for sending/not sending students to public schools, suggestions for further research.

740. ———. How can residential schools for the blind improve the socialization of pupils? *International Journal for the Education of the Blind,* Dec. 1953, Vol. 3, No. 2, pp. 222–23.

Presents problem of normal relationship between blind and sighted children. Various methods tried in the past have had little lasting help. Names some other seemingly more successful.

741. Calhoon, James R. Learning pathways. *Education of the Visually Handicapped,* Dec. 1971, Vol. 3, No. 4, pp. 106–8.

Author feels that training courses focus on impaired sense while remaining senses are ones that will have to be used for learning. This and the number of children with several impaired senses leads him to feel more interdisciplinary courses would be preferable.

742. Clark, Leslie L., Ed. *Proceedings of the West Coast Regional Conference on Research Related to Blind and Severely Visually Impaired Children.* New York: AFB, 1965, 147 pp., $2.

Information given on research techniques to uncover hidden blind population. Various causes and treatments of blindness in children presented.

Current research covered includes updating braille reading instruction, developing educational programs for multiply handicapped, developing direct translation (of print) device, measuring human sonar abilities, and state-wide program of O & M instruction in public schools. Ref.

743. Cole, Samuel J. Confidentiality policies and practices in residential schools for the blind. *New Outlook for the Blind,* Feb. 1973, Vol. 67, No. 2, pp. 52–55.

Report of 1972 NAC survey of residential schools regarding handling of written records, types of information filed, and access to student records. Need for flexible written policy suggested.

744. College of Teachers of the Blind. *Twenty-four selected articles from "The Teacher of the Blind,"* Liverpool, England: Author, 1970, 128 pp.

A reprinting of previously published articles relating to blind children including the following areas: Multiply handicapped, domestic science, needs of young children and their parents, mobility, perception, reading and books, physical education, behavior disorders, intelligence, and retinoblastoma.

745. Corder, Reginald. Educating blind children in Stanislaus County. *New Outlook for the Blind,* Dec. 1961, Vol. 55, No. 10, pp. 332–36.

Description of planning and services for visually handicapped at county level in a Calif. county of 150,000 population.

746. Council for Exceptional Children. *Special Education: Strategies for educational progress, Council for Exceptional Children selected convention papers.* Arlington, Va.: Author, 1966, 259 pp.

Selected conference papers including 2 on visual impairment.

747. ———. *Selected convention papers* (45th annual international CEC convention, St. Louis, Mo., Mar. 26–Apr. 1, 1967). Washington, D.C.: Author, 1967, 305 pp.

Presents approx. 65 papers, some in abridged or abstract form, on relevant topics, including 3 papers on visual impairment, and 5 on general concerns.

748. ———. *Visually handicapped.* Arlington, Va.: 1968, 45 pp. (Reprinted from the *CEC Selected Convention Papers, Annual International Convention, 46th, New York City, April 14–20, 1968.*)

Presentations include: Curriculum for teachers of the visually handicapped; a preparatory college for visually impaired students; prevocational planning and rehabilitation, N.J.'s organization, cooperation and coordination of programs for the visually handicapped; teacher education; and research, development trends and translation into practice of sensory aids. Includes abstracts on multiply impaired blind children.

749. ———. *Selected convention papers. Proceedings of the Annual International Convention of the Council for Exceptional Children (47th, Denver, Colorado, April 6–12, 1969).* Arlington, Va.: Author, 1969, 536 pp.

Presents abstracts of articles and complete articles, 3 of which are on topic of visually handicapped.

750. ———. *Visually handicapped—Programs: Exceptional child bibliography series.* Reston, Va.: Author, Feb. 1971, 15 pp.

Contains 53 references from *Exceptional Child Education Abstracts* concerning educational and home programming for visually handicapped children. Cites texts for parents and teachers on topics such as: Orientation and mobility, programmed instruction, legal considerations, physical education, career planning, and recreation.

751. ——. *Visually handicapped—Research: Exceptional child bibliography series.* Reston, Va.: Author, Feb. 1971, 22 pp.

Contains 81 references from *Exceptional Child Education Abstracts* on research studies of visually handicapped children including reports on screening and identification, listening abilities, braille instruction, orientation and mobility, and program evaluation.

752. ——. *Physical education and recreation: A selective bibliography.* Arlington, Va.: Author, 1972, 24 pp.

Contains 70 abstracts, some relevant to visually handicapped children.

753. ——. *Visually handicapped—programs: A selective bibliography.* Reston, Va.: Author, 1973, 19 pp., Bibliography Series No. 619.

Lists references with descriptors and abstracts. Author and subject indexes.

754. ——. *Visually handicapped—research: A selective bibliography.* Reston, Va.: Author, 1973, 21 pp., Bibliography Series No. 620.

Lists references with descriptors and abstracts. Author and subject indexes.

755. Craig, William N. Financial statement—public residential schools in the United States October 1, 1972. *American Annals of the Deaf*, Apr. 1973, Vol. 118, No. 2, pp. 284–94.

Gives tabular data from schools in 50 states concerning income, expenditures, enrollment and per capita cost for 1971–72, and 1972–73 data including full-time employees, teaching days, teacher salaries.

756. Cruickshank, William M., & Trippe, Matthew J. *Services to blind children in New York State.* Syracuse, N.Y.: Syracuse Univ. Press, 1959, 495 pp., $5.

Principle objectives of the study were to determine educational, social, and health characteristics of legally blind children under 21 years of age in N.Y. State, to determine the services and nature of the programs and to point out areas of service which might be strengthened, and to examine the existing state legislation.

757. Davis, Aurelia. Special education in Atlanta. *New Outlook for the Blind*, Dec. 1961, Vol. 55, No. 10, pp. 329–32.

Review of education of blind in Atlanta using regular public school with resource rooms and itinerant teachers. Stresses importance of community and church groups and volunteers as back-up teams and workers in enrichment programs.

758. Davis, Carl J. Confidentiality and the school counselor. *New Outlook for the Blind*, Feb. 1973, Vol. 67, No. 2, pp. 56–59.

Discussion of the counselor's (psychologist or social caseworker) responsibility to the client (student) and administration, including a discussion of the treatment of memoranda and notes and disclosures (to administration, parents, and courts).

759. Dunn, Lloyd M., Ed. *Exceptional children in the schools.* New York: Holt, Rinehart, Winston, 1963, 580 pp.

Intended as a survey text for college students in special education or as a reference for noneducators associated with the schools. Considers blind and partially sighted among other areas of exceptionality and defines these areas' prevalence, identification, characteristics, educational procedures, and resources. Lists references, films, and other resources.

760. Falls, Charles W. *Special Education Program for Nebraska's Handicapped Children, 1965–1966.* Lincoln: State Dept. of Education, Lincoln Div. Instr., 1966, 52 pp., illus.

During the 1965–66 school year in Nebr., 8,490 handicapped children received special services, and an additional 2,433 children received speech and hearing diagnoses and psychological testing services. These services cost $129.12 per pupil.

761. Fields, Helen W. How New York City educates visually handicapped children. *New Outlook for the Blind*, Dec. 1961, Vol. 55, No. 10, pp. 337–40.

Overview of this large city's dealing with problems of educating the visually handicapped. Resource rooms, itinerant teachers, guidance counselors, and role of the Bureau for the Education of the Visually Handicapped are discussed.

762. First workshop on education of blind Negro children. *New Outlook for the Blind*, Nov. 1954, Vol. 48, No. 9, pp. 332–34.

Primarily concerned with the examination of curricula and procedures of the schools for blind Negro children in the South.

763. Frampton, Merle E., & Gall, Elena D. *Special education for the exceptional. Vol. II, The physically handicapped and special health problems.* Boston: Porter Sargent, 1955, 677 pp.

Pp. 2–146 relate to blind and partially seeing. Describes physical and psychosocial characteristics and resulting educational problems. Discusses modes of education, methods and materials, parent relationships, vocational goals, and lists relevant agencies and periodicals. Bib.

764. Frampton, Merle E., & Kearney, Ellen. *The residential school, its history, contributions, and future.* New York: Institute for the Education of the Blind, 1953, 163 pp.

Detailed contrast of residential and day school programs.

765. Gall, Elena D. A demonstration program for intellectually gifted blind youth. *International Journal for the Education of the Blind*, Oct. 1967, Vol. 17, No. 1, pp. 1–7.

For a number of reasons, including the wish to focus attention on services to intellectually gifted blind youth, 15 students with IQ range 130–150 were provided a 6-week summer program. Details of this program are presented, and some of its benefits listed.

766. Ga. State Dept. of Education. *Regulations and procedures: Program for exceptional children.* Atlanta: Author, 1969, 43 pp.

Discusses support of the state dept., the responsibilities of a program for exceptional children, teacher approval, and certification. Goals presented for various exceptionalities including visually impaired.

767. Goldberg, I. Ignacy. *Selected bibliography of special education.* New York: Columbia Univ., 1967, 126 pp.

List of selected refs., pertinent to various fields of specialization, to aid the researcher in special education.

768. Grover, Edward C., et al. *Ohio programs for visually handicapped children: A report on the 1964–65 Columbus, Ohio, Study of Partially seeing.* Columbus: Dept. of Education, Div. of Special Education, 1965, 103 pp., app.

Declining enrollment in programs for partially seeing, problems of incidence, visual functioning, and multiple handicaps were investigated, including screening 23,611 students in 4th to 6th grades. IQ level and achievement reported with case histories of 36 partially seeing children. Ref.

769. Guldager, Lars. A macro-solution in special education. *New Outlook for the Blind,* Feb. 1973, Vol. 67, No. 2, pp. 72–78.

Proposes a macro-solution (described as a comprehensive system of public and private agencies in which needed services are coordinated in the most efficient and least redundant way) for the provision of services to all exceptional children in the U.S. Specific suggestions include a state coordinator for all services, a central registry, coordination of funding, and centralized certification of personnel.

770. Gumm, Mrs. Harvey. Education and general work for the blind in Idaho. *International Journal for the Education of the Blind,* Apr. 1953, Vol. 2, No. 3, pp. 158–60.

History of school for deaf and blind, examples of former students. Description of classes, adult blind, register of blind, home teaching, vocational rehabilitation, cooperating agencies.

771. Hall, William, & Sieswerda, David. *Developing exceptional programs: Workshop in the education of the exceptional child.* Tempe: Ariz. State Univ., 1966, 145 pp.

A condensation of material from the experience and ideas of workshop participants. Including visually handicapped. Bib.

772. Hanninen, Kenneth A. *Teaching the visually handicapped.* Columbus, Ohio: Charles E. Merrill, 1975, vii + 232 pp., $12.95.

Chapters on: Adjustment of blind children in school, integration into regular classes, use of severely limited vision, reading instruction, writing and spelling, listening, orientation and mobility instruction, physical education and recreation, adaptations in common curriculum areas, visually handicapped children with multiple disabilities, and the future and education of visually handicapped.

773. Hartman, Dorothy R. Philadelphia serves the visually handicapped child. *New Outlook for the Blind,* June 1957, Vol. 51, No. 6, pp. 241–44.

Describes the sight-saving classes and supporting services.

774. Hathaway, Winifred. *Education and health of the partially seeing child.* New York: Columbia Univ. Press, 1959, 201 pp.

Treats the organization of facilities and methods to provide optimum education. Covers definition of partially seeing children, methods of identification, methods of providing special educational facilities, facilities in rural areas, school health services, teacher selection and preparation, and financing.

775. **Heinsen, Arthur C., Jr.** The school vision care program. *Academic Therapy Quarterly*, Summer 1971, Vol. 6, No. 4, pp. 417–22.

A multidisciplinary approach to the vision problem is stressed with the role of the teacher, optometric consultant, school psychologist, school nurse, and parents defined. Counseling of parents and guidance in training procedures for the classroom are suggested.

776. **Henderson, Florence.** Understanding our limitations in a functional education for blind children. *New Outlook for the Blind*, Dec. 1954, Vol. 48, No. 10, pp. 347–53.

Urges positive approaches to teaching of blind child with emphasis on the child's ability, not his limitations. Gives 6 principles of learning for the blind child.

777. **Hendrickson, Walter B.** *From shelter to self-reliance: A history of the Illinois Braille and Sight Saving School.* Jacksonville, Ill.: School, 1972, x + 235 pp., $6.

This history, covering the years 1848–1970, is the story of one particular residential school, but it also offers an overview of the evolving theories concerning the education of the blind.

778. **Heslinga, K., & van 'T Hooft, F.** Medical care and pedagogical policy in a residential school for blind and partially sighted children. *Education of the Visually Handicapped*, Oct. 1969, Vol. 1, No. 3, pp. 76–79.

Discussion rather critical of physicians as to ways they provide care and do research with blind. Authors feel they do not take whole child into account.

779. **Ind. State Office of the State Supt. of Public Instruction.** *Exceptional pupils: Special education bulletin number 1.* Indianapolis: Author, 1968, 129 pp.

Bulletin overviewing Ind.'s special education of exceptional pupils.

780. **Jernigan, Kenneth.** In Tennessee we call it progress. *International Journal for the Education of the Blind*, Feb. 1953, Vol. 2, No. 2, pp. 142–43.

Describes the then-new campus and buildings of the Tenn. School for the Blind, calling them "ultra modern." Gives brief history of School's origin and progress.

781. **Jones, John W.** *Blind children: Degree of vision mode of reading.* Washington, D.C.: Govt. Printing Office, 1961, 38 pp.

Data on 14,125 legally blind school-age children were tabulated and analyzed to compile statistical information on the degree of remaining vision and mode of reading. Results revealed that less than 25% of the children are totally blind, over 60% have vision sufficient for use in instructional programs. Separate tabulations made of local and residential school registrations.

782. ————. Office of Education sponsors research conference on visually handicapped. *International Journal for the Education of the Blind*, Oct. 1961, Vol. 11, No. 1, pp. 1–3.

In response to a felt need for a total framework within which research in greater depth could be planned, OE called together special educators who identified 24 educational problems which are listed. Suggested priorities are also given.

783. Jones, John W., & Collins, Anne P. Trends in program and pupil placement practices in the special education of visually handicapped children. *International Journal for the Education of the Blind*, May 1965, Vol. 14, No. 4, pp. 97–101.

With supporting statistics, reports a survey of organizational and staff patterns, characteristics of children served, and sources of referral for programs for the handicapped nationally.

784. ———. *Educational programs for visually handicapped children.* Washington, D.C.: Govt. Printing Office, 1966, 74 pp., app., illus.

Findings of nationwide survey, conducted by Office of Education, on program and placement practices in the area of special education. Statistics on enrollment, student-teacher ratios, pupil eligibility factors, etc.

785. Jones, Morris V., Ed. *Special education programs within the States.* Springfield, Ill.: Charles C Thomas, 1968, 427 pp.

Perkins School for the Blind is discussed among 21 other special schools and diagnostic centers in the U.S.

786. Jordan, Thomas E., & Cegelka, Walter, Jr., Eds. *Exceptional Children.* New York: MSS Information Corp., 1972, 328 pp. $8.75.

Collection of readings on current issues, trends, and concepts in education; 3 are on the visually handicapped child, including 1 on psychological evaluation.

787. Kans. State Dept. of Education. *Planning for visually impaired children in Kansas schools: An administrative guide.* Topeka: Author, 1970, 13 pp.

Guide intended to aid Kans. school administrators in planning educational programs for visually impaired children in their communities. Defines children who may be served; states eligibility standards.

788. Kerr, Joseph J. Evaluating a school for the blind. *International Journal for the Education of the Blind*, June 1952, Vol. 1, No. 4, pp. 78–80.

Presents requirements a school had to meet to qualify for accreditation and membership in Middle States Association of Colleges and Secondary Schools. Included aims, self-evaluation, areas included, ratings, visiting committee and report of committee's findings.

789. Kirk, Edith C. Detroit's program for blind children. *New Outlook for the Blind*, Dec. 1965, Vol. 59, No. 10, pp. 339–41.

For 170 children in Detroit vision program shows: Proportion in relation to Detroit school population, sex and race, age at testing at vision clinic, age at entering special program, causes and extent of vision loss, intelligence, and reasons for leaving program. Implications of study discussed.

790. Kloss, Alton G. Relationship between schools for the blind and agencies for the adult blind. *International Journal for the Education of the Blind*, Oct. 1957, Vol. 7, No. 1, pp. 1–8.

Describes the program at the Western Pennsylvania School for Blind Children and how both public and private agencies help in service to children and parents.

791. Lansdown, Richard. What the research doesn't know. *Journal of Special Education*, Dec. 1969, Vol. 58, No. 4, pp. 20–24.

Discusses the problems in lack of research into the educational needs of visually impaired children including personality and social adjustment, educational methods, aptitudes, language and speech, lighting and classroom aids, print size, and employment. Brief reviews of current and past research presented under each topic.

792. Laycock, Samuel R. *Special education in Canada.* Toronto: W. J. Gage, 1963, 187 pp.

A collection of special education lectures delivered by the author under the Quance Lectures in Canadian Education (Univ. of Saskatchewan, 1963). Trends and studies of the visually handicapped are discussed. Information is presented on definitions, diagnosis, educational possibilities, and general services available.

793. Lester, Regina L. The visually handicapped child. In Robison D. Harley, Ed., *Pediatric Ophthalmology*. Philadelphia: W. B. Saunders, 1975, pp. 830–51, illus., $50.

Discusses habilitation and education of children with varied amounts of vision limitation of adventitious or congenital origin, briefly describing integrated and segregated approaches to education, recreational, and social services. Also lists agencies which provide special education, preschool and vocational counseling, and private agencies which serve on a nationwide basis.

794. Lipscomb, Nell. The case worker's role in social action. *New Outlook for the Blind*, June 1964, Vol. 58, No. 6, pp. 174–76.

Difficulties encountered and eventually overcome in establishing braille classes for blind Negro children in New Orleans.

795. Lord, F. E. Education of the physically handicapped: Review and implications. *PRISE Reporter*, May 1974, Vol. 5, pp. 1–2.

Discusses the history and issues of state support, instructional innovation, segregation, and the legislative mandate to educate all handicapped children.

796. Los Angeles Unified School District. *Status 1968: Report of the Special Education Branch, Los Angeles Unified School District.* Author, 1969, 140 pp.

Chapters on the visually handicapped are included in an overview of special education branch programs.

797. Lowenfeld, Berthold. History and development of specialized education for the blind. *New Outlook for the Blind*, Dec. 1956, Vol. 50, No. 10, pp. 401–8. Also in *Exceptional Children*, Nov. 1956.

From the school of Valentin Hauy in Paris in 1785, to residential schools, to braille classes in public schools, discusses the changes toward integration, including legislation. Education should be provided in the kind of school which is best for each individual child.

798. ———. The school psychologist and the visually handicapped child. In Monroe B. Gottsegen & Gloria B. Gottsegen, Eds., *Professional School psychology, II.* New York: Grune & Stratton, 1963, Chap. 9.

Author presents an overview of the responsibilities of the school psychologist. Also includes: A careful definition of the visually handicapped, statistics on number and types of visually handicapped children in U.S. and, the types of educational programs available to this group with a discussion of individual variables to consider in educational placement.

799. ———, **Ed.** *The visually handicapped child in school.* New York: John Day, 1973, 384 pp., $16.

Complete discussion of past and current education of visually handicapped. Chapters include: History, psychological considerations, understanding and meeting development need, psychological and educational assessment, utilization of sensory-perceptual abilities, kinds of educational programs, communication skills, special subject adjustments and skills, life adjustment, the child with additional problems, and preparation of teachers. Long list of recommended additional reading.

800. Mackie, Romaine P., et al. *Special education in the United States: Statistics 1948–1966.* New York: Teachers' Col. Press, Columbia Univ., 1969, 90 pp.

Based on public and residential schools, the report includes Office of Education statistics for 1963 and estimates for 1966. Results give indications in such areas as enrollment, gap between need and reception of special services in school-age population, nursery programs, etc. Implications of indications are considered. Specific data concern trends in the area of visual handicaps, among others.

801. Magleby, F. LeGrande, & Farley, Owen W. Education for blind children. *American Foundation for the Blind Research Bulletin 16,* May 1968, pp. 69–72.

Brief report of characteristics of 59 blind adults who had been educated in residential schools and 39 educated in day programs. Results favor residential schooling.

802. Massie, Dennis. Guidelines for research in the education of partially seeing children. *New Outlook for the Blind,* Feb. 1965, Vol. 59, No. 2, pp. 57–58.

Fifteen studies of education of partially seeing children were examined to discover the nature, significance, and implications of research in this area.

803. Merry, Ralph V. *Problems in the education of visually handicapped children.* Harvard Studies in Education series, Vol. 19. New York: Johnson Reprint Corp., 1933, 243 pp.

Considers the problems of visually handicapped elementary school children. Includes development of education for the visually handicapped; discussion of preschool, kindergarten, day classes, residential education, and sight-saving classes; health problems; intelligence and school achievement; personality and guidance problems, and problems in selecting and training teachers.

804. Meyer, Henry J. Joint agreement program in Illinois: Another effort to meet the needs of visually handicapped children. *International Journal for the Education of the Blind,* Mar. 1966, Vol. 15, No. 3, pp. 83–85.

Fairly detailed description of procedures through which selected blind children move from the residential school to schools in their home communities. Of special interest is the strong role of the residential school.

805. Misbach, Dorothy L., & Sweeney, Joan. *Education of the visually handicapped in California public schools,* Sacramento: Calif. State Dept. of Education, 1970, 95 pp.

Designed as a guide and reference for administrators and teachers of the visually handicapped in the Calif. public schools.

806. Mitchell, Paul C. The golden decade: Ten years of progress in the education of visually handicapped children. *International Journal for the Education of the Blind,* May 1958, Vol. 7, No. 4, pp. 105–9.

Professional growth of educators and improved campuses and plants are matched by expansion of the educational programs. Special services such as travel training, groups for slow learners, and increased vocational offerings are evident in many schools. An account of the vast gains in the previous decade.

807. Mont. State Dept. of Public Instruction. *Special help for special children.* Helena: Mont. State Dept. of Education, 1964, 24 pp.

A 1962 teacher survey in Mont. groups special children by type of problem. Status and problems of state's special education program summarized. Ten questions enabling local districts to evaluate their services, and suggestions to teachers and others for improving services included.

808. Mulholland, Mary E. Confidentiality and the school: Introduction. *New Outlook for the Blind,* Feb. 1973, Vol. 67, No. 2, pp. 49, 51.

An introduction to a symposium based on a Workshop on Confidentiality sponsored by the National Accreditation Council in June 1972. Explains the background of the Workshop and the schedule of the various meetings.

809. Myers, S. O. American diversity versus British compactness. *New Outlook for the Blind,* June 1954, Vol. 48, No. 6, pp. 197–200.

A British visitor compares American and British ways of educating blind children.

810. Naples, Victor J., et al. *A program for visually impaired children.* Columbus, Ohio: State Dept. of Education, Div. of Special Education, 1973, 51 pp.

Booklet explains how to organize programs for the visually handicapped according to the vision center concept which combines the outstanding features of self-contained classrooms, resource teacher plans, and itinerant teacher plans. State-sponsored services discussed.

811. National Accreditation Council. Confidentiality and the school: Workshop report. *New Outlook for the Blind,* Feb. 1973, Vol. 67, No. 2, pp. 59–61.

Report of 4 group discussions relating to the COMSTAC standards on confidentiality as they relate to the Russell Sage Foundation *Guidelines for the collection, maintenance, and dissemination of pupil records: Report of a conference on the ethical and legal aspects of school record keeping* (New York: Russell Sage Foundation, 1970, pp. 20–22). Recommendations were made that could serve as a checklist for agencies developing written policies.

812. Nezol, A. James. State organizational patterns for education of visually impaired children. *Exceptional Children*, Sept. 1974, Vol. 41, No. 1, pp. 43–44.

Brief report on survey data collected in 1973. Questionnaires sent to persons on state level most directly responsible for administering programs for visually impaired children; 41 states replied.

813. Nolan, Carson Y. Blind children: Degree of vision, mode of reading–A 1963 replication. *New Outlook for the Blind*, Sept. 1965, Vol. 59, No. 7, pp. 233–38.

Compares data from 2 studies of American Printing House for the Blind annual registrations of legally blind children with emphasis on the relationships between degree of vision and mode of reading, i.e., braille or large type. Tables and statistical data.

814. ———. A 1966 reappraisal of the relationship between visual acuity and mode of reading for blind children. *New Outlook for the Blind*, Oct. 1967, Vol. 61, No. 8, pp. 255–61.

Statistical analysis of American Printing House for the Blind records of 18,652 children served in 1966, showing visual levels related to mode of reading and grade distributions. A trend toward greater use of vision is evident.

815. ———. *Educational Research, Development, and Reference Group report on research and development activities—Fiscal 1972*. Louisville, Ky.: American Printing House for the Blind, 1972, 29 pp.

Reviews progress on projects in 5 major areas: Aural study systems, basic research in tactual perception, braille codes pilot project, educational and instructional materials, and bibliographies.

816. Nolan, Carson Y., & Ashcroft, Samuel C. The visually handicapped. *Review of Educational Research*, 1969, Vol. 39, No. 1, pp. 52–70.

Stresses necessity of research concerning measurement techniques, human engineering approaches to the development of aids and teaching materials, and evaluation of teacher and program effectiveness.

817. Nolan, Carson Y., & Bott, Joan E. Relationships between visual acuity and reading medium for blind children—1969. *New Outlook for the Blind*, Mar. 1971, Vol. 65, No. 3, pp. 90–96.

Reports 1 of a series of periodic analyses of data of the American Printing House for the Blind showing relationships between degree of vision and mode of reading in various types of school programs. Statistics show increase in multiply handicapped residential, commission, and local school enrollments with trend toward increased use of residual vision.

818. Norris, Miriam. *The school age blind child project*. New York: AFB, 1961, 55 pp., $2.

Purpose of follow-up study of 62 blind children was to further understanding of the young blind child. Seventy-one percent of the children were making satisfactory progress in school, but the others were experiencing learning problems which necessitated a change in the school placement. Many of the learning problems resulted from emotional disturbances.

819. Office of Education. *Educational programs for visually handicapped children*. Washington, D.C.: Govt. Printing Office, 1966, 74 pp.

Reports from nation-wide survey on program and placement practices for visually handicapped children from 353 special local public school programs and 54 residential schools employing 1 or more full-time teachers of visually handicapped during 1962–63.

820. Olsen, Maurice. What counts in educational services? *New Outlook for the Blind*, Jan. 1963, Vol. 57, No. 1, pp. 21–22.

Author sees the school program and the educational staff as the areas of primary importance.

821. Oregon School data on effects of RLF. *New Outlook for the Blind*, May 1959, Vol. 53, No. 5, p. 185.

Compares enrollment data of the Oregon State School for the Blind with previously printed statistics for Calif.

822. Oseroff, Andrew, & Birch, Jack W. Clearinghouse: Relationships of socioeconomic background and school performance of partially seeing children. *Exceptional Children*, Oct. 1971, Vol. 38, No. 2, pp. 158–59.

Academic achievement and economic background of 29 intermediate grade children enrolled in special educational programs for the partially seeing were studied. Results indicated that socioeconomic status was significantly related to both age-grade status and academic achievement at the 5% level of confidence.

823. Ostberg, Ann-Mari, & Lindqvist, Bengt. *Learning problems in connection with special information media for the visually handicapped—A selected bibliography.* Uppsala, Sweden: Teachers College of, 1970, 56 pp.

Bibliography on education of the blind and special sections on tactual and visual sources of information.

824. Paschalita, Sister M. Special education and the American Catholic School System. *New Outlook for the Blind*, May 1953, Vol. 47, No. 5, pp. 134–41.

Describes the typical effects of blindness upon children, the educational needs which result, and a brief history of special education in U.S. Moves into more recent development of special education facilities in parish schools and the teacher training available at Catholic Univ. of America.

825. Pascoe, Tom. The education of the visually handicapped. *Forward Trends*, Spring 1973, Vol. 17, No. 1, pp. 32–34.

Areas considered include team assessment approach to early intervention and placement, organization of schools, curriculum, and training of staff.

826. Peabody, Ralph L., & Birch, Jack W. Educational implications of partial vision: New findings from a national study. *International Journal for the Education of the Blind*, Oct. 1967, Vol. 17, No. 1, pp. 21–24.

Based on research data, describes the typical partially seeing child. Lists and discusses a few of the implications of this description for education.

827. Peeler, Egbert N. Minimum standards for schools for the blind. *International Journal for the Education of the Blind*, May 1957, Vol. 6, No. 4, pp. 88–90.

Describes why standards are needed, the AAIB Committee on Standards and Evaluation, and its questionnaire. Gives some examples of results of that questionnaire and resulting recommendations.

828. Rex, Evelyn. Educational implications of recent medical research concerning blindness. *International Journal for the Education of the Blind*, May 1962, Vol. 11, No. 4, pp. 120–25.

Although some causes of blindness are reduced, the total number of blind children is greater, many are multiply handicapped, and the need to educate them in day schools raises new challenges. Even the attitudes of educational staff and fellow students must change.

829. Ricketts, Peter. No place like home. *New Beacon*, Apr. 1974, Vol. 58, No. 684, pp. 90–91.

Blind author discusses trend to integrated education, and gives his personal reasons for wishing he had attended a day school.

830. R.I. Legis. Comm. to Study the Education of Handicapped Youth. *Education of handicapped children in Rhode Island, a report to the legislature*. R.I.: Author, Mar. 14, 1963, 160 pp.

831. Roberts, Ferne K. National recognition for accreditation of residential schools for blind students. *Exceptional Children*, May 1972, Vol. 38, No. 9, pp. 742–43.

The National Accreditation Council for Agencies Serving the Blind and Visually Handicapped (NAC) has been recognized by the Office of Education as an accrediting association. NAC developed a guide which stresses elements essential for accreditation.

832. Root, Ferne K. Today's challenges in teaching visually handicapped children. *International Journal for the Education of the Blind*, May 1965, Vol. 14, No. 4, pp. 101–5.

Four major challenges of the preceding decade are discussed: Responsibility for educational decisions; responsibility for the "silent partner" role; responsibility for the paradox of preservation—change; and responsibility for leadership.

833. Rosinger, G., et al. *An assessment of Ohio residential schools and other public school settings for educating deaf students and blind students: Final report*. Columbus, Ohio: Battelle Memorial Inst., 1969, 61 pp.

Study involving research, comparisons, consultation with experts, to determine effectiveness of 1 Ohio State residential school for the blind and 1 for the deaf, and whether or not the state should continue to operate them. Includes results, recommendations, areas for further research.

834. Rucker, Chauncy N., & Rabinstein, John E., Eds. *Exceptional children: An introduction*. New York: MSS Educational Publishing, 1969, 142 pp.

Twenty-two articles on exceptional child education intended to provide supplementary reading for undergraduate courses. Includes sections on the blind and partially sighted.

835. Scholl, Geraldine T. The education of children with visual impairments. In William M. Cruickshank & G. Orville Johnson, Eds. *Education of exceptional children and youth*. Englewood Cliffs, N.J.: Prentice-Hall, 1967, pp. 287–342.

Defines and describes visual handicaps and their effects on development of children. Reviews types of schooling, roles of teachers, variations in programming, and special areas such as braille and orientation and mobility.

836. ———. *Self-study and evaluation guide for residential schools, 1968 Edition.* New York: National Accreditation Council, 1968, 514 pp.

Designed as an instrument for school self-study, the guide sets forth evaluative criteria for determining the quality of residential educational programs for blind children.

837. ———. Accreditation: What it can mean for residential schools. *New Outlook for the Blind*, Feb. 1969, Vol. 63, No. 2, pp. 50–54.

Values, process, and philosophy of accreditation for residential schools.

838. ———. *Development of self-study instruments for use in accrediting. Final report.* Washington, D.C.: Office of Education, July 1969, 58 pp.

Staff reaction form utilized to evaluate the Self-Study and Evaluation Guide for Residential Schools. Guide was considered deficient as mechanism for describing programs for multiply handicapped and for describing role of houseparents. Overall Guide found to be appropriate and useful for describing programs. App. includes forms used.

839. ———. Fringe benefits of accreditation for residential schools. *New Outlook for the Blind*, Sept. 1971, Vol. 65, No. 7, pp. 220–23.

Benefits include reassurance to financial supporters, agencies, parents, students, and teachers that the school is a desirable institution and worthy of support. Also explores in greater detail internal fringe benefits to the school, staff, and operations.

840. ———. Confidentiality and the school: Summary of workshop reports. *New Outlook for the Blind*, Feb. 1973, Vol. 67, No. 2, pp. 62–65.

Summary of the issues raised during the workshop sessions. Covers the need for written records, sources of information, kinds of records, access to records, and the danger of no records.

841. Simpson, Dorothea. A veteran agency in a unique service. *New Outlook for the Blind*, June 1954, Vol. 48, No. 6, pp. 179–84.

How the Connecticut State Board of Education of the Blind enlarged its programs for students at all levels.

842. Tannenbaum, Abraham J. *Special education and programs for disadvantaged children and youth.* Washington, D.C.: Council for Exceptional Children, 1968, 135 pp.

Nine conference papers on topics including behavior disorders in children from deprived backgrounds, problems of perception and cognition, the disadvantaged gifted. Offers presentations from special education programs on learning disabilities, the mentally retarded, orthopedically handicapped, health impaired, visually handicapped, and those needing speech therapy.

843. Tex. Univ. Col. of Education. *Proceedings of the Second Colloquium on Exceptional Children and Youth.* Austin: Univ. of Tex. Press, 1966, 148 pp.

Presents lectures by authorities on visual impairment and summaries of discussions following each lecture.

844. Tobin, Michael J. Modern research towards improving educational opportunities for the visually handicapped. *New Beacon*, Dec. 1974, Vol. 58, No. 692, pp. 313–17.

Presents argument that fundamental/theoretical research and research that is immediately applicable in the classroom situation are complementary, and a balance must be struck between them.

845. Trapp, E. Philip, & Himelstein, Philip, Eds. *Readings on the exceptional child, research and theory.* New York: Appleton-Century-Crofts, 1962, 674 pp.

Experimental studies and critical reviews of related studies are compiled in 48 chapters on the exceptional child. Writings on the visually handicapped are included.

846. Tyler, Wilbert P. Some aspects of blindness. *International Journal for the Education of the Blind,* Dec. 1959, Vol. 9, No. 2, pp. 32–35.

Blindness restricts the individual in concepts, locomotion, and in environmental control. Emotional problems may result from blindness and the attitudes of others. The author suggests how the teacher should try to compensate.

847. Dept. of Health, Education & Welfare. *Education of handicapped children and youth: A conference report on possibilities and plans under the provisions of Title I, Elementary and Secondary Education Act of 1965 (Washington, D.C., Aug. 11 and 12, 1965).* Washington, D.C.: Author, 1965, 56 pp.

Possibilities and plans are explored in papers by directors of special education in Kans. and Calif. Describes relevant needs of handicapped and maladjusted children in Chicago's disadvantaged neighborhoods, and activities for the handicapped in the District of Columbia. Includes 24 project outlines, 5 recommendations, references to Title I, lists of Title I coordinators and key contacts.

848. Univ. of Calif. *Educational facilities for the visually handicapped.* Berkeley: Univ. of Calif. Dept. of Architecture, 1966, 217 pp.

Brief description of the work process and results of a study by 18 3rd-year students. Discusses importance of architectural form and organization to the blind child. Information accumulated and synthesized into an architectural reflection of the factors needed to develop the multiply handicapped blind child to his fullest mental and physical potential.

849. Vernon, McCay. Problems in the education of visually-handicapped children. *New Beacon,* Aug. 1973, Vol. 57, No. 76, pp. 198–200.

Recommendations of a British committee include early diagnosis and parent guidance, maximum contact with the normally sighted (though educational needs are seen to be best met in special schools), and the Optacon. Stresses independence and mobility.

850. Wanecek, Ottokar. The goal of education in the training of the blind. *International Journal for the Education of the Blind,* Oct. 1952, Vol. 2, No. 1, pp. 124–25.

Maintains that goals of education should be the same for the blind as for the sighted.

851. Watson, Charles W. The education of visually handicapped children in California. *New Outlook for the Blind,* June 1956, Vol. 50, No. 6, pp. 216–23. Also in *California Schools,* Jan. 1956.

With statistical data, gives the number of partially seeing and blind children in Calif. Discusses problems in finding the children with visual problems and classifying them. Local responsibility, financing, preschool services, and trends in education are presented. Ref.

852. Weishahn, Mel W., & Mitchell, Richard. Educational placement practices with visually disabled and orthopedically disabled children—a comparison. *Rehabilitation Literature*, Sept. 1971, Vol. 32, No. 9, pp. 263–66, 288.

Compares trends in educational placement practices for the visually and physically handicapped. Shows parallel trends toward greater integration into regular education programs, but with a lag in the development of integrating programs for the physically handicapped.

853. Yick, Margaret R. Our friends abroad. *International Journal for the Education of the Blind*, Oct. 1956, Vol. 6, No. 1, pp. 18–21.

Describes the program of affiliation between Overbrook School for the Blind and a school in France, as arranged through American Friends' Service Committee. Students, correspondence, and materials are exchanged between the 2 schools.

9. Educational Setting, Curriculum, Methods, and Materials

854. Aamoth, Lillie. Educational principles for teaching blind children. *International Journal for the Education of the Blind,* June 1954, Vol. 3, No. 4, pp. 259–61.

Advises on enlarging horizons through personality development, supportive environment, student-teacher relationships, and teacher requirements. Describes educational principles: Concreteness, unified instruction, additional stimulus, self-activity.

855. Adaptive Physical Education Task Force. *Expanding physical education services to pupils with handicapping conditions: Summary report.* Madison, Wis.: Madison Public Schools, 1974.

A report following an investigation of need to broaden the scope of physical education and recreation services to students with handicapping conditions. Sections include: Needs assessment, long-range implementation objectives, staff development and training, and overall plan for school-community recreation program.

856. AIM for the Handicapped. *AIM: Adventures in movement for the handicapped.* Dayton, Ohio: Author, 1974.

Handbook of information about Adventures in Movement for the Handicapped (AIM) and AIM techniques. Discusses organizational goals, including specific objectives in programming for blind children. Included is a specific outline for the AIM method of movement education with a breakdown of each class period in terms of basic exercises, locomotor movements, and rhythmic dance patterns or creative movements.

857. Akau, Lindo Jo. Vibration technique for blind nonspeakers. *Education of the Visually Handicapped,* May 1970, Vol. 2, No. 2, pp. 52–54.

Use of vibration technique with visually handicapped nonspeakers is described. Case history illustrates the slow process but eventual success with the method.

858. Albright, Tacy B. A brighter era for the Texas School for the Blind. *International Journal for the Education of the Blind,* Apr. 1953, Vol. 2, No. 3, pp. 154–56.

Detailed description of renovation of school including lighting, colors, brightness, and acoustics.

859. Alonso, Lou. The child with impaired vision in the regular classroom. *Seer,* Fall 1973, Vol. 74, No. 3, pp. 5–8. Reprinted from *Today's Education,* Nov. 1967.

Suggestions for classroom teachers to maximize the opportunities for visually impaired children to learn in the regular classroom.

860. Alonso, Lou, & Wessel, Janet, Eds. *Physical education and recreation for the visually handicapped: Report of the First Physical Education and Recreation Workshop for visually handicapped children and youth.* East Lansing: Mich. State Univ. Press, 1967, 223 pp.

A workshop for administrators, physical educators, special educators, and others examined physical education curricula needs of the visually handicapped. Bib.

861. American Association for Health, Physical Education, and Recreation. *Physical education and recreation for handicapped children: Proceedings of a study conference on research and demonstration needs.* Washington, D.C.: Office of Education, HEW, 1968, 91 pp.

Includes articles on the status of physical education for the visually handicapped. Presents concepts in research and demonstration needs in physical education and recreation for the physically handicapped.

862. ――――. *Physical education and recreation of the visually handicapped.* Washington, D.C.: Author, 1972, 67 pp., $2.95.

A concise booklet written primarily for physical educators and teachers in public schools.

863. American Foundation for the Blind. *The Pine Brook report: National work session on the education of the blind with the sighted.* New York: AFB, 1954, 72 pp.

Report of a conference of 20 specialists discussing trends in integrated education: Cooperative Plan, Integrated Plan, Itinerant Teacher Plan. Lists suggested classroom equipment.

864. ――――. *Itinerant teaching service for blind children: Proceedings of a national work session held at Bear Mountain, New York, August 20–24, 1956.* New York: Author, 1957, 106 pp., $1.

Itinerant teaching is considered in terms of its philosophy, the teacher, and its function. Includes discussion of equipment, books and supplies, educational placement and the teamwork approach, legislation and program administration.

865. ――――. *Industrial arts for blind students.* Author, 1960, 80 pp., $2.

Sets forth standards for curriculum, records, and the organization and equipment for the industrial arts shop.

866. ――――. *Sex education for the visually handicapped in schools and agencies. . . . Selected papers.* New York: Author, 1975, 76 pp., $3.

Collection of articles previously printed in *New Outlook for the Blind.*

867. Anderson, William. *Teaching the physically handicapped to swim.* New York: Transatlantic Arts, 1968, 84 pp.

Swimming strokes, suggested exercises, group teaching, and a typical sequence of lessons and exercises are considered, with attention given to blind and other handicapped children. Provides case histories and learner's pool plans.

868. Andrews, Francis M. Maryland School for the Blind integrates. *International Journal for the Education of the Blind*, Mar. 1955, Vol. 4, No. 3, pp. 48–49.

Describes the gradual integration of Negro and white students.

869. Anthony, Gene H. Creativity and the visually handicapped: Implications for the industrial arts. *Education of the Visually Handicapped*, Dec. 1969, Vol. 1, No. 4, pp. 122–23.

Discusses need to provide blind children with opportunities for creative expression. Emphasis on teaching of manipulative skills, development of sequence activities, and introduction of basic tools.

870. Arnheim, D.; Auxter, D.; & Crowe, W. *Principles and methods of adapted physical education*, 2nd ed. St. Louis, Mo.: C. V. Mosby, 1973, 460 pp., illus. (1st ed. 1969, 419 pp.)

Presents programs in adapting physical education. Discusses various elements of conducting programs: Organization and administration, class organization, facilities, exercise programs, an exercise for tension reduction, and adapted games and sports. Considers problems especially related to sensory disorders.

871. Ashcroft, Samuel C. Remedial program reminders. *International Journal for the Education of the Blind*, Dec. 1956, Vol. 6, No. 2, pp. 31–35.

Since remedial programs in reading and other subjects are needed, good organization is important, as is the decision on who should receive the help. Systematize; consider readiness, motivate, and use meaningful materials; remember that retention is influenced by many factors; and know when to stop.

872. ———. Cues from teaching machines for programmatic educational planning. *International Journal for the Education of the Blind*, Dec. 1962, Vol. 12, No. 2, pp. 51–54.

Principles and features of teaching machines and programming have useful applications for instruction of visually handicapped, whether implemented with auto-instructional devices or through everyday teaching practices. Makes some specific suggestions.

873. Ashford, J. Timothy, & Thurman, Alena J. The role music can play in child life. *New Outlook for the Blind*, Mar. 1955, Vol. 49, No. 3, pp. 98–101.

Music can bring joy, both emotional and intellectual, has social values especially in group singing, and helps the child to grow normally. The psychological reactions to music may be regarded as curative. Music teachers play an important role in child development.

874. Atkins, Gerald. Evaluating calculating tools for the blind. *International Journal for the Education of the Blind*, Dec. 1954, Vol. 4, No. 2, pp. 32–33.

Study of present methods for mathematical calculations and their shortcomings. Suggestions of requirements to meet ideal device.

875. Auerbach, Helen. Teaching arithmetic to the partially seeing. *International Journal for the Education of the Blind*, Dec. 1959, Vol. 9, No. 2, pp. 44–46.

Although philosophy and methods are basically the same as for children in general, describes some adaptations. Emphasis is upon understanding of principles. Encourage the child in order to build up a liking for arithmetic.

876. Avery, Constance D. A psychologist looks at the issue of public vs.

residential school placement for the blind. *New Outlook for the Blind,* Sept. 1968, Vol. 62, No. 7, pp. 221–26.

Discusses the advantages and disadvantages of both day and residential schools; in the interests of blind children, competition between the 2 forms of schooling should be replaced by cooperation.

877. **Bakker, Josina.** Communication and computation skills for blind students attending public schools. Lindenhurst, N.Y.: Board of Coop. Educational Services, Visually Impaired Program, 1972, 32 pp. Mimeo.

Services, guidelines for teachers, and curriculum outlines for Readiness for Braille Reading and Writing, Braille Reading, Braille Writing, Signature Writing, Nemeth Code and Scientific Notation, and Teaching Braille to the Adventitiously Blinded Child.

878. **Barraga, Natalie.** Social opportunities available to students in residential schools. *International Journal for the Education of the Blind,* May 1958, Vol. 7, No. 4, pp. 110–15.

Tells why social experience is an important preparation for life and gives the history of expanded social life in residential schools. Reports a study to determine the current nature and extent of social opportunities in residential schools with resulting recommendations.

879. ———. Mode of reading for low-vision students. *International Journal for the Education of the Blind,* May 1963, Vol. 12, No. 4, pp. 103–7.

Following review of the literature, describes a study of reading characteristics of a group of low-vision students who regularly use both ink print and braille. Following 6 45-minute training sessions, some gains in reading skills were found.

880. **Bateman, Barbara, & Wetherell, Janis L.** Some educational characteristics of partially seeing children. *International Journal for the Education of the Blind,* Dec. 1967, Vol. 17, No. 2, pp. 33–40.

With supporting tables, summarizes relationships found in 6 analyses of data obtained from 31 teachers about 297 partially seeing children. Some findings appear to be related to characteristics of the teachers.

881. **Bauman, Mary K., & Strauss, Susan H.** A comparison of blind children from day and residential schools in a camp setting. *International Journal for the Education of the Blind,* Mar. 1962, Vol. 11, No. 3, pp. 74–77.

Through rating procedures, children at a summer camp were evaluated on social competency, self-sufficiency, interpersonal skills, and mobility. Little clear difference was found between children from day and residential schools.

882. **Becker, Carol, & Kalina, Kenneth.** The Cranmer Abacus and its use in residential schools for the blind and in day school programs. *New Outlook for the Blind,* Nov. 1975, Vol. 69, No. 9, pp. 412–15, 417.

A number of studies are cited to show the abacus has positive effect on development of arithmetic skills and that its use in residential schools is now very widespread. Use in public schools gaining popularity.

883. **Bennette, George G.** A study of music curricula for blind students. *New Outlook for the Blind,* Jan. 1966, Vol. 60, No. 1, pp. 20–22.

Forty-five residential schools surveyed as to types of instruments taught, number of students per instrument, etc. Obtaining contemporary braille music and improving music reading ability emerged as problems.

884. Benton, Christine, & Ellis, Agnes. Teaching reading to beginning students. *International Journal for the Education of the Blind*, May 1956, Vol. 5, No. 4, pp. 88–90.

Explains program with emphasis on reading readiness: What it is, items important in development; methods used and why used; factors influencing braille reading; how braille is taught to young children. Lists recommended books.

885. Berger, Allen, & Kantz, Constance R. Sources of information and materials for blind and visually limited pupils. *Elementary English*, Dec. 1970, Vol. 47, No. 8, pp. 1097–1105.

Designed for regular classroom teachers. Lists sources, describes terminology, school problems, and braille system.

886. Bersch, Ruth J. Using experience charts in reading readiness. *International Journal for the Education of the Blind*, Oct. 1960, Vol. 10, No. 1, pp. 30–31.

Describes the development and use of experience charts based on field trips or some other sharing experience. With careful teacher guidance, the charts provide frequent repetition of words soon to be used in reading.

887. Bevans, Judith. Development of a recreational music program at Perkins School for the Blind. *International Journal for the Education of the Blind*, Mar. 1965, Vol. 14, No. 3, pp. 72–76.

The purpose of recreational music should not be merely listening or appreciation; nor should it be to produce musicians. Rather, it is to experience music and use it as a vehicle for self-expression. Programs in lower and upper schools are described.

888. ————. The exceptional child and Orff. *Education of the Visually Handicapped*, Dec. 1969, Vol. 1, No. 4, pp. 116–20. Reprinted from *Music Educators' Journal*, Mar. 1969.

A music program for the multiply handicapped blind developed by Carl Orff is described. Suggestions are made concerning musical instruments, singing, song development, and movement and dance.

889. Bidgood, Frederick E. A study of sex education programs for visually handicapped persons. *New Outlook for the Blind*, Dec. 1971, Vol. 65, No. 10, pp. 318–23.

Reports on a survey of existing educational programs in sex education available to visually handicapped persons. Results indicated that the majority of public and residential schools felt a responsibility to provide sex education for them.

890. Birch, Jack W., et al. *School achievement and effect of type size on reading in visually handicapped children.* Washington, D.C.: Office of Education, HEW, 1966, 166 pp.

Best type size was determined for each child and a standardized achievement test in appropriate type size administered. Results and conclusions presented. States implications for special education practices, vocational rehabilitation, teacher education, and research.

891. Birecree, Daniel C. Research on science and mathematics models used in teaching the blind. *International Journal for the Education of the Blind,* June 1954, Vol. 3, No. 4, pp. 265–68.

Questionnaires to schools, commercial companies, and organizations result in list with discussion of advantages and disadvantages of commercial and homemade models. Author concludes few schools have models necessary for proper teaching of science and mathematics.

892. Bischoff, Robert W. Industrial education for the visually handicapped. *Utah Eagle,* Jan. 1975, Vol. 86, No. 4, pp. 1–3.

Presents the reasons for industrial education, especially for visually handicapped youth; describes related courses at Utah School for the Blind; and lists with references certain other industrial education content.

893. Bleiberg, Robyn. Is there a need for a specially designed reading series for beginning blind readers? *New Outlook for the Blind,* May 1970, Vol. 64, No. 5, pp. 135–38.

Questionnaire sent to 101 teachers of the blind to examine need for new material to teach reading. Results showed more than ¾ of the teachers surveyed would use a new beginning reading series. Rates popularity of presently used series, notes problems in learning braille, and recommends characteristics for a new series.

894. Bourgeault, Stanley E. A discussion of the integrated or resource plan for education of the visually handicapped. *New Outlook for the Blind,* May 1960, Vol. 54, No. 5, pp. 153–58.

Responsibilities in establishing programs for visually handicapped with sighted children shown in step-by-step description of a resource program. Includes elaboration on the relationship of resource with regular teacher, and between resource and regular classroom.

895. ———. *Methods of teaching the blind: The language arts.* New York: American Foundation for Overseas Blind, 1969, 48 pp.

Following general statements about how children learn, presents very specific methods for teaching reading and writing of braille, handwriting, and effective use of reader service.

896. Bowden, M. G., & Otto, Henry J., Eds. *The education of the exceptional child in Casis School.* Austin: Univ. of Tex. Press, 1964, 158 pp.

Describes an educational program which provides for handicapped and normal children in the same school setting. Describes special services for the partially sighted.

897. Brothers, Roy J. Arithmetic computation by the blind. *Education of the Visually Handicapped,* Mar. 1972, Vol. 4, No. 1, pp. 1–8.

Evaluation of abacus on the basis of academic achievement, test scores, and SAT results.

898. ———. Classroom use of the Braille Code Recognition materials. *Education of the Visually Handicapped,* Mar. 1974, Vol. 6, No. 1, pp. 6–13.

Describes Braille Code Recognition materials and the effectiveness of the materials on the braille reading skills of students.

899. Bruce, Robert E. Using the overhead projector with visually impaired students. *Education of the Visually Handicapped,* May 1973, Vol. 5, No. 2, pp. 43–46.

Discusses advantages of using the overhead projector to teach mathematics.

900. ———. Let's go metric (A manual for teachers). *Education of the Visually Handicapped*, Dec. 1975, Vol. 7, No. 4, pp. 119–23.

Explains basic Metric System and its symbols. Gives rules for use of Metric Ladders to change units of one denomination to those of another denomination in their respective measures. Provides examples.

901. Bryan, Charles A. Secondary school sciences for the blind. *International Journal for the Education of the Blind*, Oct. 1956, Vol. 6, No. 1, pp. 11–18.

Suggestions on how to teach blind children biology, nature study, chemistry, and physics. Emphasizes learning from direct experience.

902. Bryan, Dorothy, Ed. Educating partially seeing children in the public schools. *Exceptional Children*, 1953, Vol. 19, pp. 269–72, 288.

Summary statements, of 1952 Omaha ICEC workshop on this problem, are made on (1) changes in the enrollment with possible causes, (2) varying class patterns, including possibility of combining 2 or more types of exceptionality in a single class, (3) teacher education, (4) supervisory problems.

903. Buell, Charles. Where should blind youth be educated? A survey. *Exceptional Children*, 1953, Vol. 19, pp. 304–8, 327.

Questionnaire returns from all but 2 of the residential schools for the blind in the U.S. show that ½ of the schools retain their pupils through high school, ⅓ send some pupils to public high school and 1/6 send out all pupils beyond a certain grade.

904. ———. Wrestling in the life of a blind boy. *International Journal for the Education of the Blind*, Mar. 1958, Vol. 7, No. 3, pp. 93–96.

As a sport in which the blind boy can compete on equal terms, wrestling can have broad influence upon that boy's development. Gives 2 case histories as illustrations.

905. ———. Developments in physical education for blind children. *New Outlook for the Blind*, Sept. 1964, Vol. 58, No. 7, pp. 202–6.

Comprehensive survey of programs and equipment and information about physical education for blind children. Focuses on recent gains in this field.

906. ———. Physical education for blind children in public schools. *New Outlook for the Blind*, Oct. 1967, Vol. 61, No. 8, pp. 248–54, illus.

Attitudes of school staff often exclude blind children from physical education in day school programs. Author urges active involvement and describes procedures to accomplish it. Ref.

907. ———. How to include blind and partially seeing children in public secondary school vigorous physical education. *Physical Educator*, Mar. 1972, Vol. 29, No. 1, pp. 6–8.

Discusses common attitudes toward blindness. Recommends adequate class placement of student in unmodified activities and suggests methods of instruction for use with blind children.

908. ———. *Physical education and recreation for the visually handicapped.*

Washington, D.C. American Assoc. for Health, Physical Education, and Recreation, 1973, 67 pp., $2.95.

Has 3 sections: What physical educators and recreation specialists should know about blindness, activities for visually handicapped children, and a 10-page annotated bib.

909. ————. Bibliography on physical education. Philadelphia: Assoc. for Education of the Visually Handicapped, rev. 1974, 6 pp., free. Mimeo.

Contains an annotated listing of books, articles, periodicals and newsletters, and films and slides for use in programming for visually impaired persons. Subjects treated in addition to activities include: Integration, curriculum design, and research. Books and publications available in braille and large type from the American Printing House for the Blind are listed.

910. ————. *Physical education for blind children.* Springfield, Ill.: Charles C Thomas, 1966, 224 pp. (Rev. ed., 1974, $9, paper $7.95)

Covers sports, games, relays, races, contests, achievement scales, and curricula. Mentions past and present programs in public and residential schools, recreation and leisure time activities (guide for parents).

911. Burgart, Herbert J. Art helps teach sight by touch. *School Arts*, May 1959.

Uses clay modeling as an illustration of the values of an art program. Provides advice for the ceramics teacher.

912. Burleson, Derek L. Starting a sex education program: Guidelines for the administrator. *New Outlook for the Blind*, May 1974, Vol. 68, No. 5, pp. 216–18. Also in *Sex education for the visually handicapped in schools and agencies. . . . Selected papers.* New York: AFB, 1975, $3, pp. 17–19.

An advisory committee, adequate publicity and public relations, provisions of specialized training and appropriate materials, and selection of staff are important considerations for the administrator.

913. Byrne, Susan. A design for a mobile, audio-tactile exhibition for blind and sighted school-age children. *New Outlook for the Blind*, June 1974, Vol. 68, No. 6, pp. 252–59, illus.

Design of an exhibit to be used as a playing-learning environment for children 6–11 years of age in which they are encouraged to explore independently and to communicate their feelings and impressions to their fellow students. Includes color, size, texture, and various spatial concepts.

914. Campbell, Dorothy. Blind children in the "normal" classroom. *New Outlook for the Blind*, Nov. 1955, Vol. 49, No. 9, pp. 321–24. Reprinted from *Understanding the Child*, June 1955.

Describes the integration of blind children into 2 Calif. school systems at nursery school and resource room levels. Gives examples of integrated activities, community participation, and the full acceptance of the child.

915. Carmack, Ted R. Teleteaching for the blind. *New Outlook for the Blind*, Oct. 1968, Vol. 62, No. 8, pp. 261–62.

Patterned on Teleteaching, a system of home instruction for physically handicapped students, Braille Institute, Calif., is teaching 9 blind adults braille, typing, home management, and daily living skills. The therapeutic value of reducing loneliness is also an asset.

916. Carter, V. R. Where shall blind children be educated? *International Journal for the Education of the Blind*, Dec. 1954, Vol. 4, No. 2, pp. 21–23.

Presents author's opinion on education in residential or public schools and review of facts and ideas from critics outside and inside the field. Question of residential and/or public day school undecided by many professional people.

917. Carver, Thomas R. The design and use of a light probe for teaching science to blind students. *American Foundation for the Blind Research Bulletin 16*, May 1968, pp. 79–91, illus.

Describes the evolution, design, and use of an optical light probe for use in laboratory science classes.

918. Chapman, Ann, & Cramer, Miriam. *Dance and the blind child.* New York: American Dance Guild, 1973, 17 pp., 75¢.

Written from the viewpoint of teaching 1 blind child in a class with sighted children. Contains a detailed lesson plan.

919. Cicenia, Erbert F., et al. *The challenge of educating the blind child in the regular classroom.* Albany, N.Y.: Bureau for Handicapped Children, State Dept. of Education, 1957?, 16 pp.

Pictorial story of blind children attending school with sighted children. Describes cooperative effort of school and home. Suggestions made for elementary school program with photographs illustrating activities.

920. Coffey, John L. Programmed instruction for the blind. *International Journal for the Education of the Blind*, Dec. 1963, Vol. 13, No. 2, pp. 38–44.

One unit of English and 3 of algebra were programmed and brailled, then used with 16 junior high and 16 senior high blind students, to determine relative effectiveness of 2 methods of presentation and 2 methods of response. Programmed instruction for the blind is entirely feasible.

921. Colton, F. V., & Caton, H. R. Self-styled approach to instructional design. *Audiovisual Instruction*, 1974, Vol. 19, pp. 24–30.

922. Conn. Institute for the Blind. *Business work-experience curriculum guide.* Hartford: Author, n.d., 51 pp.

Designed to facilitate the development of skills, knowledge, and attitudes necessary for successful adjustment to and participation in the business world.

923. Cool, Mr. & Mrs. John B. We selected the residential school. *International Journal for the Education of the Blind*, Mar. 1955, Vol. 4, No. 3, pp. 45–47.

Gives some pros and cons for both residential and integrated schools, and authors' specific reasons for choice of residential school for their son.

924. Coombs, Virginia H. Guidelines for teaching arts and crafts to blind children in elementary grades. *International Journal for the Education of the Blind*, Mar. 1967, Vol. 16, No. 3, pp. 79–83.

Teaching arts and crafts is discussed in terms of 5 goals with great emphasis upon realistic experience with the environment. A handskills checklist is provided.

925. Cravats, Monroe. Biology for the blind. *Science Teacher*, Apr. 1972, Vol. 39, No. 4, pp. 49–50.

Presents complete directions for a biology laboratory exercise on digestion for visually handicapped students.

926. Curtis, Charles K. Teaching geography to blind students: A plea for investigation. *New Outlook for the Blind*, June 1971, Vol. 65, No. 6, pp. 187–89, 194.

Lists many questions related to teaching geography to blind children and the paucity of answers. Recommends needed research. Ref.

927. Curtis, Charles K., & McWhannel, J. Douglas. On the use of the inquiry approach in social studies with blind children. *New Outlook for the Blind*, Sept. 1972, Vol. 66, No. 7, pp. 223–26.

Description of a project adopted by a 10th grade class at Jericho Hill School for the Blind in Canada which demonstrates that blind students can use the inquiry approach to social studies with relatively simple modifications.

928. Dajani, S. T. Teaching arithmetic to blind children. *International Journal for the Education of the Blind*, Dec. 1953, Vol. 3, No. 2, pp. 223–24.

Braille writing and former methods of teaching arithmetic are slow. Author explains new method he has developed which is faster and more accurate. He recommends it especially in the higher grades.

929. D'Alonzo, Bruno J. Puppets fill the classroom with imagination. *TEACHING Exceptional Children*, Spring, 1974, Vol. 6, No. 3, pp. 140–44.

Exceptional children, including visually impaired, can make and use puppets in class to improve language development or raise self-concept.

930. Daniel, Joseph C., Jr. Ornithology as a learning tool. *New Outlook for the Blind*, Mar. 1954, Vol. 48, No. 3, pp. 67–70.

Describes how study of birds can stimulate development of touch, smell, and hearing for the blind child. Suggests that nature study is a good tool for sensory development.

931. Daniels, Arthur S., & Davies, Evelyn A. *Adapted physical education: Principles and practice of physical education for exceptional students.* New York: Harper & Row, 1965. (3rd ed., 1975, xiii + 443 pp., illus., $12.95)

A discussion of activities for blind children is included.

932. Davidow, Mae E. *The abacus made easy.* Louisville, Ky.: American Printing House for the Blind, 1966, 88 pp.

Presents a simplified manual for teaching the Cranmer Abacus to visually handicapped students. In large print.

933. ———. *A guide for social competency: Course of study for the visually handicapped.* Louisville, Ky.: American Printing House, 1974, iii + 81 pp., free.

Covers 4 age groups from kindergarten through high school and is divided into areas of personal appearance, interpersonal relations, dining skills and table etiquette, as well as household skills and record-keeping.

934. Dawson, Yvette N. Physical education for the blind. *Rehabilitation Teacher,* Apr. 1971, Vol. 3, No. 4, pp. 15–32.

Basic teaching plans, need for individual attention and guidelines for selecting games and activities.

935. Decker, R. Joan. Creative art experience for blind children. *International Journal for the Education of the Blind,* May 1960, Vol. 9, No. 4, pp. 104–6.

Discusses the need for and value of the creative art experience for blind children. Materials must be carefully chosen with modeling, sculpture, construction, pottery, and crafts the principle subject matter.

936. DeMott, Richard M., & Fistler, Ronald. Reporting continuous progress. *Education of the Visually Handicapped,* Oct. 1973, Vol. 5, No. 3, pp. 86–92.

Describes the approach used in the Iowa Braille and Sight Saving School which is based upon observable behaviors which comprise the curriculum, objectives, tests, and graduation requirements. Considers aspects such as student awareness of expectations and teacher orientation toward goals. Includes examples of behavioral tasks and a record chart.

937. Dewey, Helen. Welcome to the gripe corner. *Education of the Visually Handicapped,* Dec. 1973, Vol. 5, No. 4, pp. 114–16.

During a successful 5-week program, 6 legally blind students were given a system of airing complaints and encouraged to use it. Students stood in "gripe corner" signalling desire to privately discuss problem with teacher or aide. Teachers and aides also used "corner."

938. Dickman, Irving R., Ed. *Sex education and family life for visually handicapped children and youth: A resource guide.* New York: AFB, 1975, x + 86 pp., $4.

Developed out of a 3-year joint project of AFB and SIECUS. Part 1 deals with historical and psychological aspects of sex education and blind persons; Part 2 contains concepts and learning activities; Part 3 lists resources for both student and teacher.

939. Dodd, Carol A. Multiply successes when introducing basic multiplication ideas to visually handicapped children. *Education of the Visually Handicapped,* May 1975, Vol. 7, No. 2, pp. 53–56.

Describes (with illustration) the teaching of basic multiplication ideas to visually handicapped children. Discusses thinking strategies as well as mastery of facts.

940. Dorward, Barbara, & Barraga, Natalie. *Teaching aids for blind and visually limited children.* New York: AFB, 1968, 132 pp., $2.75.

Intended for parents and teachers, guide details construction and use of 32 teaching aids.

941. Douglass, Sue, & Mangold, Sally. Precision teaching of visually impaired students. *Education of the Visually Handicapped,* May 1975, Vol. 7, No. 2, pp. 48–52.

Describes precision teaching not as a new method, but as a supplement to a teacher's existing program. Talks specifically about use of method with 2 blind children.

942. Drake, Helena M., & Travis, Florence. Phonetic fun with letters. *International Journal for the Education of the Blind*, May 1963, Vol. 12, No. 4, pp. 112–14.

Along with tongue-twister rhymes for each letter of the alphabet, teachers made books illustrated with real objects such as buttons, fur, spoons, etc. Full instructions for making these materials are provided.

943. Dunford, Benjamin C. What price good music? *International Journal for the Education of the Blind*, Oct. 1954, Vol. 4, No. 1, pp. 8–10.

Students should be aware of many types of music, should be exposed to these and allowed to form their own opinion. Discussion of various types of music from early times to present.

944. Dunham, Jerome, & Shelton, Howard. Machine presented audible programmed instruction for the blind. *Education of the Visually Handicapped*, Dec. 1973, Vol. 5, No. 4, pp. 117–19.

Pilot program testing feasibility of modifying programmed texts for audio presentation in academic skills training program. Explains equipment used, its use. Lists advantages and results of programmed instructions. Forty-two Ss, visually handicapped.

945. Dunkin, Donald J. Educational TV. *International Journal for the Education of the Blind*, Dec. 1962, Vol. 12, No. 2, pp. 55–57.

How to use educational television in the classroom, its values and advantages, and answers to some questions about it.

946. Eames, Thomas H. Visual handicaps to reading. *Journal of Education*, Feb. 1959, Vol. 141, No. 3, 35 pp.

List of publishers of textbooks for partially seeing children is given with a discussion of the blind or partially seeing child in school. Data of a comparative study of eye conditions collected from 3,500 records are presented in summary with a selected bib. of previous reports made by Eames.

947. Edwards, Donald H. An adventure in learning. *International Journal for the Education of the Blind*, Mar. 1965, Vol. 14, No. 3, pp. 76–79.

A full week of outdoor education, in the form of camping, is built into the total curriculum. The many advantages are listed and suggestions are made for developing such a program.

948. English, William. Wrestling in schools for the blind. *International Journal for the Education of the Blind*, Mar. 1957, Vol. 6, No. 3, pp. 68–70.

Why wrestling is a good sport for blind youth, the development of competition through regional associations, and the opportunities for contact with sighted peers.

949. ———. Cross country running. *International Journal for the Education of the Blind*, May 1957, Vol. 6, No. 4, pp. 86–87.

Describes how the Ohio State School for the Blind handles cross country running for blind youth with partially sighted partners.

950. Enis, Carol A., & Cataruzolo, Michael. Sex education in the residential school for the blind. *Education of the Visually Handicapped*, May 1972, Vol. 4, No. 2, pp. 61–64.

Reviews means by which the sighted child learns about sex to emphasize that the blind child is severely handicapped in this. Questionnaire sent to residential schools revealed that 64% have a program in sex education, but great variance was found in these programs.

951. Etier, A. Faborn. *A study to determine the effectiveness of electronically paced typewriting instruction for blind students: Final report. Project No. 2F031.* Washington, D.C.: Dept. of Health, Education & Welfare, 1973, 92 pp., app.

Results of a study undertaken to develop electronically paced instructional materials, to test the effectiveness of these materials, and to develop a training manual for teachers.

952. Evans, Rosemary, & Simpkins, Katherine. Computer assisted instruction for the blind. *Education of the Visually Handicapped,* Oct. 1972, Vol. 4, No. 3, pp. 83–85.

Discusses computer assisted arithmetic instruction for visually handicapped children in intermediate grades. Describes physical apparatus of computer terminals, methods of initiating and maintaining the child in the project.

953. Evans, Walter E. How can we improve classroom instruction? *International Journal for the Education of the Blind,* May 1960, Vol. 9, No. 4, pp. 101–3.

Describes how a workshop was used to improve classroom instruction and gives the results of an evaluation questionnaire.

954. Fait, Hollis F. *Special physical education: Adapted, corrective, development,* 3rd ed. Philadelphia: W. B. Saunders, 1972, xi + 442 pp.

Includes some material for visually handicapped children.

955. Flowers, Woodie. A sound-source ball for blind children. *American Foundation for the Blind Research Bulletin 16,* May 1968, pp. 17–39, illus.

Detailed specifications and designs for ball with evaluation, diagrams and pictures. Recommendations. Ref.

956. Forbes, John. Braille translation: The computer aids the blind. *Mitre Matrix,* Apr. 1972, Vol. 5, No. 2, pp. 22–30.

Describes a program of daily translation of classwork which allows integration into regular classes.

957. Forman, Edward. The inclusion of visually limited and blind children in a sighted physical education program. *Education of the Visually Handicapped,* Dec. 1969, Vol. 1, No. 4, pp. 113–15.

Skills necessary for the integration of visually handicapped children in sighted physical education classes with discussion of recreational activities, games, and adaptations used.

958. Foster, Mary Lou. Aid for teaching telephone dialing to blind students. *International Journal for the Education of the Blind,* Dec. 1954, Vol. 4, No. 2, p. 30.

Description of teaching dialing at the Western Pennsylvania School for Blind Children through the help of the Bell Telephone Co. Details on how it works.

959. Foulke, Emerson, & Uhde, Thomas. Do blind children need sex education? *New Outlook for the Blind,* May 1974, Vol. 68, No. 5, pp. 193–200, 209. *Also in Sex education for the visually handicapped in schools and agencies. . . . Selected papers.* New York: AFB, 1975, $3, pp. 8–16.

Preliminary report on blind adolescents' knowledge and attitudes about human sexuality, based on interviews with 18 males and 3 females. Also describes Human Sexuality Opinion Survey.

960. Franks, Frank L. Integrating gifted, visually handicapped students into senior high school classes for the gifted. *New Outlook for the Blind*, Nov. 1962, Vol. 56, No. 9, pp. 316–18.

Presents checklist to be used as guide in considering reasons for and against placement of visually handicapped students in classes for the gifted. Suggests objective information should always be supplemented with teacher judgment.

961. ———. Measurement in science for blind students. *TEACHING Exceptional Children*, Fall 1970, Vol. 3, No. 1, pp. 2–11, illus.

Brief review of research re measurement instruments. Description of 4 measurement devices adapted and/or developed by American Printing House for the Blind and discussion of concepts which can be taught using those instruments.

962. ———. Educational materials development in primary science: An introductory science laboratory for young blind students. *Education of the Visually Handicapped*, Dec. 1975, Vol. 7, No. 4, pp. 97–101.

Reports research and development of science instructional aids for young blind students, including 3 steps: (1) identification of deficit curriculum areas and concepts taught, (2) prototype development, and (3) evaluation.

963. Franks, Frank L., & Baird, Richard M. Geographical concepts and the visually handicapped. *Exceptional Children*, Dec. 1971, Vol. 38, No. 4, pp. 321–24.

Study investigated geographical concept attainment in visually handicapped students with goal of improving their map-reading skills. Testing results were an overall 83.5% correct identification of landforms and suggested that use of the 3-dimensional materials was successful.

964. Franks, Frank L., & Nolan, Carson Y. Development of geographical concepts in blind children. *Education of the Visually Handicapped*, Mar. 1970, Vol. 2, No. 1, pp. 1–8.

Seventy-five Ss tested on geographical concepts. Results showed increased repetition of terms contributed to higher overall gains. Presence of patterns of increased learning through repetition is supported.

965. ———. Measuring geographical concept attainment in visually handicapped students. *Education of the Visually Handicapped*, Mar. 1971, Vol. 3, No. 1, pp. 11–17.

To develop a measurement instrument 24 braille and 24 large-print readers were studied. On the 40–item test which was developed no significant differences were found between braille and large-print readers. The reliability of the 40-item test as an instrument to evaluate geographical concept attainment was felt to be verified.

966. Freel, Mirle E., Jr. Art for visually impaired children. *Education of the Visually Handicapped*, May 1969, Vol. 1, No. 2, pp. 44–46.

Considerations in teaching art to the blind and examples of results.

967. Freund, Colleen. Teaching art to the blind child integrated with sighted children. *New Outlook for the Blind*, Sept. 1969, Vol. 63, No. 7, pp. 205–10.

With illustrations, describes specific art projects for blind children to improve the child's confidence and feeling of integration as well as art skills.

968. Freund, Elisabeth D. New material for math instruction. *International Journal for the Education of the Blind*, Mar. 1963, Vol. 12, No. 3, pp. 94–95.

With the aid of an illustration, shows how a combination of plastic tapes and plexiglas can be used to make materials for math instruction.

969. ———. Touch and learn. *New Outlook for the Blind*, Sept. 1967, Vol. 61, No. 7, pp. 223–26.

Description and evaluation of the touch and learn center at the Overbrook School for the Blind.

970. ———. Screen pads for longhand writing. *New Outlook for the Blind*, May 1968, Vol. 62, No. 5, pp. 144–47.

Exactly how to construct and use a pad of window screening stapled to paper board in teaching script writing. With this pad, most blind persons can write at least signatures.

971. Fulker, Wilber H., & Fulker, Mary. *Techniques with tangibles: A manual for teaching the blind.* Springfield, Ill.: Charles C Thomas, 1968, 72 pp.

Description and discussion of tangible teaching apparatus, such as thermoform, models, cutaways, etc.

972. Gaver, Wayne. *Woodworking guide for visually handicapped students.* Santa Cruz, Calif.: County Office of Education, 1972, 113 pp.

Compiled to help the visually handicapped learn to work safely in the woodshop. Divided into sections on each of the principal machines found in school woodshops.

973. Geffen, Lawrence F., & Palmore, Sandra J. *Selected bibliography on mathematics for the blind.* Ypsilanti: E. Mich. Univ., Aug. 1969, 15 pp.

One hundred thirty-seven references on math presented, some in foreign languages, some with annotations. Includes historical and research material as well as methodological articles for the teacher.

974. Genensky, Samuel M. *Closed circuit TV and the education of the partially sighted.* Santa Monica, Calif.: Rand Corp., 1970, 18 pp.

Study of 50 legally blind *S*s with a wide variety of eye disorders indicated that for the legally blind CCTV is significantly more useful than purely optical aids.

975. Genensky, Samuel M.; Petersen, H. E.; Yoshimura, R. I.; et al. *Interactive classroom TV system for the handicapped.* Santa Monica, Calif.: Rand Corp., 1974, 54 pp., illus.

Description of an interactive multicamera-multimonitor CCTV system which permits the teacher to be in continuous visual communication with her partially sighted students.

976. George, Colleen, et al. Development of an aerobics conditioning program for the visually handicapped. *Journal of Physical Education and Recreation*, May 1975, Vol. 46, No. 5, pp. 39–40.

Objective was to enhance students' cardiovascular function and improve strength and endurance of the skeletal musculature. Students did achieve improved fitness.

977. Gibbons, Helen. Safety for visually impaired children. *New Outlook for the Blind*, Apr. 1962, Vol. 56, No. 4, pp. 127–30. Also in *Safety Education*, Nov. 1961.

Discusses role of the school in safety, and parts played by the administration, the school nurse, the classroom teacher, and the special teacher. Offers some guidelines for home safety.

978. Gibbons, Helen, & Hatfield, Elizabeth M. An eye report for children with visual problems for the guidance of educators. *International Journal for the Education of the Blind*, May 1964, Vol. 13, No. 4, pp. 109–16.

Reproduces and explains use and value of a standard eye report form which will provide the information needed for planning educational programs.

979. Gilmore, Florence. One public school's experiment with blind children. *New Outlook for the Blind*, Feb. 1956, Vol. 50, No. 2, pp. 42–46.

Describes the gradual growth of acceptance of blind children and their integration into a Calif. school.

980. Gissoni, Fred L. Carrying classroom notes in a bucket. *International Journal for the Education of the Blind*, Oct. 1961, Vol. 11, No. 1, pp. 20–22.

Detailed suggestions for how a student can take notes by tape recorder, later organize those notes, and easily find the items he wants.

981. ⸺⸺. Vocational significance of the abacus for the blind. *New Outlook for the Blind*, Nov. 1963, Vol. 57, No. 9, pp. 358–60.

Discusses the Cranmer Abacus. Recommends a 1-volume press braille instruction book entitled *Using the Cranmer Abacus for the blind*, and an inkprint introduction, "The Japanese abacus, its use and theory."

982. ⸺⸺. *Using the Cranmer Abacus for the blind.* Louisville, Ky.: American Printing House for the Blind, 1964, 38 pp.

Instruction manual for Cranmer Abacus.

983. ⸺⸺. The abacus explosion. *New Outlook for the Blind*, Feb. 1965, Vol. 59, No. 2, pp. 75–76.

Beginning with the first production model of the Cranmer Abacus in Sept. 1963, traces the signs of rapidly growing interest in this tool. To develop more professional literature on this tool, the Abacus Assoc. of America has been formed.

984. Governor Morehead School. *Instruction in music for visually handicapped children. Volume 1.* Raleigh, N.C.: Author, 1967, 56 pp.

Volume contains the general plan of instruction in music at the school. Covers music in the elementary grades, materials needed, choruses, individual voice instruction, piano and organ instruction.

985. Grover, Wayne. *Woodworking guide for visually handicapped students,* *a five county vocational skills training program for the blind.* Santa Cruz, Calif.: County Board of Education, 1972, 122 pp.

Industrial arts curriculum describes travel techniques and orientation in the shop, measuring devices, hand tools, and machines.

986. Grupp, James W. 2,500 miles of experiences: Summer school at IBSSS. *Education of the Visually Handicapped,* May 1970, Vol. 2, No. 2, pp. 55–57.

Description of a 6-week "total living experience" summer school program. Areas stressed were social development, cultural enrichment, and basic experiences.

987. Hadley story. *Dialogue,* Winter 1974, Vol. 13, No. 4, pp. 61–66.

The story of the Hadley School for the Blind in Winnetka, Ill.—the only correspondence school specifically designed for the general educational needs of blind and deaf-blind persons.

988. Haliczer, S. L. Physical education tests for boys. *International Journal for the Education of the Blind,* May 1959, Vol. 8, No. 4, pp. 129–33.

Detailed description of the "Decathlon" and the "Track and Field" Achievement Test" for blind boys, with record sheets, scoring system, and standards. Comparison with results for sighted students is encouraging.

989. Hall, Margaret M. The blind child in kindergarten. *New Outlook for the Blind,* Jan. 1961, Vol. 55, No. 1, pp. 11–16.

A teacher's experiences with a particular blind student in a regular kindergarten class. Teacher gives her own "ten commandments" for working with a handicapped child.

990. Harper, Florine W. Recognition of functional hearing loss by a speech therapist in a residential school for the blind. *Education of the Visually Handicapped,* Oct. 1971, Vol. 3, No. 3, pp. 87–90.

Discusses the difficulty of a speech therapist in a residential school for the blind in identifying nonorganic or functional hearing loss.

991. Hastings, James R. Industrial arts for the blind student. *International Journal for the Education of the Blind,* Dec. 1964, Vol. 14, No. 2, pp. 52–55.

Gives the purpose of industrial arts which is (1) manipulative, and (2) related information. All levels of the school program should contribute. Industrial arts is not a substitute for vocational education which is more specialized job preparation.

992. Hathaway, Donald W. World classroom. *International Journal for the Education of the Blind,* Mar. 1963, Vol. 12, No. 3, pp. 65–69.

History and current services of the Hadley School for the Blind with emphasis on its overseas services.

993. Hatlen, Philip H. Physical education for the visually handicapped. *International Journal for the Education of the Blind,* Oct. 1967, Vol. 17, No. 1, pp. 17–21.

Offers a definition of physical education and relates it to programs as observed in day and residential schools, urging more realistic handling in the day school setting.

994. Hattendorf, Janice K. An abacus update. *New Outlook for the Blind,* Apr. 1971, Vol. 65, No. 4, pp. 112–16.

Briefly reviews history of abacus use, reasons for its popularity, how Cranmer adapted the abacus for the blind, and some school programs teaching the abacus.

995. Haupt, Charlotte. Improving blind children's perceptions. *New Outlook for the Blind,* June 1964, Vol. 58, No. 6, pp. 172–73.

Problems a blind child encounters in dealing with concrete concepts, and how clay and other arts and crafts can be helpful.

996. ———. Creative expression through art. *Education of the Visually Handicapped,* May 1969, Vol. 1, No. 2, pp. 41–43.

Teacher of art to blind must pay attention to individuals, empathize with them, and be flexible.

997. Havill, Stephen J. The sociometric status of visually handicapped students in public school classes. *American Foundation for the Blind Research Bulletin 20,* Mar. 1970, pp. 57–90, app.

Evaluates the sociometric status of 63 visually handicapped children in day school programs, matched with normally seeing children. Also, the effects of such factors as grade level, sex, degree of visual loss, socioeconomic level, and school achievement.

998. Hayes, James W. Teaching popular music in schools for the blind. *International Journal for the Education of the Blind,* June 1952, Vol. 1, No. 4, pp. 105–7.

This phase many schools have ignored. Should be taught in organized course of study covering various types. Discusses talent, age to begin, amount of time. Blind can enter this competitive field and succeed.

999. Henderson, David R. *Laboratory methods in physics for the blind.* [n.p.], 1965, 74 pp.

Auditory and tactile adaptation of physics laboratory apparatus is described, together with 5 methods of drawing raised-line and indented diagrams for use in experiments. A survey of physics laboratory methods in schools for blind in the U.S. and 7 foreign countries, and 2 simple experiments for blind high school students are included.

1000. Henderson, Lois T. The best for David. *International Journal for the Education of the Blind,* May 1955, Vol. 4, No. 4, pp. 65–68.

Story written by mother about education of blind son in residential school with the tremendous advantages she feels it has given him in almost all areas. Examples given.

1001. Hildreth, Gladys J. Methods used in teaching clothing construction and selection. *International Journal for the Education of the Blind,* Oct. 1959, Vol. 9, No. 1, pp. 18–20.

Analyzes the results of questionnaires to which 9 schools responded. Lists clothing curriculum and methods used and makes 6 recommendations to improve teaching in this area.

1002. Holan, Frank V. Adapting visual aids for the blind. *New Outlook for the Blind,* Mar. 1968, Vol. 62, No. 3, pp. 96–100.

How a college instructor put into tactual form for his blind student the visual aids and tests he used in class.

1003. Holmes, Ruth V. The planning and implementation of a sex educational program for visually handicapped children in a residential setting. *New Outlook for the Blind*, May 1974, Vol. 68, No. 5, pp. 219–25. Also in *Sex education for the visually handicapped in schools and agencies. . . . Selected papers.* New York: AFB, 1975, $3, pp. 43–49.

Three levels of instruction (elementary, intermediate, and senior) gave consideration to staffing, budget, curriculum, materials, models, and communication between home and staff.

1004. Hooper, Marjorie S. The Nemeth Code—how and why. *International Journal for the Education of the Blind*, Dec. 1957, Vol. 7, No. 2, pp. 56–60.

History of the development of the Nemeth Code, why it was needed, and its application.

1005. Hordines, John. Games in physical education of the blind. *International Journal for the Education of the Blind*, Apr. 1953, Vol. 2, No. 3, pp. 160–62.

Description of various games with their playing rules, adaptations for the blind: MacCall baseball, giant volley ball, base football.

1006. ———. Trampolining for children at New York Institute for the Education of the Blind. *International Journal for the Education of the Blind*, Sept. 1953, Vol. 3, No. 1, pp. 200–203.

Describes fascination with activity, proper safety measures, teaching methods: First lesson, elementary progressive routine, intermediate progressive routine, advanced progressive routine.

1007. ———. Physical education of blind children. *International Journal for the Education of the Blind*, Mar. 1954, Vol. 3, No. 3, pp. 242–46.

Lists 12 basic needs of blind children, 5 broad goals of physical education, 20 precautions to observe in teaching this subject, class time allotment for various activities. Also provides, in list form, a cross section of a phys. ed. and recreation program, naming at least 60 possible activities, and a breakdown of activities by season.

1008. Householder, Daniel L. Industrial education for blind students. *International Journal for the Education of the Blind*, Mar. 1963, Vol. 12, No. 3, pp. 84–87.

Following a statement of the importance and place of industrial education for blind students, describes goals, operating techniques, aids and devices, teaching methods, and instructional materials.

1009. Huckins, Ross L. More science through "firsthand" experimenting. *New Outlook for the Blind*, June 1958, Vol. 52, No. 6, pp. 222–24.

Discusses science equipment and space to use it, utilizing opportunities already available, meaningful experimentation, and experiments not dangerous for the blind.

1010. Huff, Roger. Development of an enlarged abacus. *Education of the Visually Handicapped*, Oct. 1972, Vol. 4, No. 3, pp. 88–90.

Evaluates an abacus one-third larger than the Cranmer Abacus for use in mathematics by visually handicapped students.

1011. Huff, Roger, & Franks, Frank L. Educational materials development in primary mathematics: Fractional parts of wholes. *Education of the Visually Handicapped*, May 1973, Vol. 5, No. 2, pp. 46–54.

Revealed that primary level visually handicapped students had no difficulty manipulating the component parts of an instructional aid to introduce fractional parts of wholes.

1012. Hulsey, Steve. Liberating the blind student: A Del. program seems to demonstrate that with proper backup, the blind can advantageously join sighted pupils in the classroom. *American Education*, July 1973, Vol. 9, No. 6, pp. 18–22, illus.

The program offers 3 alternatives: Attendance at a residential school; enrollment in the Resource Teaching program; attendance at regular school under the itinerant teacher program. The emphasis of the article is on the last.

1013. Hurley, John M. Industrial arts for blind students. *International Journal for the Education of the Blind*, Oct. 1961, Vol. 11, No. 1, pp. 24–25.

What industrial arts is and a list of its many values for the blind student with special hints for the teacher.

1014. Hussey, S. R., & Legge, Lowell. The "Halifax Method" of arithmetical calculations. *International Journal for the Education of the Blind*, Dec. 1956, Vol. 6, No. 2, pp. 36–40.

Describes exactly how to do and/or teach the 4 fundamental operations as methods of mental calculation.

1015. Iverson, Lee A. Adequate industrial education in schools for the blind. *New Outlook for the Blind*, Dec. 1954, Vol. 48, No. 10, pp. 370–75.

Blind children need exposure to materials and objects. Part of this can be gained through industrial education. Differentiates among industrial arts, vocational education, cooperative industrial education, work experience, and arts and crafts.

1016. Jacobs, Homer L. Lessons in living at the Alabama School of Piano Technology. *New Outlook for the Blind*, Dec. 1964, Vol. 58, No. 10, pp. 331–32.

Students receive instruction in activities of daily living, mobility, communications, etc., as well as piano technology.

1017. James, Philip. A drawing board for the blind. *International Journal for the Education of the Blind*, May 1964, Vol. 13, No. 4, p. 125.

How to make a drawing board with wire window screen covered with paper. Drawing in ordinary wax crayon on this board can be felt by the blind child.

1018. Johnson, Philip R. Physical education for blind children in public elementary schools. *New Outlook for the Blind*, Nov. 1969, Vol. 63, No. 9, pp. 264–71.

Changes and modifications necessary to integrate blind children into an elementary school physical education program. Ref.

1019. Jones, Reginald L.; Lavine, Karen; & Shell, Joan. Blind children integrated in classrooms with sighted children: A sociometric study. *New Outlook for the Blind*, Mar. 1972, Vol. 66, No. 3, pp. 75–80.

Study utilizes sociometric methods to examine the acceptance of blind children integrated in classrooms with sighted in social, academic, and physical areas. Secondary question deals with the sociometric characteristics of children who show a high degree of acceptance of their blind classmates. Results show blind children tend to be less acceptable on most items than their sighted peers. Sighted who had a high degree of acceptance of blind classmates tended to be less popular children.

1020. Karterud, Halvdan. The case for Esperanto in schools for the blind. *International Journal for the Education of the Blind*, May 1961, Vol. 10, No. 4, pp. 108–11.

Urges the introduction of Esperanto into the curriculum and lists its values for blind persons.

1021. Kaufman, Abraham S. Tutoring a visually handicapped student in high school chemistry. *New Outlook for the Blind*, Dec. 1971, Vol. 65, No. 10, pp. 313–17.

Describes teacher-developed materials and techniques used by a high school teacher for tutoring a visually handicapped student in high school chemistry.

1022. Kenmore, Jeanne R. Enrichment of the primary reading program in the resource room. *New Outlook for the Blind*, Feb. 1957, Vol. 51, No. 2, pp. 56–64.

Making the reading experience "come alive" through materials, and creative thinking, while teaching basic skills.

1023. Kenyon, Eunice. Twenty-four hours a day. *International Journal for the Education of the Blind*, Oct. 1963, Vol. 13, No. 1, pp. 19–22.

Describes the many and varied needs of children in any group living setting and some of the ways in which staff can meet those needs.

1024. Kerina, Jane M. I. The segregated setting: Positive values and problems. *New Outlook for the Blind*, Sept. 1958, Vol. 52, No. 7, pp. 249–54.

First of 3 articles on early childhood. With examples from case of 1 child, argues that segregated setting provides achievable goals, promotes realistic concepts, and facilitates participation.

1025. Kilgus, Eva. Art in my grade. *International Journal for the Education of the Blind*, Oct. 1955, Vol. 5, No. 1, pp. 9–12.

Teacher of 4th-grade class with 9 children with various degrees of visual handicaps and intelligence lists art activities, and success.

1026. Kirk, Edith C. A typewriting program for visually limited children. *New Outlook for the Blind*, Feb. 1969, Vol. 63, No. 2, pp. 56–62.

Why typewriting is important for blind children and detailed discussion of the equipment, procedures, and possible problems in teaching it.

1027. Knight, John J. Teacher produced slides aid reading for low vision children. *TEACHING Exceptional Children*, Summer 1971, Vol. 3, No. 4, pp. 202–8, illus.

Slides can present the low vision child with visual information he is required to learn, yet in a size and brightness that more adequately meet his unique visual needs. Description of an automatic programmed teaching machine with a reflection box, slide projector, and tape recorder. Step-by-step instructions for slide preparation are included.

1028. Korhonen, Gloria V. Music as an educational value for the blind. *New Outlook for the Blind*, Mar. 1956, Vol. 50, No. 3, pp. 91–94.

Although blind children do not automatically have an aptitude for music, this study can increase the skills and sensitivities of the child, particularly in the areas of socialization, rhythm response, singing, instrumental performance, and listening.

1029. Kratz, Laura. *Movement without sight.* Palo Alto, Calif.: Peek Publications, 1973, 135 pp., illus., paperback.

Some of the areas discussed are posture, locomotion, fitness, individual activities, stunts, rhythms, dance, evaluation, motivation, and special methods.

1030. Krebs, C. Roselynn. The blind child in kindergarten. *New Outlook for the Blind,* Jan. 1961, Vol. 55, No. 1, pp. 8–10.

Experiences of a public school kindergarten teacher with a blind child in a regular class lead her to believe this is the proper place for the child. She mentions various schools and agencies that were helpful to her during her initial efforts.

1031. Kurzhals, Ina W. A psychological view in the education of the young blind child in a residential school. *New Outlook for the Blind,* Jan. 1954, Vol. 48, No. 1, pp. 17–22.

An experienced teacher discusses in detail how she and the residential school cope with the psychological problems of learning without vision.

1032. ———. Reading made meaningful through a readiness for learning program. *International Journal for the Education of the Blind,* May 1966, Vol. 15, No. 4, pp. 107–11.

From the beginning of reading instruction, the child must know that reading is talk written down; reading is the description of familiar objects; and reading is a way of learning. With aid of illustrations, author suggests ways to help the child know these 3 things.

1033. ———. Fashioning learning opportunities for the child with impaired vision. *New Outlook for the Blind,* May 1968, Vol. 62, No. 5, pp. 160–66.

Learning results from many aspects of the teacher-pupil relationship; provides many examples of how to make this relationship effective and positive.

1034. Lamon, William E., & Threadgill, Judy. The Papy-Lamon Minicomputer for blind children: An aid in learning mathematics. *New Outlook for the Blind,* Sept. 1975, Vol. 69, No. 7, pp. 289–94, illus.

The utilization of this adaptation of the Papy Minicomputer is primarily intended to develop an understanding of the concept of number and the fundamental operations with whole numbers through sensory exploration by the child.

1035. Lane, I. An experiment in programmed learning for the visually-handicapped. *Teacher of the Blind,* Spring 1975, Vol. 63, No. 63, pp. 73–75.

Brief description of an experiment which seems to indicate that visually handicapped children can learn from audio programming. A program of this sort may have particular value in a class having a wide range of ability, allowing the teacher to use it while engaged with an individual pupil. It is also useful for those having difficulty with braille.

1036. Langdon, J. N. Some consequences of the boarding school education of the visually disabled. *New Beacon*, Feb. 1970, Vol. 54, No. 634, pp. 32–37.

Survey of parents, teenagers, and young adults on experiences with boarding school education. Parents reported a low degree of dissatisfaction; estrangement of child from juvenile society greatest disadvantage. Former pupils evidenced a considerable degree of dissatisfaction.

1037. Larson, Richard W. Teaching orientation to blind children. *Education of the Visually Handicapped*, Mar. 1975, Vol. 7, No. 1, pp. 26–31.

Proposes a theory of the development of the concepts related to physical orientation and suggests ways in which orientation can be taught.

1038. Lefkowitz, Leon J. Evaluating physical education programs. *New Outlook for the Blind*, Apr. 1962, Vol. 56, No. 4, pp. 137–38.

Describes established criteria to be used for evaluating programs in residential schools for the blind. Examines items such as health examination, classification, student leadership, class size, time allotment, grades, facilities, equipment, corrective program, intramural program, interscholastic athletic program, professional teacher preparation, written curriculum, safety measures, insurance, and coeducational activities.

1039. Leonard, J. A. Static and mobile balancing performance of blind adolescent grammar school children. *New Outlook for the Blind*, Mar. 1969, Vol. 63, No. 3, pp. 65–72.

Comparison of balancing on a beam for 101 blind and 114 sighted youth, ages 11–20 in Great Britain. Presents and interprets complex statistical data.

1040. Levine, Helen G. *A proposed program of personal adjustment for visually handicapped pupils.* Washington, D.C.: Bureau of Elementary and Secondary Education, HEW, 1969, 60 pp.

Detailed plan to provide skills of daily living, social skills, mobility, and braille in a day school program.

1041. Levine, S. Joseph. *A recorded aid for braille music. Paper no. 3: The prospectus series.* East Lansing: Mich. State Univ. Regional Instructional Materials Center for Handicapped Children and Youth, 1968, 9 pp.

Designed to teach instrumental music through the integration of tape recordings with established methods of reading braille music and playing by ear.

1042. Lewis, Marian. A year of change to the abacus. *Education of the Visually Handicapped*, Mar. 1969, Vol. 1, No. 1, pp. 28–30.

Advantages of and training for using the adapted abacus in classrooms for the blind.

1043. ———. Must visually handicapped students be low achievers in math? *Education of the Visually Handicapped*, May 1970, Vol. 2, No. 2, pp. 60–61.

Discusses the need for more study to establish the best means for teaching mathematics concepts. Need cited for testing to differentiate between ability in reasoning and in computation, and for analyzing the apparatus used for computation when comparing test scores.

1044. ————. Teaching arithmetic computation skills. *Education of the Visually Handicapped*, Oct. 1970, Vol. 2, No. 3, pp. 66–72.

Survey of residential schools and resource rooms as to how computation is taught to the visually handicapped. Specific devices mentioned. Suggestions for the future.

1045. Lewis, Marian, & Coker, Gary. The use of abacus contests to increase interest in mathematics. *New Outlook for the Blind*, Feb. 1971, Vol. 65, No. 2, pp. 41–48.

Explores use of the abacus to supplement the mathematics program for the visually handicapped. App. details abacus contests suggested as a stimulus to learning.

1046. Lewis, Mary F. A handbell choir for blind students. *New Outlook for the Blind*, Sept. 1974, Vol. 68, No. 7, pp. 297–99.

Suggestions for establishing a handbell choir including preparing braille music.

1047. Lien, Torger L. A new helper in the weave shop. *International Journal for the Education of the Blind*, Dec. 1953, Vol. 3, No. 2, pp. 219–20.

Discusses broken warp threads problem, device to stop machine at time of break and show where break is which enables much quicker fixing.

1048. Liguori, Sister M. Building reading readiness in blind children. *New Outlook for the Blind*, Oct. 1956, Vol. 50, No. 8, pp. 295–302.

Lists ways parents and teachers can improve the child's reading readiness and eliminate retarding influences. Among the suggestions are learning to look, planned experiences, developing auditory discrimination through experiences in sound, and interpretative development.

1049. Linn, Marcia C. An experiential science curriculum for the visually impaired. *Exceptional Children*, Sept. 1972, Vol. 39, No. 1, pp. 37–43.

Adaptation and evaluation of a materials-centered experiential curriculum for elementary age visually impaired children. Classroom trials showed students made significant gains in understanding both content and process objectives of physical and life science units.

1050. ————. Providing an experience centered program for the visually-impaired child. *Teacher of the Blind*, Oct. 1975, Vol. 63, No. 4, pp. 106–11.

Describes a project in which 2 experience-oriented science programs were adapted for visually impaired children. Also, a number of activities were developed to meet specific needs of the blind.

1051. Linn, Marcia C., & Thier, Herbert D. Adapting science material for the blind (ASMB): Expectation for student outcomes. *Science Education*, Apr.–June 1975, Vol. 59, No. 2, pp. 235–46.

1052. Lloyd, Dorothy J. Learning through experiencing. *Education of the Visually Handicapped*, Mar. 1972, Vol. 4, No. 1, pp. 19–21.

Author advocates learning by tactual perception, suggesting opportunities available through flexible curriculum, study of nutrition, and attending theater.

1053. Los Angeles Unified School District. *Sequenced instructional programs in physical education for the handicapped.* Los Angeles: Author, 1970, 336 pp.

A practical guide for physical educators who have handicapped children in their classes in public schools.

1054. Lowery, Sharene. Rebound tumbling for the visually handicapped. *International Journal for the Education of the Blind*, Dec. 1960, Vol. 10, No. 2, pp. 44–48.

Outlines and gives supporting lesson plans for use of the trampoline in tumbling. Suggests solutions to special problems related to the visual handicap.

1055. McClintock, Sue. Creative dramatics with the blind. *International Journal for the Education of the Blind*, Sept. 1953, Vol. 3, No. 1, pp. 194–95.

Importance of children's play and make-believe. Creative dramatics: Need for handicapped child in learning to express himself. Explains methods of teaching in Texas School for the Blind.

1056. McCrimmon, Suella. Programmed instruction as a means of teaching blind children addition and subtraction on the abacus. *Education of the Visually Handicapped*, Oct. 1974, Vol. 6, No. 3, pp. 72–79.

Development and evaluation of an abacus program. Implications for education and further research.

1057. McGuinness, Richard M. A descriptive study of blind children educated in the itinerant teacher, resource room, and special school settings. *American Foundation for the Blind Research Bulletin 20*, Mar. 1970, pp. 1–56, app.

Study of 97 totally blind students in 4th–6th grades. Results compare itinerant, resource, and residential school effectiveness.

1058. MacLean, Ronald L. Physical education for boys at the Illinois School for the Blind. *International Journal for the Education of the Blind*, Feb. 1952, Vol. 1, No. 3, pp. 51–55.

Description of programs: Swimming classes, gymnasium, decathlon, varsity teams, including swimming, track, intramural program, football, kick-goal, blind basketball, golf, and softball. Detailed description of areas and procedures then felt to be unique.

1059. McVay, Ruth A. A crafts program for blind children. *New Outlook for the Blind*, Oct. 1966, Vol. 60, No. 8, pp. 243–44.

The author, who taught arts and crafts with blind children, explains adaptations that must be made for all blind children and presents activities and projects for 5 different achievement groups.

1060. ———. More about crafts for Detroit blind children. *New Outlook for the Blind*, June 1968, Vol. 62, No. 6, pp. 188–91.

Discusses values of a craft program in day school classes for blind children and describes some of the projects.

1061. Maloney, Elizabeth. Itinerant teaching services from the viewpoint of the private agency for the blind. *International Journal for the Education of the Blind*, Dec. 1960, Vol. 10, No. 2, pp. 51–57.

Tells what itinerant teaching is, why it has become so popular, and how a private agency for the blind relates to such a program. The agency may offer services to both children and teachers.

1062. ———. The private agency's participation in the itinerant teaching program. *New Outlook for the Blind*, Dec. 1960, Vol. 54, No. 10, pp. 367–71.

Discusses role of itinerant teacher, problems in program, and how the private agency can assist.

1063. Martin, Clessen J., & Alonso, Lou. *Comprehension of full length and telegraphic materials among blind children. Final report.* East Lansing: Mich. State Univ., 1967, 111 pp.

Tests assumption that conventional textbook prose contains words and word sequences unnecessary for comprehension. Appears to support the feasibility of telegraphic learning materials as a method of increasing the rate of information input among blind children.

1064. Martucci, Ernest A. Curtain going up. *International Journal for the Education of the Blind*, Mar. 1959, Vol. 8, No. 3, pp. 77–83.

Discusses the purposes of drama in a school for the blind and describes a new, rather unstructured way of producing a play which had very beneficial results.

1065. Mattsson, Esther. Color and design for the visually handicapped. *International Journal for the Education of the Blind*, Mar. 1963, Vol. 12, No. 3, pp. 77–79.

Describes an experimental project in water-color painting for a group of 10 pupils, all but 1 having partial vision. Teachers are urged to provide opportunities for expression in form and color.

1066. Meldrum, John. Interscholastic music festivals. *International Journal for the Education of the Blind*, May 1957, Vol. 6, No. 4, pp. 96–97.

Brief history of the music festivals, why they are so interesting and valuable, and how they are organized.

1067. ———. Is music of therapeutic value to the blind? *International Journal for the Education of the Blind*, Dec. 1959, Vol. 9, No. 2, pp. 38–40.

Produces some evidence that music represents therapy for some students but, as taught at Oklahoma School for the Blind, it is chiefly a cultural study.

1068. Mich. State Univ. *Physical education and recreation for the visually handicapped.* Lansing, Mich.: Author, 1967, 223 pp.

A report of a 2-week workshop for 60 teachers.

1069. Miller, Erdene. Helpers in the kindergarten. *International Journal for the Education of the Blind*, Mar. 1960, Vol. 9, No. 3, pp. 54–57.

Provides a number of simple suggestions which help the young child adjust to kindergarten, including braille readiness exercises.

1070. Miller, Oral O., et al. Programs for the handicapped. *Journal of Health, Physical Education, Recreation*, Apr. 1971, Vol. 42, No. 4, pp. 59–64.

Four articles deal with physical education or recreational activities including bowling for the blind, integration of visually handicapped children into a public elementary school phys. ed. program, adaptations effective in integrating blind students with sighted peers, and benefits blind children can obtain from kicking tin cans.

1071. Misbach, Dorothy L. An itinerant teaching program in the elementary grades. *New Outlook for the Blind*, Dec. 1955, Vol. 49, No. 10, pp. 366–71.

Defines the itinerant teaching activity, tells how to establish a program, and describes the importance of the Talking Book, braille writing and typing, and volunteer support services.

1072. Mooney, Muriel K. Blind children need training, not sympathy. *Music Educators Journal*, Apr. 1972, Vol. 58, pp. 56–59.

Author teaches piano, music theory, and music appreciation at a school for the blind. Article includes discussion of specific resource material available to both student and teacher.

1073. Moore, Donald D. Sex education for blind high school students. *Education of the Visually Handicapped*, Mar. 1969, Vol. 1, No. 1, pp. 22–25.

Thirty students participated in a 6-week course to discover whether formal sex education would be mastered by the visually handicapped. Analysis of the results revealed that all students learned most of the material.

1074. Moore, Mary. Development of number concept in blind children. *Education of the Visually Handicapped*, Oct. 1973, Vol. 5, No. 3, pp. 65–71.

Explained are ways sighted preschool children acquire classification skills, and presented for teachers of blind first-grade children is a hierarchically organized sequence of tasks for teaching concepts of classification, seriation, and numbers to develop proficiency in arithmetic.

1075. Morgan, Myra F. Square dancing in a school for the blind. *International Journal for the Education of the Blind*, Dec. 1956, Vol. 6, No. 2, pp. 43–44.

Tells why square dancing is an excellent activity for young people and some suggestions for handling it with blind students.

1076. Morin, Edward A. Programmed instruction: Today's challenge in educating visually handicapped. *Education of the Visually Handicapped*, Mar. 1970, Vol. 2, No. 1, pp. 8–11.

Potential of programmed instruction with visually handicapped discussed. It can meet individual needs at an accelerated pace, provide for more accurate measurement and evaluation, and involve the student directly in the learning process.

1077. Morris, June E., & Nolan, Carson Y. Materials and techniques for study. *Education of the Visually Handicapped*, Mar. 1969, Vol. 1, No. 1, pp. 8–11.

Eighteen visually handicapped students were asked their views on textbook format and study techniques in order to determine the format which would provide for the most efficient use of recorded material and to explore study techniques.

1078. ———. *Aural study systems for the visually handicapped: A task analysis. Interim progress report numbers 1–4.* Washington, D.C.: Bureau of Education for the Handicapped, 1970, 99 pp.

Reports describe systems designed to explore processes involved in aural learning by the blind and to develop an entire system of study using recorded texts.

1079. Moss, James W. Resource centers for teachers of handicapped children. *Journal of Special Education,* Winter 1971, Vol. 5, No. 1, pp. 67–71.

Describes a model of a resource center for handicapped children which will be primarily a service for teachers. The visually handicapped are to be among the children served.

1080. Mumford, D. O. Drama summer school. *Teacher of the Blind,* Winter 1974–75, Vol. 63, No. 2, pp. 48–51.

Observations and suggestions resulting from an experimental program.

1081. National Society for the Prevention of Blindness. *Helping the partially seeing child in the regular classroom.* New York: Author, 1965, 15 pp.

Checklists and recommendations are provided for behavior patterns using the health record, visual environment, and seating arrangement. Also covers use of materials and equipment.

1082. ———. *Some suggested sources of equipment and teacher aids for partially seeing children.* New York: Author, 1966, 15 pp.

Manual to assist location of educational materials and equipment.

1083. Neff, Jan. Behavior objectives and learning activities in sex education for the visually handicapped: Suggestions for a curriculum. *Sex education for the visually handicapped in schools and agencies. . . . Selected papers.* New York: AFB, 1975, pp. 50–76, $3.

Developed specifically for use with students, aged 5–21, in a residential school who are grouped according to their developmental level and potential with consideration given to chronological age wherever possible. To be used by the total school staff, in the dormitories as well as in the classroom. Materials and resources are listed.

1084. Nelson, Pauline. Teletraining. *International Journal for the Education of the Blind,* May 1961, Vol. 10, No. 4, pp. 114–16.

Use of a teletrainer obtained from telephone company helps primary students in voice control, vocabulary building, number concepts, and telephone skills.

1085. Nemeth, Abraham. Teaching meaningful mathematics to blind and partially sighted children. *New Outlook for the Blind,* Nov. 1959, Vol. 53, No. 9, pp. 318–21.

Concludes that one may not assume that objects or concepts familiar to us or to the child's classmates are also familiar to him. Teaching methods must be modified to suit the individual child.

1086. Neumann, Frederick T. A tactile-developmental technique for abacus instruction and operation. *New Outlook for the Blind,* June 1970, Vol. 64, No. 6, pp. 161–66.

Potential of the abacus as a portable arithmetical tool for the visually handicapped. Its use is described.

1087. ———. Demonstrating the relationship between three-dimensional figures and their two-dimensional representations to blind students of mathematics. *New Outlook for the Blind,* Apr. 1971, Vol. 65, No. 4, pp. 126–28.

Describes a kit of collapsible geometric figures and how to use them in teaching.

1088. Nezol, A. James. Physical education for integrated blind students: Its relationship to sociometric status and recreational activity choices. *Education of the Visually Handicapped*, Mar. 1972, Vol. 4, No. 1, pp. 16–18.

Examined the relationship of high quality physical education programs for 60 blind junior and senior high school students placed in regular classes to the social attitudes of their seeing peers and to the kind of recreational activity they favored.

1089. Nolan, Carson Y. Research in teaching mathematics to blind children. *International Journal for the Education of the Blind*, May 1964, Vol. 13, No. 4, pp. 97–100.

Detailed description of the adaptation of a mathematics curriculum developed by Schott. Brief mention of the soroban (abacus) as adapted by Cranmer.

1090. Nolan, Carson Y., & Bruce, Robert E. An experimental program in elementary mathematics for the blind. *International Journal for the Education of the Blind*, Mar. 1962, Vol. 11, No. 3, pp. 71–74.

To overcome the retardation in arithmetic so characteristic of blind children, a curriculum by Schott was adapted. Pilot study use of this curriculum and planned 3-year evaluation are described.

1091. O'Brien, Rosemary. The integrated resource room for visually impaired children. *New Outlook for the Blind*, Oct. 1973, Vol. 67, No. 8, pp. 363–68.

Discussion of the resource room in the Montgomery Co. (Md.) Public Schools, including a description of the special skills taught, the process of selecting the school within the system where the program is to be located, the criteria for admitting children to the program, and the use of staff. Notes positive effects on children involved.

1092. Ohlsen, R. L., Jr. New reform in residential schools. *Education of the Visually Handicapped*, May 1971, Vol. 3, No. 2, pp. 60–62.

Describes a program to develop independence and social skills in blind adolescents. Comparison of public school and residential school orientation and development is made by noting experiences from a summer program in which the 2 groups worked together; the adolescent from the residential program is shown to be better able to cope with social skills.

1093. Oliver, James N.; Bolt, Martha L.; Buell, Charles; et al. Physical education for the visually handicapped. *Journal of Health, Physical Education and Recreation*, June 1970, Vol. 41, No. 6, pp. 37–43.

Four articles include discussion of blindness and the child's sequence of development, softball for blind students, the school's responsibility for providing physical activities, and the integration of the sightless student into regular physical activities.

1094. Olsen, Maurice. Modern curriculum provisions for visually handicapped children. *International Journal for the Education of the Blind*, Mar. 1963, Vol. 12, No. 3, pp. 80–83.

Detailed report of a conference of 16 educational specialists defining modern curriculum trends with special attention to mathematics, low vision aids, mobility, programmed instruction, and administrative recommendations.

1095. Packard, Bruce. A technique for developing perceptual materials for the blind. *American Foundation for the Blind Research Bulletin 25*, Jan. 1973, pp. 253–55.

Brief report of tactual materials to improve cognitive functioning of congenitally totally blind children.

1096. Pearson, Kathleen. Taking a new look at physical education. *New Outlook for the Blind*, Nov. 1965, Vol. 59, No. 9, pp. 315–17.

On basis of personal observation and, especially, review of the literature, urges review of facilities and programs of physical education for blind children and a reevaluation of the philosophy which often sees these programs as unimportant. Ref.

1097. Peck, Olive. The blind student in secondary education. *Bulletin of the National Association of Secondary School Principals*, Jan. 1955.

Addressed to the principal who faces his first experience with a blind pupil in his school, the article discusses survey of school facilities, help the pupil will need, and program adjustments.

1098. Penny, J. K. Music at Henshaw's. *Teacher of the Blind*, Oct. 1975, Vol. 63, No. 4, pp. 118–20.

Music teacher's experiences with blind students in both music playing and music appreciation.

1099. Pittam, Vera G. Reading readiness. *New Outlook for the Blind*, Nov. 1965, Vol. 59, No. 9, pp. 322–24. Reprinted from *Teacher of the Blind*, Apr. 1965.

Describes important skills for reading readiness under the following headings: Tactual perception and discrimination, knowledge of left and right, ability to follow instructions, auditory perception and discrimination, listening to and retelling stories, experiential background, mental and emotional readiness, and the feeling that reading is meaningful.

1100. Ray, Wilbert S. A Skinner box recorder for the blind student. *Psychological Record*, Fall 1971, Vol. 21, No. 4, p. 527.

Describes adaptation of laboratory equipment for a blind student.

1101. Ray, Wilbert S., & McDonald, C. Edgar. The blind student and the Skinner box. *Psychological Record*, Winter 1971, Vol. 21, No. 1, pp. 35–36.

Detailed description of the modification of a Skinner box as used by a blind student in an instructional psychology laboratory.

1102. Reimer, Norman. A report of tools adapted for use of blind students. *International Journal for the Education of the Blind*, Oct. 1963, Vol. 13, No. 1, pp. 29–31.

Describes 2 tools adapted for shop use of blind students: A master square, and a combination guard and guide for a band saw.

1103. Resnick, Rose. Creative movement classes for visually handicapped children in a public school setting. *New Outlook for the Blind*, Dec. 1973, Vol. 67, No. 10, pp. 442–47.

Importance of classes to develop motor skills, posture, orientation, balance, and self-concept. Includes sample lessons and summary of techniques.

1104. Richterman, Harold. A personal adjustment and orientation program for children. *New Outlook for the Blind*, Dec. 1963, Vol. 57, No. 10, pp. 389–92.

Needs determine goals. Discusses determination of child's potential, describes curriculum, selection of children.

1105. Ricketts, Peter. Unaccustomed as I was. *New Beacon*, Nov. 1973, Vol. 57, No. 679, pp. 290–291.

Author describes experiences as blind member of integrated class in public speaking.

1106. Roades, Sue-Ann; Pisch, Lillian; & Axelrod, Saul. Use of behavior modification procedures with visually handicapped students. *Education of the Visually Handicapped*, Mar. 1974, Vol. 6, No. 1, pp. 19–26.

Reports 2 case studies.

1107. Roderick, Martha M. Exceptional children develop through art expression. *New Outlook for the Blind*, Apr. 1956, Vol. 50, No. 4, pp. 134–39. Originally published in *Educational Leadership*, Feb. 1956.

How an art studio within a public school stimulates creativity and self-expression in normal and exceptional children. Tells of the work of some specific children, and shows pictures of some work by blind children.

1108. Rogow, Sally. Puppetry as an aid in language development. *New Outlook for the Blind*, Oct. 1965, Vol. 59, No. 8, pp. 272–74.

Puppetry, a form of creative dramatics, is an integrating experience, mentally and emotionally stimulating to the children. A project with 3 groups of blind children is described.

1109. Romine, Nicholas M. Arts and crafts. *International Journal for the Education of the Blind*, Feb. 1952, Vol. 1, No. 3, pp. 68–69.

Discusses necessity and importance of working with hands from early beginning of man down to present development of arts and crafts of all types, importance of arts and crafts in every school for the blind, relevance to leisure time and criminal records.

1110. Rupard, Betty W. Corrective physical education at the Virginia School. *International Journal for the Education of the Blind*, Feb. 1953, Vol. 2, No. 2, p. 144.

Briefly describes the program begun at the School for the Deaf and Blind, its goals and basic procedures.

1111. Russo, Richard J. Corrective and recreational gym classes for the blind. *New Outlook for the Blind*, May 1969, Vol. 63, No. 5, pp. 147–51.

How physical education, and especially calisthenics, can begin with a conditioning routine, move into team games, and where needed become a corrective program.

1112. Sanborn, Leland C. The partially sighted child in a school for the blind. *New Outlook for the Blind*, June 1963, Vol. 57, No. 6, pp. 191–94.

The New York State School for the Blind describes their residential school program for nearly 200 students. Discusses many facets of comprehensive program.

1113. Schiff, William. Research on raised line drawings. *New Outlook for the Blind*, Apr. 1965, Vol. 59, No. 4, pp. 134–37.

Reviews importance of diagrams in many books and, therefore, need for tactile diagrams. Reports evaluation of discriminability of "tactile arrow" as directional symbol.

1114. Schiff, William, & Isikow, Herbert. Stimulus redundancy in the tactile perception of histograms. *International Journal for the Education of the Blind*, Oct. 1966, Vol. 16, No. 1, pp. 1–11.

To evaluate relative effectiveness of different ways of presenting graphic content of texts, experimental histograms were varied in bar-length, regularity of histogram, tactile quality of information indicating bar-length, and redundancy of stimulus information. Forty blind high school students matched for IQ served as *S*s. Practical results of findings are discussed. Ref.

1115. Schindele, Rudolf. The social adjustment of visually handicapped children in different educational settings. *American Foundation for the Blind Research Bulletin 28*, Oct. 1974, pp. 125–44.

Visually handicapped students in regular school were compared with those in residential schools and with a control group of sighted students. Generally negative findings show far less difference between visually handicapped and sighted than had been expected.

1116. Schmidt, Edna H. Teaching reading by use of word games. *International Journal for the Education of the Blind*, Dec. 1958, Vol. 8, No. 2, pp. 46–50.

Word games are a pleasant way to give the child practice in reading. Details are provided for games which provide vocabulary recognition, improving phonetic skills, recognition of certain braille contractions, and some which serve multiple purposes.

1117. Scholl, Geraldine T. *The principal works with the visually impaired.* Washington, D.C.: Council for Exceptional Children, 1968, 70 pp.

Guidelines for principals of regular schools who are planning for selection, placement, and integration of visually handicapped children. Reviews residential and day schools and lists regional Special Education Instructional Materials Centers.

1118. ————. The psychosocial effects of blindness: Implications for program planning in sex education. *New Outlook for the Blind*, May 1974, Vol. 68, No. 5, pp. 201–9. Also in *Sex education for the visually handicapped in schools and agencies . . . Selected papers.* New York: AFB, 1975, $3, pp. 20–28.

Selected factors in developmental process are described and related to program planning. Also discussed are variables related to blindness and to individual characteristics.

1119. Seamons, Gloria. *Swimming for the blind.* Provo, Utah: Brigham Young Univ., 1966, 42 pp.

Presents program of swimming instruction for the blind. Discusses program organization, facilities, equipment, aids, personnel, instruction, objectives. Outlines master program of 52 lessons. Bib.

1120. Sennet, Edith L. Creative writing and the blind child. *Education of the Visually Handicapped*, Oct. 1969, Vol. 1, No. 3, pp. 81–85.

Techniques to use in teaching creative writing to blind. Importance of this subject to make child feel a part of his environment.

1121. Shaw, George. The piano and its care. *International Journal for the Education of the Blind*, Apr. 1953, Vol. 2, No. 3, pp. 156–57.
Detailed information on care.

1122. Shepherd, Louis T., Jr., & Simons, Gene M. Music training for the visually handicapped. *Music Educators Journal*, Feb. 1970, Vol. 56, No. 6, pp. 80–81.
Problems faced by blind students of music described including explanation of braille music and the difficulties associated with its use. Suggestions to aid students to become professional musicians are made.

1123. Shumway, H. Smith. Wyoming visually handicapped children attend public school. *New Outlook for the Blind*, May 1964, Vol. 58, No. 5, pp. 142–44.
Detailed information about how Wyo. deals with its blind and visually handicapped children. How school attendance decisions are made, preparation of school for blind student, and use of supplementary tutoring and materials.

1124. Sibert, Katie N. Symposium—Self-image: A guide to adjustment. An itinerant teacher's aims. *New Outlook for the Blind*, Mar. 1961, Vol. 55, No. 3, pp. 82–4.
Describes work of and materials used by an itinerant teacher. Several case examples are given.

1125. ———. The use of eye reports by an educator. *International Journal for the Education of the Blind*, Mar. 1966, Vol. 15, No. 3, pp. 78–81.
Discusses how eye reports can aid educator in at least 7 ways: School placement, program planning, educational procedure, social guidance, vocational guidance, in securing financial assistance, and in research and statistical studies.

1126. Silver, Ruth. Auditory training for the multiply handicapped visually impaired child. *DVH Newsletter*, Summer 1974, Vol. 19, No. 1, p. 12.
Teaching suggestions designed for classroom implementation. How to utilize sounds made by toys, environmental sounds, and speech. Activities intended to teach awareness, localization, and discriminations of sounds.

1127. ———. Responding to sound through toys, the environment, and speech. *TEACHING Exceptional Children*, Winter 1975, Vol. 7, No. 2, pp. 38–44.
Practical suggestions for developing in the multiply handicapped preschool child awareness of sounds, discrimination, localization, and simple response patterns. Suggests how to start with easy discriminations of words, move to more complex with use of memory.

1128. Simon, Janet D. A course in spoken communication for high school students who are visually handicapped. *Education of the Visually Handicapped*, May 1974, Vol. 6, No. 2, pp. 41–43.
Background survey in 49 residential schools prompted development of this pilot course designed to improve ability in spoken, receptive, and nonverbal communications. Gives components of typical lesson plan. Pilot project had positive results.

1129. Simpkins, Katherine. An auditory training program for kindergarten through third grade. *Education of the Visually Handicapped*, Oct. 1971, Vol. 3, No. 3, pp. 70–73.

Curriculum guide. Results favorable with environmental sounds, doubtful with language.

1130. Sinclair, D. Art teaching for the blind. *Teacher of the Blind*, Spring 1975, Vol. 63, No. 3, pp. 65–72.

Discusses art teaching and the benefits blind students receive—releasing inner tensions, development of manipulatory skills, body awareness, development of imagination and sensitivity, and development of logical thinking and positive movement.

1131. Skinner, Dorothea E. The partially sighted child in the regular classroom . . . *Special Education in Canada*, Mar. 1970, Vol. 44, No. 3, pp. 26–28.

Answers questions about the partially sighted child including: Definition of limited vision and visual acuity, indications of clumsiness, changes in the physical setting, recommended books about eye health, psychological difficulties, large print materials, placement, completion of assignments, and blackboard needs.

1132. Smith, Benjamin. The role of the private school for the blind in the education of blind and multi-handicapped blind children. *Lantern,* June 1972, Vol. 41, No. 3, pp. 14–18.

Notes the advantages and disadvantages of public and private education for visually and multi-handicapped children with emphasis on the role of the private school. Acknowledges that neither meets all the needs of the handicapped child.

1133. ———. Problems the public schools face. *Lantern,* Feb. 1973, Vol. 42, No. 2, pp. 3–9.

Reports difficulties of visually handicapped children who have been transferred from public school to Perkins School for the Blind.

1134. Spar, Harry J. Itinerant teaching as a method of educating blind children. *New Outlook for the Blind*, Feb. 1956, Vol. 50, No. 2, pp. 51–55.

Argues against segregated braille classes and for itinerant teaching support in regular classes. Gives the status of itinerant teaching in N.Y. State.

1135. Starkovich, Paul. "The Oregon Plan" for 1963 inaugurates a tape-recording project. *New Outlook for the Blind*, May 1963, Vol. 57, No. 5, pp. 157–59.

Discusses the advantages of the state-wide recording program which will issue playback machines and recorded materials to all qualified blind students in grades 10–12.

1136. Stephens, Thomas M., & Birch, Jack W. Merits of special class, resource, and itinerant plans for teaching partially seeing children. *Exceptional Children*, 1969, Vol. 35, No. 6, pp. 481–85.

Reviews pertinent literature re advantages and disadvantages of 3 organizational schemes for education of partially seeing children. Findings of recent studies are compared with stated advantages for each pattern.

1137. Struve, Nancy L.; Thier, Herbert D.; Hadary, Doris; et al. The effect of an experimental science curriculum for the visually impaired on course objectives and manipulative skills. *Education of the Visually Handicapped*, Mar. 1975, Vol. 7, No. 1, pp. 9–14.

Study to determine effect of the Science Curriculum Improvement Study on manipulative skills and to investigate the relationship between improved manipulative skills and progress on the content, process, and logical thinking objectives of the adapted SCIS program.

1138. Stubbs, Mabel. Meeting the needs of adjustment. *International Journal for the Education of the Blind*, Mar. 1963, Vol. 12, No. 3, pp. 69–70.

Brief description of a class for pupils with special educational problems with the purpose of bringing each class member to his appropriate grade level in each subject.

1139. Suffolk Co. Board of Cooperative Educational Services. *Communication and computation skills for blind students attending public schools.* Dix Hills, N.Y.: Author, 1972, 34 pp.

Evaluative and instructional procedures used by itinerant teachers to teach readiness for braille reading and writing, as well as braille reading and writing, signature writing, Nemeth Code, and scientific notation.

1140. Sullivan, Martha G. *Understanding children who are partially seeing: A classroom teacher's guide.* Seattle, Wash.: Bernie Straub, 1974, 34 pp., $1.50.

Explains the nature and effect of various types of visual loss, discusses the classroom setting (seating, lighting, etc.) and the use of special equipment, material, and methods.

1141. Svaldi, Vincent F., & Romig, Dennis A. A busy and exciting summer for visually handicapped youth. *Education of the Visually Handicapped*, Dec. 1969, Vol. 1, No. 4, pp. 124–26.

Summer program emphasized vocational, on-the-job training, and independent mobility skills. These as well as the skills involved in physical education, home economics, home mechanics, and communication are discussed.

1142. Sykes, Kim C., et al. *Creative arts and crafts for children with visual handicaps.* Louisville, Ky.: American Printing House for the Blind, 1974, 48 pp.

Teaching guide gives instructions for 23 projects thought to be appropriate for use with visually handicapped children.

1143. Tabler, Cecelia. Results of a two-year language study. *International Journal for the Education of the Blind*, Mar. 1960, Vol. 9, No. 3, pp. 59–62.

Upon discovering unsatisfactory achievement in the language area, the Mo. School for the Blind entered upon a 2-year remedial program. Statistical evidence of the success of this program is provided.

1144. Tait, Perla E. Believing without seeing: Teaching the blind child in a "regular" kindergarten. *Childhood Education*, Mar. 1974, Vol. 50, No. 5, pp. 285–91.

Practical advice on general handling as well as specific suggestions to aid the teacher in making games and activities meaningful to the visually handicapped child.

1145. Taylor, William, Jr. I went to public school. *New Outlook for the Blind*, Jan. 1956, Vol. 50, No. 1, pp. 19–21.

Day schooling helps the individual come to terms with the psychological environment of the sighted but to do this it is important to integrate the child maximally; merely going to day school will not accomplish this without effort. Hiring fellow students as readers and guides helps.

1146. Thier, Herbert D. Laboratory science for visually handicapped elementary school children. *New Outlook for the Blind*, June 1971, Vol. 65, No. 6, pp. 190–94.

Describes a Univ. of California project, Adapting Science Materials for the Blind. A laboratory approach is stressed, with observation, manipulation of materials, and development of language skills to describe and explain events.

1147. Thomas, T. V. Teaching by television at Homai College. *New Outlook for the Blind*, Oct. 1968, Vol. 62, No. 8, pp. 259–60.

A school for the blind in New Zealand is using TV to enlarge material so that partially sighted children can learn from pictures and diagrams. Procedures are described.

1148. Thompson, R. Paul. A music program for visually handicapped children. *New Outlook for the Blind*, Feb. 1957, Vol. 51, No. 2, pp. 43–55.

Details the curriculum of a total music program K-6 under the following headings: (1) Whole-child music experience; (2) Music experience areas; (3) The Instrumental Plan—teaching music reading through playing; (4) The Vocal Plan—teaching music reading through singing.

1149. Thurrell, Richard J. Special problems of motivation in the blind student. *International Journal for the Education of the Blind*, Dec. 1966, Vol. 16, No. 2, pp. 45–48.

The blind child is asked to learn social skills that begin and remain largely "for sighted others." This paper deals with motivation for such learning.

1150. Tinsley, Tuck. The use of Origami in the mathematics education of visually impaired students. *Education of the Visually Handicapped*, Mar. 1972, Vol. 4, No. 1, pp. 8–11.

Explains that Origami, Japanese paper-folding, can supplement mathematics instruction of blind and partially sighted persons. Three sample diagrams present guidelines for folding an altitude, finding the sum of the angles of a triangle, and folding an angle bisector.

1151. Tobin, Michael J. The attitudes of non-specialist teachers towards visually handicapped pupils. *Teacher of the Blind*, Jan. 1972, Vol. 60, No. 2, pp. 60–64.

Brief report on a survey of 80 British teachers.

1152. Tobin, Michael J.; Clarke, D.; Lane, I.; et al. Programed learning for the blind: Some exploratory studies. *Education of the Visually Handicapped*, Mar. 1970, Vol. 2, No. 1, pp. 11–23.

Six studies briefly described: programed instruction for teaching braille (2 programs), development and construction of a braille teaching machine, use of a branching program to teach social studies, testing a science program, and evaluating the effectiveness of braille and audio presentation of programed materials.

1153. Tobin, Michael J.; Norris, Norma; & Irving, Rita. Teaching English to the visually handicapped. *Teacher of the Blind*, July 1973, Vol. 61, No. 4, pp. 104–13.

Practicing teachers in Great Britain cooperated by means of seminars, conferences, individual interviews, and detailed teaching diaries in the year-long investigation which formed the basis of the report of which this article is the summary.

1154. Toft, C. Rural studies for the visually handicapped in schools. *Teacher of the Blind*, Apr. 1972, Vol. 60, No. 3, pp. 97–106.

Description of the study plan for a course aimed at developing understanding, appreciation, and use of various aspects of rural environment for personal and social well-being. Course includes agriculture, horticulture, field and laboratory biology, rural crafts, and natural history.

1155. Tombaugh, Dorothy. Laboratory techniques for the blind. *American Biology Teacher*, May 1972, Vol. 34, No. 5, pp. 258–60.

The author has had 6 blind students in sophomore biology and describes variations in laboratory procedure which have insured full participation by these students.

1156. Tonkovic, Franjo. An approach to the problem of integrated education of blind children. *International Journal for the Education of the Blind*, May 1967, Vol. 16, No. 4, pp. 115–19.

Relates integration/segregation to the attitudes of society and the place blind persons hold within a given society. Integration has a historical logic.

1157. Torbett, David S. A humanistic and futuristic approach to sex education for blind children. *New Outlook for the Blind*, May 1974, Vol. 68, No. 5, pp. 210–15. Also in *Sex education for the visually handicapped in schools and agencies . . . Selected papers*. New York: AFB, 1975, $3, pp. 29–34.

Sex education programs must take into account the sexual negativism of American culture, especially in relation to touch. Teachers and parents need help with their own insecurities so they can better educate their children.

1158. Trump, J. Lloyd. An image of the curriculum of the future. *International Journal for the Education of the Blind*, Oct. 1963, Vol. 13, No. 1, pp. 23–26.

To keep up with all fields of knowledge, the organization and setting of the curriculum must change, with learning centers and materials centers more important. Flexibility and technology will be the keynotes.

1159. Univ. of the State of N.Y. *Adapting materials for educating blind children with sighted children*. Albany, N.Y.: Author, n.d., 40 pp.

Illustrates specific materials which can be adapted for use by blind children who are integrated with sighted children. Includes discussion of tactile books, puzzles, braille readiness materials, experience charts, workbooks, flashcards, self-teaching activities, word wheels, and manipulative aids.

1160. van 'T Hooft, F., & Heslinga, K. Sex education of blind-born children. *New Outlook for the Blind*, Jan. 1968, Vol. 62, No. 1, pp. 15–22. Also in *Sex education for the visually handicapped in schools and agencies . . . Selected papers*. New York: AFB, 1975, $3, pp. 1–7.

Discusses special problems of blind children learning about sexuality. Recommends sex education before sexual feelings appear.

1161. Vermey, Geerat J. Observations on raised-line drawings. *Education of the Visually Handicapped*, May 1969, Vol. 1, No. 2, pp. 47–52.

Discussion of various methods of producing raised-line drawings. Difficulties in interpretation of illustrations. How to teach use of braille illustrations.

1162. Vernon, McCay. Integrated education of the visually handicapped. *Teacher of the Blind*, Winter 1974–75, Vol. 63, No. 2, pp. 36–42.

Discusses with caution the proposal for the integrated education of all visually handicapped children by the Dept. of Education and Science Committee on the Education of the Visually Handicapped.

1163. Vodola, Thomas. *Individualized physical education program for the handicapped child.* Englewood Cliffs, N.J.: Prentice-Hall, 1973, 308 pp.

Book is useful for teachers of the multi-handicapped.

1164. Walter, Marion. Use of geoboards to teach mathematics. *Education of the Visually Handicapped*, May 1974, Vol. 6, No. 2, pp. 59–62.

Students played geoboard games to learn to make geometric designs, copy patterns, find areas of simple shapes, at the Halifax School for the Blind where the boards were effective in teaching geometric concepts to 3rd- and 10th-grade children.

1165. Ward, Ted, et al. *Workshop training kits. Vol. 1.* East Lansing: Mich. State Univ., Regional Instructional Materials Center for Handicapped Children and Youth, 1973, 206 pp.

This volume presents 4 kits for development of teacher skills to be used with severely handicapped children, and 6 kits for training personnel to instruct inservice teachers. Kits include a task analysis game for sequential teaching. 3 reinforcement mystery games, and activity involving charting behavior, all for use with the deaf-blind.

1166. Ware, Paul D. Casting a blind student in a high school play. *New Outlook for the Blind*, Feb. 1968, Vol. 62, No. 2, pp. 48–49, illus.

How a blind high school student was accepted as just another member of the cast.

1167. Wargo, William D. *Industrial arts for the visually handicapped.* Tallahassee: Fla. State Univ., 1971, 59 pp., app., illus.

Report on the significance of industrial arts for visually handicapped elementary school children. Includes objectives, methodology, project illustrations, bench plans, and observation records.

1168. ———. The Astoria Park program of industrial arts for visually handicapped children. *Man/Society/Technology*, May–June 1973, Vol. 32, No. 8, pp. 311–14.

Describes a public elementary school program established as a follow-up to a demonstration pilot program concerned with concepts and technology for teachers of the visually handicapped. Emphasizes the contributions industrial arts training makes to the development of feelings and personality.

1169. Waterhouse, Edward J. Arithmetic aids for the blind. *International Journal for the Education of the Blind*, Dec. 1955, Vol. 5, No. 2, pp. 25–29.

Discusses various aids and devices for use in teaching and doing arithmetic. Includes discussion of arithmetic patterns/processes used by blind people. Offers suggestions from blind boys and girls seeking to accomplish arithmetic computation.

1170. Weckler, Judy L. A part to play. *International Journal for the Education of the Blind*, Oct. 1964, Vol. 14, No. 1, pp. 13–19.

Rather full discussion of the benefits of drama, whether a curriculum subject or a drama club. With the Drama Club at Perkins School for the Blind as an illustration, details the steps in putting on a play.

1171. Weisgerber, Robert A. Individualizing for the handicapped child in the regular classroom. *Education Technology*, Nov. 1974, Vol. 14, No. 11, pp. 33–35.

Presents checklist to help regular teachers determine whether they are prepared to meet handicapped students' needs and to individualize instruction.

1172. ———. Planning for the individualization of learning with blind students. *Education of the Visually Handicapped*, Dec. 1975, Vol. 7, No. 4, pp. 112–15.

Describes elements important in individualized learning suggestions for implementing an individualized approach, and design of necessary instructional materials.

1173. Wexler, Abraham. *Experimental science for the blind: An instruction manual based on a variety of devices.* London: Pergamon, 1961, 97 pp., illus.

Detailed manual for practical science experiments with full descriptions of novel devices used in these experiments.

1174. Wheeler, R. H., & Hooley, A.M. *Physical education for the handicapped.* Philadelphia: Lea & Fiberger, 1969, 352 pp.

Seven pages devoted to the visually impaired.

1175. Wienke, Phoebe. Blind children in an integrated physical education program. *New Outlook for the Blind*, Mar. 1966, Vol. 60, No. 3, pp. 73–76.

Author strongly favors integrated phys. ed. Discusses benefits, classroom teacher's role in implementing program, adaptations required for hockey, volleyball, basketball.

1176. Willenberg, Ernest P. Safety education for exceptional children. *Safety Education*, Feb. 1961, pp. 7–8, 29–30.

Seeks to establish that handicapped children face unique hazards and that there is a relationship between the classification of the impairment and the type of hazard. Discusses safety education for the mentally, physically, aurally, and visually handicapped.

1177. Williams, Martha G. "Experience days" for partially seeing children. *New Outlook for the Blind*, Oct. 1965, Vol. 59, No. 8, pp. 288–90.

Details how to enlarge the experience of a partially seeing child in a 1-day tour of simple but stimulating experiences and some follow-up activities.

1178. Williams, Mrs. Frank N. Enriched mathematics for the blind. *International Journal for the Education of the Blind*, Mar. 1955, Vol. 4, No. 3, pp. 50–52.

Cultural education in mathematics, music, literature, history and social studies furnish educational background essential for life's well being. Enriched mathematical teaching includes objectivity, real contacts (shopping, paying jobs, budgetting, etc.).

1179. Willoughby, Doris, et al., Eds. *Your school includes a blind student.* Chatsworth, Calif.: National Federation of the Blind, Teachers Div., 1974, 34 pp., free. (Braille $4.85.)

Addressed to the regular classroom teacher with no prior experience with blindness.

1180. Wilson, Myrle P. Braillewriters for beginners. *International Journal for the Education of the Blind*, Oct. 1955, Vol. 5, No. 1, pp. 13–14.

Experiment with beginners and first graders involving heterogeneous group of 13, ages 7–11, with one retarded aged 13. Revealed that braillewriter is easier than slate, which children prefer, effective in teaching and writing. Presents techniques: Correct fingering, rhythm, sequence for new letters of alphabet, spelling, writing names.

1181. Winkley, William M. Public high school or residential high school for blind students? *Education of the Visually Handicapped*, Dec. 1972, Vol. 4, No. 4, pp. 120–22.

Evaluated programs in several states in terms of academic preparation of blind students for college. Found no significant differences in college performance between the 2 groups (28 residential school graduates and 95 integrated graduates), suggesting that factors other than academic quality should be considered in determining placement.

1182. Witcher, Clifford M. The teaching of mathematics to the blind. *Mathematics Teacher*, May 1955.

Historical survey of the means by which blind persons have been taught mathematics, various teaching devices, and braille mathematical notation.

1183. Wolinsky, Gloria F. Some thoughts on curriculum development for the very young handicapped children. *Education of the Visually Handicapped*, Dec. 1972, Vol. 4, No. 4, pp. 112–19.

Three dimensions, learning, biological characteristics, nurturance, presented in a schematic form illustrate how time and the child cross these dimensions and how growth is an interactive process.

1184. Woodcock, Charles C. A slick trick in woodworking. *International Journal for the Education of the Blind*, Dec. 1956, Vol. 6, No. 2, pp. 44–45.

An excellent way to finish furniture or any wooden object, and a way which blind students can usually handle independently, is a combination of paint and wax. Instructions are provided.

1185. ———. A sensory stimulation center for blind children. *Phi Delta Kappan*, Apr. 1974, Vol. 55, No. 8, p. 541.

Suggests the development of sensory stimulation centers for blind children which would be a highly developed play space to teach concepts and develop muscular activities.

1186. Wright, Rosalind. A self-discovery venture for visually handicapped children. *International Journal for the Education of the Blind*, Dec. 1968, Vol. 18, No. 4, pp. 124–26.

Outlines content of a sex education program for 4th-, 5th-, and 6th-grade visually handicapped students.

1187. Wyder, Frank T.; Wilson, Milton E., Jr.; & Frumkin, R. M. Information as a factor in perception of the blind by teachers. *Perceptual and Motor Skills,* 1967, Vol. 25, No. 1, p. 188.

1188. Young, Edna H., & Hawk, Sara S. *Moto-kinesthetic speech training.* Stanford, Calif.: Stanford Univ., 1955, 176 pp.

Discusses the application of moto-kinesthetics to speech problems with regard to blindness. Analyzes blindness as specific problem area.

10. Tactual Maps, Charts, and Drawings

1189. Bailey, Jane L. Meaningful maps for the blind and seeing. *New Outlook for the Blind*, Mar. 1956, Vol. 50, No. 3, pp. 77–83.

Suggestions to teachers for helping the blind child to use maps effectively.

1190. Bentzen, Billie L. Production and testing of an orientation and travel map for visually handicapped persons. *New Outlook for the Blind*, Oct. 1972, Vol. 66, No. 8, pp. 249–55, illus.

Describes development of tactual map of a school campus utilizing a progression of details. A travel test using 6 proficient blind travelers shows that such a map can facilitate travel for a proficient traveler who receives no information about the area other than the map.

1191. Berlá, Edward P. Behavioral strategies and problems in scanning and interpreting tactual displays. *New Outlook for the Blind*, Oct. 1972, Vol. 66, No. 8, pp. 277–86.

Based on pseudomap mailing followed by telephone interview of 12 blind adults who were skilled in use of tactual materials. Discussion of 1- and 2-handed scanning, horizontal vs. vertical scan, hand and finger utilization, areal vs. point symbols, tracking, orientation, directional orientation, and keys.

1192. ———. Strategies in scanning a tactual pseudomap. *Education of the Visually Handicapped*, Mar. 1973, Vol. 5, No. 1, pp. 8–19.

Study compared effectiveness of brief instructions in various strategies. Concludes that training blind students to scan a map vertically produces the most accurate and consistent performance.

1193. Berlá, Edward P., & Butterfield, Lawrence H., Jr. Teachers' views on tactile maps for blind students: Problems and needs. *Education of the Visually Handicapped*, Dec. 1975, Vol. 7, No. 4, pp. 116–18.

A questionnaire to teachers defined difficulties in using tactile maps with blind students. Results are discussed under following headings: Conceptual and experiential prerequisites to map reading, materials used for maps, map symbology and design, and inspection and use of tactile maps.

1194. Berlá, Edward P., & Murr, Marvin J. Searching tactual space. *Education of the Visually Handicapped*, May 1974, Vol. 6, No. 2, pp. 49–58.

Compares effectiveness of training in 3 different tactual map reading search patterns with 144 braille readers in grades 4–12. Two-handed vertical scanning technique proved superior to other techniques examined.

1195. ———. The effects of tactual noise on locating point symbols and tracking a line on a tactile pseudomap. *Journal of Special Education*, 1975, Vol. 9, pp. 183–90.

1196. Chang, Carolyn, & Johnson, Daniel E. Tactual maps with interchangeable parts. *New Outlook for the Blind*, Apr. 1968, Vol. 62, No. 4, pp. 122–24.

Using Valcro [sic], a portable tactual map or chart with interchangeable pieces can serve many mobility students in different locations. Detailed instructions given.

1197. Craven, Roger W. The use of aluminum sheets in producing tactual maps for blind persons. *New Outlook for the Blind*, Nov. 1972, Vol. 66, No. 9, pp. 323–30, illus.

Description of how an aluminum alloy sheet (a photo-offset plate from a printing office) and improvised tools can be used to make a master copy of a map for Thermoform reproduction. Discussion of braille map-making in general. Feels that some of the techniques can be applied to other kinds of illustrations as well.

1198. ———. Making embossed maps as a hobby. *New Beacon*, Mar. 1973, Vol. 57, No. 671, pp. 58–62.

Author describes methods of making inexpensive, clear maps, charts, diagrams for the blind with the aid of Thermoform machine.

1199. Foster, R. B. A technique for map-makers. *New Beacon*, Mar. 1973, Vol. 57, No. 671, pp. 62–63.

Suggests method for greatly enlarging picture of area to be mapped, without losing accuracy, prior to adding tactual elements. Implications for mobility instruction.

1200. Gill, J. M. Tactual mapping. *American Foundation for the Blind Research Bulletin 28*, Oct. 1974, pp. 57–80.

General info. about tactual maps as well as discussion of various methods of production. Bib.

1201. Gill, J. M., & James, G. A. A study of the discriminability of tactual point symbols. *American Foundation for the Blind Research Bulletin 26*, June 1973, pp. 19–34.

One hundred ninety-four visually handicappel *S*s employed in test of 30 symbols intended for use on diagrams and tactual maps. Thirteen symbols met discriminability criteria.

1202. ———. Mobility maps: The choice of symbols. *New Beacon*, Feb. 1974, Vol. 58, No. 682, pp. 35–38.

Discusses production of mobility maps. Presents chart of 24 symbols used in mobility map-making.

1203. Gilson, Charles; Wurzburger, Berdell; & Johnson, Daniel E. The use of the raised map in teaching mobility to blind children. *New Outlook for the Blind*, Feb. 1965, Vol. 59, No. 2, pp. 59–62.

Describes the advantages and some disadvantages of the raised map with brief case studies as illustrations. Two maps are reproduced.

1204. Groves, Paul A., & Wiedel, Joseph W. Tactual mapping: Problems of design and interpretation. *International Journal for the Education of the Blind*, Mar. 1968, Vol. 18, No. 1, pp. 10–16.

Initial research was done to design and produce large-scale orientation and mobility maps. The successful mobility map provides just sufficient information to meet specific movement requirements of the blind person. The research objective is a manual of map design and reproduction for mobility instructors.

1205. James, G. A., & Gill, J. M. Mobility maps for the visually handicapped: A study of learning and retention of raised symbols. *American Foundation for the Blind Research Bulletin 27,* Apr. 1974, pp. 87–89.

Ability to retain and use 14 tactual symbols and to read a tactual map was examined with 25 visually handicapped children. Utility of the symbols themselves and their feasibility regarding tactual map reading was recorded.

1206. ———. A pilot study on the discriminability of tactile areal and line symbols for the blind. *American Foundation for the Blind Research Bulletin 29,* June 1975, pp. 23–31, illus.

Eight tactile areal and 17 linear symbols for use on maps and graphics were produced on Braillon and tested for discriminability in separate sets by the method of paired comparisons. Sixty-two blind English schoolboys were *S*s. Five areal and 10 linear symbols met the criteria for discrimination suggested by Nolan and Morris (1971).

1207. James, Grahame. Problems in the standardisation of design and symbolisation in tactile route maps for the blind. *New Beacon,* Apr. 1972, Vol. 56, No. 660, pp. 87–91.

Examines problems involved in producing standardized designs and symbols for tactile route maps for the blind. Three major symbol types are line, point, and areal or texture.

1208. ———. A kit for making raised maps. *New Beacon,* Apr. 1975, Vol. 59, No. 696, pp. 85–90, illus.

Describes development of kit for making tactual maps cheaply and without complicated machinery. It is suggested that symbols in the kit form a national standard in United Kingdom.

1209. James, Grahame, & Swain, Richard. Learning bus routes using a tactual map. *New Outlook for the Blind,* May 1975, Vol. 69, No. 5, pp. 212–17.

A new map-making kit was used to produce a tactual map of a section of a city, including 2 bus routes. After training, 4 blind adults completed both map-reading evaluation and use of the map in travel.

1210. Leonard, J. Alfred, & Newman, R. C. Three types of "maps" for blind travel. *Ergonomics,* 1970, Vol. 13, No. 2, pp. 165–79.

Three route maps are described, and results of an experiment with 29 blind *S*s show that with any 1 at least half the *S*s were able to complete an unfamiliar route without additional instructions.

1211. ———. Three types of maps for blind travel. *Rehabilitation Teacher,* Feb. 1972, Vol. 4, No. 2, pp. 9–27.

Report of study of 1 static and 3 portable route maps used by 29 persons undergoing a 4-week training course with guide dogs. Portable maps were: Disc with braille information, tape cassette, and memory. Static map used to instruct subjects in use of the portable maps.

1212. Mandola, John. A theoretical approach to graphic aids for the blind. *International Journal for the Education of the Blind*, Mar. 1968, Vol. 18, No. 1, pp. 20–24.

After describing graphic aids for the blind, points out perceptual problems in models and similar aids and the many assumptions in their use, assumptions unsupported by research. Urges continued investigation of the value of using such models.

1213. Morris, June E., & Nolan, Carson Y. Minimum sizes for areal type tactual symbols. *International Journal for the Education of the Blind*, Dec. 1963, Vol. 13, No. 2, pp. 48–51.

Minimum outer dimensions were established for 7 discrete areal type tactual symbols reproduced in vacuum-formed plastic. Grade differences were found in students' ability to recognize symbols as dimensions diminished.

1214. Mumford, D. O. The Leicester map project. *New Beacon*, Sept. 1972, Vol. 56, No. 665, pp. 231–33.

Discusses tactual maps and their use in mobility. The following information should be on a useful map: Distinction between side and main roads, dual carriageways, zebra crossings, traffic light intersections, roundabouts, churches, public parks, schools, and bus terminals.

1215. Nolan, Carson Y. Relative legibility of raised and incised tactual figures. *Education of the Visually Handicapped*, May 1971, Vol. 3, No. 2, pp. 33–36.

Sixty-nine braille readers in grades 4–12 were used in a study to determine if legibility and figure quality of incised symbols differ from the qualities of raised symbols. Conclusion was that use of incised figures in tactual nonverbal displays seriously slows down reading speed and should be avoided.

1216. Nolan, Carson Y., & Morris, June E. *Improvement of tactual symbols for blind children. Final report.* Louisville, Ky.: American Printing House for the Blind, 1971, 88 pp.

Reports pair-comparison studies of elements in maps and their effective application in actual maps. Legibility, map design, and map user training are closely interrelated and play critical roles in the blind person's ability to use tactual maps.

1217. Report of meeting on embossed maps. *Teacher of the Blind*, Apr. 1972, Vol. 60, No. 3, pp. 110–16.

Summary of a meeting re improved methods of producing maps and diagrams, including the flexibility made possible by the Thermoform machine.

1218. Rosenberg, Frances. How to do raised-line drawings. *California Transcriber*, Fall 1974, Vol. 16, No. 3, 8 pp.

1219. Schiff, William; Kaufer, Lane; & Mosak, Sandra. Informative tactile stimuli in the perception of direction. *American Foundation for the Blind Research Bulletin 14*, Mar. 1967, pp. 65–94, illus. Also in *Perceptual and Motor Skills*, 1966.

Reports 3 experiments using a new directional symbol. As diagrams became more complex, the new symbol was more efficient and preferred.

1220. Sherman, John C. Maps the blind can see. *Journal of Geography,* Sept. 1955.

Describes the goals for a research program related to improved maps for the blind.

1221. ———. Needs and resources in maps for the blind. *New Outlook for the Blind,* Apr. 1965, Vol. 59, No. 4, pp. 130–34. Reprinted from *Surveying and Mapping,* Dec. 1964.

Lists a few of the varied maps needed by blind people and difficulties in producing them. Pressing needs are maps for nonbraille readers, and more research.

1222. Wiedel, Joseph W. *Development and standardization of symbols and improvements in the design of tactual illustrations for the blind.* College Park: Univ. of Md., Dept. of Geography, July 1967, 20 pp.

Reports on the results of a pilot study dealing with the design of large-scale mobility maps that can be reproduced in substantial quantity at modest cost. Three methods evaluated in the study—Thermoform, silk screening, and thermocraft.

1223. ———. Tactual maps for the visually handicapped: Some developmental problems. *New Outlook for the Blind,* Mar. 1969, Vol. 63, No. 3, pp. 80–88.

With illustrations, describes studies of maps and, especially, map symbols. Symbols should be at a minimum, clearly keyed, and highly contrasting.

1224. Wiedel, Joseph W., & Groves, Paul A. Designing and producing tactual maps for the visually handicapped. *New Outlook for the Blind,* Sept. 1969, Vol. 63, No. 7, pp. 196–201, illus.

Discusses planned research on design and production of large-scale maps meeting certain guidelines.

1225. ———. *Tactual mapping: Design, reproduction, reading and interpretation.* College Park: Univ. of Md., 1972, 116 pp., app., $2.50.

Report on findings of a research project conducted to design easily reproduced large-scale maps for use by the blind. Bib.

11. Higher Education and Follow-up of Students

1226. Adair, Elly. Mobility, physical education and the total academic experience of the blind college student. *Rehabilitation Teacher*, June 1974, Vol. 6, No. 6, pp. 15–23.

Discussion by a peripatologist of the many special problems faced by the blind college student.

1227. Ark. Enterprises for the Blind. *College preparation of blind prospective college students: Final report.* Little Rock: Author, 1967, 108 pp., illus.

Two groups of college-bound blind students were studied—1 group given 10 weeks of precollege preparation. Follow-up indicated positive results, although degree was not always great. Recommendations for future and implications for guidance personnel in colleges.

1228. Asenjo, J. Albert, & Axelrod, Seymour. A survey of vocational objectives of blind college students in the U.S. *New Outlook for the Blind*, Jan. 1957, Vol. 51, No. 1, pp. 9–16.

Summarizes information gathered via questionnaires from 493 blind college students about their vocational objectives. Since 30% had chosen teaching, data was also collected concerning opportunities for employment as teachers for blind persons.

1229. Ashcraft, Carolyn. An inquiry into attitudes of college students toward the blind. *International Journal for the Education of the Blind*, May 1966, Vol. 15, No. 4, pp. 114–16.

An attitude scale was given to 41 sighted students in a college guidance course. A generally positive attitude prevailed.

1230. Buell, Josephine. Rehabilitation status of former students of the California School for the Blind. *New Outlook for the Blind*, May 1955, Vol. 49, No. 5, pp. 169–73.

Analyzes the employment or other status of 199 former pupils of the school. Interprets some implications of results. Tables.

1231. ———. Employment status of former pupils of the California School for the Blind. *Exceptional Children*, 1956, Vol. 23, pp. 102–3.

Study shows that over a 25-year period (1927–51) of the 77% of the graduates studied, 75% were gainfully employed although nearly 25% of this group were working in subsidized occupations.

1232. Carter, Burnham. How to use educational recordings effectively—A survey of blind college students. *New Outlook for the Blind*, Nov. 1962, Vol. 56, No. 9, pp. 332–34.

Reports findings of survey done to assist preparation of manual for blind college students and to discover how/if they could compete with sighted peers. Includes information on students' characteristics, study methods, reading practices, materials used, social participation.

1233. Condon, Margaret E. Blind college students in New York State. *New Outlook for the Blind*, June 1961, Vol. 55, No. 6, pp. 211–15.

Detailed discussion of requirements and facilities for blind college students at N.Y. State Colleges. Specific mention of certain schools and number of blind students.

1234. Cripwell, Tessa. Open to all. *New Beacon*, Dec. 1975, Vol. 59, No. 704, pp. 316–17.

An encouraging account of study at the Open Univ., a correspondence program with one week of summer school on campus.

1235. Fitting, Edward A. Rehabilitation status of former students at the Michigan School for the Blind. *New Outlook for the Blind*, Jan. 1955, Vol. 49, No. 1, pp. 21–26.

Gives results of a follow-up of 60 graduates and 24 nongraduates of the Michigan School for the Blind, reporting chiefly in 3 areas: Marital status, social adjustment, and vocational adjustment.

1236. Gust, Tim, et al., Comp. *References concerning administrative, attitudinal and architectural access to higher education for the handicapped, Vol. 3, No. 8.* Pittsburgh, Pa.: Univ. of Pittsburgh, 1969, 12 pp.

Lists 94 references concerning administrative and attitudinal aspects and 87 concerning architectural design for the handicapped.

1237. Hull, Vernon. A pre-college conference for blind students. *International Journal for the Education of the Blind*, Oct. 1962, Vol. 12, No. 1, pp. 27–28.

An early model for pre-college evaluation and orientation conferences, what they include and how they are managed.

1238. Kumpe, Roy. Preparation of blind prospective college students. *International Journal for the Education of the Blind*, Oct. 1968, Vol. 18, No. 3, pp. 79–81.

Summarizes a project to demonstrate value of additional preparation of blind high school graduates before entering college.

1239. ———. College preparation of blind prospective college students. *New Outlook for the Blind*, Nov. 1968, Vol. 62, No. 9, pp. 286–88.

Based on research sample of 102 *S*s divided into experimental and control groups, shows that precollege training program has value.

1240. Leavitt, Glenn. Time, money, and students with visual limitations. *New Outlook for the Blind*, Oct. 1971, Vol. 65, No. 8, pp. 271–75.

Suggestions made for ways visually handicapped college students can improve their methods of study and increase their learning efficiency.

1241. McGill, William O., & Frish, Edith. Helping blind students to prepare for college. *New Outlook for the Blind*, June 1960, Vol. 54, No. 6, pp. 219–21.

Describes a college preparatory program run by the Chicago Lighthouse for the Blind in the summer of 1959 which dealt with adjustments necessary for all students entering college and special adjustments perhaps necessary for the blind student. Main areas of concern were: Understanding college procedures, practice in effective study methods, personal-social development.

1242. Mahan, Guy H. Special provisions for handicapped students in colleges. *Exceptional Children*, Sept. 1974, Vol. 41, No. 1, pp. 51–53.

Responses of 994 4-year colleges re admission policies and facilities for handicapped students, including blind. Handicapped students were accepted by about 75%, of which 25% had special facilities. Suggests how handicapped can increase chances of college success and how college policies and facilities might be improved for the handicapped.

1243. Massey, B. C.; Selby, James; Draper, Tom; et al. Experiences at college: The joys and difficulties encountered. In American Assoc. of Workers for the Blind, *Blindness 1971*. Washington, D.C.: Author, 1971, pp. 95–119.

A series of short papers by college students covering precollege background, undergraduate days, specific effects of blindness, communication problems and solutions, and a summary of the experiences of 1 student.

1244. Potts, Philip C. The story of AFB scholarships. *New Outlook for the Blind*, Mar. 1959, Vol. 53, No. 3, pp. 104–7.

Brief history of AFB scholarships, beginning in 1925, characteristics of students served, their current employment status, and some accomplishments of program.

1245. Prisuta, Richard. *A follow-up study of auditorially, visually, and orthopedically handicapped pupils in Cincinnati.* Pittsburgh, Pa.: Pittsburgh Univ., 1970, 137 pp.

Investigation for use in future educational planning for handicapped children. Includes aurally, visually, and physically handicapped public school graduates. Findings show the majority of the handicapped pupils capable of successful occupational adjustment to unskilled and semiskilled jobs; however, impractical school experiences were not marketable enough to provide economic stability.

1246. Rawls, Rachel F., & Rawls, Horace D. *A study of the visually handicapped graduates of the Governor Morehead School.* Raleigh, N.C.: Governor Morehead School, 1968, 80 pp., app., illus.

Assesses social adjustment of graduates in order to evaluate philosophy and programs of school.

1247. Reed, Alice E., & Cantoni, Louis J. Employment status of handicapped college graduates. *New Outlook for the Blind*, Nov. 1966, Vol. 60, No. 9, pp. 266–68.

Report on a study of employment status of 53 disabled graduates (9 blind).

1248. Rossi, Peter, Jr., & Fagan, John. A summer program for college bound students. *Education of the Visually Handicapped*, May 1974, Vol. 6, No. 2, pp. 44–48.

Describes 1-month residential summer program for visually handicapped high school students, providing precollege preparation and experience on an actual campus. Elaborates on some of the program courses. Notes benefits, counseling activities, informal evaluation potential.

1249. Rusalem, Herbert. The importance of an occupational choice in the college adjustment of blind students. *International Journal for the Education of the Blind*, Dec. 1961, Vol. 11, No. 2, pp. 33–36.

The blind student who has made realistic vocational decisions by the time he enters college will feel less distraction, more direction in his studies, better decision-making at crucial college choice points, and a more favorable relationship with his state rehabilitation agency.

1250. ———. *Guiding the physically handicapped college student.* New York: Columbia Univ., 1962, T C Series in Special Education.

The ramifications of working with physically disabled college students, including blind and partially sighted, are explored. Suggests ways to improve service to them. Bib.

1251. Russell, Dojelo C. College preparation for blind students. *International Journal for the Education of the Blind*, Mar. 1964, Vol. 13, No. 3, pp. 79–84.

Detailed description of the 1963 summer course for the college bound at Southwest Rehabilitation Center for the Blind, and plans for the 1964 course.

1252. Scholl, Geraldine T.; Bauman, Mary K.; & Crissey, Marie S., Proj. Dirs. *Final report: A study of the vocational success of groups of the visually handicapped.* Ann Arbor: Univ. of Mich., Nov. 1969, xiv + 209 pp., app.

Purpose of project to examine factors that seem to contribute to vocational success. Findings showed a high percentage unemployed; those employed had annual income below median for general population and were in a narrow range of occupations. Variables showing statistical relationship to vocational success include IQ, sex, other disabilities, travel ability, and level of education.

1253. Shlensky, Ronald. Issues raised in group process with blind pre-college students. *Adolescence*, Winter 1972, Vol. 7, No. 28, pp. 427–34.

Describes a precollege preparatory course for blind students offered by a rehabilitative agency, especially the 1 hour a week of group work with a psychiatrist. Two groups comprised of about 8 *S*s met for 5–7 weeks. Issues raised by the *S*s are discussed under 2 categories: General, and blind-related. Universal nature of the problems is stressed.

1254. Smith, Clyde R. *An analysis of the effectiveness of a college preparatory program for the visually impaired.* Washington, D.C.: Rehabilitation Services Admin., HEW, 1969, 181 pp.

Tests administered to 27 participants in a 9-week summer program to determine its effectiveness. Results indicated that self-concept was a significant variable in discriminating between the 2 groups and in predicting students likely to persist through the freshman year. Attrition greatest among the 18 controls.

1255. ———. A look at a college orientation program for the visually impaired. *Education of the Visually Handicapped*, Dec. 1970, Vol. 2, No. 4, pp. 116–20.

The college preparatory program at Arkansas Enterprises for the Blind is examined. The 9-week summer course is designed to help the high school graduate solve the personal, social, and academic problems he will encounter as a college student. Includes academic instruction, orientation and mobility, techniques of daily living, communicative skills, social skills, and counseling.

1256. ———. The relationship between self-concept and success in the freshman year of college. *New Outlook for the Blind*, Mar. 1972, Vol. 66, No. 3, pp. 84–89.

Through use of the Tennessee Self-Concept Scale and a semantic differential scale, 45 students entering their freshman year in college were tested. Results showed "nonpersisting" students have poor psychological defenses, are more confused in their self perceptions, have lower self-esteem, have a more inconsistent self-concept, have more defenses, show more deviant or maladjusted tendencies, and have low personality integration scores.

1257. Snider, Harold. A reading room for visually-handicapped students. *New Beacon*, Jan. 1974, Vol. 58, No. 681, pp. 10–13.

The author, a blind graduate student at Oxford Univ. in Great Britain, describes design and implementation of the reading room: Publicizing the need of blind individuals at the university level, raising funds, supervising construction.

1258. Spungin, Susan J., Ed. *Precollege programs for blind and visually handicapped students.* New York: AFB, 1975, 30 pp.

Informative articles on preparation for integration into college community. Topics include: Precollege programs and curriculum, psychosocial evaluation, and independent living.

1259. Stocker, Claudell S. This is the way we do it in Kansas. *Rehabilitation Teacher*, Oct. 1974, Vol. 6, No. 10, pp. 11–21.

History and description of the college preparatory program at the Kansas Rehabilitation Center for the Blind.

1260. Stromer, Walter F. College professors' reactions to blind students. *New Outlook for the Blind*, June 1968, Vol. 62, No. 6, pp. 192–95.

Summarizes responses of 25 college professors to a questionnaire about problems they might have had with blind students and the degree of responsibility shown by blind students for getting help as needed.

1261. Thiele, H. W. The occupational achievements of a group of blind persons. *Occupational Psychology*, Jan. 1954, Vol. 28, pp. 40–56.

A survey of the achievements of 219 *S*s indicates wider range of employment than had been supposed. Suggestions for increasing this range. Summary of Ph.D. thesis at Univ. of London.

12. Teachers and Other Staff, Their Training, Handbooks, etc.

1262. Abel, Georgie Lee. *Resources for teachers of blind with sighted children.* New York: AFB, 1954, 58 pp., app.

Manual of resources and equipment for use of teachers in public schools.

1263. ———. Teachers of blind children seek professional improvement. *New Outlook for the Blind,* Nov. 1955, Vol. 49, No. 9, pp. 333–38.

The content and popularity of summer courses shows the great interest of teachers in professional improvement.

1264. ———. Professional education for teachers of the visually handicapped in a teacher education center. *International Journal for the Education of the Blind,* May 1962, Vol. 11, No. 4, pp. 105–12.

How standards set by professional organizations, conferences, and governmental influence helped to develop high quality training programs for teachers of the visually handicapped.

1265. ———, **Comp.** *Resources for teachers of blind with sighted children,* rev. ed. New York: AFB, 1957, 58 pp.

1266. American Assoc. of Instructors of the Blind. *The houseparent in a school for the blind.* Philadelphia: Author, 1958, 119 pp.

A compilation of lectures and discussions during a 2-week institute at North Carolina School for the Blind. Discusses in detail the role, functions, and kinds of information needed by the houseparent.

1267. ———. *Report on the Midwest Administrators Workshop on Houseparents, March 2–5, 1960.* St. Louis, Mo.: Author, 1960, 258 pp.

Reports in detail papers and discussions on all aspects of the houseparent's role.

1268. American Association of Instructors of the Blind & American Foundation for the Blind. *An institute for houseparents of visually handicapped children: Proceedings.* New York: AFB, 1957. Mimeo.

A large collection of papers and summaries of papers presented at Washington Univ., St. Louis, Mo., July 8–19, 1957. Topics include role and qualifications of the houseparent, information about the development of children, and special problems with the blind child.

1269. Anderson, Robert M., Comp. & Ed. *Proceedings of the first Conference on Professional Laboratory Experiences in Special Education (Normal, Illinois, May 9–10, 1969).* Normal: Ill. State Univ., Nov. 1969, 43 pp.

Includes group discussions on visually handicapped children and a summary of the university student-teaching program.

1270. Andrews, Francis M. The housemother. *International Journal for the Education of the Blind*, May 1957, Vol. 6, No. 4, pp. 98–99.

The housemother is one of the most important staff in the residential school. Her long and busy day described, her many and varied responsibilities.

1271. Arensman, Dorothy. The role of the teacher for visually handicapped in vision assessment. *Education of the Visually Handicapped*, Mar. 1975, Vol. 7, No. 1, pp. 5–8.

Identifies procedures and materials helpful to teacher in such assessment, with explanation of suggested report form.

1272. Ashcroft, Samuel C.; Harley, Randall K.; & Hart, Verna. Development of leadership personnel in visually handicapped. *Education of the Visually Handicapped*, Dec. 1971, Vol. 3, No. 4, pp. 109–10.

Summarizes conclusions regarding training professionals to work with the visually handicapped. Suggests reexamination of degree levels and personnel needs. Recommends cooperation in research, between staffs of agencies and through consulting teams.

1273. Ashcroft, Samuel C., & Henderson, Freda. *Programmed instruction in braille.* Pittsburgh, Pa.: Stanwix House, 1963, 358 pp.

An easy means for sighted teachers to master braille through small sequential increments which develop simultaneous reading and writing skills. Self-tests are provided.

1274. Aylor, Kay E. Seeing better with blindfolds. *American Education,* May 1972, Vol. 8, No. 4, pp. 35–38, illus.

As part of a new teachers program at the Univ. of N. Colorado, students are required to use a blindfold in a variety of situations and environments. Graduates of the program will be "dual competency teachers for the blind," qualified to teach mobility skills as well as academic subjects.

1275. Barlow, Merrill M. Houseparent not housekeeper. *International Journal for the Education of the Blind*, Dec. 1955, Vol. 5, No. 2, pp. 41–43.

How houseparents may advance their professional abilities and services while retaining sympathy and understanding for the children in their care. Suggests helpful reading material.

1276. Blessing, Kenneth R., Ed. *The role of resource consultant in special education.* Washington, D.C.: Council for Exceptional Children, 1968, 131 pp.

After an overview by the editor, 8 positional papers consider the resource consultant's role in various special education areas including 2 contributions in the area of the visually impaired.

1277. Bourgeault, Stanley E. Self-imposed limitations in creative teaching. *International Journal for the Education of the Blind*, May 1963, Vol. 12, No. 4, pp. 115–16.

How can we create a climate in which the creative capacities of all teachers can be released? Factors favoring rigidity are: Strict adherence to certain techniques of materials presentation, "pet" techniques, too quick casting aside of techniques that fail, idealizing objectives, and stereotyping children.

1278. Bowers, Robert A. Some considerations for future teacher preparation. *New Outlook for the Blind*, Dec. 1963, Vol. 57, No. 10, pp. 384–88.

Suggests 8 needs in future teacher preparation for consideration and discusses each.

1279. Briggs, Beverly M. High school speech assistants in a residential school for the blind. *Education of the Visually Handicapped*, Dec. 1974, Vol. 6, No. 4, pp. 119–24.

Pros and cons of using high school students to assist with younger children. Training of assistants must be adequate. Then program can benefit both assistant and younger student.

1280. Cauffman, Josef. So you want to teach the blind. *International Journal for the Education of the Blind*, Dec. 1954, Vol. 4, No. 2, pp. 28–29.

Author looks beyond formal qualifications and certifications of teacher. His first requisite is love of children, giving security and understanding. Notes differences between sentimentality and love.

1281. College of Teachers of the Blind. *Handbook for school teachers of the blind*. Bristol, England: Author, 1961, 284 pp.

After a lengthy discussion of the psychology of blindness, gives specific suggestions for dealing with children of various ages in basic and special studies. Chapters on history and legislation, the eye, and apparatus.

1282. Council for Exceptional Children. *Special education: Teacher education directory, 1968–1969*. Washington, D.C.: Author, 1969, 104 pp.

A resource for the Council for Exceptional Children provides knowledge about programs and personnel in special education for students in the field, agencies, professionals, and to increase communication between professionals and the general public. Indexes list university programs, levels of study available, faculty biographical information, degrees or certification offered.

1283. Davis, Alice H.; Michelotti, Anna S.; & Coulson, John R. *Special services provided for the visually handicapped in Indiana County*. Indiana, Pa.: Indiana Co. Schools, 1970, 29 pp. Mimeo.

Handbook for administrators and teachers of children who might be considered visually handicapped. Purposes: To alert staff to the various diseases, handicaps, and behaviors; to explain program objectives; to describe services available in Indiana Co.; and to assemble general information associated with the program for the visually handicapped.

1284. Dunn, Lloyd M.; Geer, William C.; & Godwin, Winifred L. A look at the need for teachers of the blind in the south. *International Journal for the Education of the Blind*, May 1955, Vol. 4, No. 4, pp. 74–79.

Discusses 1954 study to determine shortage of trained educators for special education: Method of collecting information, growth of special education, prevalence of blindness, teachers in residential schools, supply and demand for teachers, salaries, recruitment, specialized preparation of teachers, training programs, summary of findings, recommendations.

1285. Farlow, J. The role of the houseparent. *Teacher of the Blind*, Oct. 1975, Vol. 63, No. 4, pp. 111–18.

Discusses skills needed by child care staff, problems in staff training, and proposes remedies.

1286. Frampton, M. E. A study of salary and wages. *International Journal for the Education of the Blind*, June 1954, Vol. 3, No. 4, pp. 262–65.

Summarizes findings of study of salaries and wages paid in 34 residential and 13 public schools in the U.S. Tables show initial salaries and increments, minimum, maximum, and type of employee—teachers, psychologists, kitchen help, laundresses, etc. Concludes there are wide differentials and cites need for some specialized personnel.

1287. Glass, Rowena. What, then, is a houseparent? *Florida School Herald*, May 1974, Vol. 73, No. 9, pp. 1–3.

A houseparent describes some of the problems she encounters and the variety of roles she fills as a dormitory teacher.

1288. Gorder, Genevieve, et al. *Instruction guide for teachers of the blind.* Seattle: Seattle Public Schools, Administrative and Service Center, 1968?, 33 pp.

Information on objectives, needs, classroom management (primary and intermediate) and course of study in addition to curricula information. Includes vocabulary of terms relating to the eye.

1289. Griggs, Norman J. Our obligations in teaching. *International Journal for the Education of the Blind*, Mar. 1955, Vol. 4, No. 3, pp. 55–57.

John Dewey's ideas on education: Learning is active, not passive, concerned with future as well as present life of child; child is seeker of experience. Educators of blind must supplement normal experiences. Teachers of blind must have humility, patience, justice, and truthfulness.

1290. Haynes, Roy. The role of a blind teacher. *International Journal for the Education of the Blind*, Dec. 1955, Vol. 5, No. 2, pp. 40–41.

Author suggests that blind teachers can help blind pupils meet problems realistically; parents and children often talk more easily with blind teachers than with sighted teachers. All positions cannot be filled satisfactorily by the totally blind; should be decided by given situation. Blind teachers' own accomplishments should help motivate pupils.

1291. Heisler, William T. Teacher training within a residential school program. *International Journal for the Education of the Blind*, May 1962, Vol. 11, No. 4, pp. 112–16.

Describes the general plan and content of a training program for teachers of the blind as organized cooperatively between a residential school and a university. Overseas students and training for teachers of the deaf-blind are included.

1292. Hill, Otter J. Classroom supervision. *International Journal for the Education of the Blind*, Feb. 1952, Vol. 1, No. 3, pp. 55–58.

Presents guidelines for supervision of classroom teachers and housemothers. Includes list to guide supervisors observations, suggestions on working relationships with those supervised, classroom visits and follow-up. Discusses administration ratings.

1293. The houseparent as a person. *International Journal for the Education of the Blind*, Mar. 1959, Vol. 8, No. 3, pp. 83–88.

This is the 1st chapter of a manual developed at an institute for houseparents. Describes the good houseparent in terms of emotional stability, emotional adaptability, spiritual balance, personal appearance, and education.

1294. Huff, Roger, et al. *Special problems, special solutions: Handbook for teachers of the visually handicapped.* Atlanta: Ga. State Dept. of Education, 1969, 51 pp.

Discusses definitions and standards of eligibility for the special education program, organization of the program, acquisition of special materials, the instructional materials reference centers, requirements for teacher certification, and job descriptions for all personnel.

1295. Ill. State Office of the Supt. of Public Instruction. *Special education teacher approval procedures.* Springfield: Dept. of Special Education, 1968, 32 pp.

Presents state's minimum training requirements for approval of school social workers and school psychologists and teachers in various areas including those of blind and partially sighted.

1296. Ind. Dept. of Public Instruction, Div. of Special Education. *A career for tomorrow . . . Special education.* Indianapolis: Author, 1967, 31 pp.

Presents summary of various special education careers, lists of Indiana colleges offering training for such careers, descriptions of characteristics and educational needs of those served by special education professionals. Provides photographic illus.

1297. Jones, John W. The professional preparation of educators of visually handicapped children before and after the start of federal grants. *International Journal for the Education of the Blind*, Oct. 1966, Vol. 16, No. 1, pp. 16–18.

Provides details of evidence that more educators are receiving professional preparation in more states, including preparation of teachers for the deaf-blind.

1298. Jones, Ulysses S.; Rasmussen, Emma; Woolly, J. M.; et al. The houseparent in the residential school. *New Outlook for the Blind*, June 1955, Vol. 49, No. 6, pp. 191–212.

Abstracts of papers from a symposium with the following titles: Our feelings concerning houseparents, the housemother and the institution team, teachers and parents—a joint responsibility, the houseparent's role in home-school relations, a school nurse looks at houseparents' problems, and selected bibliography.

1299. Kenmore, Jeanne R. Educating teachers for blind children. *New Outlook for the Blind*, May 1960, Vol. 54, No. 5, pp. 165–68.

Discusses early sources of teachers for the blind, in-service training and meetings, newer approaches and sources with related controversy on issues of teacher training. Discusses lack of national standards, and presents guidelines for selection of a teacher-training program.

1300. Ky. State Dept. of Education. *Proceedings of the State Conference for Teachers of Exceptional Children.* Frankfort, Ky.: Author, 1968, 107 pp.

Proceedings in Louisville, Ky. (Sheraton Hotel, Oct. 25–26), include addresses on the parents of the handicapped child, student evaluation in special education, and on total family involvement in the education of the handicapped. Group reports are provided on the visually handicapped.

1301. Kuhn, Judith. A comparison of teacher's attitudes toward blindness and exposure to blind children. *New Outlook for the Blind*, Dec. 1971, Vol. 65, No. 10, pp. 337–40.

Study sought to determine whether regular elementary school teachers working in a school with a resource room for blind children would indicate more positive attitudes toward blindness. Results indicated that the 2 groups of teachers did not differ significantly in their attitudes to blind children.

1302. Lydon, William T., & McGraw, M. Loretta. *Concept development for visually handicapped children: A resource guide for teachers and other professionals working in educational settings*, rev. ed. New York: AFB, 1973, 69 pp., $2.

Originally developed at Oak Hill School (Connecticut) for its own use, this revised edition contains a framework and suggestions for integrating concept development into the educational curriculum for blind children from kindergarten on.

1303. McDonald, Kay, et al. The blindfold experience. *Education of the Visually Handicapped*, Oct. 1973, Vol. 5, No. 3, pp. 84–86.

Twelve sighted advisors in a precollege orientation program for visually handicapped students wore blindfolds for mobility, equipment, and eating activities after which they showed significantly increased sensitivity and ability to work with the blind students.

1304. Mackie, Romaine P., & Dunn, Lloyd M. *Teachers of children who are blind*. Washington, D.C.: Govt. Printing Office, 1955, 109 pp.

Reports competencies and experiences needed by such teachers, including the results of a study of the opinions of teachers themselves.

1305. Manaster, Al; Pillar, Judith; Drell, Alice; et al. Training of non-clinical professionals in group therapy techniques. *New Outlook for the Blind*, Jan. 1967, Vol. 61, No. 1, pp. 16–20.

Procedures and values of training teaching staff to act as co-therapists.

1306. Mayadas, Nazneen S. Houseparents' expectations: A crucial variable in the performance of blind institutionalized children. *New Outlook for the Blind*, Feb. 1975, Vol. 69, No. 2, pp. 77–83, 85.

The author contends that it is of utmost importance that houseparents be selected carefully and receive continued training. They must become familiar with the world of the blind, and blind and sighted together must determine behavioral expectancies for the blind child. The expectations of "significant others" tend to shape performance.

1307. Miller, I. N. Development and preparation of teaching manuals. *New Outlook for the Blind*, Mar. 1964, Vol. 58, No. 3, pp. 73–75.

Various situations in which teaching manuals are needed and one agency's procedure in writing them.

1308. Napier, Grace D., & Weishahn, Mel W. *Handbook for teachers of the visually handicapped*. Washington, D.C.: Office of Education, HEW, 1970, 117 pp.

Designed to aid the inexperienced teacher. Includes discussion of acquisition of materials and services; suggestions for utilizing the services of a resource or itinerant teacher; techniques in the area of orientation and mobility; common visual impairments. Bib.

1309. N.Y. State School for the Blind. Improving contributions of houseparents to care, education and welfare of visually handicapped children and youth. Batavia, N.Y.: Author, 1973, 26 pp. Mimeo.

Summaries of presentations at a houseparent training conference, May 25–27, 1973. Topics include: Attitudes of houseparents, living skills program, social privileges, table manners, concept development, discipline, and staff interrelationships.

1310. Pelone, Anthony J. *Helping the visually handicapped child in a regular class.* New York: Teachers Col. Press, Columbia Univ., 1957, 99 pp., app., $1.75.

Practical information concerning regular class placement of partially sighted and blind children is presented. Includes discussion of eye conditions and resulting limitations and use of optical aids.

1311. Petrucci, Dorothy. All teachers of the blind should know braille. *International Journal for the Education of the Blind,* Oct. 1957, Vol. 7, No. 1, pp. 8–11.

Describes an in-service training class in braille for the teachers at the Iowa Braille and Sight-Saving School, and its benefits.

1312. Pierce, Esther I. An ambassador of good will. *International Journal for the Education of the Blind,* Mar. 1963, Vol. 12, No. 3, pp. 70–71.

The houseparent's functions described with emphasis on interpersonal relationships.

1313. Powers, W. R. Bootstrap pulling. *International Journal for the Education of the Blind,* Oct. 1960, Vol. 10, No. 1, pp. 13–16.

A houseparent responds to recommendations of the institute on houseparents held in St. Louis, summer 1957. Lists what houseparents expect of school administrators in terms of educational programs, rewards, improved working conditions, and recognition.

1314. Quigley, Helen, et al. *Instruction guide for teachers of the partially seeing.* Seattle: Seattle Public Schools, 1968, 31 pp.

Provides information on needs and characteristics, class organization, and course of study. Includes curriculum adaptations at the primary, intermediate, junior, and senior high school levels.

1315. Rawls, Rachel F., & Peeler, E. N. Pre-employment training for houseparents. *International Journal for the Education of the Blind,* Mar. 1967, Vol. 16, No. 3, pp. 83–87.

Describes a month-long pre-employment training program for houseparents under Bureau of Apprenticeship Training funding. Discusses staff, daily program, and costs.

1316. Riordan, Mary. *Teaching objectives for the itinerant resource teacher of visually limited students.* Phoenix, Ariz.: Creighton School Dist. #14, 1973, 19 pp.

The manual presents objectives and proficiency levels for the development of communication, living, and social skills for students from kindergarten through grade 12.

1317. Rocco, Joyce, & Rocco, Frank. Should houseparents assist in mobility training? *New Outlook for the Blind*, Nov. 1964, Vol. 58, No. 9, pp. 288–89.

Report of a workshop presented to houseparents to enable them to better assist students in mobility. Both presenters and houseparents were enthusiastic.

1318. The role of houseparents. *New Outlook for the Blind*, May 1954, Vol. 48, No. 5, pp. 161–62.

First regional houseparents' conference and its results.

1319. Scholl, Geraldine T. In-service education for houseparents. *New Outlook for the Blind*, Mar. 1956, Vol. 50, No. 3, pp. 84–87.

Describes the job content and conditions of the typical houseparent, prescribes training, and reports results of such training at Michigan School for the Blind.

1320. ———. *Teacher preparation for visually handicapped children: A look into the future.* Ann Arbor: Mich. Univ., 1967, 6 pp.

Reviews trends in visually impaired educational programming and the implications for teacher education. Considers the changing role of residential schools including possible roles as diagnostic and remedial treatment centers.

1321. Sowell, Mary H. A handbook for teachers in schools for the blind. *International Journal for the Education of the Blind*, Oct. 1956, Vol. 6, No. 1, pp. 2–4.

Addressed to the potential teacher of visually handicapped children, discusses need for positive attitude, special aspects of classroom preparation, expectations for pupil accomplishments, curriculum, and blindisms.

1322. Tenn. State Dept. of Education. *Proceedings of a Special Study Institute for Tennessee Educators of Visually Handicapped Pupils (Louisville, Kentucky, April 21–23, 1969).* Nashville: Author, 1969, 63 pp.

Presents the proceedings of Institute held to provide public day school personnel with an opportunity to study methods of locating, acquiring, and utilizing materials for visually handicapped students.

1323. Walker, Don L. The residential school as a student teaching center. *International Journal for the Education of the Blind*, Mar. 1961, Vol. 10, No. 3, pp. 70–73.

Describes how a cooperative arrangement between the Iowa Braille and Sight Saving School and Iowa State Teachers College made the residential school a laboratory for the professional education of public school teachers, with benefits to all involved.

1324. Washington, Pauline S. Reactions and observations of a teacher of visually handicapped children. *New Outlook for the Blind*, June 1963, Vol. 57, No. 6, pp. 195–97.

The teacher should share notes on her daily observation of students with other specialized members of the school's "team" for assistance with individual prognosis and curriculum planning, etc.

1325. Weishahn, Mel W. Study of graduates in the education of the visually disabled. *Exceptional Children*, Apr. 1972, Vol. 38, No. 8, pp. 605–12.

Results of questionnaire study of characteristics of graduates with masters degrees in education of visually disabled.

1326. Wilcox, Everett. Characteristics, training, and performance of house-parents. *International Journal for the Education of the Blind*, May 1959, Vol. 8, No. 4, pp. 117–25.

Gives results of a 1955 study to determine the nature of the house-parent's position on the institution staff, the administrative policy on selection and performance of houseparents, training available to houseparents, and characteristics of successful houseparents.

1327. Wooldridge, Lillian, et al. *Techniques for daily living: Curriculum guides.* Jacksonville: Ill. Braille and Sight Saving School, 1970, 205 pp.

Designed for cottage parents, provides guides and explicit directions for teaching wide range of daily living skills.

13. Factors in Vocational Choice and Vocational Training in General

1328. American Foundation for the Blind. *National conference on career education.* New York: Author, 1973, 42 pp., app. Mimeo.

Leaders in special education, rehabilitation, and vocational education from 10 states discuss career education for blind and visually handicapped in each state and develop individual plans of action. Includes "Some issues surrounding the state of the art in career education in general and particularly for blind and visually handicapped persons," by John E. Uxer.

1329. Arthur, Julietta K. *Employment for the handicapped; a guide for the disabled, their families, and their counselors.* Nashville: Abingdon Press, 1967, 272 pp.

Presents vocational information and advice on such topics as the nature of disability and its implications, sources of help, preparing to work, job opportunities. Provides names and addresses of resourceful organizations, agencies, periodicals, and other publications.

1330. Bast, Bernard A. A predictive study of employability among the visually impaired with the California Psychological Inventory. Ann Arbor: Univ. of Michigan, 1971, xiii + 150 pp. Dissertation.

Relates California Psychological Inventory to personality differences between groups of employed and unemployed blind. $Ss = 51$ visually impaired males employed full time for a min. of 2.8 years and 50 visually impaired males who were unemployed for at least 2.7 years. The results may provide a useful approach to employment prediction.

1331. Bauman, Mary K. Foundations for vocational choice in grades 1–9. *Education of the Visually Handicapped*, May 1971, Vol. 3, No. 2, pp. 40–45.

Discusses importance of gradual exposure of blind students to both concepts of job content and concepts of work habits and standards.

1332. ———. Guided vocational choice. *New Outlook for the Blind*, Oct. 1975, Vol. 69, No. 8, pp. 354–60.

Reviews the special attention which should be given to certain factors in client's history, tests and work samples which might be used in guidance and importance of experience. Closes with current state of the art summary. Ref.

1333. Borchert, Charles R. Blind trainees succeed in industry. *New Outlook for the Blind*, Feb. 1967, Vol. 61, No. 2, pp. 44–46. Reprinted from *Rehabilitation Record*, Sept.–Oct. 1966.

Briefly describes the process and success of vocational training of blind clients alongside sighted students in a trade-technical school.

1334. Buell, Charles. Vocational preparation of students. *New Outlook for the Blind,* Apr. 1954, Vol. 48, No. 4, pp. 113–18.

Results of a questionnaire sent to placement personnel in order to determine strengths and weaknesses of young blind people seeking employment.

1335. Burke, Edward H. Guidance needs of the visually handicapped. *International Journal for the Education of the Blind,* Oct. 1954, Vol. 4, No. 1, pp. 16–17.

Based on New York City experience, discusses individualized counseling, making teachers guidance conscious, articulation among various school levels, and the counselor as a liaison.

1336. ⸺. Symposium—Self-image: A guide to adjustment. Guidance re-examined. *New Outlook for the Blind,* Mar. 1961, Vol. 55, No. 3, pp. 97–98.

The role of the guidance counselor for the visually handicapped in public school. Works with child, parents, teachers, and other agencies.

1337. Cargill, Floyd. Careers conference in a residential school for the blind. *International Journal for the Education of the Blind,* Oct. 1957, Vol. 7, No. 1, pp. 26–30.

What a careers conference is and how to run it, including sample program, nature of speakers, and outline for occupational information.

1338. Carroll, Lillian R., & LaBarre, Alfred H. A cooperative vocational guidance course for visually impaired students-clients. *New Outlook for the Blind,* Apr. 1974, Vol. 68, No. 4, pp. 163–69. Also in *Florida School Herald,* Jan. 1974.

Describes course in daily living skills, job-hunting techniques, and explores literature on vocations. Bib.

1339. Chambers, Gerald. A work-study program at the Maryland School for the Blind. *International Journal for the Education of the Blind,* Dec. 1967, Vol. 17, No. 2, pp. 57–58.

A work program was initiated for youngsters unlikely to graduate and/or needing transition from classroom to job. Details how the program functioned and its results.

1340. Clark, Gary M. Problems in vocational rehabilitation of the visually handicapped. *New Outlook for the Blind,* Jan. 1966, Vol. 60, No. 1, pp. 22–27.

Discusses necessary prevocational adjustment and obstacles to it, problems in getting and holding a job, shortcomings of traditional preparatory programs, recommendations for meeting existing problems.

1341. Clayton, Isaac P. An expanded program in prevocational education at the Maryland School for the Blind. *Education of the Visually Handicapped,* Oct. 1971, Vol. 3, No. 3, pp. 80–81.

Brief description of program for academically below-average student.

1342. Coker, D. Gary. The development of a vocational program in a residential school for the visually handicapped. *New Outlook for the Blind,* Jan. 1974, Vol. 68, No. 1, pp. 25–28.

Discussion of vocational education programs based on experiences at the Tennessee School for the Blind which has an open-enrollment work experience program that is correlated with classroom work.

1343. Conn. Institute for the Blind. *Manual for a work-experience program.* Hartford: Author, 1970, 122 pp., app.

Detailed description of a comprehensive program of vocational rehabilitation services at the Oak Hill School.

1344. Crawford, Fred L. Occupational information and the school guidance program. *International Journal for the Education of the Blind*, Dec. 1963, Vol. 13, No. 2, pp. 45–47.

Both group and individual guidance are needed. Sources of occupational information, motivating students, and an outline of information students should seek about occupations are provided. Cooperation with vocational rehabilitation counselors is recommended.

1345. ———. *Career planning for the blind: A manual for students and teachers.* New York: Farrar, Straus, & Giroux, 1966, 189 pp.

The text includes information on careers, labor market, occupational choice, etc. A practical book.

1346. Dauwalder, Donald D. *Education, training, and employment of the blind.* Pittsburgh: W. Pa. School for Blind Children, 1966, 224 pp. + 23-pp. app.

With support of much tabular data, presents results of complex surveys of residential and day school programs, industrial arts and vocational education, employment, placement and guidance, and the status of high school graduates.

1347. Davis, Carl J. A contemporary guidance program. *New Outlook for the Blind*, Nov. 1957, Vol. 51, No. 9, pp. 416–18.

Describes the program at Perkins School, including staff functions and how individual needs are met.

1348. ———. Guidance and vocational counseling. *International Journal for the Education of the Blind*, Mar. 1958, Vol. 7, No. 3, pp. 78–83.

What constitutes a guidance program, how it functions, and how and why guidance is different in schools for the blind. Consultation with teachers, observation of the students over many years, building a realistic self-image in the students, and providing good occupational information are significant factors.

1349. ———, Ed. *Guidance programs for blind children: A report of a conference, April, 1959.* Watertown, Mass.: Perkins School for the Blind, 1959, 142 pp.

This record of the proceedings of the conference presents primary aspects of a guidance program with principles and procedures which could be applied to all blind pupils whether in residential schools or in day school situations.

1350. Derganc, Mildred. Summer high school program at the Lighthouse. *New Outlook for the Blind*, June 1964, Vol. 58, No. 6, pp. 185–87.

Description of a 4-week program of vocational evaluation for teenagers. Program is felt to be very worthwhile if properly staffed and planned.

1351. Ferson, Regis F. Vocational guidance at the Western Pennsylvania School. *New Outlook for the Blind*, Jan. 1955, Vol. 49, No. 1, pp. 6–15.

Objective, up-to-date occupational information is much needed, especially in braille. Audio-visual aids and relating the classroom to life should be added to formal guidance procedures. Social skills should be emphasized. Individual conferences, some use of alumni resources, and follow-up are vital. Ref.

1352. Finkle, Louis J. A work-study program for residential schools for the blind. *Education of the Visually Handicapped*, May 1971, Vol. 3, No. 2, pp. 52–54.

Possibility of using work-study concept in residential schools is discussed. Ways and means of efficiently implementing the program are considered.

1353. Hoskins, Len. Florida's industrial training laboratory for blind persons. *New Outlook for the Blind*, Mar. 1974, Vol. 68, No. 3, pp. 119–23.

Description of the course with examples of the specific kinds of training. The Laboratory has a Job Simulation Division and an Electronics Training Course which includes training in more than mechanical areas.

1354. Huber, Dennis J. Learn to earn: A school work-experience program. *New Outlook for the Blind*, May 1973, Vol. 67, No. 5, pp. 219–21.

Students at the Western Pennsylvania School for the Blind are provided part-time work experience in a sheltered workshop. Article includes guidelines by which the program is operating and the plans for modifying and improving it.

1355. Klinkhamer, George E. The implications of career education for visually handicapped students. *New Outlook for the Blind*, May 1973, Vol. 67, No. 5, pp. 207–9, 215.

Summary of the needs of handicapped persons for career education, the value of employment to the individual and to society, the role of federal funding, and possible approaches to career education. In conclusion stresses "need for mutual planning by all concerned agencies toward meeting the career education needs of visually handicapped students."

1356. McAulay, John H. *Vocational schools as training facilities for blind workers.* New York: AFB, 1954, 95 pp.

Provides basic information about offering vocational training to blind persons in general vocational schools.

1357. Md. School for the Blind. *A vocational education program for blind children and youth. Phase I final report.* Baltimore: Md. State Dept. of Education, Div. of Vocational-Technical Education, Aug. 1972, 73 pp.

Discusses a pilot program in response to survey findings of occupational opportunities and employment history of adults who attended the Maryland School. Provides results of 128 employer interviews identifying skills and visual abilities required for jobs in a variety of fields.

1358. Pumo, Benjamin J. Stepping back to get ahead in career planning. *New Outlook for the Blind*, Nov. 1968, Vol. 62, No. 9, pp. 277–81.

Describes Careers Unlimited program of Metropolitan Society for the Blind, Detroit. Tells how the program meets 3 goals: Dissemination of information, community involvement, and program development for the blind student in public school.

1359. ————. Prevention of vocational disabilities through comprehensive planning. *New Outlook for the Blind*, Feb. 1970, Vol. 64, No. 2, pp. 53–59.

Explores role of the vocational consultant, need for improved use of existing resources and the interdisciplinary approach, immediate and future demands which must be met, an occupational information center program, the conference held on Careers Unlimited, and vocational disability prevention.

1360. Raskin, Nathaniel J. *Vocational counseling of blind students.* New York: AFB, 1955, 24 pp.

Results of a questionnaire survey undertaken to evaluate existing vocational counseling procedures and the relationship between the school and the state rehabilitation agency.

1361. Routh, Thomas A. *Rehabilitation counseling of the blind.* Springfield, Ill.: Charles C Thomas, 1970, 85 pp.

The author advances some suggestions to rehabilitation counselors so that they may adequately assist blind persons in determining suitable, practical, and feasible vocational objectives.

1362. Russell, Gene H. *Evaluation document, a five-county vocational skills training program for the blind.* Santa Cruz, Calif.: Santa Cruz Co. Board of Education, 1972, 63 pp.

Evaluates inservice training of the regular instructors, and a 2-year program designed to encourage skill development of the students of junior high, secondary, and junior college level. Among 6 conclusions after evaluation is positive finding on integration of blind in regular programs. Nine recommendations.

1363. ————. *Project document, a five-county vocational skills training program for the blind.* Santa Cruz, Calif.: Santa Cruz Co. Board of Education, 1972, 180 pp.

Presents ideas, techniques, and written documents of a 3-year program, including technical and living skills and work experience, to provide vocational skills and counseling to blind students in grades 7–14. Includes 35 sample forms, lists of local resources utilized, and suggested equipment.

1364. Russell, Gene H., & Butler, David M. The Five-County Vocational Skills Training Program, 1970–1972. *New Outlook for the Blind*, Sept. 1973, Vol. 67, No. 7, pp. 301–8.

California students were integrated successfully in public school vocational programs with help of a skills specialist experienced in teaching the visually handicapped.

1365. Sevransky, Paul. The process of vocational development—Implitions for counseling male blind college students. *New Outlook for the Blind*, Dec. 1967, Vol. 61, No. 10, pp. 333–38.

After discussing the characteristics and reasons for vocational indecision and vocational immaturity in general, states that there is a high incidence of vocational immaturity in blind youth. Lists how rehabilitation should try to cope with this.

1366. Spurrier, Eugene. A work-study program for students in a residential school for the blind. *New Outlook for the Blind*, Dec. 1968, Vol. 62, No. 10, pp. 319–20.

Brief description of joint project of residential school, state agency, and private agency to provide work-study experience for academically slow students.

1367. Stubbins, Joseph, & Nall, Erika, Comps. *Workshops for the handicapped: An annotated bibliography, No. 5.* Los Angeles: Calif. State Col., 1968, 60 pp. (Avail. National Assoc. of Sheltered Workshops and Homebound Programs, Washington, D.C., $1.)

Lists 127 annotated references to work experience programs from July 1967–July 1968, and 22 references pertinent to standards and evaluation. Includes articles describing federal programs in actual workshops and those in schools and hospitals.

1368. Tremble, Judith T., & Campbell, Lawrence F. A diversified cooperative work-experience program for blind and multiply handicapped blind students. *New Outlook for the Blind*, May 1973, Vol. 67, No. 5, pp. 216–19.

A description of a program at Oak Hill School (Conn.) which provides both individualized classroom preparation for the world of work and carefully selected placements in part-time jobs on and off campus. Curriculum includes academic subjects, work skills development, training in specialty areas, and on-the-job services during the work experience phase.

1369. Urban, Stanley J., & Tsuji, Thomas, Eds. *The special needs student in vocational education: Selected readings.* New York: MSS Information Corp., 1974, 286 pp., $13 cloth, $7.50 paper.

Thirty-one articles treat various aspects of vocational education for the disadvantaged, including the visually handicapped, in this book of readings for graduate students, vocational educators, and teacher educators. Lists instructional materials centers and community resources for the handicapped.

1370. Uxer, John E. Career education and visually handicapped persons: Some issues surrounding the state of the art. *New Outlook for the Blind*, May 1973, Vol. 67, No. 5, pp. 200–206.

The philosophy of career education is contrasted with the specific program approaches used in implementing it. Presents an overview of national career education and highlights of Texas programs. Discusses problems in this field and urges development of effective life preparation and adjustment programs.

1371. Vedovatti, Philip G., & Wright, Charles. A work-experience program at the Montana School for the Deaf and Blind. *New Outlook for the Blind*, Dec. 1968, Vol. 62, No. 10, pp. 321–22.

Cooperation between the Montana School and the state agency provides a work-experience program for 5 visually handicapped boys. Practical reading, applied mathematics, social skills, shop courses and physical education are coordinated with jobs in the community.

1372. Viskant, Kathryn; Rex, Evelyn; & Livers, David. Vocational counseling of the visually handicapped in Illinois high schools. *New Outlook for the Blind*, Oct. 1969, Vol. 63, No. 8, pp. 251–54.

Questionnaires were sent to high school guidance counselors and special teachers to study vocational counseling services for the visually handicapped. Information received showed that visually handicapped students are treated the same as sighted classmates, but that counselors are not aware of positions open to the visually impaired.

1373. Weishan, Robert J. Toward involving the total community in career education. *New Outlook for the Blind*, Nov. 1973, Vol. 67, No. 9, pp. 415–19, 421, 423.

Through a PR program, each segment of the community—parents, businessmen and others—can be made aware of the roles it can play in a career education program including planning, decision-making, and helping to teach about jobs, life styles, and adult roles.

1374. Welsch, Rosemary A. Pre-vocational guidance and counseling of visually handicapped youth in the Chicago public schools. *New Outlook for the Blind*, Nov. 1966, Vol. 60, No. 9, pp. 279–82.

Gives background on guidance program development since 1913. Discusses program for high school students, efforts to promote students' prospective thinking about his place in the workaday world after graduation, etc.

1375. Woal, S. Theodore. A career education program for visually handicapped students. *Vocational Guidance Quarterly*, 1975, Vol. 23, No. 2, pp. 172–73.

Describes inclusion of visually handicapped students in program of self- and career-awareness for elementary level students. Braille transcriptions of career booklets, visits from employed individuals, and field trips to firms employing handicapped workers are part of the program.

1376. Wolfe, Eldon. A work experience program. *International Journal for the Education of the Blind*, Oct. 1958, Vol. 8, No. 1, pp. 32–34.

To meet the needs of students who need concrete learning experiences, the Michigan School for the Blind developed a work experience program chiefly centering in work at the school. From this students learned skills they could use at home, and student attitudes were greatly benefited.

1377. Wolfe, Harvey E. Career education: A new dimension in education for living. *New Outlook for the Blind*, May 1973, Vol. 67, No. 5, pp. 193–99.

Discussion of recommendations of the National Advisory Council on Vocational Education, the goals established by the U.S. Office of Education and the efforts of AFB's National Task Force on Career Education. Description of 4 career education models—school-based, employer-based, home community-based, and residential-based.

1378. Working party for the partially sighted. The partially-sighted school leaver (Report). *Teacher of the Blind*, Autumn 1974, Vol. 62, No. 1, pp. 9–16.

Discussion of careers education program in England, and the feeling that there should be more provision specifically for the partially sighted. Statistics for 285 school leavers show the numbers entering 30 different occupations and 5 categories of further education.

1379. Wurster, Marion V. Career education in 1975. *New Outlook for the Blind*, Apr. 1975, Vol. 69, No. 4, pp. 155–59.

Discusses what is happening to insure that blind and visually handicapped students have equal access to the growing literature on learning about and preparing for the world of work, with focus on efforts of Ohio State Univ., the State of Texas, and AFB.

1380. Young, Earl B., Ed. *Vocational education for handicapped persons: Handbook for program implementation.* Washington, D.C.: Office of Education, HEW, 1969, 131 pp.

Discusses considerations in planning vocational education for the hearing impaired, visually impaired, and physically handicapped.

14. Rehabilitation: General

1381. Andrews, Francis M. Rehabilitation and schools for the blind. *New Outlook for the Blind*, Feb. 1955, Vol. 49, No. 2, pp. 53–55.

Relates the work of the State Dept. of Rehabilitation (Md.) to students and graduates of the residential school. Gives some follow-up figures and concludes that the rather successful record would not have been possible without cooperation between school and Dept. of Vocational Rehabilitation.

1382. Branscombe, Martha. The changing role of non-governmental organizations in planning rehabilitation programs. *New Outlook for the Blind*, Jan. 1965, Vol. 59, No. 1, pp. 13–14.

Points out the change from local rehabilitation services to the international interests and efforts of such nongovernmental organizations as American Foundation for Overseas Blind and Royal Commonwealth Society for the Blind. Suggests 5 special roles such organizations might play.

1383. Carnes, G. D.; Hansen, Carl E.; & Parker, Randall M., Eds. *Readings in rehabilitation of the blind client. Conference proceedings: Vocational planning for the blind client.* Austin: Univ. of Tex., 1971, 121 pp.

Collection of papers presented to provide essential information for new counselors in state commissions for the blind and generate a planning orientation to their rehabilitation efforts.

1384. Carroll, Thomas. Rehabilitation of the visually impaired. *Optometric Weekly*, July 1974, Vol. 65, No. 25, pp. 644–49.

Identifies 6 areas of research need including areas of nonophthalmic medical aspects, devices to improve mobility. Makes 8 recommendations and suggestions to the National Institute of Neurological Diseases and Blindness.

1385. Cull, John G., & Hardy, Richard E., Eds. *Rehabilitation techniques in severe disability: Case studies.* Springfield, Ill.: Charles C Thomas, 1974, 238 pp., $10.75.

Presents 14 readings as resource data for rehabilitation classes and new personnel in rehabilitation programs to promote relevant discussion. Discussion questions and suggested readings follow each section. Included among case studies are several on visual impairment, diabetes, diabetes with blindness.

1386. Daum, Henry. Rehabilitation teamwork: Public welfare and community resources. *New Outlook for the Blind*, Feb. 1958, Vol. 52, No. 2, pp. 43–49.

Discusses agency cooperation to provide the blind client with a fuller life, more self-sufficiency, and improved adjustment.

1387. Dishart, Martin. Family adjustment in the rehabilitation plan. *New Outlook for the Blind*, Nov. 1964, Vol. 58, No. 9, pp. 292–94. Reprinted from *Journal of Rehabilitation*, Jan.–Feb. 1964.

Discusses positive aspects of teaching a disabled client the best ways to put other people at ease and how to perceive and accept their feelings about his disability.

1388. Gallagher, William F. The challenge of change—Piecemeal versus total rehabilitation. *New Outlook for the Blind*, Feb. 1964, Vol. 58, No. 2, pp. 33–35.

Author views rehabilitation as a total effort divided into 4 major stages: Physical, social, emotional, and vocational. The important goals of each stage are discussed.

1389. Gorthy, Willis C. Rehabilitation—a state responsibility. *New Outlook for the Blind*, Dec. 1955, Vol. 49, No. 10, pp. 356–63.

Increased funding from the government calls for more sound philosophy, study of the needs of the handicapped, and better planning. Outlines the elements in an adequate state plan for rehabilitation.

1390. Gruber, Kathern F., & Voorhees, Arthur L., Eds. *The Grove Park Report: Principles underlying nonmedical vocational and rehabilitation preparation services for blind persons.* New York: AFB, 1961, 40 pp., $2.

An outgrowth of a conference in 1960, this book sets forth principles for personal adjustment training, prevocational training, vocational training, training of vending stand operators, training for transcribing machine operators, and homemaking.

1391. Hood, Clare. Gathering, screening, and interpreting medical information. *New Outlook for the Blind*, Mar. 1965, Vol. 59, No. 3, pp. 95–97.

Why an agency needs and how it should use careful analysis of medical and ophthalmological information about each client.

1392. Hunt, Joseph. Impact and potential of rehabilitation. *New Outlook for the Blind*, Oct. 1959, Vol. 53, No. 8, pp. 275–80.

On the basis of both earnings and the observed confidence and well-being of blind people, states the gains made through rehabilitation over the years. Lists goals for the future with suggestions on reaching them.

1393. Knowles, Lyle. Successful and unsuccessful rehabilitation of the legally blind. *New Outlook for the Blind*, May 1969, Vol. 63, No. 5, pp. 129–36.

On the basis of rehabilitation agency records, 245 successful and 210 unsuccessful blind clients were compared on a series of personal characteristics. Statistical data shows the relative importance of these characteristics to rehabilitation.

1394. McPhee, William M., & Magleby, F. LeGrande. Vocational rehabilitation in Montana. *New Outlook for the Blind*, Sept. 1961, Vol. 55, No. 7, pp. 259–64.

The vocational adjustment of clients termed rehabilitated and non-rehabilitated are compared. Factors which influenced successful vocational adjustment are brought out.

1395. MacFarland, Douglas C. The blind and the visually impaired. In James F. Garrett & Edna S. Levine, Eds., *Rehabilitation practices with the physically disabled.* New York: Columbia Univ. Press, 1973, pp. 433–60.

After brief demographic and historical sections, reviews the special rehabilitation needs and services to satisfy those needs.

1396. Magers, George. A sequential plan for services. *New Outlook for the Blind,* Dec. 1961, Vol. 55, No. 10, pp. 355–59.

Detailed plan for working with visually handicapped as outlined and implemented by State of Nevada over a period of several years. Use of referral and contractual services in sequence.

1397. Muldoon, John F. Work and motivation of the difficult blind client. *New Outlook for the Blind,* Jan. 1967, Vol. 61, No. 1, pp. 21–29.

There are 3 major obstacles to rehabilitation of difficult blind clients: Client-centered, counselor-centered, and community-centered. Suggests theoretical backgrounds and solutions. Ref.

1398. Platt, Philip S. Ten years of cooperative rehabilitation activities—operations and results. *New Outlook for the Blind,* Oct. 1957, Vol. 51, No. 8, pp. 357–63.

Detailed analysis of data on 501 trainees sent to the Lighthouse, New York City, for evaluation, prevocational, and vocational training services. Lists some of the benefits to the blind people served.

1399. Rabinoff, George W. Coordination of education with welfare and medical services. *New Outlook for the Blind,* May 1964, Vol. 58, No. 5, pp. 146–49.

History of, goals for, and means of rehabilitation. Need for education about physically handicapped on several fronts.

1400. Rambo, Douglas. Adult education classes for blind and visually handicapped prison inmates. *New Outlook for the Blind,* Nov. 1972, Vol. 66, No. 9, pp. 303–6.

A description of the classes provided for blind and partially sighted inmates at the Main Tennessee State Penitentiary and the volunteer program there for large-print typing, tape recording, and brailling of educational materials for blind persons in the state.

1401. Reid, Ellen. *Factors influencing vocational rehabilitation of the blind.* New York: AFB, Oct. 1960, 238 pp., $3.

Study describes rules, policies, and procedures of a state commission for the blind; seeks ways to identify factors affecting rehabilitation success and to alter unfavorable factors during rehabilitation; and seeks ways to identify and fill the unmet needs of blind clients.

1402. Robinson, Robert L. The blinded veteran of the Vietnam War: A profile. *New Outlook for the Blind,* Nov. 1971, Vol. 65, No. 9, pp. 287–90.

Discusses the problems of the newly blinded, and often multiply handicapped, Vietnam veteran. The role of the Blinded Veterans Assoc. as a possible motivating force is mentioned.

1403. Rusalem, Herbert. *Coping with the unseen environment: An introduction to the vocational rehabilitation of blind persons.* New York: Teachers' Col. Press, 1972, xi + 361 pp., $11.50.

Written about the seriously visually handicapped person; discusses vocational aptitude, interests, counseling, education, rehabilitation, and schools for the visually handicapped. Addressed to rehabilitation workers who have minimal preparation and experience in working with the blind.

1404. Smith, Geoffrey. The role of workshops. *New Beacon*, Feb. 1973, Vol. 57, No. 670, pp. 30–31.

With the postwar trend toward integration of the blind, what philosophy should be held by and on segregated/sheltered workshops? Suggestions.

1405. Thomas, Robert E. The main stream of rehabilitation. *New Outlook for the Blind*, Mar. 1962, Vol. 56, No. 3, pp. 77–81.

Briefly discusses history of rehabilitation from 1920 to 1962, professional training of rehabilitation workers, public relations, the home teacher's role, and implications of vocational rehabilitation.

1406. U.S. Dept. of Health, Education & Welfare. *A study of factors affecting the social and psychological integration of the blind into the normal working environment. Final report on Social and Rehabilitation Service: Project 19–P–58386–F.* Washington, D.C.: Author, 1971, 291 pp., app.

Conclusions based on study of 6 major factors: (1) fundamentals of rehabilitation, (2) education of the blind, (3) vocational rehabilitation of the blind in general and their employment, (4) vocational rehabilitation of specific groups of the blind, (5) preparation of sighted working environment to accept blind worker, and (6) aid to employed blind persons in their family social life. Bib.

1407. Upshaw, McAllister. The community and its agency. *New Outlook for the Blind*, June 1961, Vol. 55, No. 6, pp. 191–98.

Very comprehensive overview of need for and work of rehabilitation service center. Guide to agency self-examination is included.

1408. Whitten, E. B. Public understanding of rehabilitation. *New Outlook for the Blind*, Sept. 1956, Vol. 50, No. 7, pp. 254–57.

Points out the conflict in the public mind between claims for independence through rehabilitation and claims for special privileges; this must be resolved within the field itself. Public education is continuous, with workers and blind persons both contributing.

1409. Williams, Desley R. The changing world of the blind. *Australian Occupational Therapy Journal*, 1967, Vol. 14, No. 4, pp. 30–44.

Discusses the rehabilitation of the blind in terms of the psychological implications of blindness, a plan of occupational therapy and adaptation to daily living, and the attitudes of others in the community.

1410. Wright, George N., & Trotter, Ann B. *Rehabilitation research.* Madison: Univ. of Wis., 1968, 674 pp.

Chap. 10, Visual Disorders, describes 4 research projects: Development of a Personnel Selection Battery, coordinated by J. Tiffin; Interest Testing of the Blind through Automated Methods, W. M. Cannon; Optical Aids, C. B. Dolan; and Techniques for Placing the Blind in Competitive Industry, R. D. Williams.

1411. Wyant, Dennis R. Blinded Vietnam era veterans in search of work. *New Outlook for the Blind*, Nov. 1975, Vol. 69, No. 9, pp. 410–11.

Questionnaire revealed that few veterans were utilizing available resources and that training was needed in resumé preparation, job-seeking procedures, and interview techniques.

15. Rehabilitation Personnel, Their Functions, and General Methods

1412. American Foundation for the Blind. *Workers for the blind—How well are they paid?* New York: Author, 1967, 21 pp.

Salary schedules determined through a survey of workers who spent at least half their time in direct service for the legally blind. Findings reported, presented in chart and graph form.

1413. Anderson, Jean W. Home teachers are teachers. *New Outlook for the Blind*, May 1965, Vol. 59, No. 5, pp. 169–72.

Addressing the long controversy over whether home teachers are really social workers, author defends position that they are teachers. Ref.

1414. Ark. Rehabilitation Research & Training Center. *Conference Proceedings: Training conference—Improving rehabilitation services for the blind through staff relationships.* Univ. of Ark./Ark. Rehab. Services, July 1974, 20 pp.

The purpose of the training was to improve client services through increased understanding and improved working relationships between and among blind, partially sighted and sighted coworkers.

1415. Baker, Mary R. Approaches to a differential use of staff. *New Outlook for the Blind*, Oct. 1966, Vol. 60, No. 8, pp. 250–54.

The author considers the particular decisions necessary to differentiate tasks of professional social worker from tasks which can be performed by persons without professional education, and what different on-the-job training is necessary for the social work assistant.

1416. Baumann, Hannah. Selective placement by a state employment service. *New Outlook for the Blind*, Feb. 1958, Vol. 52, No. 2, pp. 56–59.

Discusses criteria and approach in making placements, flexibility encouraged to meet individual needs, overcoming prejudice, orientation assistance offered, vocational opportunities and the future.

1417. Blank, H. Robert. Countertransference problems in the professional worker. *New Outlook for the Blind*, June 1954, Vol. 48, No. 6, pp. 185–88.

"Countertransferences are those reactions of the worker to the client determined by unconscious conflict in the worker, which, if unrecognized, will interfere with his professional functioning." Gives illustrations and suggests remedies.

1418. ———. Blind spots in the professional worker about blindness. *New Outlook for the Blind*, May 1958, Vol. 52, No. 5, pp. 173–76.

Discusses countertransferance problems caused by unconscious conflicts about blindness in the professional worker. Such problems may lead the counselor, etc., to attribute any client's personality problem to blindness simply because the client is blind.

1419. ———. The multidisciplinary treatment and research team. *New Outlook for the Blind*, Apr. 1960, Vol. 54, No. 4, pp. 115–18.

States that the multidisciplinary team is a positive move towards breaking down the centuries-old isolation that has characterized many areas of work with the blind. Discusses major obstacles to optimal interdisciplinary collaboration, and need to understand and overcome them. Presents model plan for good teamwork.

1420. ———. The challenge of rehabilitation. *New Outlook for the Blind*, June 1962, Vol. 56, No. 6, pp. 203–8.

Discusses the multidisciplinary rehabilitation team, relative roles of team members, the counselor and the psychotherapist, communication in rehabilitation.

1421. ———. Reactions to loss of body parts—Some research priorities in rehabilitation. *New Outlook for the Blind*, May 1968, Vol. 62, No. 5, pp. 137–43.

Because prevention is the best treatment for psychological problems resulting from blindness, professional workers must be taught what psychological reactions to expect and how to help family and client deal with them. Ref.

1422. Clay, Frances. Toward competence in serving the blind. *Journal of Rehabilitation*, 1960, Vol. 26, No. 2, pp. 14–16, 24.

The counselor's role in working with the blind client is discussed.

1423. ———, **Ed.** *Vocational rehabilitation counseling with the blind through the use of social casework methods.* (Proceedings: Institute Held for Vocational Rehabilitation Counselors with the Blind, Memphis, Nov. 30–Dec. 2, 1959). Washington, D.C.: Dept. of Health, Education & Welfare, 1960, 28 pp.

Proceedings of Institute designed to help vocational rehabilitation counselors of the blind incorporate the basic philosophy and concepts of social work into their own counseling techniques.

1424. Connor, Gordon B. An educator looks at attitudes. *New Outlook for the Blind*, May 1963, Vol. 57, No. 5, pp. 153–56.

Discusses the problem of workers with the handicapped understanding their own motives/attitudes, and developing attitudes that will make their work most rewarding for themselves and their clients/students.

1425. Crawford, Fred L. The blind counselor in a general rehabilitation agency. *New Outlook for the Blind*, Mar. 1964, Vol. 58, No. 3, pp. 71–72.

Author feels that many of the objections to having blind counselors in general rehabilitation agencies have no sound basis in fact. He thinks agencies for the blind should be active in improving this situation and rehabilitation centers and colleges should examine their practices.

1426. Cummings, Francis J. Blind professional personnel on agency staffs. *New Outlook for the Blind*, Mar. 1956, Vol. 50, No. 3, pp. 95–98. Also in AAWB convention *Proceedings*, 1955.

Author reports the responses of 8 leading agency executives to his questions about blind personnel on agency staffs, including statements of problems and recommendations.

1427. Dechaine, Lucy. The blind social worker and the client-worker relationship. *New Outlook for the Blind,* Nov. 1972, Vol. 66, No. 9, pp. 315–19.

Author discusses her blindness as it relates to her job as a social caseworker. Covers client reactions of disbelief, overt and covert rejection, overprotection, over-solicitousness, testing and acceptance. States that blindness itself is not a handicap in casework; it becomes a handicap when the social worker is uncomfortable about it and is unable to deal with whatever problems it produces.

1428. Devereaux, Jane. Social casework and vocational adjustment. *New Outlook for the Blind,* June 1957, Vol. 51, No. 6, pp. 249–53.

How social caseworkers and vocational specialists can work together in a rehabilitation agency.

1429. Diehl, William H. The role of the placement counselor in rehabilitation: His problems, fears, and solutions. *New Outlook for the Blind,* June 1970, Vol. 64, No. 6, pp. 167–68.

Problems of a rehabilitation counselor working with the visually handicapped enumerated. Role of counselor supervisor suggested as a possible reason for counselor difficulty.

1430. Dimock, Marshall. The challenge of being an administrator. *New Outlook for the Blind,* Sept. 1962, Vol. 56, No. 7, pp. 229–32.

Responsibilities, characteristics, and challenges of an administrator described.

1431. Dover, Frances. Use of casework concepts in help to blind people. *New Outlook for the Blind,* Oct. 1963, Vol. 57, No. 8, pp. 287–95.

Discusses historical perspective, distinctive features, principles and methods, need for professional knowledge and skill, multidisciplined approach, case recording, adjustive process.

1432. ———. The case study approach in an agency for the blind. *New Outlook for the Blind,* Nov. 1971, Vol. 65, No. 9, pp. 298–306.

The psychosocial approach in social casework is described as a process through which information about a person and his situation is obtained and examined systematically to arrive at a realistic plan of help.

1433. Ehrhardt, Earl O. Staff development and efficiency. *New Outlook for the Blind,* Sept. 1955, Vol. 49, No. 7, pp. 241–46.

Against a background of concepts used in industrial management, describes autocratic management, paternalistic management, and democratic management. Discusses a number of management principles which can be useful in an agency for the blind.

1434. Finestone, Samuel; Lowry, Fern; Whiteman, Martin, et al. *Social casework and blindness.* New York: AFB, 1960, 157 pp., $2.75.

Eight papers consider social casework with the blind including basic assumptions in casework and the implications of blindness for the caseworker, diagnostic and treatment processes, psychological appraisal of blindness, sociological appraisal of blindness, the family in rehabilitation of the blind, and the relationship of the caseworker to the community.

1435. Gallagher, William F. Diagnosis in depth. *New Outlook for the Blind,* Dec. 1966, Vol. 60, No. 10, pp. 293–95.

Comments on confusion in definition of "diagnosis." Cites counselor's need for back-up team, new evaluation methods, and cooperative planning for the client.

1436. Gilmartin, Thomas. The role of the training supervisor. *New Outlook for the Blind,* Apr. 1957, Vol. 51, No. 4, pp. 131–35.

Supervisor's role viewed as development of adequate staff, coordination and planning, holding staff group sessions, and controlling staff load.

1437. Goodman, William. An interrelated approach to teaching visually handicapped children and mobility education. *Exceptional Children,* Feb. 1970, Vol. 36, No. 6, pp. 445–49.

Discusses training a professional to serve as both mobility teacher and regular teacher: Preparation and responsibilities, advantages, and unresolved questions.

1438. Graham, Milton D. Problems of recruiting professional personnel through fellowship and research grants. *New Outlook for the Blind,* Apr. 1960, Vol. 54, No. 4, pp. 119–24.

Urges that fellowships be set up on a national or regional level, encouraging students to enter careers in the area of work for/with the blind. Offers philosophical guidelines for a rational aid program, suggestions on practical implementation. Discussion of standards and academic standing of those already in the field.

1439. Greenwood, Ernest. Attributes of a profession. *New Outlook for the Blind,* May 1960, Vol. 54, No. 5, pp. 169–78.

The author maintains that all professions possess (1) systematic theory, (2) authority, (3) community sanction, (4) ethical codes, and (5) a culture in significantly greater quantity than do nonprofessional occupations. The article sets out to fully describe these 5 attributes.

1440. Handel, Alexander F. Let's all be counted. *New Outlook for the Blind,* Sept. 1955, Vol. 49, No. 7, pp. 237–40.

Describes a planned survey of the status of professional, administrative, and technical personnel serving blind persons. Pleads for cooperation.

1441. Jones, Eddie B., & Mann, V. S. Upgrading counselor training in Mississippi. *New Outlook for the Blind,* Mar. 1964, Vol. 58, No. 3, pp. 89–90.

Arrangements made with State Univ. to improve professional skills of counselor in rehabilitation of blindness.

1442. Kunce, Joseph T.; Iacono, Carmine U.; & Miller, Douglas E. Determination of caseload feasibility. *Journal of Applied Rehabilitation Counseling,* 1974, Vol. 5, No. 4, pp. 215–19.

Demonstrates the predictability of vocational outcomes of rehabilitation clients by the use of specific prediction rules. Demonstration of rules' application.

1443. Ortof, Murray E. Efficient staffing of agencies for blind persons. *New Outlook for the Blind,* Feb. 1965, Vol. 59, No. 2, pp. 52–53.

Recruitment is complicated by the community image of the agency for the blind, sometimes by lack of professional atmosphere, working conditions, and the tendency of schools of social work to direct their students into certain kinds of agencies. Lists solutions in terms of efficient use of personnel, staff training and development, etc.

1444. Potter, C. Stanley. The team approach to rehabilitation. *New Outlook for the Blind*, Dec. 1961, Vol. 55, No. 10, pp. 347–52.

A psychologist speaks to physicians urging them to make referrals to rehabilitative agencies and detailing practical problems relating to visual loss. Some history of society's attitude toward blindness is given. Steps and services included in rehabilitation process are discussed.

1445. Roberts, Alvin. Some thoughts on home teaching supervision. *New Outlook for the Blind*, June 1966, Vol. 60, No. 6, pp. 169–73.

Cites move toward professionalization of home teaching. To use existing staff with inadequate academic training or experience, competent supervision is requisite. Lists 6 recommendations for supervisors.

1446. ————. Establishing realistic case loads for rehabilitation teachers. *New Outlook for the Blind*, Feb. 1975, Vol. 69, No. 2, pp. 62–63, 85, 87.

A suggested formula for teachers providing home instruction, based on ·a 2-week teaching cycle, established the number of hours available for instruction by subtracting travel time and preparation time from the total number of hours in the teaching cycle.

1447. Rusalem, Herbert. A follow-up study of professional trainees. *New Outlook for the Blind*, Jan. 1957, Vol. 51, No. 1, pp. 31–33.

Questionnaires to 24 graduates of an IHB-OVR professional training program show the values and suggested changes but, most of all, reflect the interest of administrators in better trained personnel.

1448. ————. The status of home teaching as a profession. *New Outlook for the Blind*, Sept. 1960, Vol. 54, No. 7, pp. 240–46.

While social work and psychology have progressed as professions, home teaching has actually regressed. It has variable standards and lacks specificity of content. Job analysis criteria and sociological criteria of a profession are listed, with some suggestions for the future of home teaching.

1449. Stark, Sidney. The role of the rehabilitation counselor. *New Outlook for the Blind*, Apr. 1957, Vol. 51, No. 4, pp. 135–39.

Details the role of the counselor in a rehabilitation center, especially relating to evaluation and to the prevocational period in the client's experience.

1450. Stern, Mildred F. The use of supervision. *New Outlook for the Blind*, Feb. 1968, Vol. 62, No. 2, pp. 50–55.

With special application to home teachers, discusses the supervisory process as education, administration, and enabling, the latter being to help the supervisee do his work to the best of his ability.

1451. Tickton, Sidney G. *Professional and technical workers for the blind: How much are they paid?* New York: AFB, 1958, 36 pp.

Mid-1950s report comparing salaries of professional and technical workers providing specialized services for the blind with those of persons in other occupations and industries.

1452. Ward, Allan L. The response of individuals beginning work with blind persons. *New Outlook for the Blind*, Jan. 1973, Vol. 67, No. 1, pp. 1–5. (also in *Outlook's* Offprint Series, 15¢)

Report of a 3-year program at Arkansas Enterprises for the Blind in which 90 interns were questioned about their reactions to working with blind persons. Suggestions are given for coping with the negative reactions. It was concluded that explaining, in advance, the likelihood of negative reactions and holding frequent individual and group discussions during the internship helps to alleviate these feelings.

1453. Watson, Frances. Interviewing: Some techniques. *New Outlook for the Blind*, June 1961, Vol. 55, No. 6, pp. 199–203.

Describes stages a newly blinded person will often go through and interview techniques that are helpful to the counselor.

1454. Weiss, Viola W. Client-worker relationship—Key to counseling. *New Outlook for the Blind*, Jan. 1962, Vol. 56, No. 1, pp. 10–14.

Discusses in detail the relationship between client and worker, stressing that the important elements in the relationship are empathy, respect, and patience.

1455. Wile, Eva. The team approach in a rehabilitation agency for the blind. *New Outlook for the Blind*, Feb. 1970, Vol. 64, No. 2, pp. 33–37.

Origin, stages of implementation, models of the approach, composition of the team, roles and responsibilities of team members, and the central role of the rehabilitation counselor discussed.

16.   Life and Work Adjustment Services, Centers, and Staff

1456. Allwein, Herman. Home teaching of the adult blind. *Rehabilitation Record*, Mar.–Apr. 1972, Vol. 13, No. 2, pp. 7–10.

1457. American Foundation for the Blind. *A step-by-step guide to personal management for blind persons.* New York: Author, 1970, 239 pp. (2nd ed. 1974, 120 pp., $3.50; braille, American Printing House for the Blind, $6.)

Instructional procedures provided in areas of hygiene, grooming, clothing, and cosmetics. Techniques provided for various aspects of homemaking, and additional guidelines in etiquette, gestures, table manners, telephone dialing are given. Includes information on equipment. Ref.

1458. ————. *Rehabilitation centers for the blind and visually impaired: The state of the art 1975: Final report of the National Workshop on Rehabilitation Centers, St. Louis, Missouri, May 19–22, 1975.* New York: Author, 1975, 72 pp.

Detailed report of the St. Louis Workshop which was organized to consider and deal with recent changes and developments in the area of blindness which effect rehabilitative work with the visually impaired.

1459. ————. *Rehabilitation teaching for the blind and visually disabled: The state of the art 1975. Final report of the National Workshop on Rehabilitation Teachers, St. Louis, Missouri, June 9–12, 1975.* New York: Author, 1975, 79 pp., app.

Report on workshop conducted to develop guidelines and curriculum for professional preparation and in-service training programs for rehabilitation teachers. Bib.

1460. Arndt, Hilda C. Case recording: A service to blind clients. *New Outlook for the Blind*, Feb. 1963, Vol. 57, No. 2, pp. 52–55.

Discusses the primary purpose of a case record, how it can be developed for maximum use, resistance to case recording, and use of the case record.

1461. Arndt, Hilda C., & Brown, W. Neil. Supervising rehabilitation teachers —Summary of a national institute. *New Outlook for the Blind*, June 1967, Vol. 61, No. 6, pp. 169–80.

Summarizes papers and discussions during the institute under the following: Nature and purpose of supervision, the teaching-learning process, communication, orderly approach to service, case records, staff development, and evaluation.

1462. Barr, Ruth L. New technique helps blind write. *Seer,* Spring 1972, Vol. 43, No. 1, pp. 13–16. Reprinted from *Science,* July 3, 1971.

A new polyethylene paper improves usefulness of raised-line characters as tested with 20 blind and 30 blindfolded sighted *S*s.

1463. Becker, Velma R. Teaching handwriting—A home teaching skill. *New Outlook for the Blind,* Dec. 1963, Vol. 57, No. 10, pp. 406–8.

Describes development of a Handwriting Manual and Work Book.

1464. Bindt, Juliet. Modern trends in the education of the adult blind. *New Outlook for the Blind,* June 1953, Vol. 47, No. 6, pp. 178–82.

Discusses 10 reasons why blind people are becoming more integrated into society and how home teachers contribute to this integration and acceptance.

1465. Bloom, Jean; Match, Elmer; & Rowe, Mary A. Integration of the visually limited into a comprehensive rehabilitation center. *New Outlook for the Blind,* Sept. 1969, Vol. 63, No. 7, pp. 193–95.

Discusses integration of 29 visually limited clients with other disability groups in a center for vocational evaluation, results and implications.

1466. Bridges, William V. The role of the home teacher. *New Outlook for the Blind,* Dec. 1960, Vol. 54, No. 10, pp. 375–78.

Discusses the home teacher's role in the area of casework services, specialized services, community involvement, and public relations.

1467. Brown, Adele. *So what about sewing.* Large type ed. 3 vols. Chicago: Catholic Guild, 197–, $8.

The author, a blind homemaker, has developed her own techniques for both hand and machine sewing.

1468. Brown, Charles C. Preparing the client and his family for referral to a rehabilitation center. *New Outlook for the Blind,* Mar. 1966, Vol. 60, No. 3, p. 96.

Describes counselor's role, types of interviews, types of information which should be exchanged.

1469. Buell, John A. Situation signature: A case study. *Rehabilitation Teacher,* June 1974, Vol. 6, No. 6, pp. 9–13.

Detailed description of the equipment and method used by the author in teaching one of his students to sign her name.

1470. Carroll, Thomas J. New techniques in training the blind. *Journal of the Association for Physical and Mental Rehabilitation,* Jan.–Feb. 1956.

Lists 20 losses connected with the physical loss of sight itself. Illustrates new rehabilitation techniques by describing the work at St. Paul's Rehabilitation Center.

1471. ———. Home teaching—Whence and whither. *New Outlook for the Blind,* Dec. 1956, Vol. 50, No. 10, pp. 388–92.

With some historical background, this is an inspirational discussion of the services provided by home teachers.

1472. Coffin, Nerine. Report from Syracuse Lighthouse. *New Outlook for the Blind,* Dec. 1963, Vol. 57, No. 10, pp. 409–10.

A program to teach the blind basic techniques of daily living.

1473. Coughlan, Barbara C. Social work aspects of home teaching. *New Outlook for the Blind,* Jan. 1962, Vol. 56, No. 1, pp. 1–3.

Discusses history and development, principles of social work, how the home teacher uses it.

1474. Crawford, Frances. Present-day concepts and practices of rehabilitation teaching. *New Outlook for the Blind,* Apr. 1971, Vol. 65, No. 4, pp. 120–25.

With emphasis on individual differences among clients and importance of developing potentials of each client, suggests methods and techniques for the modern rehabilitation teacher.

1475. Cull, John G., & Hardy, Richard E. *Counseling strategies with special populations.* Springfield, Ill.: Charles C Thomas, 1975, xiv + 341 pp., $12.95.

In a book dealing with counseling problems of many special groups, one chapter is: Special Considerations in Counseling Blind and Severely Visually Impaired Persons.

1476. Dale, Verda M., & Uhlinger, Susan J. *Resources in home economics for the blind homemaker.* Amherst, Mass.: Author, 1969, 23 pp., 50¢.

Provides home economists with sources of information about blindness and teaching home economics to blind persons. Indicates whether each reference is available in braille, record, tape, or print.

1477. Dauterman, William L. The scope and limitations of the rehabilitation center for the adult blind. *New Outlook for the Blind,* Jan. 1953, Vol. 47, No. 1, pp. 16–21.

In relation to the Kansas Rehabilitation Center for the Adult Blind, describes personnel and plant, purposes, and services and benefits expected for the client. Limitations appear in the distance from the client's home, too much is expected by referring counselors, some factors in client cannot be changed, and limitations in funding and staff time.

1478. DeForest, Robert A. Can a blind person learn first aid? *New Outlook for the Blind,* Nov. 1969, Vol. 63, No. 9, pp. 262–63.

Tells how 12 blind adults used touch, smell, and hearing to succeed in a pilot first aid course.

1479. Dickinson, Raymond M. The discipline of home teaching. *New Outlook for the Blind,* Dec. 1956, Vol. 50, No. 10, pp. 393–400.

History of home teaching from its establishment in 1882 to present status. Defines the home teacher in 10 ways. Discusses duties and remuneration, but a major factor is the spirit of service through professional human relationship.

1480. ———. Why do we need home teachers? *New Outlook for the Blind,* Sept. 1963, Vol. 57, No. 7, pp. 263–67.

Defines home teacher of today as a professional teacher-counselor. The job of the home teacher has changed from maid-of-all-work to professional practitioner with a specific function for which specific training is needed.

1481. Dickman, Irving R. *Living with blindness.* New York: Public Affairs Pamphlets, 1972, 28 pp., 25¢. Also avail. from AFB.

Discusses major causes of blindness, prevention, services and resources for the blind, steps in rehabilitation, and remaining problems.

1482. ———. *Independent living: New goals for disabled persons.* New York: Public Affairs Pamphlets, 1975, 28 pp., 35¢. Also avail. from AFB.

Ways of providing handicapped persons the opportunity to choose alternative ways of living.

1483. Dishart, Martin. A study of the effectiveness of psychological services for the blind. *New Outlook for the Blind,* Dec. 1960, Vol. 54, No. 10, pp. 351–56.

Study evaluated effectiveness of counseling services received by 60 blind adults at the Columbia Lighthouse. Points out that services cannot be assumed to be positively effective simply because they exist, that in fact they may be harmful. Areas of study include: Adjustment counseling, group counseling, family counseling. Discusses study's validity, testing, findings, conclusions.

1484. Dykema, Dorothy. The role of the instructor-counselor as applied to home teaching. *New Outlook for the Blind,* Mar. 1965, Vol. 59, No. 3, pp. 81–85.

Reviews literature on whether any teacher should be a counselor as well, and more specifically whether the home teacher should be a counselor. If the dual role is assumed by 1 worker, adequate preparation for both aspects of the role are important.

1485. Finestone, Samuel. Blind people and the community. *New Outlook for the Blind,* Mar. 1959, Vol. 53, No. 3, pp. 85–88.

How the home teacher assists the blind person to participate fully in the community.

1486. Finnis, Jane. Problems of being visually handicapped. *New Beacon,* Oct. 1973, Vol. 57, No. 678, pp. 254–58.

A visually handicapped person discusses 4 problem areas: Employment and career advancement, complications in daily living activities, social relationships with sighted persons, participation in running one's own affairs. Several possible advantages of the impairment are also mentioned.

1487. Freedman, Saul. Home teaching potentials in the rehabilitation process. *New Outlook for the Blind,* Nov. 1966, Vol. 60, No. 9, pp. 285–88.

Discusses status of home teaching as a profession, improvements in the field, home teacher's role in the rehabilitation team, and ways in which agencies can capitalize on the home teacher.

1488. ———. Work and its emotional implications. *New Outlook for the Blind,* Dec. 1967, Vol. 61, No. 10, pp. 323–27, 338.

Recognizes the psychological meanings of work for many individuals but urges complete rehabilitation prior to placement, returning to former employment if possible, and effective, meaningful placement free from the stereotypes of occupations for the blind.

1489. ———. The rehabilitation center's responsibility: Preparation and placement. *New Outlook for the Blind,* Jan. 1970, Vol. 64, No. 1, pp. 1–5.

With placement as the goal, broadly defined, the center must include evaluation, adjustment training, vocational training, family involvement, and responsibility to the community.

1490. Freyberger, Patricia E. Comparative methods in teaching cooking to the congenitally vs. the adventitiously blind adult. *New Outlook for the Blind,* May 1971, Vol. 65, No. 5, p. 149–51, 154.

Defines the 2 kinds of blindness, materials and methods used in teaching cooking with both, and makes general recommendations.

1491. Fuller, Gloria J.; Hillier, Elizabeth; McKinney, Florence; et al. Prerecorded instructions for teaching food preparation skills. *New Outlook for the Blind*, Dec. 1975, Vol. 69, No. 10, pp. 457–60.

Describes setting up the program and results of pilot study. Specific tips and recommendations for preparation of tapes given. Found some can indeed learn through use of prerecorded instructions.

1492. Gillispie, George M. Rehabilitation centers a necessity? *Braille Forum*, July–Aug. 1975, Vol. 14, No. 1, pp. 5–6.

Summary of a conference held in St. Louis, Mo., which concluded that rehabilitation centers are considered a necessity if services are to be complete and all-encompassing.

1493. Hardy, Richard E. Providing counseling services to blind and severely visually impaired persons. In John G. Cull & Richard E. Hardy, Eds., *Vocational rehabilitation: Profession and process.* Springfield, Ill.: Charles C Thomas, 1972, pp. 396–405.

After a general statement about the nature of counseling, enlarges on rehabilitation counseling for this special population, with emphasis on the importance of developing independence in the client.

1494. Harrison, Letha M. Script writing for the blind. *Education of the Visually Handicapped*, May 1970, Vol. 2, No. 2, pp. 61–62.

Indications from a questionnaire are that there is an interest in teaching script writing and a need for a new method of instruction. Suggests use of clock concept for positioning and direction with raised-line paper used for spacing.

1495. Hayes, Harry E. Life adjustment services for the blind. *Journal of Rehabilitation*, 1959, Vol. 25, pp. 7–9, 13.

The rehabilitation center is discussed as a fundamental element in adjustment. Case sketches provided.

1496. Holdsworth, J. Rehabilitation techniques for the newly blind. *Australian Occupational Therapy Journal*, 1967, Vol. 14, No. 4, pp. 45–47.

A program is delineated suggesting self-help techniques and mobility techniques. Suggests ways of minimizing psychological frustration.

1497. Jenkins, Caroline. You don't have to see to manage a home. *Tennessee Public Welfare Record*, Oct. 1971, Vol. 34, No. 5, pp. 102–5, 120.

Outlines the 10-week home management course for blind housewives at A. P. Mills Industries for the Blind.

1498. Johnson, Suzanne. Factors influencing the acceptance by rehabilitation clients of instruction in script writing and typewriting. *New Outlook for the Blind*, Nov. 1970, Vol. 64, No. 9, pp. 281–84.

Study of factors in student decisions to accept instruction in script writing vs. typewriting shows the former to be more popular.

1499. ———. Community resources used by the rehabilitation teacher. *New Outlook for the Blind*, Feb. 1972, Vol. 66, No. 2, pp. 56–58.

Suggests that agencies serving the blind have been reluctant to utilize resources in the community that are available to all citizens. Describes the resources—educational, material, recreational—that were used during one year to point out what is available.

1500. Jones, Sally. *Sewing techniques for the blind girl,* rev. ed. Albany, Calif.: Orientation Center for the Blind, 1972, 16 pp., illus. (Originally published in 1963.)

1501. Jordan, John F., & Hunter, William F. Counseling the blind. *International Journal for the Education of the Blind,* Oct. 1961, Vol. 11, No. 1, pp. 4–9.

With brief historical background, discusses some of the theoretical assumptions, practical problems, procedures, and methodology involved in counseling the blind. An operational approach to counseling is tentatively outlined.

1502. Kaarlela, Ruth. Home teaching—A description. *New Outlook for the Blind,* Mar. 1966, Vol. 60, No. 3, pp. 80–83.

Attempts to describe context in which Western Michigan Univ.'s home teacher training is offered. Lists items to encourage considering home teaching as a single professional area.

1503. ———. The emerging role of the rehabilitation teacher. *Rehabilitation Teacher,* Feb. 1970, Vol. 2, No. 2, pp. 21–27.

Summarizes history of the role of rehabilitation teachers and discusses the current role as it relates to other professional disciplines instructing the blind.

1504. Kossick, Rodney J. The establishment of a blind rehabilitation center in a rural state. *New Outlook for the Blind,* Apr. 1969, Vol. 63, No. 4, pp. 103–5.

Description of a full-time adjustment-training program including description of the students' daily schedule. Special diet considerations given for diabetic students. Students learned the skills necessary to function without sight, achieved a realistic concept of their abilities and limitations and an intellectual understanding and better emotional acceptance of the handicap while acquiring independent mobility.

1505. Kumpe, Roy. Southwest Rehabilitation Center for the Blind. *New Outlook for the Blind,* Nov. 1953, Vol. 47, No. 9, pp. 271–74.

History, operation, and success of the Center, with 3 illustrative case histories.

1506. Laurence, Marilyn. The Self-Reliance Institute: Filling the gap in work experience. *New Outlook for the Blind,* May 1973, Vol. 67, No. 5, pp. 221–25.

Describes program of an intensive summer program which prods achievement through heightening self-awareness and self-esteem.

1507. Leavitt, Glenn S. Teaching oral-aural communication skills in a rehabilitation center for the blind. *New Outlook for the Blind,* Dec. 1973, Vol. 67, No. 10, pp. 448–53.

Using tape and cassette recorders, talking book machines and telephones, students at the Michigan Rehabilitation Center learn oral-aural communication skills, including listening, conversation, use of playback-recording devices, techniques of aural reading, and knowledge of the sources of recorded reading material.

1508. Loeb, Gladys E. Braille labeling and managing food and supplies for the blind homemaker. *Rehabilitation Teacher,* Nov. 1971, Vol. 3, No. 11, pp. 11–28.

Written by a blind homemaker, article describes methods of storing and marking food containers for identification with a braille labeling system.

1509. Ludden, Richard T. Chaplain service in a voluntary rehabilitation and training center for the blind. *New Outlook for the Blind,* Oct. 1970, Vol. 64, No. 8, pp. 256–57.

Describes role of chaplain as part of the program of psychosocial services of the center.

1510. MacDonald, D. A. My area. *New Beacon,* Oct. 1973, Vol. 57, No. 678, pp. 261–62.

Author relates his experiences as home teacher and resource worker in the Outer Hebrides and Skye.

1511. MacFarland, Douglas C. The importance of family attitudes in vocational rehabilitation. *New Outlook for the Blind,* Dec. 1957, Vol. 51, No. 10, pp. 443–45.

Shows, with aid of 2 case studies, the importance of good family attitudes to successful rehabilitation. Lack of training in family counseling and lack of time prevent most rehabilitation counselors or home teachers from handling problems in family attitudes, so it is recommended agencies consider hiring a family work specialist.

1512. McKay, Evelyn C. The historical role of the home teacher. *New Outlook for the Blind,* May 1965, Vol. 59, No. 5, pp. 167–68.

Reviews changing roles of home teachers, 1885 to present, but basic function of bringing hope, skills, and independence to blind people has not changed.

1513. Maleson, Annette. Housekeeping: The work that is never done. Introduction and chapter one on bed making. *Rehabilitation Teacher,* Oct. 1972, Vol. 4, No. 10, pp. 21–28. Part of series.

Hospital technique is recommended and explained.

1514. ———. Housekeeping: The work that is never done. Chapter two: Laundering. *Rehabilitation Teacher,* Nov. 1972, Vol. 4, No. 11, pp. 25–39. Part of series.

Gives hints on braille labeling of the machine and clothes sorting. Compares washers, laundries, and detergents.

1515. ———. Housekeeping: The work that is never done. Chapter three: Ironing. *Rehabilitation Teacher,* Dec. 1972, Vol. 4, No. 12, pp. 17–36. Part of series.

1516. ———. Housekeeping: The work that is never done. Chapter four: House cleaning. *Rehabilitation Teacher,* Jan. 1973, Vol. 5, No. 1, pp. 3–22. Part of series.

Gives techniques on dusting, polishing, using the vacuum cleaner.

1517. ———. Housekeeping: The work that is never done. Chapter five: The kitchen. *Rehabilitation Teacher,* Feb. 1973, Vol. 5, No. 2, pp. 3–22. Part of series.

Discusses kitchen organization and food preparation steps, including use of stove.

1518. ———. Housekeeping: The work that is never done. Chapter six: Cooking. *Rehabilitation Teacher,* Mar. 1973, Vol. 5, No. 3, pp. 17–31. Part of series.

Discusses ways of applying heat to food, compares various types of cookware for ease of use.

1519. ———. Housekeeping: The work that is never done. Chapter seven: Coffee and tea. *Rehabilitation Teacher*, Apr. 1973, Vol. 5, No. 4, pp. 17–30. Part of series.

Considers making tea and coffee.

1520. ———. Housekeeping: The work that is never done. Chapter eight: Cooking III. *Rehabilitation Teacher*, May 1973, Vol. 5, No. 5, pp. 13–22. Part of series.

Describes specific techniques such as using a dull table knife as a sensor and turning over food in a skillet.

1521. ———. Housekeeping: The work that is never done. Chapter nine: Cooking IV. *Rehabilitation Teacher*, June 1973, Vol. 5, No. 6, pp. 27–38. Part of series.

Presents procedure for preparing breakfast of fruit juice, eggs, bacon, toast, and coffee.

1522. ———. Housekeeping: The work that is never done. Chapter ten: Cooking V. *Rehabilitation Teacher*, July 1973, Vol. 5, No. 7, pp. 21–34. Part of series.

Discusses broiling, roasting, and pot roasting, and preparation of meat, poultry, fish, casseroles, salads, starchy foods, and canned vegetables.

1523. ———. Housekeeping: The work that is never done. Ultimate goals— I. *Rehabilitation Teacher*, Mar. 1974, Vol. 6, No. 3, pp. 3–16. Part of series.

Gives specific instructions on techniques for entertaining guests.

1524. ———. Housekeeping: The work that is never done. Ultimate goals— II. *Rehabilitation Teacher*, Apr. 1974, Vol. 6, No. 4, pp. 3–17. Part of series.

Gives suggestions for developing eating skills.

1525. ———. Housekeeping: The work that is never done. Cooking for company. *Rehabilitation Teacher*, July 1974, Vol. 6, No. 7, pp. 5–20. Part of series.

Tips on menus, baking, and how to approach entertaining.

1526. Manaster, Al. The theragnostic group in a rehabilitation center for visually handicapped persons. *New Outlook for the Blind*, Oct. 1971, Vol. 65, No. 8, pp. 261–64.

Discusses the use of theragnostic groups (nondirective group interaction in which the interaction can not only have therapeutic effects for the participant but can also provide to the staff members diagnostic information about the client) at a rehabilitation center.

1527. Marcone, Ted. Some thoughts on evaluation training. *New Outlook for the Blind*, Sept. 1954, Vol. 48, No. 7, pp. 213–17.

Use of training to evaluate both the client and his goals requires very individualized programs which respect the client's wishes and personality. The teacher must be flexible, adaptable, resourceful, and devoted to his work.

1528. Marks, Anna S., & Marks, Robert A. *Teaching the blind script-writing by the Marks method.* New York: AFB, 1956, 23 pp., $2.

Gives detailed directions for learning to use the Marks Writing Guide. The manual is also distributed with each Guide sold by AFB Aids and Appliances Div.

1529. Meehan, Linda. Activities of daily living: A program in life-orientation. *Florida School Herald*, Apr. 1975, Vol. 74, No. 8, pp. 1–3.

School's student "Diners Club" is described. All students, divided into groups, compete to achieve the most improved eating skills, table manners, social skills, and independence.

1530. Meyers, Mary M. Underestimation is predetermination. *Rehabilitation Teacher*, Aug.–Sept. 1973, Vol. 5, Nos. 8–9, pp. 21–31.

Detailed description of the author's experiences in teaching blind clients to make macramé bags and belts.

1531. Miller, William H. Group counseling with the blind. *Education of the Visually Handicapped*, May 1971, Vol. 3, No. 2, pp. 46–51.

Basic principles are given. Importance of counselor's attitude about blind stressed. Problems a counselor may face, particularly counselee's need to accept his handicap, are explored. Structuring of group counseling for the blind is detailed.

1532. Morrison, Marie. Homemaker program for blind women. *New Outlook for the Blind*, May 1963, Vol. 57, No. 5, pp. 168–69.

Comments from blind homemakers inspired the Columbus Assoc. for the Blind to contact local community resources in an effort to help. Describes program devised and response.

1533. Morrison, Mary. The other 128 hours a week: Teaching personal management to blind young adults. *New Outlook for the Blind*, Dec. 1974, Vol. 68, No. 10, pp. 454–459, 469.

Areas of personal management discussed include signature writing, shopping, money management, and using a calendar.

1534. Needham, Walter E.; DeL'Aune, William R.; & Fry, Gilbert W. Patients' expectations in a residential rehabilitation center. *New Outlook for the Blind*, Nov. 1975, Vol. 69, No. 9, pp. 399–401, 406.

Blind persons entering a rehab. center have a variety of expectations which may change during their stay. Suggests that therapists be sensitive to patients' expressed desires and deal with them in a constructive manner within the program's resources.

1535. Nelson, John P. Making of a will. *Braille Forum*, May–June 1975, Vol. 13, No. 6, pp. 20–21.

Briefly discusses the problems involved in the making and signing of a will by a blind person.

1536. Nelson, Nathan. Rehabilitation centers, An appraisal. *New Outlook for the Blind*, Mar. 1958, Vol. 52, No. 3, pp. 83–86.

Discusses the principal problem facing rehabilitation centers and some pertinent questions. Also discusses prevocational unit services, costs and prices in operation of centers, and team approach to the whole person.

1537. Office of Vocational Rehabilitation. *Rehabilitation centers for blind persons: Report of Seminar, New Orleans, Louisiana, February 1956.* Washington, D.C.: Govt. Printing Office, 1956, 43 pp.

A report on proceedings and conclusions of seminar conducted primarily to develop specific principles and standards for the administration and operation of rehabilitation centers. Participants included 17 persons with extensive experience in various areas of rehabilitation center administration and operations.

1538. Pirozzi, Dorothy. *The art of makeup for the visually handicapped.* New York: Assoc. for the Blind, 1973, 24 pp., $1.25.

Large print booklet of helpful hints based on author's own experiences both as a blind woman and as a teacher of blind women.

1539. Potts, Judy. The role of occupational therapy with the visually handicapped. *Canadian Journal of Occupational Therapy,* Spring 1975, Vol. 42, No. 1, pp. 21–24.

Gives statistics re visually handicapped population of Canada and describes therapist's involvement in teaching use of specific techniques and aids for activities of daily living.

1540. Rahn, Constance H. *Home economics guide for visually handicapped students, a five county vocational skills training program for the blind.* Santa Cruz, Calif.: Board of Education, 1972, 196 pp.

This curriculum guide discusses foods, grooming, home management and child care, sewing, and major appliances. App. includes a discussion of orientation and mobility, and a list of of consumer publications.

1541. Richterman, Harold. The place of the rehabilitation center in the rehabilitation counseling process. *New Outlook for the Blind,* Apr. 1958, Vol. 52, No. 4, pp. 117–22.

Defines "rehabilitation center" and discusses qualifications more important than its size. Defines "rehabilitation counselor" as part of a team. Other discussion includes procedure determined by findings of caseworker, rehabilitation appraisal, training, coordination of services, placement, follow-up. Client's needs evaluated in terms of center's programs.

1542. Ricketts, Peter. For appearance's sake. *New Beacon,* Dec. 1975, Vol. 59, No. 704, pp. 313–14.

Suggestions for shopping for clothing.

1543. Rives, Louis H., Jr. A study of home teacher functions and training needs. *New Outlook for the Blind,* June 1960, Vol. 54, No. 6, pp. 224–25.

Outlines the goals of a study to be undertaken by AAWB through a grant from the Office of Vocational Rehabilitation. The study was to provide recommendations on what the functions and responsibilities of home teachers should be, and to develop a curriculum to prepare individuals to discharge those functions and responsibilities.

1544. Roberts, Edna S. Teaching the Continental method of eating to blind persons. *New Outlook for the Blind,* Apr. 1974, Vol. 68, No. 4, pp. 170–73.

Eighteen blind and visually handicapped persons participated in this study to determine how well they could learn the Continental method of eating. Thirteen mastered the method extremely well.

1545. Rouse, Dorothy D.; Gruber, Kathern F.; & Bledsoe, C. W. Occupational therapy for blind patients. *American Journal of Occupational Therapy,* Sept.–Oct. 1956, Vol. 10, No. 5, pp. 252–53.

Occupational therapy for blind patients cannot be reduced to a formula.

1546. Sausser, Doris P. The role of the rehabilitation teacher—A national point of view. *New Outlook for the Blind*, June 1967, Vol. 61, No. 6, pp. 181–84.

Following a brief history of home teaching, discusses salary levels, standards, and the current evolution into rehabilitation teaching.

1547. Schaeffer, Joseph N. *Comprehensive adjustment services for the blind: Final report.* Detroit: Rehabilitation Institute, 1969, 26 pp., app.

Results of research and demonstration project conducted over a 5-year period, established the feasibility of an adjustment training program for blind adults carried out in a general rehabilitation hospital.

1548. Schwab, Lois O. *Proceedings of training institute for rehabilitation teachers of the blind teaching the newly blinded homemaker (Lincoln, Nebraska, July 12–17, 1970).* Lincoln: Neb. Univ., Dept. of Home Economics, 1970, 47 pp.

Presents 9 papers on topic. Explains way different sources work together toward homemaker rehabilitation, future services and vocational opportunities for the blind, relationship between rehabilitation teacher and home economist.

1549. Snyder, Therese, & Kesselman, Marcia. Teaching English as a Second Language to blind people. *New Outlook for the Blind*, June 1972, Vol. 66, No. 6, pp. 161–66.

Explanation of the program to teach English as a Second Language at the Catholic Guild for the Blind in New York City. Aural-oral approach is used in small groups or on a one-to-one basis depending on the ability and education of the students in the program. Case histories cited.

1550. Soyer, David. Blind persons as individuals of integrity and responsibility. *New Outlook for the Blind*, Nov. 1963, Vol. 57, No. 9, pp. 353–58.

Discusses the techniques used in casework treatment of several clients, results of each, and basis for treatment plan. Wherever diagnostic thinking warrants it, the client should be encouraged to take responsibility for his own development and to move away from the agency.

1551. ————. The right to fail. *New Outlook for the Blind*, Jan. 1965, Vol. 59, No. 1, pp. 27–32.

With illustrative case reports, discusses the principle that self-determination is basic to casework. Agencies too strongly challenge the aspirations of blind clients without consideration for the client's own aspirations. Attitudes of workers may actually dampen the aspirations of their clients; lists 3 ways this can occur. Ref.

1552. Stark, Mary L. Restoration and habilitation of handwriting skills to adults in a rehabilitation center setting. *New Outlook for the Blind*, Dec. 1970, Vol. 64, No. 10, pp. 330–39.

Suggestions to develop or improve handwriting skills. Instructional materials described and availability given.

1553. Stern, Mildred F. Coordination of casework—Rehabilitation teaching services. *New Outlook for the Blind*, Jan. 1971, Vol. 54, No. 1, pp. 25–30. Reprinted from *Rehabilitation Teacher*, Feb. 1970.

Concerns of the social worker and the rehabilitation teacher are elucidated, emphasizing their separate roles and responsibilities in addition to the need for teamwork.

1554. Stocker, Claudell. A new approach to teaching handwriting to the blind. *New Outlook for the Blind,* June 1963, Vol. 57, No. 6, pp. 208–9.

Discusses method used for several months at the Kansas Rehabilitation Center for the Blind which has proven to be successful.

1555. Takemoto, Yasuko. Scriptwriting training at Ho'opono. *New Outlook for the Blind,* Feb. 1964, Vol. 58, No. 2, pp. 61–62.

Detailed information on how one agency teaches script writing to the totally blind. Emphasis on positive effect success has on students.

1556. Thume, Lyle. Symbols of blindness. *New Outlook for the Blind,* June 1957, Vol. 51, No. 6, pp. 245–47.

How to recognize and deal with a rehabilitation center trainee's resistance to such symbols of blindness as the white cane.

1557. ———. Rehabilitation for whom? *New Outlook for the Blind,* Jan. 1960, Vol. 54, No. 1, pp. 22–25.

Discusses the trend in rehabilitation centers of accepting widely heterogeneous groups of blind persons, maintaining that though many of these group members have been considered beyond help, they have made progress in the centers. Presents idea that much "pioneer work" useful in general rehabilitation has been done in work with the blind, and must continue in work with those who have "multiple problems."

1558. ———. Can rehabilitation centers serve students from residential schools? *International Journal for the Education of the Blind,* Dec. 1961, Vol. 11, No. 2, pp. 37–39.

The author believes that graduates of residential schools have a specific body of needs that can often be met in a rehabilitation center even when they have some travel facility. One possible need is gradual transition from the protective school environment to the freedoms and responsibilities of adult society.

1559. ———. Implications of an integrated adjustment training service for blind adults. *New Outlook for the Blind,* Nov. 1969, Vol. 63, No. 9, pp. 272–74.

Reports 5 years' experience with a prevocational adjustment training program in a general rehabilitation center. Advantages and disadvantages of the integrated program are discussed.

1560. Tobias, Jerry V. Binaural recordings for training the newly blind. *Perceptual and Motor Skills,* 1965, Vol. 20, No. 2, pp. 385–91.

Tests showed that *S*s trained by listening to binaural recordings behaved more cautiously and listened to their surroundings with greater attention than *S*s given no previous experience of any kind. Indicates that recorded training material provides an early step toward rehabilitation for the newly blind.

1561. Urena, Manuel. Rehabilitation centers for the blind: What are they, and what should they do? *Braille Monitor,* Feb. 1975, pp. 74–81.

Briefly covers the history of rehabilitation centers showing that what the author regards as increased standardization in recent years has sacrificed the individual's benefits to some extent. Suggests guidelines for restoring more individualized service.

1562. Utrup, Robert G. Home mechanics for the visually impaired: Part I. *Rehabilitation Teacher,* May 1974, Vol. 6, No. 5, pp. 31–42. Reprinted from manual of same title, pub. by the Graduate College, Univ. of Mich., 1973?

Describes need for and benefits of organized home mechanics program, lesson format. Presents lessons on using adhesives, cleaning drains.

1563. ————. Home mechanics for the visually impaired: Part II. *Rehabilitation Teacher*, June 1974, Vol. 6, No. 6, pp. 25–34.

Presents comprehensive lessons on faucet repair, use of fire extinguishers, flush tank maintenance, fuse box repair.

1564. ————. Home mechanics for the visually impaired: Part III. *Rehabilitation Teacher*, July 1974, Vol. 6, No. 7, pp. 25–34.

Presents lessons in glazing (installing glass windows, etc.), hammer selection and use, hand sanding.

1565. ————. Home mechanics for the visually impaired: Part IV. *Rehabilitation Teacher*, Aug. 1974, Vol. 6, No. 8, pp. 3–32.

Lesson plans for instruction in use of handsaws, hangers (such as nails, toggle bolts), pliers, wrenches, and for sharpening and painting. Each topic section includes lesson activities, lists of needed materials, tactual aids, questions and answers, procedures, safety notes.

1566. ————. Home mechanics for the visually impaired: Part V. *Rehabilitation Teacher*, Sept. 1974, Vol. 6, No. 9, pp. 15–32.

Presents 3 detailed lesson plans on nails and woodscrews, screwdrivers, knife sharpening.

1567. ————. Home mechanics for the visually impaired: Part VI. *Rehabilitation Teacher*, Oct. 1974, Vol. 6, No. 10, pp. 3–10.

Presents detailed lesson plans for wiring a push-pull plug and a lamp socket. Includes safety precautions, purchasing information, tool list, references.

1568. Viskant, Kathryn. Cooperative homemaking program in Illinois. *Rehabilitation Teacher*, Jan. 1970, Vol. 2, No. 1, pp. 19–29.

Agency cooperation results in blind persons having tutors who conduct classes in cooking, sewing, and other homemaking skills. Orientation is provided to staff and coordinators.

1569. Voorhees, Arthur L. Counseling the blind. *Vocational Guidance Quarterly*, Winter 1954–55, Vol. 3.

There is little need to vary from generally good counseling techniques in order to counsel blind persons but the counselor should be sensitive to certain factors as listed.

1570. Waffa, Joseph. Fencing as an aid to the habilitation or rehabilitation of blind persons. *New Outlook for the Blind*, Feb. 1963, Vol. 57, No. 2, pp. 39–43.

The sport is invaluable for developing physical qualities of endurance and stamina, posture, dexterity, and balance; quick and accurate actions or reactions.

1571. Webb, Lillian J. Effective case recording in the rehabilitation teacher program. *New Outlook for the Blind*, Apr. 1968, Vol. 62, No. 4, pp. 127–30.

Complete, flexible case recording, adapted to its individual purpose, can make rehabilitation teaching more effective. Specific suggestions are given.

1572. Webb, Nancy C. The use of myoelectric feedback in teaching facial expression to the blind. *American Foundation for the Blind Research Bulletin 27*, Apr. 1974, pp. 231–62.

Five adult blind *S*s were trained to produce facial expressions through provision of auditory feedback of their facial activity by transducing myoelectric signals from facial muscles into sound.

1573. Wheeler, Jane G. Teaching the concept of the diagonal during handwriting lessons for the congenitally blind. *New Outlook for the Blind*, Oct. 1970, Vol. 64, No. 8, pp. 249–55.

Discusses the difficulty of the congenitally blind in visualizing diagonal lines in terms of teaching handwriting skills. Includes lesson plans.

1574. Widerberg, Lloyd, & Kaariela, Ruth. *Techniques for eating: A guide for blind persons.* Kalamazoo: W. Mich. Univ., School of Graduate Studies, 1969, 10 pp.

For persons working with the blind. Presents general suggestions and specific techniques in precise steps.

1575. ———. *Basic components of orientation and movement techniques.* Kalamazoo: W. Mich. Univ., Instit. of Blind Rehab., 1970, 19 pp., $1.

Intended for rehabilitation teachers, guide describes the areas of orientation and movement which are part of rehabilitation teaching of the blind.

1576. Williams, Marie S. Programs for blind diabetic clients at a rehabilitation center. *New Outlook for the Blind*, Nov. 1975, Vol. 69, No. 9, pp. 402–6.

Program developed in response to individual needs includes ongoing cooperation with local diabetes groups, services of a nurse-consultant, use of a diabetic profile sheet, development of housing and medical resources and of teaching kits for insulin measurement and urine testing. Stresses uniqueness of each diabetic client.

1577. Wilson, Edouard L. Programming individual and adjunctive therapeutic services for visually impaired clients in a rehabilitation center. *New Outlook for the Blind*, Sept. 1972, Vol. 66, No. 7, pp. 215–20.

Explanation of mild, acute, and chronic emotional reactions to onset of blindness and discussion of individual psychotherapy and adjunctive techniques (group therapy or psychodrama) as used at the New York Assoc. for the Blind. Cites 3 types of psychotherapy and 9 basic processes used and explains methods of working with groups. States that a rehabilitation agency can offer a comprehensive therapy program.

1578. Winters, Kris. First report of the Alameda County Placement Project for the Blind. *New Outlook for the Blind*, Feb. 1966, Vol. 60, No. 2, pp. 39–42.

Describes project need, procedure, goals, and conclusion: Many clients have prevocational rehabilitation needs which, unmet, preclude gainful employment.

1579. ———. The Alameda County Placement Project: A final report. *New Outlook for the Blind*, Mar. 1969, Vol. 63, No. 3, pp. 73–79.

Reports an intensive rehabilitation project with blind clients with limited potential, incomplete education, emotional problems, and past histories of chronic illness. Describes staff, procedures, and project cost.

1580. Woodring, Jesse, & Gregg, Nancy J. Occupational therapy in the rehabilitation of the blind. *American Journal of Occupational Therapy,* May–June 1955.

Principles of occupational therapy are applied in prevocational training at the Minneapolis Society for the Blind.

1581. Yank, Berit. A new approach to adjustment training for blinded individuals. *New Outlook for the Blind,* Dec. 1968, Vol. 62, No. 10, pp. 313–18.

Nebraska's 3-week adjustment training program included skills of daily living, orientation and mobility, communication skills and homemaking. Describes program participants, staff, equipment used, teaching techniques, and planned social events in the program. Reports favorable results and problems.

1582. Yeadon, Anne. *Toward independence: The use of instructional objectives in teaching daily living skills to the blind.* New York: AFB, 1974, xxvi + 96 pp., $4.

An explanation of what instructional objectives are, how to develop them, and how to use them in teaching blind persons. Illustrated by a daily living skills class developed around instructional objectives.

1583. Yerby, Alonzo S. Planning the rehabilitation center. *New Outlook for the Blind,* Jan. 1956, Vol. 50, No. 1, pp. 22–26.

The rehabilitation center must coordinate a wide range of services which are listed. The kinds of disabilities to be served also determines the organization. An arrangement of components is suggested, but it is recommended that planners make a critical analysis of existing centers, also.

1584. Yoder, Norman M. Apartment living for rehabilitation clients during training. *New Outlook for the Blind,* Jan. 1975, Vol. 69, No. 1, pp. 32–33.

At the Cleveland Society for the Blind, trainees are expected to apply skills learned there to problems of daily life encountered in the adjacent apartment building where they live during training.

17. Specific Occupations and Relevant Training, Placement, Attitudes Related to Employment

1585. **Abels, H. Leola, & Cantoni, Louis J.** Employability of blind dictaphone operators. *New Outlook for the Blind,* Jan. 1965, Vol. 59, No. 1, pp. 33–34.

Compares 10 unemployed and 10 employed dictaphone operators. The employed were better educated, more intelligent, older, spent less time in training as dictaphone operators, required fewer training situations, needed fewer agency dollars, and were better adjusted emotionally.

1586. **Alford, Milton M.** Placing a blind diabetic as a computer programmer. *New Outlook for the Blind,* Feb. 1969, Vol. 63, No. 2, pp. 45–48.

Through detailed story of one man, tells problems and successes in placing a blind diabetic.

1587. **Allen, Gordon W.** Sheltered employment—a symposium: Planning sheltered employment services at the community level. *New Outlook for the Blind,* Sept. 1957, Vol. 51, No. 7, pp. 298–303.

Describes some of the problems of planning sheltered employment services and how government can participate through the Office of Vocational Rehabilitation.

1588. **Altman, Anne, & Baumann, Hannah.** Finding jobs for the blind. *New Outlook for the Blind,* Feb. 1956, Vol. 50, No. 2, pp. 47–51. Reprinted from *Employment Security Review,* Sept. 1955.

A project to demonstrate placement of blind workers involved evaluation of present methods, development of new methods, and preparation of a manual and training guide for Employment Service personnel. Problems found in workers and staff are discussed.

1589. **American Assoc. of Workers for the Blind.** *Contemporary papers, Volume IV: Employment of the blind: I.R.S. Conference and other papers.* Washington, D.C.: Author, 1969, 30 pp.

Report of Washington Conference on the Employment of the Blind, Feb. 1969; papers on new careers by George A. Magers, and automation by Louis H. Rives, Jr.

1590. **American Foundation for the Blind.** *The Middletown Lighthouse for the Blind: A survey.* New York: Author, 1957, 52 pp.

A study and evaluation of a workshop for blind persons which includes training and residential facilities for its patrons.

1591. ———. *Visually handicapped workers in service occupations in the food service and lodging industries.* New York: Author, 1967, 12 pp., free.

Summaries given for 20 types of jobs. Visual requisites stated for all.

1592. ————. *The employment of visually handicapped persons in hotels and motels. Regional conference, Delaware, New Jersey, New York, Pennsylvania, June 23–25, 1969.* New York: Author, 1969, 21 pp., app.

Proceedings of conference to determine why few visually handicapped persons are employed in hotels and motels and to plan procedures to develop more such employment opportunities.

1593. ————. *Visually handicapped workers in recreation services.* New York: Author, 1969, 16 pp.

Presents guidelines for the selection, training, and placement of blind and visually handicapped in the field of recreation.

1594. Ark. Enterprises for the Blind. *Training blind persons to work as taxpayer service representatives for Internal Revenue Service: Final report of a demonstration project from March 1967 through May 1971.* Little Rock: Author, 1971, 92 pp., app.

Demonstration project to determine feasibility of training blind for this job. Compared successful and unsuccessful trainees. Program was successful in placing workers. Positive implications for other related jobs.

1595. Arms, Wallace R. Braille bookkeeping. *New Outlook for the Blind,* Sept. 1972, Vol. 66, No. 7, pp. 209–13.

Experiment shows feasibility of braille bookkeeping but lists problems.

1596. ACM Committee on Professional Activities of the Blind. *The blind in computer programming: An international conference.* Washington, D.C.: Dept. of Health, Education & Welfare, 1969, 148 pp., app.

Presents papers concerned with problems of selection, training, and employment of blind persons as professional workers in computer programming.

1597. Baker, Larry D. Authoritarianism, attitudes toward blindness, and managers: Implications for the employment of blind persons. *New Outlook for the Blind,* Sept. 1974, Vol. 68, No. 7, pp. 308–14.

High authoritarians tend to hold more negative attitudes toward the blind and they also hold or aspire to important decision- and policy-making positions in organizations. Review of the literature and suggestions for needed research.

1598. Baker, Larry D.; DiMarco, Nicholas; & Scott, W. E. Effects of supervisor's sex and level of authoritarianism on evaluation and reinforcement of blind and sighted workers. *Journal of Applied Psychology,* 1975, Vol. 60, No. 1, pp. 28–32.

Findings show blind workers are rewarded significantly more than sighted workers for identical performance and no significant main effects occurred for level of authoritarianism and sex; 120 Ss, ½ male, ½ female.

1599. Barrett, Walter. A private agency's program for independent vending stand operators. *New Outlook for the Blind,* Jan. 1958, Vol. 52, No. 1, pp. 11–16.

Discusses in detail the newstand phase of the program as well as the placement of operators at cigar and candy concessions and small candy stores. The goal is to establish in business those who are capable of functioning successfully with little or no help from the agency.

1600. Barry, Franklyn S. The teacher in Room 18. *New Outlook for the Blind*, Oct. 1964, Vol. 58, No. 8, pp. 257–59. Reprinted from *N.Y. State Education*, May 1964.

Report of experiences with a public school hiring a blind elementary school teacher. Situation is seen through eyes of the teacher, administrators, fellow teachers, students, and their parents.

1601. Bauman, Mary K. *Characteristics of blind and visually handicapped people in professional, sales, and managerial work.* Harrisburg, Pa.: Office for the Blind, Dept. of Public Welfare, 1963, 116 pp.

Statistical analysis and interpretation of personal data collected through interviews with 434 blind workers in the above occupations. Similarities and differences among subgroups are shown. Graphs, tables, and statistical data presented.

1602. Bauman, Mary K., & Yoder, Norman M. *Placing the blind and visually handicapped in professional occupations.* Harrisburg, Pa.: Office for the Blind, Dept. of Public Welfare, 1962, 254 pp.

Based on interviews with 434 workers across U.S., describes how blind people function in the fields of mathematics, science, law, religion, teaching, social service, rehabilitation, medicine, music, the verbal arts, and business.

1603. ———. *Placing the blind and visually handicapped in clerical, industrial and service fields.* Harrisburg, Pa.: Office for the Blind, Dept. of Public Welfare, 1967, 331 pp.

Following introductory chapters on placement in general, describes jobs, and how those jobs are done by blind people, as reported by 752 blind people interviewed in all parts of U.S. Briefly describes characteristics of sample group.

1604. Berger, Gertrude. The blind teacher, creativity, and the multi-sensory classroom. *New Outlook for the Blind*, Sept. 1972, Vol. 66, No. 7, pp. 230–32.

Author suggests that the blind teacher, utilizing a multi-sensory approach to classroom instruction in lieu of visual stimuli, has a more creative approach which "frees the imagination and develops skills which are broader than those seen in a traditional academic curriculum."

1605. Berkeley, Selma G., & Jackson, Barbara E. *Your career as a medical secretary transcriber.* New York: John Wiley, 1975, xi + 194 pp., $6.95, paperback.

An informative text for the interested person. Included is a chapter on the opportunities for the visually impaired.

1606. Bischoff, Robert W. Problems of employment for the visually handicapped. *Utah Eagle*, Mar. 1974, Vol. 85, No. 6, pp. 1, 7–9.

Lists some of the more frequent problems of young people seeking first employment with suggestions to alleviate the problems.

1607. Black, Bertram J. Sheltered employment—a symposium: The sheltered workshop—a challenge to social welfare. *New Outlook for the Blind*, Sept. 1957, Vol. 51, No. 7, pp. 293–98.

Lists kinds of sheltered workshops, their potential for offering varied services, the role of the social worker in the workshop, and briefly describes the Altro Workshops in New York City. Proposes that sheltered workshops be regarded as "foster work" programs.

1608. Black, Donald E. The hiring policies of selected Iowa businesses and industries with respect to employment of blind persons. Ann Arbor, Mich.: University Microfilms, 1970, 173 pp., $10. Dissertation.

Report based on tabulation of questionnaire responses by 84 small and 57 large businesses. Also includes survey of 27 blind males re their evaluation of the industrial arts training program.

1609. Blind persons as social workers and rehabilitation counselors. *New Outlook for the Blind*, Oct. 1967, Vol. 61, No. 8, pp. 266–68.

Through a question and answer sequence, responds to doubts that blind persons can function as social workers and rehabilitation counselors.

1610. Blind X-ray technicians outperform those with sight. *Cross-Reference*, Aug. 1971, Vol. 1, No. 8, pp. 10–11.

Brief report on a 6-mo. training program in medical and industrial x-ray processing in S.C.

1611. Brady, John, & Wuenschel, Raymond J. Principles and techniques of placement. *New Outlook for the Blind*, May 1958, Vol. 52, No. 5, pp. 177–81.

Discusses placement service, the qualified disabled applicant, the employer, the job, and community resources as aids to placement.

1612. Branson, Helen K. Preparing the blind for hospital jobs. *New Outlook for the Blind*, Nov. 1962, Vol. 56, No. 9, pp. 335–37.

A visually handicapped nurse discusses employment of similarly handicapped people in over 50 Los Angeles medical institutions: Contractual arrangements for training; types of positions held; strength and limitations; preparing and placing the blind in such position.

1613. ———. A remedial reading experiment. *New Outlook for the Blind*, Nov. 1963, Vol. 57, No. 9, pp. 350–52.

Discusses some observations on the influence of a blind counselor working with sighted children in a remedial reading project.

1614. Branson, Helen K., & Branson, Ralph. Should blind persons teach in the public schools? *New Outlook for the Blind*, May 1964, Vol. 58, No. 5, pp. 153–56.

A totally blind couple's experiences in teaching in a public high school. Helpful suggestions are given.

1615. Busse, Larry L., & McElroy, Arthur A. The blind can chart. *TEACHING Exceptional Children*, Summer 1975, Vol. 7, No. 4, pp. 116–17.

Describes techniques used to train a legally blind teacher to chart student progress on 6-cycle graph paper.

1616. Carroll, Terrence E. Sin, sloth, and sheltered employment. *New Outlook for the Blind*, Mar. 1966, Vol. 60, No. 3, pp. 90–92.

Discusses the ideology of work, and the "work ethic," relative to sheltered workshops and changes which should be made in them.

1617. Chappell, J. Hiram. The blind man on the farm. *New Outlook for the Blind*, May 1953, Vol. 47, No. 5, pp. 142–47.

The number of blind persons in agricultural occupations is far below the number to be expected on the basis of population statistics. Reviews possible reasons for this and ways to attack the problem.

1618. ————. *Counselors guide: How to analyze the rehabilitation needs of blind persons on the farm.* Washington, D.C.: Office of Vocational Rehabilitation, Rehabilitation Service Series No. 160 (rev.), 1954.

Lists rural occupations in which blind persons have succeeded, suggestions for the counselor, and lists of agencies and organizations which provide services to farmers.

1619. ————. The outlook in piano tuning for qualified blind persons. *New Outlook for the Blind,* Dec. 1959, Vol. 53, No. 10, pp. 366–71.

Argues that piano tuning is a very profitable vocation, that failures of blind people in tuning resulted largely from poor or inadequate training, and challenges the schools to provide better training. Believes more schools may be needed.

1620. Chevion, Dov, & Schiff, Yehuda. *Research on rehabilitation of blind and visually handicapped in operating data-processing machines. Report No. 5, on training of the blind in computer-programming.* Jerusalem: Ministry of Social Welfare, 1967, 49 pp.

Details of methods and aids used in above training.

1621. Chouinard, Edward L. Sheltered employment—a symposium: Sheltered workshops—past and present. *New Outlook for the Blind,* Sept. 1957, Vol. 51, No. 7, pp. 279–86.

Early origins and history of workshops from the middle ages to present.

1622. Cimino, Anthony. Let's pull all strings but stay well-tempered. *International Journal for the Education of the Blind,* Mar. 1956, Vol. 5, No. 3, pp. 58–60.

Discusses piano tuning as a profession for blind people and studying for that profession.

1623. Clark, Robert P. Business Enterprises Education Program: A course for supervisors. *New Outlook for the Blind,* Mar. 1974, Vol. 68, No. 3, pp. 128–29, 131.

Instructors in educational psychology and guidance, management, marketing, accounting, food science, institution administration, etc., participated in a trial course. Results show the course can increase proficiency of supervisors.

1624. Clay, Henry. Greenhouse and nursery training for the blind. *International Journal for the Education of the Blind,* Mar. 1962, Vol. 11, No. 3, pp. 69–70.

A research project at the Georgia Academy for the Blind culminated in a 33-page instructional manual and a film showing how to train blind persons to grow bedding plants, cut flowers, bulbs, shrubs, and fruit trees.

1625. Clayton, Isaac P. Career opportunities for visually handicapped persons in Maryland. *New Outlook for the Blind,* May 1973, Vol. 67, No. 5, pp. 210–15.

Report of 1972 survey of 478 employers to determine number of blind employees, jobs held, and employer attitudes; also, survey of 343 former students regarding current employment, employment success, and reaction to goals of project.

1626. Coen, James P.; Nooe, Dick C.; Plummer, Ralph; et al. The social worker with visual impairment. *New Outlook for the Blind*, Dec. 1964, Vol. 58, No. 10, pp. 311–15. Reprinted from *Social Casework*, Jan. 1964.

Report of experiences of 3 blind social workers. Includes information on necessary training, orientation, relationships with other staff members, use of reader services, work with groups, and relationships with clients.

1627. Collier, Boy N., Jr. Teaching: A vocation for the handicapped? *Vocational Guidance Quarterly*, Sept. 1971, Vol. 20, No. 1, pp. 48–51.

Survey conducted to determine entry restrictions into the teaching profession for those with diabetes, epilepsy, visual, or auditory handicaps. Persons with diabetes or epilepsy were found to be virtually eliminated from employment in the education field more than persons with visual or auditory handicaps.

1628. Committee on Professional Activities of the Blind of the Assoc. for Computing Machinery. *The selection, training, and placement of blind computer programmers.* St. Louis, Mo.: Author, 1966, 45 pp.

Report designed as a guide for teacher concerned with education of computer professionals, employer of those in this field, rehabilitation worker, and blind person interested in this profession.

1629. Committee on the Employment of Blind Persons as Professional Workers. *Blind persons as social workers and rehabilitation counselors.* New York: Author, 1967, 9 pp.

Presented in question and answer format, urges qualified blind persons be trained and placed as social workers and rehabilitation counselors. Maintains that blind trainees can meet same eligibility requirements and standards and can function in same way as sighted colleagues.

1630. Crawford, Fred L., & Lirtzman, Sidney. *Counseling and placement of blind persons in professional occupations: Practice and research.* New York: N.Y. Assoc. for the Blind, 1966, 160 pp.

Summary of results of a 3-year study on placement of blind persons in professional work with an analysis of employer attitudes toward blindness and an outline of current standards for hiring workers in 25 professional occupations. Bib.

1631. Cronin, Robert. I give IQ tests without looking. *New Outlook for the Blind*, May 1970, Vol. 64, No. 5, pp. 142–47.

Description of problems encountered by a blind school psychologist with creative solutions to the problems in terms of adapting tests and relationships with the children.

1632. Cross, Kenneth. Public school teaching as a career for the blind: Mythology and methodology. *New Outlook for the Blind*, Feb. 1972, Vol. 66, No. 2, pp. 43–49.

In light of own experience, discusses teaching as a profession for blind people including suggestions regarding hiring interview, use of visual aids, and correcting papers.

1633. Dent, Oran B. An investigation of attitudes toward work adjustment of the blind. *New Outlook for the Blind*, Dec. 1962, Vol. 56, No. 10, pp. 357–62.

Reports on study investigating attitudes toward job-holding and work adjustment abilities of the blind in job situations where their actual competency has been demonstrated. Discussion of procedure, results. Four hundred *S*s. Nonblind rated more favorably than blind. The higher the job's social status, the better the adjustment.

1634. Dept. of Special Education & Rehabilitation. *Business Enterprises Education Program: Course guide.* Nashville: Univ. of Tenn., 1973, 501 pp.

Course guide for manpower development and training in business enterprise programs.

1635. DeRuyter, John. The training of blind computer programmers. *New Outlook for the Blind*, Jan. 1968, Vol. 62, No. 1, pp. 7–10, 23.

Success of a blind paraplegic as a computer programmer led a business school to establish a program of training in programming for the blind. Describes selection of students, training techniques, tools needed, and placement.

1636. Dickey, Thomas W., & Vieceli, Louis. A survey of the vocational placement of visually handicapped persons and their degree of vision. *New Outlook for the Blind*, Feb. 1972, Vol. 66, No. 2, pp. 38–42.

Results of survey of 225 graduates of Job Development and Placement Course. Relates professional and nonprofessional jobs to 3 levels of vision.

1637. Dodge, Helen, & Ward, John P. Opportunities for blind professional people: Two examples. *New Outlook for the Blind*, Jan. 1958, Vol. 52, No. 1, pp. 17–20.

Part 1 discusses qualifications of the blind music therapist and how they can counter problems and utilize assets. Part 2 discusses teaching political science and the development of an efficient, low cost, lightweight tape recorder as a boon to research efforts.

1638. Durfee, S. B. The status of piano technology. *International Journal for the Education of the Blind*, May 1959, Vol. 8, No. 4, pp. 137–39.

Functions and knowledge needed by a piano technician sets him apart from the mere tuner. Answers questions about the training and employment of technicians and urges an increase in this kind of training in schools for the blind.

1639. Feintuch, Alfred. Sheltered workshops: A conceptual framework. *New Outlook for the Blind*, Feb. 1959, Vol. 53, No. 2, pp. 69–72.

Contribution of sheltered shops centers in: (1) relief from social isolation, (2) improved communication, (3) better work habits, (4) the client's improved confidence in his ability to meet industrial standards, and (5) greater effectiveness of vocational and psychological counseling when integrated with sheltered shop programs.

1640. Finnis, Jane. The other side of the mike. *New Beacon*, Mar. 1973, Vol. 57, No. 671, pp. 64–66.

The blind author, working as a free-lance interviewer aired on BBC, describes how she established herself in her job and how she carries out her work.

1641. First workshop on industrial homework. *New Outlook for the Blind*, May 1954, Vol. 48, No. 5, pp. 153–56.

Describes the workshop and details its recommendations for providing work to blind persons at home.

1642. Foote, Charles W. Skilcraft: A new sales program. *New Outlook for the Blind*, Dec. 1957, Vol. 51, No. 10, pp. 475–76.

Reasons for adopting the Skilcraft trademark for blind-made products, how it will be developed and used, and anticipated advantages.

1643. Freund, Elisabeth D. Tasters and smellers in the food and fragrance industry: A limited new job possibility for the blind. *Rehabilitation Record*, Mar.–Apr. 1973, Vol. 14, No. 2, pp. 6–9.

Describes job opportunities in quality control in the above industries.

1644. Friedensohn, Oscar. A look at vending stand operation: Patterns and trends. *New Outlook for the Blind*, Jan. 1966, Vol. 60, No. 1, pp. 1–3.

Questionnaires returned by 34 states reporting number of stands, number of blind operators/assistants, income distribution. Findings and interpretations of the informal study given.

1645. Fries, Emil B. Present and future status of piano tuning and servicing as a vocation for the blind. *New Outlook for the Blind*, Nov. 1962, Vol. 56, No. 9, pp. 322–26.

Author feels this is promising field for properly trained blind people. Describes program at the Piano Hospital and Training Center in Vancouver, Wash. Discusses agencies' role in preparing and assisting students to receive training in piano tuning.

1646. Gallagher, William F., Ed. *Selection, training, and placement of qualified blind teachers in teaching positions in the public school systems at both the elementary and the secondary grade levels.* New York: N.Y. Assoc. for the Blind, 1967, 45 pp.

This report of the National Training Institute, New York, May 1967, is intended for school, college, and placement bureau officials. Gives guidelines for the selection, training, and placement of blind teachers which are the result of group workshops.

1647. ————. *Employment of qualified blind teachers in teaching positions in the public school systems at both the elementary and the secondary grade levels.* Washington, D.C.: Social and Rehabilitation Service, HEW, 1969, 80 pp.

Proceedings of an institute including a paper on the importance of employing blind teachers and papers on teaching grades 5 & 6, general science in grades 7–9, math, Spanish, physics, and chemistry. Also discusses the availability of qualified blind teachers, job seeking, and administration considerations.

1648. Gildea, Robert A. Guidelines for training blind computer programers. *New Outlook for the Blind*, Nov. 1970, Vol. 64, No. 9, pp. 297–300.

Describes selection criteria, training objectives and techniques, and the procedures of placement.

1649. Goodpasture, R. C. Workshops work! *New Outlook for the Blind,* May 1963, Vol. 57, No. 5, pp. 164–67.

Discusses NIB, and evidence that workshops work.

1650. Greater Detroit Society for the Blind. *Occupational information library for the blind.* Detroit: Author, 1974, $53. (A card catalogue.)

1651. Grossberg, Sidney H., & Beyer, Barbara L. Field instruction with blind students. *Social Work Education Reporter,* Dec.–Jan. 1972, Vol. 20, No. 1, pp. 60–63.

Discusses special problems faced by the blind social work student. Possible solutions are suggested.

1652. Gunderson, Robert. Radio theory and practice for the blind. *International Journal for the Education of the Blind,* June 1952, Vol. 1, No. 4, pp. 89–93.

Briefly discusses problems involved in teaching radio and electronics to the blind: A lack of relevant braille literature and of specialized measuring instruments. Lists and describes 19 pieces of equipment developed or found suitable and relevant braille magazines.

1653. Hadley School for the Blind. *National training institute on special and technical secretarial occupations for the blind.* Winnetka, Ill.: Author, 1971, 11 pp.

Proceedings of 4-day institute, held in Chicago, May 1971, on career opportunities for visually handicapped secretaries. General topics include psychological testing, educational needs, job placement, employer attitudes, office aids and interpersonal skills necessary for successful visually handicapped secretaries, a laboratory demonstration, and a research project.

1654. Hallenbeck, Charles E. Curriculum standards in the United States for training blind persons in computer occupations. *New Outlook for the Blind,* June 1973, Vol. 67, No. 6, pp. 266–71.

Summary of experience in U.S. in training and employing blind persons in computer operations. Training in specialized facilities compared with training in integrated educational institutions. Recommendations for continued progress.

1655. Handel, Alexander F. Sheltered employment—a symposium: Introduction. *New Outlook for the Blind,* Sept. 1957, Vol. 51, No. 7, pp. 278–79.

Brief introductory overview of the functions and services of workshops.

1656. Hardy, Richard E. Music as a professional occupation for the blind. *New Outlook for the Blind,* May 1966, Vol. 60, No. 5, pp. 155–57.

Presents brief historical background on blind persons as musicians/entertainers. Discusses error of assuming any blind child would do well in music field, and vocational opportunities in that field. Lists 4 points essential for successful musical careers.

1657. ————. Relating psychological data to job analysis information in vocational counseling. *New Outlook for the Blind,* Sept. 1969, Vol. 63, No. 7, pp. 202–4.

Guidelines for the counselor relating job knowledge to client needs so that possible problems and possible solutions are considered.

1658. Harkness, Charles A. Nondebilitating diseases and industrial hiring practices. *Vocational Guidance Quarterly*, Sept. 1971, Vol. 20, No. 1, pp. 52–55.

Survey conducted in the fall of 1969 of industrial hiring practices as they related to diabetes, epilepsy, hearing loss, and visual deficit. Results suggested that insurance companies and their restrictions served as justification for tendency of businesses not to hire people with nondebilitating diseases.

1659. Hewitt, Brian. Integration in teaching a manual skill. *New Beacon*, Oct. 1975, Vol. 59, No. 702, pp. 260–62.

An instructor in piano tuning compares results of training blind tuners in segregated and integrated settings and concludes that as presently organized, manual skills are better taught by specialist staff in the segregated setting.

1660. Huntington, Edward F. Can a blind person be a successful teacher? *New Outlook for the Blind*, Jan. 1967, Vol. 61, No. 1, pp. 6–7.

Studied, through questionnaires and interviews, attitudes of school administrators to employing blind teachers. Successful and problem work assignments for blind teachers were identified.

1661. ———. *Administrative considerations in the employment of blind teachers.* New York: Lighthouse for the Blind, 1972, 96 pp., $1.50.

Data shows that none of the anticipated concerns was a serious problem for blind teachers.

1662. Hyde, James F., Jr. *Law as a profession for the blind.* New York: AFB, 1954, 67 pp.

Series of articles covering various aspects of the legal profession compiled to afford information and guidance to the blind individual who wishes to enter this field. Articles included are based on individual personal experiences.

1663. Jacobs, Abraham. Sheltered employment—a symposium: Vocational rehabilitation of the blind. *New Outlook for the Blind*, Sept. 1957, Vol. 51, No. 7, pp. 286–92.

The economic, social, and psychological benefits of rehabilitation are enhanced by its recognition of individual differences and by 12 points which the author calls "a blind individual's Bill of Rights."

1664. Johnson, Carl A. Concession stand operation in a centrally-managed program. *New Outlook for the Blind*, Sept. 1955, Vol. 49, No. 7, pp. 247–51.

Describes the vending stand program of the Cleveland Society for the Blind as an example of a centrally managed business enterprise program. Agency and operator set policy jointly, there is a manual of operations, and standards are high. Improvement is constantly sought.

1665. ———. Toward greater opportunities in business enterprises. *New Outlook for the Blind*, June 1960, Vol. 54, No. 6, pp. 215–18.

Discusses formation of the American Business Council for the Blind, purpose of which is to achieve more uniform success in the vending stand business for employable blind people. Discusses purposes of business enterprises, need for national planning, ABCB's structural provision for communication, need to keep up with the times, control of administrative and overhead costs.

1666. Johnson, Hugh D. Refreshment stand operation. *International Journal for the Education of the Blind*, Feb. 1952, Vol. 1, No. 3, p. 60.

As a successful field of employment, schools for the blind should give training in this vocation. Description of 2 stands in Maryland School for the Blind, types of training with detailed information.

1667. Kenmore, Jeanne R. Helping blind persons to find and prepare for employment. *New Outlook for the Blind*, Mar. 1973, Vol. 67, No. 3, pp. 111–15.

Four kinds of job market surveys are recommended for discovering possible occupations. The role of schools in promoting the success of blind youngsters when they enter the job market is discussed. The role of the placement officer is emphasized as are the roles of agencies and government. Examples are drawn from many countries around the world.

1668. Kleber, C. C. Special workshops—History and development. *New Outlook for the Blind*, Oct. 1956, Vol. 50, No. 8, pp. 303–6.

From the first workshop at Perkins School for the Blind in 1842, traces the history and discusses the influence of National Industries for the Blind.

1669. Kruger, Irving J. Homebound employment for the blind and visually handicapped in New Jersey. *New Outlook for the Blind*, Dec. 1972, Vol. 66, No. 10, pp. 345–48.

Discussion of need for homebound employment, examples of homebound workers. Describes Craftshop Program, Wholesale Products Program, and chair-caning and rush-seating program. Points out problems and high costs in operating such a program.

1670. Larkin, Charles N. Sociological considerations in placement of blind workers. *New Outlook for the Blind*, Nov. 1963, Vol. 57, No. 9, pp. 360–61.

Discusses estimating possible success of a placement.

1671. Lasley, Jim. Farming by touch. *Lion*, Nov. 1971, Vol. 54, No. 5, pp. 17–18.

The story of how a legally blind farmer works his 250-acre tobacco farm in N.C.

1672. Lindberg, Gene. Training eyes to speed up with words. *New Outlook for the Blind*, Mar. 1953, Vol. 47, No. 3, pp. 75–77.

Work and background of a teacher of communications skills.

1673. Link, Harry J. Placement and employment of the visually impaired: State of the art and identification of unmet needs. *New Outlook for the Blind*, Sept. 1975, Vol. 69, No. 7, pp. 320–24.

Describes vocational rehabilitation and other federal legislation that has opened jobs, naming areas which have attracted visually impaired persons. Two surveys of unmet needs indicate need for more placement, more real work skills, and early career education.

1674. Litwiller, Clifford. Why special courses for tuning instructors of the blind. *New Outlook for the Blind*, Apr. 1957, Vol. 51, No. 4, pp. 145–48.

With quotations from graduates, justifies the course for tuning instructors at Roosevelt Univ., Chicago.

1675. Loban, L. N. Group insurance and the handicapped. *Blind Californian,* Fall 1974, Vol. 15, No. 2, pp. 23–26.

A report prepared for the Governor's Committee on Employment of the Handicapped based on questionnaire replies from 14 insurance companies operating in Calif. in the fields of group medical and group life insurance.

1676. Maas, Melvin J. Changing attitudes toward employment of the blind. *New Outlook for the Blind,* Mar. 1958, Vol. 52, No. 3, pp. 86–88.

Informal questionnaire to state agencies for the blind disclosed a somewhat more encouraging climate for employment with a reduction of old prejudices of employers.

1677. McCauley, W. Alfred. *The blind person as a college teacher.* New York: AFB, 1961, 88 pp.

Questionnaire study undertaken to ascertain how blind persons actually perform as college teachers, the degree of administrative acceptance of these teachers, and the problems they encounter in entering this profession.

1678. ———. Blind persons in college teaching. *New Outlook for the Blind,* Jan. 1961, Vol. 55, No. 1, pp. 1–7.

Blind college teachers and those who hire them were questioned. Reports results and implications.

1679. McCollom, M. A. Is super seniority a must? *New Outlook for the Blind,* Apr. 1957, Vol. 51, No. 4, pp. 149–51.

The issue of job seniority in an industry and placement of blind workers with some advice on dealing with this objection on the part of employers.

1680. MacFarland, Douglas C. Some guides to placement procedure. *New Outlook for the Blind,* Apr. 1954, Vol. 48, No. 4, pp. 100–104.

Detailed discussion of how to approach and relate to a potential employer in order to place a blind worker.

1681. ———. *A study of work efficiency of blind and sighted workers in industry.* New York: AFB, 1956, 58 pp.

Study showed no significant differences between the blind and the sighted in 6 factors determining work efficiency, in annual earnings, in production rating, in days absent, and in safety records. Intelligence test scores of the blind were significantly higher.

1682. McGreal, Thomas L., & Wiseman, Dennis. The blind teacher in the educational job market. *New Outlook for the Blind,* Feb. 1973, Vol. 67, No. 2, pp. 80–83.

Gives specific suggestions for the blind applicant for a teaching position, including obtaining a personal interview, filing application forms and other pertinent data, and preparing for and conducting the interview. States that if these suggestions are followed and if state and federal associations serving the blind publicize the abilities of blind workers, opportunities for employment will improve.

1683. McKae, Doug. Jay Birch, 20/20 scouter. *Scouting*, Sept. 1974, Vol. 62, No. 6, pp. 62, 100.

The story of Jay Birch, a Scouting professional for 7 years before losing his sight in 1970; he has successfully continued in his chosen career.

1684. Macmillan, Maurice. Promoting employment. *New Beacon*, Aug. 1972, Vol. 56, No. 664, pp. 203–4.

Discusses development of specialized aids, equipment, and social services which increased employment opportunities for the blind in Great Britain.

1685. Margolin, Morris. Blind physicians and the practice of medicine. *New Outlook for the Blind*, June 1959, Vol. 53, No. 6, pp. 199–205.

Reviews and in some ways enlarges upon an article about blind physicians written by Arthur and Virginia Keeney and published in *Archives of Ophthalmology*, June 1950. Provides suggestions on how a blind person can function as a physician and describes their limitations.

1686. Milan, Kurt. The sky's the limit. *Rehabilitation Record*, Mar.–Apr. 1973, Vol. 14, No. 2, pp. 11–12.

The story of a totally blind young man who earned a bachelor's degree in meteorology and obtained employment as an instructor of meteorology at the National Weather Bureau.

1687. Murr, Arthur C. The position of civil service in vocational rehabilitation of the blind. *New Outlook for the Blind*, Nov. 1958, Vol. 52, No. 9, pp. 339–42.

Discusses the government's selective placement program conducted by the U.S. Civil Service Commission, applicant qualifications, relationship to the President's Committee on Employment of the Physically Handicapped, and the field coordinator's role in "Operation Understanding."

1688. National Accreditation Council. *Self-study and evaluation guide for sheltered workshops.* New York: AFB, 1968, 213 pp.

Designed as an instrument for a sheltered workshop for the blind which operates as an independent agency rather than as part of a larger multiservice organization. Provides forms and evaluation procedures for major aspects of administration and for workshop service programs.

1689. New York Assoc. for the Blind. *Conference to promote the employment of blind persons in U.S. Civil Service occupations: October 8–9, 1964.* New York: Author, 1964, 35 pp.

Discussion of a pilot program to bring about more employment opportunities for the blind under Civil Service.

1690. ———. *Selection, training, and placement of qualified blind teachers in teaching positions in the public school systems at both the elementary and the secondary grade levels: Report on National Training Institute held at the Lighthouse, May 2–4, 1967.* New York: Author, 1967, 45 pp.

Results of conference held to promote an interest in and awareness of blind teachers by school administrators, teacher training and placement bureau personnel, rehabilitation counselors.

1691. ———. *Employment of qualified blind teachers in teaching positions in the public school systems at both the elementary and the secondary* *grade levels: Report on the Regional Training Institute held at the Lighthouse March 18–19, 1969.* New York: Author, 1969, 74 pp.

Report from institute to inform school administrators, placement personnel, and rehabilitation counselors that blind teachers can successfully assume the duties of teachers in public school programs.

1692. Nezol, A. James. A pilot course to assist blind potential teachers. *New Outlook for the Blind,* Sept. 1975, Vol. 69, No. 7, pp. 317–19.

Included practicum experiences, a Practical Approaches Laboratory, mock lessons, materials preparation workshop, lecture-demonstrations, mock interviews, conferences, and exercises in problem-solving. While the 6 students in this pilot course gained in skill and confidence, it is felt that much more needs to be done.

1693. Nichols, W. H. Blind persons in data processing: The attitude of industry. *New Outlook for the Blind,* Nov. 1970, Vol. 64, No. 9, pp. 293–96.

Discusses the attitudes of top, middle, and line management toward the visually handicapped. Roles which agencies play in overcoming negative attitudes are discussed, and the advantages of a blind programmer are emphasized.

1694. Nyquist, Ewald B. The importance of employing blind teachers in the public schools. *New Outlook for the Blind,* Jan. 1971, Vol. 65, No. 1, pp. 1–6.

Discussion of evaluation of teacher candidates, teacher preparation programs, and the qualities of a good teacher. Factors preventing the hiring of blind teachers and progress in their employment also examined.

1695. Olsen, Carl E., & Held, Marian. Sheltered employment—a symposium: The industrial workshop—destination unlimited. *New Outlook for the Blind,* Sept. 1957, Vol. 51, No. 1, pp. 303–8.

Describes and defends the kind of workshop which is a permanent employment objective, with the Lighthouse Industries in New York City as an example.

1696. O'Neill, George J. Crisis & challenge at VBI. *Lion,* Sept. 1974, Vol. 57, No. 3, pp. 14–15.

Story of the Volunteer Blind Industries in Morristown, Tenn., a project of the Lions Club that serves the blind of 21 counties of the state.

1697. Oswald, Hedwig. Blind employees succeeding as job information specialists. *Blind Californian,* Fall 1974, Vol. 15, No. 2, pp. 29–33.

The training and placement of blind persons in Federal Job Information Centers, where they handle questions concerning all facets of federal employment.

1698. Owens, Aleta R. Our student teacher was blind. *New Outlook for the Blind,* Sept. 1955, Vol. 49, No. 7, pp. 264–67.

An impressive story of the success of a blind student teacher and how he changed the attitudes of his students.

1699. Palacios, May H.; Newberry, Lawrence A.; & Bootzin, Richard R. Predictive validity of the interview. *Journal of Applied Psychology,* 1966, Vol. 50, No. 1, pp. 67–72.

Describes interview as a valid and reliable instrument for job placement and vocational success. Interviews of 144 blind adults were data for study.

1700. Parker, Tom. A look at "workshops" for the blind in Russia. *Braille Forum*, Sept.–Oct. 1974, Vol. 13, No. 2, pp. 16–21.

An abridged version of a report to the members of the National League of the Blind (England) following a visit to Russia by several members of the League.

1701. Parsons, Patricia. Life's a jigsaw puzzle. *New Beacon*, Nov. 1972, Vol. 56, No. 667, pp. 284–86.

A blind British secretary describes her lengthy struggle for increased responsibility and her resultant professional achievement.

1702. Penny, Margaret. Training of blind shorthand-typists. *International Journal for the Education of the Blind*, June 1952, Vol. 1, No. 4, pp. 81–84.

Describes and illustrates the braille scale for typists, stating that, in combination with development of teaching methods, the foundation for "blind" typing was laid and admirably built upon. Details typist's methods, briefly discusses then-current relevant employment trends.

1703. Pinner, Janet I. Are the sheltered workshops doing their job? *New Outlook for the Blind*, Jan. 1956, Vol. 50, No. 1, pp. 12–15.

Shops have been teaching job know-how, but the quality of teaching has varied. Also important to motivate, develop good work habits, and make placement effort. Points out some weaknesses in sheltered shop movement.

1704. Preuss, Bernard F. Rural rehabilitation for the blind in Missouri. *New Outlook for the Blind*, Mar. 1953, Vol. 47, No. 3, pp. 67–74.

Following a statement of philosophy and description of prevocational evaluation and training, outlines 9-month course of study of the Vocational Rehabilitation Agricultural Training Center. Reviews some details of operation, factors in success or failure, and general statement of results.

1705. *Proceedings of the National Symposium on Employment of the Visually Impaired in Secretarial Fields.* Washington, D.C.: Visually Impaired Secretarial Transcribers Assoc., 1974?

Dec. 1973 conference workshops covered finding a secretarial job, adapting job skills to overcome the problems presented by the visual handicap, demonstrating abilities, and advancing in position.

1706. Raithel, John B., & Rieman, Edward A. Switchboard operation—A national survey. *New Outlook for the Blind*, Dec. 1961, Vol. 55, No. 10, pp. 352–55.

Information relating to a national survey of progress made on switchboard operation by visually impaired. Problems encountered. Equipment used. State-by-state breakdown.

1707. Read, Harry. Labor's philosophy regarding special employment services. *New Outlook for the Blind*, Jan. 1956, Vol. 50, No. 1, pp. 8–11.

States the CIO position that rehabilitation and vocational training or retraining should be a continuous process with the workmen's compensation system. Lists problems in the employment of the handicapped, labor's insistence on safeguards, belief in pay rate in sheltered work based on industry, and the dignity of the individual.

1708. Rice, Ronald G.; Muthard, John E.; & Dumas, Neil S. The recruitment, selection, and training of blind vending stand operators. *New Outlook for the Blind*, Dec. 1970, Vol. 64, No. 10, pp. 325–29.

Study conducted to determine if there was need for nationwide validation of selection battery for visually handicapped vending stand operators. Felt that an empirically derived test battery would probably not materially improve the rehabilitation record.

1709. Routh, Thomas A. Employment for the blind. *New Outlook for the Blind*, Apr. 1955, Vol. 49, No. 4, pp. 139–40.

Discusses just what "full employment" should mean for blind people.

1710. Rowley, Harold. A new profession for the blind? *Braille Forum*, July–Aug. 1975, Vol. 14, No. 1, pp. 9–13.

Author's experience of becoming a paralegal which he feels is an opening for the blind, although he points out it is still in a pioneer stage.

1711. Royston, Richard D., & Yoder, Norman M. The third generation—A challenge to the blind. *New Outlook for the Blind*, Jan. 1968, Vol. 62, No. 1, pp. 11–14.

More sophisticated computers require higher levels of programming than did early equipment. Discusses implications for training blind programmers.

1712. Rusalem, Herbert. Desirable characteristics of blind candidates for work for the blind. *New Outlook for the Blind*, May 1956, Vol. 50, No. 5, pp. 176–80.

Blind candidates for employment in work with the blind should have: Good travel and orientation, good communication tools, a clear vocational goal, previous work experience, success in handling their own blindness, and good personal management.

1713. ———. Personal attributes for blind entry workers. *New Outlook for the Blind*, June 1957, Vol. 51, No. 6, pp. 236–40.

In work for the blind, employers seek the following personal attributes in addition to academic preparation: Independence, appropriate attitudes toward themselves, the community, and the agency, no desire for special privileges, mental health, and good work habits.

1714. ———. Attitudes toward blind counselors in state rehabilitation agencies. *Personnel and Guidance Journal*, 1961, Vol. 39, pp. 367–72.

There are few opportunities for blind counselors in agencies serving both blind and sighted. Attitudes may change with research.

1715. ———. The sheltered workshop of the 1960's. *New Outlook for the Blind*, June 1963, Vol. 57, No. 6, pp. 200–205.

Workshops may be entering a critical phase in use of several kinds of contracts and prime manufacturing. Long-range planning and social action are important, and consumer's views must be heard.

1716. Ruscio, Thomas J. *Rehabilitation of the legally blind: A case study approach to vending stand and other placements. Proceedings of a regional training institute, Springfield College, Oct. 25–26, 1973.* Springfield, Mass.: Springfield Col., 1973, 168 pp.

Includes papers on placement, especially in vending stands, while procedures for placement appear in 4 detailed case studies.

1717. Rusk, Howard A. Home employment for the disabled. *New Outlook for the Blind*, Nov. 1955, Vol. 49, No. 9, pp. 331–32.

Special projects were planned in Vt. and Ala. to bring home employment to blind people. Although the federal government can give support, the primary responsibility must lie in each community.

1718. Sabeston, May. The blind teacher in the school for seeing children. *International Journal for the Education of the Blind*, Mar. 1960, Vol. 9, No. 3, pp. 73–76. Reprinted from *New Beacon*, Oct. 1959.

A blind teacher of music tells how she handles her classes, methods and special materials used.

1719. Sakata, Robert, & Sinick, Daniel. Evaluation of prospective vending stand operators. *New Outlook for the Blind*, May 1964, Vol. 58, No. 5, pp. 144–45.

Authors feel time and money is wasted training vending stand operators who do not complete the course. They detail a specific course of evaluation for potential trainees including both standardized tests and practical experience.

1720. Scheffel, Robert R. *New careers in rehabilitation: The rehabilitation aide project.* Richmond: Va. Comm. for the Visually Handicapped, 1974, 43 pp., app.

Project determined feasibility of utilizing trained aides to provide specific aspects of orientation, mobility, and rehabilitation teaching services to selected blind and visually handicapped individuals, especially the geriatric blind.

1721. ———. The rehabilitation aide project. *New Outlook for the Blind*, Mar. 1975, Vol. 69, No. 3, pp. 116–20.

Follow-up study of program to determine feasibility of utilizing trained paraprofessionals to provide specific aspects of orientation and mobility and rehabilitation teaching services to selected visually handicapped persons.

1722. Schiff, Yehuda. The blind in the computer age. *New Outlook for the Blind*, Jan. 1968, Vol. 62, No. 1, pp. 1–6, illus.

The status of services for the blind in Israel, with detailed discussion of the training and employment of computer programmers.

1723. Scott, Robert A. The factory as a social service organization: Goal displacements in workshops for the blind. *Social Problems*, 1967, Vol. 15, No. 2, pp. 160–75.

Describes the process of goal displacement in sheltered workshops for the blind and analyzes its impact on the employment problem for the blind in general.

1724. Septinelli, Anthony E. Imagination and ingenuity—Keys to placement. *New Outlook for the Blind*, Nov. 1956, Vol. 50, No. 9, pp. 354–58.

How to place blind workers in jobs, including vending stands.

1725. Shapir, Ezra. *Research on rehabilitation of blind and visually handicapped in operating IBM punch-card machines.* Report No. 3. Jerusalem: Ministry of Social Welfare, 1966, 76 pp.

With many diagrams and illustrations, provides details of methods and materials involved in training for the above.

1726. Shell, Claude I. Selling—Another role for the placement counselor. *New Outlook for the Blind*, Feb. 1968, Vol. 62, No. 2, pp. 33–37.

Details how the counselor must be a salesman, first of himself, then of his client, and finally of the concept that a visually handicapped person can be a good employee.

1727. Sterling, Theodor D., & Bauman, Mary K. Employment potential for the blind in computer related fields. *International Journal for the Education of the Blind*, Oct. 1965, Vol. 15, No. 1, pp. 7–11.

Describes several aspects of computer work in which blind people can succeed. Cost factor of employing the blind is small; blind and sighted programmers work at about the same speed. Reports a training program for blind programmers and suggests some implications for education of the blind.

1728. Sterling, Theodor D.; Lichstein, M.; Scarpino, F.; et al. Computer work for the blind. *Journal of Rehabilitation*, 1964, Vol. 30, No. 6, pp. 20–21.

Skills, background, and necessary training for the varying levels of computer programming are delineated.

1729. Stone, J. R. Industry looks at the blind. *International Journal for the Education of the Blind*, Dec. 1958, Vol. 8, No. 2, pp. 52–58.

Industry expects of workers production, quality, and harmonious relationships with fellow workers; workers want from industry security, recognition, and acceptance by fellow workers. Blind employees fit well into this pattern. Refutes some objections to blind employees.

1730. Stout, Thomas H. CAMA board operator: A new employment opportunity for visually handicapped persons. *New Outlook for the Blind*, Oct. 1970, Vol. 64, No. 8, pp. 258–59.

Describes a new position in the telephone system.

1731. Stromer, Walter F. On the teaching of speech. *International Journal for the Education of the Blind*, May 1956, Vol. 5, No. 4, pp. 91–93.

Article by blind college teacher and public speaker. Speech correction; learning how to speak effectively; references to personal experiences and impressions rather than those of others; gestures and eye contacts discussed.

1732. Swope, Burton. Blind rope maker. *Braille Monitor*, Aug. 1975, pp. 320–21.

Describes the manufacturing business of a blind rope maker.

1733. Tate, Terry. Blind programmers at Rolls Royce—Newsletter 1, July 1974. *American Foundation for the Blind Research Bulletin 29*, June 1975, p. 227.

Reprint of brief report. Mentions equipment used.

1734. Thomason, Bruce, & Barrett, Albert M. *Opportunities for blind teachers in public schools: A report on legal aspects, policies and practices affecting their employment.* New York: AFB, 1961, 39 pp.

Questionnaire study undertaken to clarify employment situation of blind persons as public school teachers. Attempts a state-by-state compilation of factual information related to the problem.

1735. Townsend, M. Roberta. A program for industrial homework. *New Outlook for the Blind*, Sept. 1953, Vol. 47, No. 7, pp. 206–10.

Guidelines for developing an industrial homework program in terms of program content, agency, nature of the clients, staff, products and markets. Homework should be a planned part of total rehabilitation with necessary supporting services.

1736. ———. Sheltered employment—a symposium: Vermont pilot study on industrial homework. *New Outlook for the Blind*, Sept. 1957, Vol. 51, No. 1, pp. 309–15.

Reports a 2-year project of research and demonstration on the practicability of offering regular employment to the homebound disabled person in a rural state.

1737. A training and employment opportunity for blind persons with the Social Security Administration: Teleservice representative. *New Outlook for the Blind*, Jan. 1974, Vol. 68, No. 1, pp. 19, 24.

A job description.

1738. Trapny, Karl. The Austrian program for the professional training of the blind to operate telephone switchboards. *International Journal for the Education of the Blind*, Oct. 1952, Vol. 2, No. 1, pp. 118–21.

Describes the origin of this occupation for the blind, requirements and selection of applicants, training involving theory, practice, and on the job, the final examination, a report on employed operators, and discussion of how placements are found.

1739. Tung, Ta Cheng. Poultry raising by the blind in Taiwan. *New Outlook for the Blind*, Apr. 1959, Vol. 53, No. 4, pp. 141–43.

Briefly describes status of blind in Taiwan, followed by fairly detailed description of poultry raising as an occupation.

1740. U.S. Dept. of Health, Education & Welfare, Rehabilitation Services Admin. *Guidelines for the selection, training, and placement of blind persons in information service expediting.* Washington, D.C.: Author, 1975, 101 pp., app.

Guidelines resulting from a conference held to facilitate development of counseling and training programs which will enable the visually handicapped to enter this profession.

1741. Va. Commission for the Visually Handicapped. *Correlating services available to farmers.* Richmond: Author, 1963, 13 pp.

Demonstration project concludes blind person can operate farm independently from financial and work performance viewpoint if community agencies cooperate in supplying technical and financial assistance geared to his special problems.

1742. ———. *To assess the proficiency of the blind as tape duplicator operators: A final report.* Richmond: Author, 1968, 22 pp.

Study concludes that blind can successfully function in this job in most settings. A guide for training is included.

1743. Veterans Administration. Occupations of totally blinded veterans. *Employment Security Review*, 1956, Vol. 23, No. 9, pp. 14–16.

Statements on the employment of several hundred totally blinded veterans, arranged according to occupation.

1744. Walker, I. Constance. Computer programmer training for the blind and visually impaired: A case for quality standards and professionalism. *American Foundation for the Blind Research Bulletin 24*, Mar. 1972, pp. 95–112, app.

Describes standards and training methods for visually handicapped computer programmers.

1745. Ward, Allan L., & Knoch, Elmo A., Jr. Training blind persons to work as taxpayer service representatives. *New Outlook for the Blind*, Mar. 1972, Vol. 66, No. 3, pp. 81–83.

Description of the training of taxpayers assistors in a cooperative effort by Arkansas State Rehabilitation Services, Arkansas Enterprises for the Blind and the Internal Revenue Service from March 1967 thru May 1971. At the end of 1971, 60 visually handicapped persons were working for IRS in 35 states.

1746. Weadon, Connie P. The social worker's role in the public school education of visually handicapped children. *Education of the Visually Handicapped*, Dec. 1972, Vol. 4, No. 4, pp. 122–34.

A blind social worker discusses her experiences. Notes varied students' responses to her as a blind person, counseling needs of the visually handicapped students, schools' needs to learn more about available services.

1747. Whittenbury, Anne. American experiment. *New Outlook for the Blind*, Jan. 1963, Vol. 57, No. 1, pp. 22–24.

Author tells her experience in coming to U.S. to demonstrate how successfully a blind physical therapist can perform all aspects of physiotherapy. As a result of this experience, the OVR has tried to open the job to the American blind.

1748. Wilson, Edouard L. Assessing the readiness of blind persons for vocational placement. *New Outlook for the Blind*, Feb. 1974, Vol. 68, No. 2, pp. 57–60.

The relationship of work to the needs of clients is explored. Evaluation, training, and counseling as needed are recommended. Also discussed are problems related to unrealistic goals.

1749. Winters, Kris. Employment in hospital darkrooms. *New Outlook for the Blind*, Nov. 1966, Vol. 60, No. 9, pp. 269–72.

Discusses history of the darkroom, typical darkroom work areas, training for such work, trainee selection, job information, placement problems, placement and follow-up. Concludes that the field has many opportunities.

1750. Witcher, Clifford M. Industry asks: Are blind machinists safe? *American Machinist*, Mar. 1955.

Describes a training program for machinists that was 100% accident-free and some tools that permit accurate work by touch.

1751. Yarnold, A. W. The X-ray darkroom—A new approach. *Chronicle*, Dec. 1971, Vol. 11, No. 3, pp. 12–15.

Outlines the adaptations made in darkroom procedures in a hospital in New Zealand that enabled a blind person to perform the work.

1752. Young, William R. Problems of placement. *International Journal for the Education of the Blind*, Mar. 1961, Vol. 10, No. 3, pp. 73–74.

Abstract of a talk on placement of blind workers, valuable chiefly for its clear listing of aims of training in industrial arts and aims of specific vocational training.

1753. Zimin, Boris. The education and employment of blind mathematicians in computer centers in the Soviet Union. *New Outlook for the Blind,* Dec. 1968, Vol. 62, No. 10, pp. 307–8.

Briefly describes government support for blind students in Russia, with special focus on the mathematician-programmer and computer engineer.

1754. Zimmerman, A. Alfred. Development in the darkroom. *Journal of Rehabilitation,* Sept.–Oct. 1958.

Describes X-ray film development as an occupation based on experience in Calif.

18. Libraries, Instructional Materials Centers, Books, Tapes

1755. Alonso, Lou; Lappin, Carl; & Calovini, Gloria. Three centers form a consortium providing information and materials for educators and administrators of visually handicapped children. *Exceptional Children*, 1968, Vol. 34, No. 6, pp. 461–66.

Describes the services and outlets within these centers.

1756. American Foundation for the Blind. *Recording science texts for the blind.* New York: Author, 1957, 40 pp.

General instructions, plus specific explanations and examples, for readers of science texts.

1757. American Library Assoc. *Standards for library services for the blind and visually handicapped.* Chicago: Author, 1967, 54 pp.

Report dealing with large print, braille, and recorded materials. Services at national and local levels, as well as facilities, are discussed.

1758. American Printing House for the Blind. Educational research, development and reference group: Report on research and development activities —Fiscal 1975. Louisville, Ky.: Author, 1975, 21 pp. Mimeo.

Briefly describes research conducted and development in FY 1975 and that planned for FY 1976.

1759. Andrews, Joseph L., & Stern, William B. Law books for the blind. *Law Library Journal*, Mar. 1955.

Discusses importance of assistance to blind persons in law libraries and includes a bibliography of law books in braille and on Talking Book records.

1760. Benham, Thomas A. Science for the blind in recordings. *New Outlook for the Blind*, Oct. 1954, Vol. 48, No. 8, pp. 288–90.

Describes a program to determine the feasibility of putting science on records for use of the blind. If the pilot run is successful, complete technical books would be presented.

1761. Bledsoe, Thomas A. General Catalog of Volunteer-produced Textbooks at the American Printing House for the Blind. *International Journal for the Education of the Blind*, Oct. 1962, Vol. 12, No. 1, pp. 13–16.

Thanks to increased productivity of volunteer transcribers and efficient reporting, this catalog has grown to about 10,000 entries. Details how to use it as either borrower or depositor.

1762. Boelke, Joanne, Comp. *Library service to the visually and physically handicapped: A bibliography.* Minneapolis: ERIC Clearinghouse on Library & Information Sciences, 1969, 18 pp.

Selective annotated bibliography covers library service to the blind, partially sighted, and physically handicapped who are unable to use conventional printed materials. One hundred nineteen citations published from 1964 to summer 1969. Three sections: Background reading, state and local programs, library materials.

1763. Borgersen, Richard. Improving recording techniques. *New Outlook for the Blind*, Nov. 1965, Vol. 59, No. 9, pp. 308–12.

Detailed description of how to improve volunteer recordings. Discusses content specifications, equipment and its optimal use, and procedures.

1764. Bray, Robert S. The specialized needs of braille readers. *New Outlook for the Blind*, Dec. 1960, Vol. 54, No. 10, pp. 372–74.

Lists and responds to 4 broad questions about these needs.

1765. ————. The growth of a library service for blind persons. *New Outlook for the Blind*, Apr. 1964, Vol. 58, No. 4, pp. 111–14.

History of library service for the blind as provided by the government. Details work of the Div. for the Blind of the Library of Congress.

1766. Breuel, John W. The status of talking book research. *New Outlook for the Blind*, Oct. 1960, Vol. 54, No. 8, pp. 289–92.

Describes research and development of the type interesting to consumers, and cites the role of AFB in encouraging improved materials at reasonable prices for blind people.

1767. Carter, Burnham. Educational recordings: What standards should govern them? *New Outlook for the Blind*, Sept. 1962, Vol. 56, No. 7, pp. 247–51.

Discusses learning by listening, guidelines for evaluating a potential reader, "proofreading" the recordings, proper handling of texts which may include diagrams, footnotes, etc., and recording conditions.

1768. ————. The pocket book machine: An experiment in gaining time. *New Outlook for the Blind*, Apr. 1964, Vol. 58, No. 4, pp. 115–16.

Information on a small, portable disc playing machine more convenient for blind student. It allows scanning and is variable in speed.

1769. Delta Gamma Foundation. *Library aids and services available to the blind and visually handicapped.* Columbus, Ohio: Author, 1972, 40 pp.

Gives over 100 sources of reading materials available from libraries and publishers in record, tape, braille, or large-print form. Includes subject, title, content, age or grade level, availability for regional libraries, and price.

1770. Eakin, William M., & McFarland, Thomas L. *Type, printing, and the partially seeing child.* Pittsburgh: Stanwix House, 1960, 16 pp.

Discusses large-type materials. Printing terms defined and large type, clear type, and type face legibility demonstrated. Considers problems in standardization.

1771. Educational Materials Coordinating Unit. *Rates and standards.* Springfield, Ill.: State Office of Supt. of Public Instruction, 1969, 95 pp.

Recommends operating regulations for Unit in area of handproduced educational materials.

1772. Field, Gilbert. Recorded and braille textbooks: Everything the blind student needs to know (Recording for the Blind). *New Outlook for the Blind*, Apr. 1974, Vol. 68, No. 4, pp. 151–56.

Full instructions for using this service which provides tape-recorded textbooks to blind students. Has 23,000-title Master Tape Library and records new books on request.

1773. Fla. Instructional Materials Center for the Visually Handicapped. *Florida Instructional Materials Center for the Visually Handicapped: Services and procedures 1974.* Tallahassee: Fla. State Dept. of Education, 21 pp.

1774. Fonda, Gerald. An evaluation of large type. *New Outlook for the Blind*, Dec. 1966, Vol. 60, No. 10, pp. 296–98.

Discusses purposes of large type and population for which it was developed, disadvantages of large type, situations in which its use is indicated. Table on relation of visual acuity and reading distance for 8-, 12-, and 18-point type.

1775. Franzel, Adeline. A public relations plan for better library services. *New Outlook for the Blind*, Apr. 1964, Vol. 58, No. 4, pp. 101–3.

How to reach and motivate those blind people who do not now use the library.

1776. Gallozzi, Charles. Libraries for the blind. *New Outlook for the Blind*, May 1956, Vol. 50, No. 5, pp. 171–73.

Gives the history, growth, and some of the criticisms of libraries for the blind.

1777. Gartner, John N. Large type reading materials for the visually handicapped. *New Outlook for the Blind*, Oct. 1968, Vol. 62, No. 8, pp. 233–39.

Despite the fact that large numbers of older visually handicapped people could effectively use large print books, few adult books appeared on the commercial market until very recently. Describes increasing involvement of publishers and the kinds of books older readers want.

1778. Gilkeson, Ellen A. Reading Guidance in the primary grades. *International Journal for the Education of the Blind*, Feb. 1952, Vol. 1, No. 3, pp. 58–59.

Bringing books and children together. Develop readers who can and will read good books. Reading readiness (attained through richness of experience with other children, adults, and things in environment) is reached at various rates. Reading program in terms of individual children.

1779. Gore, George V., III. *The establishing and maintaining of a material and textbook center for visually handicapped students.* Working Paper, Vol. 1, No. 2. New York: Columbia Univ., 1969, 9 pp.

Needs in establishing a material resource center for the visually handicapped discussed. Describes physical layout, space utilization and equipment, general administrative policies, funding needs, staff responsibilities, material handling, record keeping, and cooperation between staff and volunteer workers.

1780. Haycraft, Howard. Books for the blind: A postscript and an appreciation. *New Outlook for the Blind*, Apr. 1964, Vol. 58, No. 4, pp. 106–10.

Condensed and updated from *American Library Association Bulletin*, Oct. 1962.

Information on talking and braille books: Who is eligible for them, how they are recorded, the role of volunteers in this field, and how books are selected. Author challenges librarians to increase reader use.

1781. ——. *Books for the blind and physically handicapped.* 4th ed. Washington, D.C.: Library of Congress, 1972, 20 pp.

Discusses extent and aspects of library services available at the Div. for the Blind and Physically Handicapped of the Library of Congress and at regional libraries. Covers future programs, the large-print revolution, and useful sources.

1782. Hunsicker, Marya. When the blind begin to read. *Library Journal*, Nov. 15, 1972, Vol. 97, No. 20, pp. 3817–18.

Author has found that there are many suitable books available in public libraries for visually limited children as most books for beginning readers are in large type. She has prepared a selected reading list of large-print titles for legally blind children, grades 1–3. Type size is given for each title.

1783. Instructional Materials Reference Center for Visually Handicapped Children. *Commercial aids that may be used or adapted for visually handicapped.* Louisville, Ky.: American Printing House for the Blind, 1969, 128 pp.

A catalogue of teaching aids with brief descriptions, source, and price.

1784. ——. *Educational aids for visually handicapped*, 2nd ed. Louisville, Ky.: American Printing House for the Blind, 1971, 83 pp.

Catalogue of aids with brief description, source, and price.

1785. ——. *The Central Catalog.* 5th ed. Louisville, Ky.: American Printing House for the Blind, 1973, 677 pp.

Source of information for transcribers, school administrators, teachers, librarians, students, parents, and workers for the blind. Contains alphabetical listing by subject area of books listed in the catalog of volunteer-produced braille, large-type, and recorded textbooks.

1786. Jones, Myrtis. A library catalog in braille? Yes! *International Journal for the Education of the Blind*, Mar. 1962, Vol. 11, No. 3, pp. 79–81.

How the Arkansas School for the Blind developed a library catalog in braille and the values in doing this.

1787. ——. School library services to visually handicapped children. *International Journal for the Education of the Blind*, Mar. 1965, Vol. 14, No. 3, pp. 79–82.

Through analysis of responses to questionnaire sent to residential schools and departments of education (33 returned), describes library services under following headings: Physical plant, resources, staff, organization of materials, services, and finances. A poverty of materials and services is found.

1788. Josephson, Eric. The needs of blind readers. *New Outlook for the Blind*, Feb. 1960, Vol. 54, No. 2, pp. 58–62.

Concerned with the reading interests of the blind and available library services, this article presents a brief history and survey of condition of these services, as well as an AFB plan for a nationwide survey of reading needs, and an outline of additional areas in which research is needed.

1789. ———. A report on blind readers. *New Outlook for the Blind*, Apr. 1964, Vol. 58, No. 4, pp. 97–101.

Findings of a study of reading among blind people. Broken down as to vital statistics and compared to sighted readers. Ease of use of regional libraries and suggestions for the future are also discussed.

1790. Kaulfuss, Edward. Where are our girlie books? *New Beacon*, May 1974, Vol. 58, No. 685, pp. 119–21.

Blind author states that sighted people receive information on sex in many ways of which blind people are deprived, and even formal sex education for the blind is inadequate, thus leading to unfortunate consequences.

1791. Kimbrough, B. T. Their readers don't have to be Jewish. *Dialogue*, Winter 1973, Vol. 12, No. 4, pp. 73–74.

The story of the Jewish Braille Institute of America in New York City which has the world's largest collection of braille and recorded Jewish-related reading material.

1792. Korb, Alfred. The tape cassette system proposed by the Library of Congress. *New Outlook for the Blind*, Apr. 1964, Vol. 58, No. 4, pp. 117–19.

Plan proposed by Library of Congress for a talking book system utilizing tapes.

1793. Landau, Robert A., & Nyren, Judith S., Eds. *Large type books in print*. New York: Bowker Co., 1970, 193 pp.

A compilation of large-type materials currently available including general reading and reference works and textbooks. Includes publisher and price info. as well as suggested grade levels.

1794. Lappin, Carl W. The Instructional Materials Reference Center for the Visually Handicapped: Report on center activities and available services. *Education of the Visually Handicapped*, Oct. 1972, Vol. 4, No. 3, pp. 65–70.

Describes growth of program, structure within American Printing House for the Blind, Central Catalog, and how services are obtained.

1795. ———. The Instructional Materials Reference Center for the visually handicapped: Research, development, and dissemination/distribution function. *Education of the Visually Handicapped*, Dec. 1972, Vol. 4, No. 4, pp. 101–6.

Reviews the IMRC's recent, current, and projected activities related to definition of need and development or adaptation of materials.

1796. ———. At your service—The Instructional Materials Reference Center for the Visually Handicapped. *TEACHING Exceptional Children*, Winter 1973, Vol. 5, No. 2, pp. 74–76.

Describes the services of the IMRC: Information, development of additional materials, and demonstration of methods of use of materials. Explains Central Catalog service which annually lists titles of volunteer-produced books in braille, large type, and recorded form.

1797. Lende, Helga. Survey of library service for the blind. *New Outlook for the Blind*, Dec. 1957, Vol. 51, No. 10, pp. 466–72.

A study of specialized services, nationwide, by eminent librarians lists problems and recommendations under the headings: Financial, organization, staff, physical conditions, records, book selection, communication, talking book machines, technical problems, publicity, and further study needed.

1798. Levine, Helen G., & Lass, Muriel C. Recorded and braille textbooks: Everything the blind student needs to know (National Braille Association). *New Outlook for the Blind*, Apr. 1974, Vol. 68, No. 4, pp. 153–56.

Full instructions for using this service which provides textbooks in braille. Scientific and mathematical tables are also available in braille.

1799. Library of Congress, Div. for the Blind and Physically Handicapped. *1972 Directory of library resources for the blind and physically handicapped.* Washington, D.C.: Author, 1972, 27 pp.

Details, by state and territory, the national program of free mail library service, describes qualifications for service and instructions for its use.

1800. ———. *Volunteers who produce books: Braille—Large type—Tape.* Washington, D.C.: Author, 1973, xviii + 65 pp., free. (Also in braille.)

Updates the 1970 edition. Lists volunteer groups and individuals who transcribe and record books and other materials for blind and physically handicapped persons.

1801. ———. *Talking books: Adult: 1972–1973*, Washington, D.C.: Author, 1974, 191 pp.

Catalog lists approx. 1,140 fiction and nonfiction titles, with annotations, in numerous categories. Order blanks included.

1802. McNally, Harold J. *The readability of certain type sizes and forms in sight-saving classes.* New York: AMS Press, 1972, vi + 71 pp., $10. (Originally published by Columbia Univ., 1943.)

1803. Morris, Effie L. Service to blind children in the New York Public Library. *New Outlook for the Blind*, May 1960, Vol. 54, No. 5, pp. 159–65.

Following brief history of library services to children, discusses special ways to meet responsibilities to blind children.

1804. Mylecraine, Mary. Library serves blind students. *Music Journal*, Nov. 1971, Vol. 29, No. 9, pp. 13–15, illus.

Describes the collection and services of the Music Services Unit of Library of Congress, Div. for the Blind and Physically Handicapped.

1805. National Accreditation Council. *Standards for production of reading materials for the blind and visually handicapped.* New York: Author, 1970, 60 pp.

Following a section on general policies, details the standards for large-print materials, recorded materials, and tactile materials.

1806. National Braille Assoc. *Tape recording—A manual for the recording of educational materials.* Midland Park, N.J.: Author, 1971, 21 pp.

Manual intended to instruct volunteers how to produce the best possible tape recordings of educational materials for use by the visually handicapped. Suggestions relate to open-reel rather than cassette tape recorders.

1807. ———. *Guidelines for the administration of groups producing reading materials for the visually handicapped.* Midland Park, N.J.: Author, 1975, 109 pp. (Avail. from Library of Congress, Div. for the Blind & Physically Handicapped, free.)

Written primarily for beginning volunteer transcribing groups, has section on general administrative guidelines, as well as sections on braille, large type, and tape recording.

1808. National Society for the Prevention of Blindness. *Guidelines for the Production of Material in Large Type.* New York: Author, 1965.

Instructions are given for type, paper, and format in the production of large-type materials by typewriter. Techniques of direct and indirect offset printing, photographic enlargement, and microfilming are described. Six agencies which provide information on large type are listed.

1809. Nolan, Carson Y. Readability of large types: A study of type sizes and type styles. *International Journal for the Education of the Blind*, Dec. 1959, Vol. 9, No. 2, pp. 41–44.

Reports a study of type face and size, using as subjects 264 children with varying amounts of vision, in grades 4–12. With supporting statistical data, results show that 18-point type is read as rapidly as 24-point type and that common textbook type is read more rapidly than an experimental type.

1810. ———. A study of pictures for large type textbooks. *International Journal for the Education of the Blind*, Mar. 1960, Vol. 9, No. 3, pp. 67–70.

Since simple reproduction of pictures enlarged through the photo-offset process is unsatisfactory, this study evaluated 4 combinations of black and white. Legibility of 5 methods for reproducing illustrations was judged by 40 visually handicapped children.

1811. ———. Legibility of ink and paper color combinations for readers of large type. *International Journal for the Education of the Blind*, Mar. 1961, Vol. 10, No. 3, pp. 82–84.

Size discrimination thresholds were obtained through repeated measurement of 12 large-type readers using targets printed in combinations of 2 ink and 5 paper colors. No significant differences in legibility were found.

1812. ———. Teacher preference for types of illustrations in large type books. *International Journal for the Education of the Blind*, May 1961, Vol. 10, No. 4, pp. 112–14.

This followup on an earlier study of methods of picture reproduction sent questionnaires to 50 teachers. Traced pictures in outline form with areas blacked in for contrast were regarded more legible.

1813. Nolan, Carson Y., & Morris, June E., Comps. Bibliography of research on large type reading. Louisville, Ky.: American Printing House for the Blind, 1971, 5 pp. Mimeo.

Includes studies of the reading process, large print, use of closed-circuit TV systems, and some reading aids.

1814. Ovenshire, Ruth, Comp. *Reading materials in large type. Reference circular.* Washington, D.C.: Library of Congress, 1973, 16 pp.

Lists commercial and volunteer producers of large-type materials and large-type books for reference and a variety of special needs.

1815. Overbeay, Donald W., & Eisnaugle, Evelyn. The central registry: Ohio's plan for service to visually handicapped children. *International Journal for the Education of the Blind,* Dec. 1965, Vol. 15, No. 2, pp. 50–51.

A center for educational materials or a record of where such materials are available was based in the residential school but planned to serve all visually handicapped students in Ohio.

1816. Prentiss, Sam. *Improving library services to the blind, partially sighted, and physically handicapped in New York State: A report prepared for the Assistant Commissioner for Libraries.* Albany: Univ. of the State of New York, Jan. 1973, 102 pp., app.

Described is the present status of library service to the blind and partially sighted in New York State, and recommended are improvements through state legislation and cooperative efforts of public and private libraries and agencies.

1817. Reading with your ears. *Exceptional Parent,* Dec.–Jan. 1972, Vol. 1, No. 4, pp. 28–29.

Describes programs of National Braille Press and Library of Congress for providing records, tapes, or cassettes of books to persons unable to use standard printed material. Talking Book program detailed.

1818. Rubir, Barbara. *A professional approach to large print and those who use it.* Berkeley: Calif. Transcribers and Educators of the Visually Handicapped, 1968, 33 pp.

A selected, annotated bibliography.

1819. Samuels, Gertrude. 'Open windows' for the blind. *International Journal for the Education of the Blind,* Mar. 1960, Vol. 9, No. 3, pp. 70–72.

Using the case record of a particular blind person as an illustration, tells the services and benefits of Recording for the Blind.

1820. Sloan, Louise L., & Habel, Adelaide. Reading speeds with textbooks in large and in standard print. *Sight-Saving Review,* Summer 1973, Vol. 43, No. 2, pp. 107–11.

Report on a study to obtain comparative measures of reading speed for both types of print when optical reading aids suitable for each size are used.

1821. Smith, W. J. A talking magazine. *New Beacon,* May 1973, Vol. 57, No. 673, pp. 121–22.

Author discusses conception and implementation of "talking magazine" for the blind, need for more such projects.

1822. Swank, R. C. *Library service for the visually and physically handicapped: A report to the California State Library.* Sacramento: Calif. State Library, 1967, 87 pp.

Objectives of study were to review library services to the blind and physically handicapped and to suggest long-term planning for improving services in Calif. Recommends state-wide network for library service.

1823. Sykes, Kim C. A comparison of the effectiveness of standard print and large print in facilitating the reading skills of visually impaired students. *Education of the Visually Handicapped*, Dec. 1971, Vol. 3, No. 4, pp. 97–105.

Study investigated whether standard print is equally or more effective than large print in determining reading ability of the visually impaired. It was concluded that under optimum reading conditions, both legally blind and visually impaired high school students perform as well on standard print as on large print on measures of comprehension and reading speed.

1824. ———. Print reading for visually handicapped children. *Education of the Visually Handicapped*, Oct. 1972, Vol. 4, No. 3, pp. 71–75.

Author feels that increased reading demands and the increasing integration of visually handicapped with sighted children necessitate print reading instruction. Discusses sight utilization with functional use of vision and reviews relevant reading materials for different ages.

1825. Traubitz, Gretchen. Library objectives in a school for the blind. *International Journal for the Education of the Blind*, May 1956, Vol. 5, No. 4, pp. 73–77.

Seven objectives for the library as an integral part of both academic and recreational programs.

1826. Trosch, Carol. Recording textbooks for the blind. *New Outlook for the Blind*, Sept. 1958, Vol. 52, No. 7, pp. 261–62.

Discusses technique of recording at slow speed and in multiple copies, and a procedure in use in which the reading is first recorded on tapes, then transcribed to discs at 16⅔ rpm. This method has improved the quality and quantity of recording.

1827. Va. Commission for the Visually Handicapped. *A pilot demonstration of the use of the British Tape Program in Maryland and Virginia, and a comparison with the Talking Book and current American Tape Program: Progress report.* Richmond: Author, 1964, 9 pp.

Demonstrates overwhelming acceptance of a tape cassette in preference to current Talking Books. Found general satisfaction with British Tape cassette and machine. American and British tapes are not interchangeable because of the engineering designs, and project was discontinued.

1828. Wash, Luba M. A teacher looks at the talking book. *International Journal for the Education of the Blind*, Dec. 1954, Vol. 4, No. 2, pp. 24–27.

Educative value in talking books including all recorded materials, operas, concerts, drama, etc. Presents number of libraries in country furnishing audio service.

1829. Wolf, Carolyn, & Miller, Joan. Hartwick serves blind. *American Libraries*, Dec. 1971, Vol. 2, No. 11, pp. 1193–94.

Discusses services the library at Hartwick Col. (New York) has been able to offer its 4 legally blind students.

1830. Wolf, James M. Talking tapes for blind leprosy patients. *New Outlook for the Blind*, Dec. 1964, Vol. 58, No. 10, pp. 329–30.

Lists 5 main causes of blindness in leprosy cases. Report of a high school project in the Canal Zone to produce tapes in English and Spanish for students blinded by leprosy. Braille is impossible for many because of hand involvement of the disease.

19. Vision Utilization, Optical Aids, and Low Vision Clinics

1831. Adams, Sherrill, et al. Visual training (low vision seminar). *Low Vision Abstracts*, Spring–Fall 1974, Vol. 2, No. 1, pp. 1–8.

Outlines 8 visual training concepts: Open cue searching, visual motor coordination, visual memory, tracking and fixation, maximal use of peripheral vision, distinction of foreground from background, discrimination of shape and position, perception of distance and depth.

1832. Anooshian, Linda J.; Warren, David H.; & Apkarian-Stielau, Pat. Progress after visual restoration: Two preliminary case reports and a request for communication. *American Foundation for the Blind Research Bulletin 27*, Apr. 1974, pp. 310–12.

Reports on perceptual training for persons who have recovered vision after a long period of blindness.

1833. Ashcroft, Samuel C., et al. *Study II, Effects of experimental teaching on the visual behavior of children educated as though they had no vision.* Nashville: Geo. Peabody Col. for Teachers, 1965, 35 pp.

Objectives of study to confirm that a short period of experimental teaching enhances visual behavior of partially sighted children as shown by significant increases in visual discrimination test scores and increase in recorded near-vision acuity as determined by an ophthalmologist. Significant gains confirmed positive findings of an earlier experiment.

1834. Barnes, Frances J. Let's call it "sight utilization." *New Outlook for the Blind*, Mar. 1963, Vol. 57, No. 3, pp. 97–98.

Negative implications of "sight saving" and "sight conservation" programs in our schools can breed and foster misconceptions regarding use of the eyes. Ophthalmologists are seeking to overcome misconceptions by saying use whatever vision you have to the maximum.

1835. Barraga, Natalie. *Increased visual behavior in low vision children.* New York: AFB, 1964, 180 pp., $2.50.

Examines the effect that specialized instruction with appropriate print materials can have on the visual behavior of children with very little remaining vision. Includes visual discrimination test, daily lesson plans, materials for instruction, and rating sheet.

1836. ———. Teaching children with low vision. *New Outlook for the Blind*, Dec. 1964, Vol. 58, No. 10, pp. 323–26.

Partially sighted children who had been educated as though they had no vision took part in an experiment which indicated that in a specialized short-term setting they could be helped to more fully utilize their remaining vision.

1837. Brady, J. P., & Lind, D. L. Experimental analysis of hysterical blindness. *Archives of General Psychiatry*, 1961, Vol. 4, pp. 331–39.

Describes application of operant conditioning technique to the assessment of behavior of a patient whose condition was diagnosed as hysterical blindness. Technique is utilized to demonstrate that patient's behavior is controlled by visual stimuli.

1838. Brazelton, Frank A., et al. A symposium on the rehabilitation of the partially sighted. *American Journal of Optometry and Archives of American Academy of Optometry*, Aug. 1970, Vol. 47, No. 8, pp. 585–87.

Describes a symposium basically clinical in orientation, emphasizing optometric care, in which the aim is fitting the visually handicapped for as normal a life as possible rather than isolating them.

1839. Cunningham, Suzanne A., & Reagan, Cora Lee. *Handbook of visual perceptual training.* [n.p.], 1972, 120 pp., illus.

1840. DeAngelis, Gerard J. The client and "vision rehabilitation." *New Outlook for the Blind*, June 1959, Vol. 53, No. 6, pp. 211–15.

Based on the vision rehabilitation program at the Industrial Home for the Blind, discusses philosophy, problems, and procedures of a low vision service.

1841. Dzik, David. An optometric evaluation of a totally blind adult (age 21). *Journal of the American Optometric Association*, Dec. 1972, Vol. 43, No. 13, pp. 1350–53.

On the basis of 1 examination, states that optometric vision training therapy, with modifications, can be used to rehabilitate and teach a blind person preacademic visual skills.

1842. Eakin, Marian E. Low vision. *Optometric Weekly*, Nov. 1974, Vol. 65, No. 38, pp. 1055–56.

Stresses importance of referrals to low vision clinics while suggesting ways optometrists can help partially sighted persons.

1843. Egi, Jane, & Takemoto, Yasuko. *Low vision clinic for individuals who are severely visually handicapped.* Honolulu: Dept. of Social Services, Voc. Rehab. & Services to the Blind Div., Sept. 1967, 42 pp.

1844. Espinosa, Ricardo. Low vision: Examination procedures. *Optometric Weekly*, Sept. 1970, Vol. 61, No. 37, pp. 29–33.

Fourth in a series dealing with methods and procedures in the management of low vision. This article describes the following examination procedures: Distance and near visual acuity, ophthalmoscopy, retinoscopy, trial frame refraction, ophthalmometer readings, and cover and fusion tests for binocularity.

1845. Faye, Eleanor E. *The low vision patient: Clinical experience with adults and children.* New York: Grune & Stratton, 1970, 237 pp., $9.75.

Papers concerning definitions of subnormal vision include discussions of the subnormal-vision patient, low vision refraction, and the low vision lens. App. includes chapters on supplementary reading, statistical analysis of 6,000 patients, equipment, setting up a clinic, and a glossary.

1846. Faye, Eleanor E., & Hood, Clare M. Low vision services in an agency: Structure and philosophy. *New Outlook for the Blind*, June 1975, Vol. 69, No. 6, pp. 241–48.

A full discussion of the operation of such a service based on the Low

Vision Service of the New York Assoc. for the Blind, including descriptions of the examination itself, follow-up and training services, and the aid loan system.

1847. ———, **Eds.** *Low vision: A symposium marking the 20th anniversary of the Lighthouse Low Vision Service.* New York: Lighthouse for the Blind, 1975, 306 pp.

Based on a multidisciplinary symposium covering: New technology of lenses, recent medical and surgical advances, neuro-ophthalmological defects, problems of the child, vocationally bound adult, the elderly, models of low vision clinics.

1848. Fields, Julie E. Sensory training for blind persons. *New Outlook for the Blind*, Jan. 1964, Vol. 58, No. 1, pp. 2–9.

Detailed discussion of necessity for training other senses in blind person. Analysis of remaining senses and detailed description of methods of training these to operate at optimum efficiency.

1849. Finn, William A.; Gadbaw, Patricia D.; Kevorkian, Gregory A.; et al. Increased field accessibility through prismatically displaced images. *New Outlook for the Blind*, Dec. 1975, Vol. 69, No. 10, pp. 465–67.

Describes use of Fresnel press-on prism lenses to optically move objects from areas of visual field loss to areas of useful vision, thereby making objects with potential hazard more visually accessible.

1850. Fonda, Gerald. Guide to the use of optical aids. *International Journal for the Education of the Blind*, Oct. 1960, Vol. 10, No. 1, pp. 12–13.

After noting when hand magnifiers are indicated, lists and describes aids for distance and aids for near vision. Suggests some implications for education.

1851. ———. *Management of the patient with subnormal vision.* St. Louis, Mo.: C. V. Mosby, 1970, 167 pp., $13.

Intended primarily for ophthalmologists, book deals with managing patients who are partially sighted. Discussion of optical and visual aids and residual vision and type and braille reading.

1852. ———. Ways to improve vision in partially sighted persons. *Geriatrics*, May 1975, Vol. 30, pp. 49–52, illus.

Description of visual aids to improve distant and near vision. Briefly touches on importance of illumination as well as patient motivation.

1853. Fonda, Gerald; Thomas, Henry; & Gore, George V., III. Educational and vocational placement and low-vision corrections in albinism: A report based on 253 patients. *Sight-Saving Review*, Spring 1971, Vol. 41, No. 1, pp. 29–36.

Primarily concerned with use of visual aids to increase effectiveness of vision in albinism. Data is presented in 2 age groups: Under 23 years of age; 23 and older. With aids, most were able to use standard print.

1854. Freudenberger, Herbert J., & Robbins, Irving. Characteristics of acceptance and rejection of optical aids in a low-vision population. *American Journal of Ophthalmology*, Apr. 1959, Vol. 47, No. 4, pp. 582–84.

Concludes that success with optical aids depends on personality makeup.

1855. Friedman, Dagmar B.; Tallman, Carter B.; & Asarkof, John E. Comprehensive low vision care: Part one. *New Outlook for the Blind,* Mar. 1974, Vol. 68, No. 3, pp. 97–103. Part two, May 1975.

The program of vision rehabilitation at Boston Univ. Medical Center is described. Using an array of optical, mechanical, and electronic devices, plus additional professional consultation, the staff focused their attention on the specific visual problems of the patient and the associated psychological, social, and economic difficulties which limited his activities.

1856. Friedman, Dagmar B.; Kayne, Herbert L.; Tallman, Carter B.; et al. Comprehensive low vision care: Part two. *New Outlook for the Blind,* May 1975, Vol. 69, No. 5, pp. 207–11. Part one, Mar. 1974.

Innovative programs of social service and counseling integrated into a multidisciplinary approach to low vision care at Boston Univ. Medical Center.

1857. Geldhof, Marcel G. Relation between print size, test distance, and corresponding Snellen acuity rating: A mathematical approach. *Optometric Weekly,* Nov. 1974, Vol. 65, No. 39, pp. 33–36.

Explains derivation of mathematical expression reported to show relationship between print size, reading distance, and corresponding Snellen acuity rating.

1858. Gettes, Bernard C. Optical aids for low vision. *International Journal for the Education of the Blind,* Mar. 1959, Vol. 8, No. 3, pp. 98–100.

Describes the contributions made by new devices, the Conoid Lenses of David Volk, M.D., and charts by Keeler. Experience at Wills Eye Hospital, Philadelphia, shows that more patients are helped with strong reading corrections than with any other device.

1859. Gibbons, Helen. Low-vision aids—The educator's responsibility. *International Journal for the Education of the Blind,* May 1963, Vol. 12, No. 4, pp. 107–9.

Educators need better understanding of low-vision aids and have a responsibility to encourage use of such aids where appropriate.

1860. Goodlaw, Edward I. Homework for low vision patients. *American Journal of Optometry and Archives of American Academy of Optometry,* 1968, Vol. 45, No. 8, pp. 532–38.

A procedure is described which facilitates patient adaptation to their optical aids.

1861. Gordon, Arnold H.; Silberman, Clare; Mintz, Morris J.; et al. Why a low vision clinic? *New Outlook for the Blind,* Feb. 1964, Vol. 58, No. 2, pp. 54–57.

Discussion of positive aspects of running a low vision clinic with an ophthalmologist, an optometrist, a social worker, and a teacher or counselor. Several case histories given.

1862. Hagberg, Carolyn L. *A descriptive study of the use of low vision optical aids as viewed by clients of Minnesota State Services for the Blind.* Minneapolis: Dept. of Special Education, Univ. of Minn., 1968, 84 pp.

Study of frequency of use of optical aids suggests that a team approach might help individuals make more effective use of those aids.

1863. Heeren, Ethel. Helping people with impaired vision. *Optometric Weekly,* Oct. 1974, Vol. 65, No. 37, pp. 1024–27.

Presents ways in which optometrists may help visually handicapped people meet psychological and practical needs. Notes practical and attitudinal difficulties.

1864. Hellinger, George. Vision rehabilitation through low vision centers. *New Outlook for the Blind,* Nov. 1967, Vol. 61, No. 9, pp. 296–301.

Defines vision rehabilitation, its benefits in vocational, personal, and educational areas, and the services of low vision centers.

1865. Hitz, John B. *Final report: Optical Aids Clinic, December 1, 1963— November 30, 1966.* Milwaukee: Marquette Univ. School of Medicine, 1967, 33 pp., app., illus., $1.

Demonstration project to provide optical aids to low vision clients. Plan for educating public/private organizations and professionals about vision problems. Bib.

1866. Hoover, Richard, & Kupfer, Carl. Low vision clinics: A report. *American Journal of Ophthalmology,* Aug. 1959, Vol. 48, No. 2, pp. 177–187.

Data on 841 cases from 7 low vision clinics.

1867. Huelsman, Charles B., Jr. Six concepts of vision. *School Health Review,* Nov. 1970, Vol. 1, No. 4, pp. 29–31.

Six concepts reviewed in historical order: Blindness, acuity, binocularity, vision skills (accommodative and convergence skills, motility), perception, and meaning or significance.

1868. Jankolovitz, Arthur, & Sutton, Mark R. Subnormal vision rehabilitation: Cases from the low vision clinic. *Optometric Weekly,* Mar. 1974, Vol. 64, No. 11, 6 pp.

Twelve cases of children and adults, 3–73 years of age, treated in low vision clinic, are described to illustrate use of low vision aids for rehabilitation of partially sighted persons.

1869. Jose, Randall T.; Cummings, Janice; & McAdams, Loretta. The model low vision clinical service: An interdisciplinary vision rehabilitation program. *New Outlook for the Blind,* June 1975, Vol. 69, No. 6, pp. 249–54.

An optical aid must be an integral part of the rehabilitation program for the whole person. Describes the potential contributions of other staff such as technician, social worker, mobility instructor, communication specialist, psychologist, etc.

1870. Jose, Randall T., & Springer, Donald. Optical aids: An interdisciplinary prescription. *New Outlook for the Blind,* Jan. 1973, Vol. 67, No. 1, pp. 12–18. (Also in *Outlook*'s Offprint Series, 15¢.)

Successful use of optical aids relates to optometrist and other professionals who provide training and follow-up, as shown by informal study of 25 patients. Possible value of optical aid for mobility often overlooked.

1871. Jose, Randall T., & Watson, Gale. Hope for the hopeless. *Optometric Weekly,* June 1975, Vol. 66, No. 20, pp. 553–57.

Training program at Vocational Rehabilitation Service, Talladega, Ala., to insure patients' maximal benefit from optical aids dispensed.

1872. Kaine, Patricia A. *Low Vision Clinic for advancing use of optical aids: Final report.* Cleveland: Cleveland Society for the Blind, 1963, 57 pp., app., illus.

Results of program designed to help visually handicapped make maximum use of residual vision, increase their employability, and stimulate cooperation and coordination of state and community services for the blind.

1873. Karb, Donald R. Preparing the visually handicapped person for motor vehicle operation. *American Journal of Optometry and Archives of American Academy of Optometry,* Aug. 1970, Vol. 47, No. 8, pp. 619–28.

Considers the possibilities of motor vehicle operation by persons wearing telescopic lenses.

1874. Kederis, Cleves, & Ashcroft, Samuel C. The Austin Conference on Utilization of Low Vision. *Education of the Visually Handicapped,* May 1970, Vol. 2, No. 2, pp. 33–38.

Report of working conference. Outlines types of children who will be served and the program provisions that have been made for them.

1875. Kelleher, Dennis. Educational background and considerations of low vision aids: Review of related literature. *American Foundation for the Blind Research Bulletin 27,* Apr. 1974, pp. 99–109.

Particularly concerned with the bioptic telescope system (telescopic spectacles), discusses development of low vision aids, relevance to educational needs, psychological considerations. Reports studies and criticism.

1876. ———. [Randall T. Jose, Ed.] Teaching the low vision patient—A new optometric area of responsibility. *Optometric Weekly,* July 1975, Vol. 66, No. 24, pp. 11–13.

Role of teacher/counselor in training patients in correct use of their low vision aids pointed out. Contributions teacher/counselor can make to prescribing optometrist noted in editorial commentary.

1877. Kerstein, Joseph J., Ed. Low vision services in the United States. *Sight-Saving Review,* Winter 1973–74, Vol. 43, No. 4, pp. 223–26.

Examines survey procedures used in compiling directory of 114 facilities in the U.S. which provide low vision aid services for the partially sighted. Notes survey does not include ophthalmologists and optometrists offering low vision care, evaluation, information. Tables list services by geographic division, state, type, and sources of referrals.

1878. Lawrence, G. Allen. Life planning for the partially seeing. *Exceptional Children,* 1957, Vol. 23, pp. 202–6.

Emphasis on need for qualified diagnosis, consideration, and treatment of eye disorders.

1879. Little, Regina. Getting the most out of visual aids. *New Outlook for the Blind,* Apr. 1965, Vol. 59, No. 4, pp. 141–44.

Casework followup of low vision clinic clients studied reasons for not using optical aids and ways to teach clients effective use of residual vision.

1880. Low vision developments. *Rehabilitation Teacher,* Jan. 1975, Vol. 7, No. 1, pp. 33–35.

By prescribing low vision aids and teaching clients to use adapted materials (large print in good contrast with background), optometrists can help patients use their remaining vision more effectively.

1881. Lowrey, Austin. Plan for a low vision clinic. *New Outlook for the Blind*, Oct. 1965, Vol. 59, No. 8, pp. 275–77.

Outlines design for a model eye care center devoted to preserving and improving remaining vision.

1882. Mann, James W. Optical aids service and its implications for education. *New Outlook for the Blind*, Feb. 1961, Vol. 55, No. 2, pp. 65–67.

Discussion of optical aids for those with some residual vision, with a plea for emphasis on what a person can be enabled to see rather than on what he cannot.

1883. Marg, Elwin, et al. Design for a phosphene visual prosthesis. *Optometric Weekly*, Jan. 1971, Vol. 62, No. 1, pp. 1–6, illus.

Describes the technical design for a phosphene visual prosthesis including descriptions of the external and internal circuits and the electrodes fitted to the surfaces of the visual cortex.

1884. Meyerson, Lee. The visually handicapped. *Review of Educational Research*, 1953, Vol. 23, pp. 476–91.

A discussion by 105 researchers on the subjects of correctable or partially correctable visual impairments, partial vision, and blindness.

1885. Mims, Forrest M. An infrared seeing aid: Inquiry reply and brief description. *American Foundation for the Blind Research Bulletin 27*, Apr. 1974, pp. 302–3.

Copy of a letter and specifications for a prototype of an optical aid.

1886. Minner, C. B. Some predilections in optical aids services. *New Outlook for the Blind*, June 1963, Vol. 57, No. 6, pp. 197–200.

Discusses the predilections which seem to be possible hindrances to a more effective, more comprehensive, and more fully satisfying application of optical aids services.

1887. Mintz, Morris J.; Gaynes, Ernest M.; & Gordon, Arnold H. *Low vision clinic: Final report.* Detroit: Sinai Hospital of Detroit, Dec. 1966, 50 pp.

1888. National Society for the Prevention of Blindness. *Directory of low vision aids facilities in the United States.* New York: Author, 1974, 19 pp. Supplement to *Sight-Saving Review*, Winter 1973–74, Vol. 43, No. 4.

1889. Newman, Julian D., Ed. *A guide to the care of low vision patients.* St. Louis, Mo.: American Optometric Assoc., 1974, 343 pp., app., $10.

Papers cover basic low vision examination, eye pathology, mechanics and philosophy of prescribing, systems of aids, psychological and sociological factors, and questions most asked by low vision patients.

1890. Optometric Extension Program. *Optometric child vision care and guidance: A series of papers released by the Optometric Extension Program to its membership 1966–67.* Duncan, Okla.: Optometric Extension Program Foundation, 1967, 114 pp.

Deals with the diagnosis and treatment of early learning problems and their relation to visual development in a series of 12 articles. Optometric viewpoint expressed is that vision is learned. Outlines methods of remedial therapy.

1891. Ritter, Charles G. Questions and answers on low vision. *New Outlook for the Blind*, Dec. 1957, Vol. 51, No. 10, pp. 446–53.

Defines terms and various appliances related to low vision. Points out the importance of matching the low vision aid with the individual characteristics of the client.

1892. Robertson, Clara H. Services to children reported by optical aids clinics. *International Journal for the Education of the Blind*, Dec. 1963, Vol. 13, No. 2, pp. 59–61.

Of 42 functioning optical aids clinics, 26 responded to a questionnaire survey. Findings show growing service to children.

1893. Rosenberg, Robert. A survey of magnification aids to low vision. *Journal of the American Optometric Association*, June 1973, Vol. 44, No. 6, pp. 628–35.

Survey of established methods and newer methods such as closed-circuit television.

1894. Rosenbloom, Alfred A., Jr. Prognostic factors in low vision rehabilitation. *American Journal of Optometry and Archives of American Academy of Optometry*, Aug. 1970, Vol. 47, No. 8, pp. 600–605.

Determined the extent to which a patient continues to use a low vision aid.

1895. Rosenbloom, Alfred A., Jr., & Jose, Randall T. The role of the low vision assistant in the care of visually impaired persons. *New Outlook for the Blind*, Jan. 1975, Vol. 69, No. 1, pp. 20–24.

Suggests a number of functions in which qualified paraprofessionals can be used to decrease the manpower shortage so that better service is available to all visually impaired persons.

1896. Rusalem, Herbert. "IHB Optical Aids Survey"—A review of research. *New Outlook for the Blind*, Dec. 1957, Vol. 51, No. 10, pp. 454–56.

Report on the first 500 persons who received service from the optical aids program of Industrial Home for the Blind, Brooklyn. Concludes that in any population of partially seeing individuals, a substantial number would probably benefit from such service.

1897. Salmon, Peter J. Improving vision among the blind. *Sight-Saving Review*, 1953, Vol. 23, No. 3, pp. 136–38.

Studies show that about 50% of persons classified as blind have some remaining sight. Suggests optical aids that can provide for improvement of the remaining vision.

1898. Schiller, Vera. Coordination of a low vision clinic. *New Outlook for the Blind*, Nov. 1967, Vol. 61, No. 9, pp. 302–3.

Briefly describes just how the low vision clinic of Industrial Home for the Blind, Brooklyn, functions with the author, as liaison between client, professional staff, and other services of the agency.

1899. Silver, Robert. Using residual vision. *New Outlook for the Blind*, Mar. 1965, Vol. 59, No. 3, pp. 93–94.

Defines residual vision by a series of examples. Effective training of people with such differing characteristics requires understanding the diagnosis, prognosis, and capabilities of specific patient.

1900. Sloan, Louise L. *Recommended aids for the partially sighted.* 2nd ed. New York: National Society for the Prevention of Blindness, 1971, 64 pp., illus., $2.

Explanation of recommended optical and electromechanical aids for the partially sighted includes a nontechnical discussion of basic optical principles.

1901. ———. Optical magnification for subnormal vision: Historical survey. *Bulletin of Prosthetics Research,* Spring 1972, pp. 177–90, illus.

Focuses particularly on developments since 1946 and covers telescopic reading aids, reading spectacles of high power, hand-held magnifiers, stand magnifiers, projection magnifiers, and closed-circuit TV readers. Touches on examination procedures for prescription of aids.

1902. Sloan, Louise L.; Habel, Adelaide; & Ravadge, Frederick. Basic test kit for selection of reading aids for the partially sighted. *American Journal of Ophthalmology,* Dec. 1974, Vol. 78, No. 6, pp. 1014–21.

Description of the contents of a basic test kit of nonspectacle reading aids with information as to use, manufacturers, and suppliers.

1903. Sloan, Louise L., & Jablonski, Maria D. Reading aids for the partially blind: Classification and measurement of more than two hundred devices. *AMA Archives of Ophthalmology,* Sept. 1959, Vol. 62, pp. 465–84.

Equivalent dioptric power, extent of useful field of vision, and other optical characteristics are summarized for spectacle aids, and stand and hand magnifiers.

1904. Spurney, Robert V. Low-vision aids for partially sighted persons. *American Journal of Ophthalmology,* Jan. 1973, Vol. 75, No. 1, pp. 133–35.

Description of a recent innovation at the Low Vision Clinic, Cleveland Society for the Blind. A plastic spectacle frame-liner has been devised which permits spectacle-borne optical aids to be used interchangeably in frames of varying shapes and sizes.

1905. Tanner, Wilson P. Adaptation of vision following cataract removal. *New Outlook for the Blind,* Nov. 1971, Vol. 65, No. 9, pp. 281–86.

Author describes his visual experiences after undergoing surgery for cataract removal on both eyes.

1906. Taugher, Philip J. A simple and well-accepted low vision aid. *Sight-Saving Review,* Winter 1972–73, Vol. 42, No. 4, pp. 209–12.

Discusses high-plus lenses which permit the patient to scan with his naked vision to orient himself and then look directly through the axis of the lens.

1907. Tobin, Michael J. A study in the improvement of visual efficiency in children registered as blind. *New Beacon,* Mar. 1972, Vol. 56, No. 659, pp. 58–60.

Teaching materials developed by Barraga used with low vision students with positive results. Visual Efficiency Scale was also used and low areas concentrated upon.

1908. Univ. of Tenn. Col. of Medicine, Dept. of Ophthalmology. *Vocational rehabilitation of the legally blind and visually handicapped through establishment of an optical aids clinic.* Memphis: Author, 1969, 15 pp.

1909. Valvo, Alberto. *Sight restoration after long-term blindness: The problems and behavior patterns of visual rehabilitation.* New York: AFB, 1971, 54 pp., illus., $4.

Discusses 6 cases of visual re-education after sight was recovered through the surgical technique osteo-odonto-kerato-prosthesis. Persons blind from birth did not recover complete visual integration because of inability to adjust to the visual structure of the external world.

1910. Weiss, Sidney. Optical aids for children with subnormal vision. In Robison D. Harley, Ed., *Pediatric Ophthalmology.* Philadelphia: W. B. Saunders, 1975, pp. 900–922, illus., $50.

Recommends procedure for history taking and examination, with descriptions and illustrations of various charts for testing vision. Briefly explains basic theory and methods of correction of subnormal vision. Describes and illustrates optical aids to improve distance and near vision. Some mention of psychoeducational aspects of low vision.

1911. Wolfe, Earl. *Optical Aids Clinic: Final report, February 1, 1960–January 31, 1963.* Charleston: W. Va. Div. of Voc. Rehab., 1963, 42 pp., app.

Concludes that low vision clinic can be helpfully located in rehabilitation center, schools for the blind and/or medical center. Closer work with opticians and greater publicity about clinic is helpful.

1912. Zoom lens—New hope for the partially blind. *Science Digest,* Apr. 1973, Vol. 73, No. 4, pp. 38–39.

Brief story on the multidirectional telescopic-lensed glasses invented by Dr. William Feinbloom, an optometrist with degrees in physics and biophysics.

20. Medical and Ophthalmological Factors, Causes of Blindness, Genetic Counseling

1913. American Assoc. of Workers for the Blind. *Contemporary papers, Volume V. Diabetes and blindness: Implications for rehabilitation services.* Washington, D.C.: Author, 1969, 22 pp.

Papers by: Edward Ricketts, Aran Safir, Thomas E. Caulfield, Saul Freedman, & W. E. Milton.

1914. American Foundation for the Blind. *Blindness and diabetes, helping the blind diabetic gain independence.* New York: Author, 1967, 12 pp., free.

A large print pamphlet outlining what blind diabetics should know about their disease and blindness.

1915. ——. *Blindness and diabetes.* New York: Author, 1975?, 16 pp.

Pamphlet outlining what the blind diabetic and those associated with him/her should know about the disease and blindness.

1916. Arbit, Jack. Evaluation of the minimal brain damage syndrome in blind children. In Proceedings of the Conference on New Approaches to the Evaluation of Blind Persons. New York: AFB, 1970, pp. 133–46. Mimeo.

A discussion of the evaluation of the syndrome in question. Includes tables and charts.

1917. Bachelis, Leonard A. Developmental patterns of individuals with bilateral congenital anophthalmos. *New Outlook for the Blind*, Apr. 1967, Vol. 61, No. 4, pp. 113–19.

With supporting statistics, reports a study of 24 cases of congenital anophthalmos in New York State. Suggests that early, comprehensive diagnostic evaluations are important to identify and treat possible additional handicaps.

1918. Bailey, Pearce. Clinical success with three eye conditions. *New Outlook for the Blind*, June 1955, Vol. 49, No. 6, pp. 222–24.

Describes recent gains in the detection, prevention, and treatment of retrolental fibroplasia, uveitis, and glaucoma.

1919. Bender, L., & Andermann, K. Brain damage in blind children with retrolental fibroplasia. *Archives of Neurology*, 1965, Vol. 12, No. 6, pp. 644–49.

Study of 22 children, who were hospitalized because it was thought their retarded development might be a form of autism caused by sensory and emotional deprivation, revealed evidence of brain damage in utero before their premature births.

1920. Birecree, Daniel C. A layman's report on retrolental fibroplasia. *International Journal for the Education of the Blind*, Dec. 1955, Vol. 5, No. 2, pp. 32–36.

Offers explanation and description of eye condition, and initial realization that it was associated with incubator oxygen. Presents conflicting ideas among clinical teams doing research. Discusses the RLF-caused increase in blind children and its implications. Tables showing frequency by years; class distribution at New York State School for the Blind; percentages in school and various classes.

1921. Bleck, Eugene E., & Nagel, Donald A., Eds. *Physically handicapped children—A medical atlas for teachers.* New York: Grune & Stratton, 1975, xiv + 304 pp., illus., $15.

Medical information written for layman. Gives definition, etiology, incidence, prognosis, and educational implications for each condition covered. Has chapter on visual disorders.

1922. Blind child's bluff. *Emergency Medicine*, Nov. 1973, Vol. 5, No. 11, pp. 257–58.

How to recognize and deal with benign post-traumatic transient cerebral blindness syndrome.

1923. Case, Samuel; Dawson, Yvette; Schartner, James; et al. Comparison of levels of fundamental skill and cardio-respiratory fitness of blind, deaf, and non-handicapped high school-age boys. *Perceptual and Motor Skills*, June 1973, Vol. 36, No. 3, Part 2, pp. 1291–94.

To secure data useful to the design of therapeutic physical education programs for blind and deaf children, selected sections of tests were administered to assess possible performance differences.

1924. Chalkley, Thomas. *Your eyes: A book for paramedical personnel and the lay reader.* Springfield, Ill., Charles C Thomas, 1974, 122 pp., illus., $4.75.

Chapters covering the anatomy of the eye, optics and refractive errors as well as visual acuity measurements, individual parts of the eye, and the more common diseases which affect each. Glossary.

1925. Chang, Charles C. Symposium—Self-image: A guide to adjustment II. Brain injury—diagnosis and treatment. *New Outlook for the Blind*, Nov. 1961, Vol. 55, No. 9, pp. 302–5.

Role of pediatrician in dealing with brain-injured patient. How to deal with parents, child himself, and community at large.

1926. Cullin, Irene C. Techniques for teaching patients with sensory defects. *Nursing Clinics of North America*, Sept. 1970, Vol. 5, No. 3, pp. 527–37.

Covers dynamics of learning. Teaching patient with glaucoma. Preparing patient for hospitalization. Teaching the blind patient. Teaching a patient after eye surgery.

1927. Dye, Arthur M. Insulin self-care for blind diabetic patients. *New Outlook for the Blind*, Oct. 1963, Vol. 57, No. 8, pp. 307–8.

Tells how an 80-year old blind woman was successfully taught to administer her own injections, an example of a clinic educational program. Discusses staff training for work with blind diabetics and need for caseworker involvement.

1928. Eichhorn, Mary M. Inherited metabolic disease and the eye. *Sight-Saving Review*, 1971, Vol. 41, No. 2, pp. 55–64.

Discusses nature of inborn errors of metabolism and some specific inherited metabolic diseases which cause eye disease or poor vision including galactosemia, Tay-Sachs disease, Fabry's disease, homocystinuria, Marfan's syndrome, and Wilson's disease.

1929. Farley, Annette D. Counselling retinal detachment patients: A review of research and practice: July 1965–June 1971. *Sight-Saving Review*, Fall 1972, Vol. 42, No. 3, pp. 157–75.

Report on a 6-year study conducted at the Eye and Ear Hospital in Pittsburgh. The ages of patients ranged from 3 mos. to 88 yrs.; a section of the report concerns special problems of various age groups. Emphasizes role of medical social worker as part of therapeutic team.

1930. Finestone, Samuel, & Gold, Sonia. *The role of the ophthalmologist in the rehabilitation of blind patients.* New York: AFB, 1959, 75 pp.

Findings indicate that ophthalmological practice has a greater potential for rehabilitative influence than is currently being exercised.

1931. Fulton, Mary; Schweezer, Diane; Ruhland, Florence; et al. Helping diabetics adapt to failing vision. *American Journal of Nursing*, Jan. 1974, Vol. 74, No. 1, pp. 54–57.

Stresses importance of adjustment to diabetes, reaction to visual deterioration, extent of visual impairment, family relationships, and motor sensory perception. Considering these factors information is given on equipment for administering insulin, exercise, and diet.

1932. Geer, William C. Status of research in chemistry of vision. *New Outlook for the Blind*, June 1955, Vol. 49, No. 6, pp. 225–27.

Supported by specific data on 1954 grants, argues that too little funding is being given to research related to the chemistry of the eye.

1933. Grim, Rosemary A. Mr. Edwards' triumph. *American Journal of Nursing*, Mar. 1972, Vol. 72, No. 3, pp. 480–81.

Home nursing taught blind diabetic to inject his own insulin.

1934. Harris, Michael G., & Heyman, Steven E. Ocular albinism: A review of the literature. Part II. *Optometric Weekly*, Feb. 15, 1973, Vol. 64, No. 7, pp. 31–37.

Discusses 9 of 12 ocular characteristics including photophobia, amblyopia, and translucent iris. Stresses value of carrier identification for family planning, recommends vision care methods for infants and older ocular albino population.

1935. Henrich, Laura J. Medical social work with eye patients. *New Outlook for the Blind*, Feb. 1957, Vol. 51, No. 2, pp. 65–69.

Interpreting eye facts to diminish shock and anxiety, preparing for surgery, helping with decisions, and providing psychiatric consultation when needed. Practical considerations and emotional support must adjust to the reality of each patient's need.

1936. Hiles, David A. Strabismus in brain damaged children. *Seer*, Fall 1975, Vol. 46, No. 3, pp. 9–12.

Discusses the characteristics and implications of acute and chronic malalignment of the eyes, their possible relationship to central nervous system defects, and possible treatments.

1937. Johnson, Samuel B. Satellite eye clinic: Mississippi Delta. *Sight-Saving Review*, Spring 1974, Vol. 44, No. 1, pp. 11–17.

An approach to providing ophthalmological services to disadvantaged persons in rural areas on a continuing basis.

1938. Jolly, Elizabeth. Genetic counseling with specific reference to visual problems. *New Outlook for the Blind*, Mar. 1967, Vol. 61, No. 3, pp. 69–72. Reprinted from *Sight-Saving Review*, Fall 1966.

Describes need for genetic counseling and how the Genetic Consultation and Counseling Service, Contra Costa Co., Calif., functions. Urges integration of clinical genetic teaching into medical schools, promoting the concept of prevention among medical students, and informing the public of the value of genetic counseling.

1939. Judge, C., & Chakanovskis, Johanna E. The Hallermann-Streiff syndrome. *Journal of Mental Deficiency Research*, June 1971, Vol. 15, No. 2, pp. 115–20.

Case study of a 12-year-old boy presented. Syndrome described as consisting of proportionate dwarfism, beaked nose, small mouth, dental abnormalities, and severe vision problems. Includes review of literature.

1940. Kantrow, Abraham H. Counseling service for diabetics. *Sight-Saving Review*, Summer 1967, Vol. 37, No. 2, pp. 73–77.

Considers loss of vision in diabetics, control and psychological acceptance of diabetes. Reviews the role of vocational counseling and services, evaluation of group counseling sessions, and reports on work done.

1941. Lowenfeld, Berthold. Observations on incidence and effects of retrolental fibroplasia. *New Outlook for the Blind*, Jan. 1959, Vol. 53, No. 1, pp. 15–19.

Based on statistics of the Field Services for Preschool Children in S. Calif., reports the number of preschool children blind from RLF and other causes. Comments upon the resulting increase in children without useful vision at the residential school.

1942. ———. The impact of retrolental fibroplasia. *New Outlook for the Blind*, Dec. 1963, Vol. 57, No. 10, pp. 402–5.

Discusses incidence of RLF. Author feels strongly that accompanying neurological defects rather than psychogenic factors are responsible for problems other than blindness seen in people with RLF. Cites study to support this belief.

1943. Miller, Irving. *Resistance to cataract surgery.* New York: AFB, 1964, 110 pp., $2.50.

Of special interest to physicians, nurses, and medical social workers, outlines some of the factors that prevent individuals from seeking medical service and offers suggestions for counseling these persons.

1944. Myers, Julian S., Ed. *An orientation to chronic disease and disability.* New York: Macmillan, 1965, 486 pp.

Aimed at graduate students and professional workers in fields where medical knowledge is necessary but normally not included in formal education. Each disease or disability is defined, diagnostic aids specified, and treatment outlined. Included are visual handicaps as well as hearing impairments, emotional disturbances, and aspects of mental retardation.

1945. National Society for the Prevention of Blindness. *Teaching about vision.* New York: Author, 1972, 71 pp., $2.

Designed as a teaching guide and reference tool for the classroom teacher, health educator, and health service personnel involved with the eye health education of children. Explains growth of the eye and development of visual functions and dysfunctions.

1946. ————. The spittin' image. *Sight-Saving Review,* Fall–Winter 1974, Vol. 44, No. 3, pp. 135–42.

An article that provides basic information as well as possibilities for prevention of blindness by utilizing prenatal genetic diagnosis and genetic counseling. Written with the specialist in mind.

1947. Neel, J. V., et al. The effects of parental consanguinity and inbreeding in Hirado, Japan: III. Vision and Learning. *Human Heredity,* 1970, Vol. 20, No. 2, pp. 129–55.

Investigates the effect of parental consanguinity, age, and sex on defects of the eye and ear.

1948. Nevin, Norman C. The genetics of severe visual handicap in childhood. *Teacher of the Blind,* Autumn 1973, Vol. 62, No. 1, pp. 4–15.

A discussion of inherited causes of blindness.

1949. Parmelee, Arthur H., Jr.; Fiske, Claude E.; & Wright, Roger H. The development of ten children with blindness as a result of retrolental fibroplasia. *American Foundation for the Blind Research Bulletin 1,* Jan. 1962, pp. 64–88. Reprinted from *A.M.A. Journal of Diseases of Children,* Aug. 1959.

Detailed developmental record of 10 children over 4–5 years, with individual histories.

1950. Phillips, Cyril. Interviewing the blind child. *Diseases of the Nervous System,* 1967, Vol. 28, No. 11, pp. 727–30.

Describes a clinical examination method for use with blind children.

1951. Pimantel, Albert T., et al. *Symposium on Usher's Syndrome.* Washington, D.C.: Gallaudet Col., 1973, 65 pp.

Presents papers, reviews, recommendations, including overview of Usher's Syndrome, genetic and ophthalmologic aspects, diagnosis, family reaction, early identification, determination of curriculum and program needs in schools for the deaf and blind.

1952. Punnett, Hope H., & Harley, Robison D. Genetics in pediatric ophthalmology. In Robison D. Harley, Ed., *Pediatric Ophthalmology.* Philadelphia: W. B. Saunders, 1975, pp. 10–58, illus., $50.

Discusses sources of chromosomal and other abnormalities as well as basic genetic mechanisms relating to the eye. Lists characteristics and inheritance patterns of ocular changes in pediatric syndromes and of developmental ocular abnormalities.

1953. Riviere, Maya. *Classification of impairment of visual function.* New York: Rehabilitation Codes, 1970, 87 pp.

Final report on a project to develop a descriptive classification for impairment of visual function, differentiated from defects of vision. Provides a means of interpreting the clinicians' examination reports in terms of the individual's needs for and response to service throughout the rehabilitation process.

1954. Robb, Richard M. Observations on a child's eyes. *Sight-Saving Review*, Summer 1970, Vol. 40, No. 2, pp. 67–72.

Early appearance and development of the eye is discussed including ophthalmologic aspects of the newborn examination. Describes common childhood eye problems including inflammations and ocular misalignment. Early testing for visual acuity is recommended.

1955. Roeske, Nancy A. Improving blind children's scholastic and social performance with medication. *Education of the Visually Handicapped*, Dec. 1969, Vol. 1, No. 4, pp. 105–13.

Mellarie administered to 28 children who presented serious learning and behavior problems to evaluate effects on behavior. Sixteen showed significant improvement; children with behavioral disorders showed most marked gain. Blindisms of 14 ceased while on medication. Neurotic and passive-aggressive children did not improve.

1956. Rubella and the eye specialist. *Sight-Saving Review*, Winter 1970–71, Vol. 40, No. 4, pp. 211–18.

Discusses ocular defects associated with congenital rubella including cataracts, unusually small eyeball size, lesions of the retina, and clouding of the cornea. Summarizes status of development of the rubella vaccine and status of the rubella control program.

1957. Seamon, Florence W. Nursing care of glaucoma patients. *Nursing Clinics of North America*, Sept. 1970, Vol. 5, No. 3, pp. 489–96.

Causes, types, therapy, and nursing care of glaucoma.

1958. Seeman, Bernard. *Your sight: Folklore, fact and common sense.* Boston: Little, Brown, 1968, 242 pp.

Practical book on eyesight intended as a handbook for the layman. Covers near- and farsightedness, glaucoma, effects of aging, cataract, detached retina, retinopathy, strabismus, amblyopia, and hazards to the eye's exterior. Explains types of corrective lenses; services and special aids for the blind and partially sighted summarized.

1959. Selman, Jay E. Rubella: Medical aspects. *Education of the Visually Handicapped*, Mar. 1972, Vol. 4, No. 1, pp. 22–25.

Outlines medical aspects of rubella to highlight factual information concerning questions frequently asked and knowledge said to be needed by teachers and child care workers.

1960. Shaw, John A. Blindness syndromes. *New Beacon*, July 1975, Vol. 59, No. 699, pp. 169–71.

A physician's discussion of blindness as part of more general medical syndromes, such as aging, diabetes, neurological disorders, trauma, etc.

1961. Silverman, William A. Prematurity and retrolental fibroplasia. *New Outlook for the Blind*, Sept. 1970, Vol. 64, No. 7, pp. 232–36.

Explores issues and unsolved problems related to RLF. Reported cases of RLF and hospital policies regarding oxygen administration to premature infants are cited.

1962. Simmons, R. E. Current opthalmological attitudes toward rehabilitation of patients with loss of vision. *New Outlook for the Blind*, Dec. 1966, Vol. 60, No. 10, pp. 299–302.

Author suggests that attitude and approach of physician who must inform the patient of his visual condition may be a neglected significant factor in patient's subsequent adjustment to blindness. Discusses survey rating ophthalmologists on concern for patient as whole individual, and awareness of need to refer blind patients for rehabilitation. Questionnaires and results included.

1963. Spivey, Bruce E. Ophthalmic skills for the nonophthalmic physician. *Sight-Saving Review*, Winter 1973–74, Vol. 43, No. 4, pp. 195–200.

Results and implications of a study regarding development of the educational objectives for a complete curriculum in ophthalmology for medical school graduates capable of general practice.

1964. Stamford, Bryant A. Cardiovascular endurance training for blind persons. *New Outlook for the Blind*, Sept. 1975, Vol. 69, No. 7, pp. 308–11.

Cardiovascular endurance training (CVET) is discussed and a chair-stepping exercise program is described. Presents evidence that supports CVET as capable of: (1) producing adequate levels of physical fitness, (2) reducing to some degree the probability of coronary heart disease, (3) reducing the effects of anxiety accompanying unguided blind mobility.

1965. Tasman, William. Retrolental fibroplasia. *Seer*, Summer 1975, Vol. 46, No. 2, pp. 6–7.

Discussion of this cause of visual impairment and the fact that, despite present knowledge of the association of oxygen with RLF, the condition continues to occur and is difficult to prevent.

1966. Vernon, McCay. Overview of Usher's Syndrome: Congenital deafness and progressive loss of vision. *Volta Review*, Feb. 1974, Vol. 6, No. 2, pp. 100–105.

Implementation of prevention programs and provision of research funds is urged. With genetic screening and counseling, early identification of affected children, and biochemical research both arrest and prevention of the visual aspect of Usher's Syndrome, affecting up to 6% of children in programs for the hearing impaired, seems feasible.

1967. Vincent, Pauline A. Patients' viewpoint of glaucoma therapy. *Sight-Saving Review*, Winter 1972–73, Vol. 42, No. 4, pp. 213–21.

Discusses the differences, according to age, sex, education, and information on their condition, among 62 glaucoma patients in following their doctors' eye-drop prescriptions.

1968. Wagner, Elizabeth M. Maternal rubella: A general orientation to the disease. *New Outlook for the Blind*, Apr. 1967, Vol. 61, No. 4, pp. 97–105, 112.

Gives the early history of measles, German measles, and attitudes toward them prior to identification of maternal rubella. Reports studies of rubella and its effects and interprets relevant statistics. Ref.

1969. Weckroth, Johan; Miettinen, Pentii; & Weckroth, Eila. The light permeability of the retina: Experiments with blind, color-blind, and seeing subjects. *American Foundation for the Blind Research Bulletin 29*, June 1975, pp. 123–43.

Fourteen blind, 12 color blind, and 12 Ss with no sign of color defect were used to determine the sensation when the receptors of the retina were forced to rely for their orientation exclusively on the light reaching them from the background of the eye.

1970. Werner, Georges H.; Latte, Bachisio; & Contini, Andrea. Trachoma. *American Foundation for the Blind Research Bulletin 19*, June 1969, pp. 107–21.

Describes trachoma, where it is found, incidence, and efforts to control it.

1971. Whittington, T. H. The eyes and eyesight in diabetes. *Nursing Times*, Sept. 23, 1971, Vol. 67, No. 38, pp. 1171–73.

Discusses ways in which diabetes affects vision.

1972. Yankauer, Alfred; Jacobziner, Harold; & Schneider, David M. The rise and fall of retrolental fibroplasia in New York State. *New Outlook for the Blind*, May 1956, Vol. 50, No. 5, pp. 165–70.

Supported by tables and graphs, shows the history of the increase and diminishing of RLF in N.Y. after a peak in 1953.

1973. Zacharias, Leona. Retrolental fibroplasia. *American Foundation for the Blind Research Bulletin 15*, Jan. 1968, pp. 159–61. Reprinted from *Journal of Pediatrics*, Jan. 1964.

Discusses evidence that then recent reappearance of RLF proves that use of supplementary oxygen is accompanied by risk of severe ocular damage, some of which could be avoided.

21. Assessment: Tests and Testing and Other Evaluation

1974. American Foundation for the Blind. *Bibliography: Assessment and evaluation for the school age visually handicapped child.* New York: Author, 197–, 5 pp.

Selected bibliography.

1975. ————. *Assessment for the educational readiness of the child with visual impairments: Three workshops.* New York: Author, 1974, 80 pp., app.

Report on workshops. Emphasis on techniques, adaptations, and information necessary for effective assessment of school-aged, visually impaired children. Bib.

1976. Avery, Constance D., & Streitfeld, Julian W. An abbreviation of the Haptic Intelligence Scale for clinical use. *Education of the Visually Handicapped,* May 1969, Vol. 1, No. 2, pp. 37–40.

Tested 32 blind and partially sighted *S*s to evaluate a shortened version of HIS; found it sufficiently accurate.

1977. Bateman, Barbara. Psychological evaluation of blind children. *New Outlook for the Blind,* June 1965, Vol. 59, No. 6, pp. 193–96.

Reviews standardized and informal assessment techniques. Urges emphasis on purpose of examination and individual characteristics of the child as guides to flexible examinations.

1978. Bauman, Mary K. *A manual of norms for tests used in counseling blind persons.* New York: AFB, 1958, 40 pp.

Presents norms for aptitude and personality tests for, or adapted for, the blind; also, guidelines for interpretation.

1979. ————. What is a test? *New Outlook for the Blind,* Apr. 1962, Vol. 56, No. 4, pp. 122–26.

Discusses standard materials administered in a standard way, standard conditions, standard measurements of results, standard comparisons, standard population, and test interpretation.

1980. ————. Group differences disclosed by inventory items. *International Journal for the Education of the Blind,* May 1964, Vol. 13, No. 4, pp. 101–06.

Groups of 150 nonresidential and 150 residential students are compared in their responses to items on the Adolescent Emotional Factors Inventory. Responses are also compared on the basis of sex.

1981. ————. *Tests used in the psychological evaluation of blind and visually handicapped persons,* and *A manual of norms for tests used in* *counseling blind persons.* Washington, D.C.: American Assoc. of Workers for the Blind, 1968, 66 pp.

Reprints a manual of norms originally published in 1958. Reports results of current questionnaires to psychologists across U.S. about what tests they are using with blind persons and how they rate those tests.

1982. ———. Clinical interpretation of personality inventories. *Education of the Visually Handicapped,* Oct. 1971, Vol. 3, No. 3, pp. 82–87.

Presents clinical interpretations of the Adolescent Emotional Factors Inventory. AEFI measures sensitivity, somatic symptoms, social competency, attitudes, adjustment, and includes a validation scale.

1983. ———. Psychological and educational assessment. In Berthold Lowenfeld, Ed., *The visually handicapped child in school.* New York: John Day, 1973, pp. 93–115.

Reviews role of psychologist, problems in test administration and interpretation, and specific measures of learning ability, aptitude, achievement, social competency, manual dexterity, personality, and interest.

1984. ———. An interest inventory for the visually handicapped. *Education of the Visually Handicapped,* Oct. 1973, Vol. 5, No. 3, pp. 78–83.

Uses for, and history of, interest inventories. How present test was developed and is administered. Differences in interests between males and females. Test is reliable and was developed to have construct validity.

1985. ———. Blind and partially sighted. In Milton T. Wisland, Ed., *Psychoeducational diagnosis of exceptional children.* Springfield, Ill.: Charles C Thomas, 1974, pp. 159–89.

Provides background about blindness, suggestions for the testing procedure, and descriptions of tests. Lists publishers of the mentioned tests. Ref.

1986. Bauman, Mary K.; Platt, Henry; & Strauss, Susan. A measure of personality for blind adolescents. *International Journal for the Education of the Blind,* Oct. 1963, Vol. 13, No. 1, pp. 7–12.

After listing some of the difficulties in personality testing, introduces a questionnaire for blind adolescents. Subscales measure 8 facets of personality, attitudes about blindness, and validation. Results compare students in residential and integrated classes. Total N 439.

1987. Bell, Victoria H. An educator's approach to assessing preschool visually handicapped children. *Education of the Visually Handicapped,* Oct. 1975, Vol. 7, No. 3, pp. 84–89.

Following discussion of reasons for and possible gains from evaluation, and the assessment environment (very familiar to child), describes specific instruments of formal assessment and areas of informal assessment. Included are assessment of motor development, vision, communication, self-help skills, and social-emotional responses. Guidelines for teacher assessment and interpretation of results. Ref.

1988. Breger, Ilana. Some structural variables in auditory projective testing. *Journal of Projective Techniques and Personality Assessment,* 1969, Vol. 33, No. 5, pp. 414–18.

Thirty blind and 30 sighted males, comparable in age and intelligence, were asked to tell stories in response to 8 selected auditory stimuli. The perceived pleasantness of auditory projective stimuli as related to emotional tone, RT, and length of stories was studied.

1989. ————. Initial notes on content in auditory projective testing. *Journal of Projective Techniques and Personality Assessment*, 1970, Vol. 34, No. 2, pp. 125–30.

Uses a comparative approach to study content in auditory projective testing. The tone of the projective response is discussed in terms of stimulus properties, nature of the auditory modality, and the particular contributions of the auditory method in personality assessment.

1990. ————. Perceived pleasantness: A stimulus variable in auditory projective testing. In Proceedings of the Conference on New Approaches to the Evaluation of Blind Persons. New York: AFB, 1970, pp. 55–58. Mimeo.

A report on psychodiagnostic testing with blind clients where the author observed the negative tone of the projective response to the auditory projective technique.

1991. Brewer, Paul W. A follow-up study evaluating the effectiveness of psychological examinations administered to adult blind at the start of their vocational rehabilitation. *American Psychologist*, Aug. 1954, Vol. 9, No. 8, p. 339.

1992. Brothers, Roy J. Arithmetic computation: Achievement of visually handicapped students in public schools. *Exceptional Children*, Apr. 1973, Vol. 39, No. 7, pp. 575–76.

Describes use of braille, abacus, and cubarithm board with the Stanford Achievement Test with 263 students in 4th, 6th, and 8th grades.

1993. Bullard, Bonnie M., & Barraga, Natalie. Subtests of evaluative instruments applicable for use with preschool visually handicapped children. *Education of the Visually Handicapped*, Dec. 1971, Vol. 3, No. 4, pp. 116–22.

Lists subtests of evaluative instruments which can be used with preschool blind children and those which are applicable for use with preschool children with impaired but useful vision.

1994. Carlson, B. Robert; Gallagher, Patricia; & Synoveck, Sue. Assessment of the motor ability of visually impaired children. *Perceptual and Motor Skills*, 1970, Vol. 30, No. 3, pp. 1009–10.

Eighteen residential lower-elementary visually impaired children were given the Brace Motor Ability Test. Residual vision had no effect on gross motor ability. Males performed better than females.

1995. Carney, Carolyn. Adaptations of psychological testing for use by the blind. *Journal of School Psychology*, June 1972, Vol. 10, No. 2, pp. 221–23.

A blind psychological examiner describes the adaptations of projective personality and intelligence tests which enabled her to administer them independently.

1996. Chase, Joan B., & Rapaport, Irene N. A verbal adaptation of the Draw-A-Person techniques for use with blind subjects: A preliminary report. *International Journal for the Education of the Blind*, Dec. 1968, Vol. 18, No. 4, pp. 113–15.

Adaptation was administered to 75 blind *S*s. Related procedures with sighted *S*s suggest congruence with regular administration of this test. Ref.

1997. Claassen, Robert. Tests for the blind. *International Journal for the Education of the Blind,* Oct. 1954, Vol. 4, No. 1, pp. 12–15.

Discussion of various tests including verbal tests and performance tests. Includes description of various tests: Kohs (adaption), marble diagrams, toy assembly, symbol-o's. Describes materials needed and testing procedures.

1998. Clark, Leslie L., & Jastrzembska, Zofja S., Eds. Proceedings of the Conference on New Approaches to the Evaluation of Blind Persons. New York: AFB, 1970, iii + 174 pp., $3. Mimeo.

Summarized proceedings of a conference held Apr. 1968 to examine present state of testing and evaluation of blind and visually impaired persons. In addition to tests and methods, the conference dealt with how evaluation procedures fit into educational and rehabilitation procedures, ethical considerations, and utilization of information obtained.

1999. Clawson, Lavere E. A study of the Clawson Worksample Tests for measuring the manual dexterity of the blind. *New Outlook for the Blind,* June 1968, Vol. 62, No. 6, pp. 182–87.

Five worksamples and 2 dexterity tests were studied with from 43 to 109 blind adults. Statistical evidence of validity and interest relationships is provided. The author concludes that worksamples can be standardized and used as objective tests.

2000. Clegg, Gordon D. A study of the Tactual Discrimination Test for measuring tactual ability of the visually handicapped. *American Foundation for the Blind Research Bulletin 25,* Jan. 1973, pp. 259–60.

Brief report of a sorting test consisting of 56 pieces of sandpaper of varied grits. Author believes that, with more development, test could predict client's tactual potential for braille.

2001. Coveny, Thomas E. A new test for the visually handicapped: A preliminary analysis of the reliability and validity of the Perkins-Binet. *Education of the Visually Handicapped,* Dec. 1972, Vol. 4, No. 4, pp. 97–101.

Concludes that both forms of the P-B have a high degree of internal consistency, and that the rather large standard deviations associated with the P-B may have implications for interpreting scores.

2002. Cowen, Emory L.; Underberg, Rita P.; & Verrillo, Ronald T. The development and testing of an attitude to blindness scale. *Journal of Social Psychology,* Nov. 1958, Vol. 48, pp. 297–304.

Describes development of a 30-item scale of attitudes toward blindness and the correlation of its results with antiminority and proauthoritarian attitudes.

2003. Cratty, Bryant J., & Sams, Theressa A. *The body image of blind children.* New York: AFB, July 1968, 70 pp., $2.50.

Ninety children evaluated by a body image survey form to develop an assessment device. Conclusions were that body image may be reliably assessed and that there were significant intragroup differences which have educational implications. Bib.

2004. Cull, Eoline C. Development and analysis of some tactual measures of intelligence for adolescent and adult blind. *American Foundation for the Blind Research Bulletin 18*, Dec. 1968, pp. 23–24.

Reports pilot testing of a measure of tactual discrimination with 30 sighted and 30 blind persons.

2005. Cundick, Bert P.; Crandell, John M., Jr.; & Hendrix, Lee. A new method for the group testing of blind persons. *New Outlook for the Blind,* Nov. 1974, Vol. 68, No. 9, pp. 398–403.

Verbal presentation of tests via prerecorded cassette tapes and a specially designed tactual answer board were tested experimentally. Results are not significantly different from those obtained via visual test-taking.

2006. Currie, Lawrence E. Work evaluation of the visually impaired: A perspective. *New Outlook for the Blind,* Dec. 1975, Vol. 69, No. 10, pp. 443–44, 446.

Defines work evaluation and describes Clawson Work Sample Test which was designed to reflect actual jobs in industry. Stresses consideration of individual differences and needs. Also discusses situational assessment.

2007. Curtis, W. Scott. The development and application of intelligence tests for the blind: A research utilization conference. Athens: Univ. of Ga., Aug. 1972, iv + 49 pp. Mimeo.

Discusses development, use, availability, and future planning for selected tests and their relation to psychological, educational, and vocational counseling.

2008. Dauterman, William L. *Manual for the Stanford Multi-Modality Imagery Test.* New York: AFB, 1972, ix + 47 pp., $2.

Details standardization studies for the Test which measures the blind person's ability to use imagery in solving mobility and other daily living problems. Methods for recording, scoring, and interpreting are presented. Indexes on testing the deaf-blind *S* and on the blind examiner are included.

2009. Dauterman, William L.; Shapiro, Bernice; & Suinn, Richard M. Performance tests of intelligence for the blind reviewed. *International Journal for the Education of the Blind,* Oct. 1967, Vol. 17, No. 1, pp. 8–16.

Provides the history, description, and some evaluation of performance tests recorded in the literature. Special problems of performance testing of partially sighted are discussed. The same types of tests keep appearing over the years but often prove too difficult or expensive to mass-produce. Ref.

2010. Dauterman, William L., & Suinn, Richard M. *Stanford-Ohwaki-Kohs Tactile Block Design Intelligence Test for the Blind.* Part One of Final Report. Palo Alto: Stanford Univ. School of Medicine, 1966, 72 pp., illus.

Six hundred thirty blind *S*s 14 yrs. and older were used in refining and standardizing the nonverbal performance Ohwaki-Kohs Block Design Test for use in the U.S. Results indicated statistically significant correlations at the .001 level between the Stanford-Kohs and the WAIS, and between the Stanford-Kohs and the Ohwaki-Kohs tests. On a retest of 50 *S*s a test-retest reliability coefficient of .86 was reported. Bib.

2011. ————. *Manual for the Stanford-Kohs Block Design Test for the*

Blind. Part three of final report, VRA Grant RD 1625-S-65. Palo Alto, Calif.: Stanford Univ. School of Medicine, 1966, 49 pp., illus.

Description of test, instructions for administration, scoring and interpretation, and relevant statistical data. Ref.

2012. Davidson, Terry. Braille tests with tactual "response buttons" allow for unaided test-taking. *New Outlook for the Blind,* Apr. 1973, Vol. 67, No. 4, pp. 158–60, illus.

Describes making, use, and scoring of a reusable answer sheet which provides the blind person with a means of checking back over and correcting responses if desired.

2013. Davis, Carl J. The assessment of intelligence of visually handicapped children. *International Journal for the Education of the Blind,* Dec. 1962, Vol. 12, No. 2, pp. 48–54.

Describes the verbal and performance measures of intelligence currently available with brief suggestions for their use.

2014. ———. New developments in the intelligence testing of blind children. In Proceedings of the Conference on New Approaches to the Evaluation of Blind Persons. New York: AFB, 1970, pp. 83–103. Mimeo.

This is a report of research with current intelligence tests and their development. Data is not limited to the U.S. Ref.

2015. Davis, Carl J., & Nolan, Carson Y. A comparison of the oral and written methods of administering achievement tests. *International Journal for the Education of the Blind,* Mar. 1961, Vol. 10, No. 3, pp. 80–82.

Describes ways in which administration of the Stanford Achievement Tests have varied from standard when used with blind students. Reports a study of scores based on oral and written administration of one section, Word Meaning. Substantial differences were found for the 2 forms of administration.

2016. Dean, Sidney I. Adjustment testing and personality factors of the blind. *Journal of Consulting Psychology,* 1957, Vol. 21, No. 2, 171–77.

Test results suggest that "the blind are not paranoid or depressed as a group; a finding at variance with previous assumptions."

2017. ———. Manifest anxiety and test taking distortion of the blind. *Journal of Consulting Psychology,* 1957, Vol. 21, No. 3, p. 276.

Brief report.

2018. Denton, L. R. Intelligence test performance and personality differences in a group of visually handicapped children. *Bulletin of the Maritime Psychological Association,* Dec. 1954.

Interim Hayes-Binet Intelligence Test and Wechsler Verbal Scale were administered to 56 blind students, ages 6–16 and ranging in school placement from kindergarten to grade 8.

2019. Dishart, Martin. Testing the blind for rehabilitation using a psychological profile. *New Outlook for the Blind,* Jan. 1959, Vol. 53, No. 1, pp. 1–14.

Suggests and provides a detailed example of a "psychological profile" which gives (1) individual testing information, (2) comparison with norms for the sighted, and (3) a report form which, it is said, the counselor can clearly understand. Uses tests of intelligence, personality, manual dexterity, and achievement.

2020. Domino, George. A non-verbal measure of intelligence for totally blind adults. *New Outlook for the Blind,* Oct. 1968, Vol. 62, No. 8, pp. 247–52.

After a brief review of non-verbal intelligence tests used with blind persons, reports use of D 48, a test which contains 44 problems, each a series of dominoes defining a principle of progression. D 48 and several other tests were administered to 30 blind males, ages 20 to 46. Results with D 48 and correlations among tests are given.

2021. Eaves, Linda, & Klonoff, Harry. A comparison of blind and sighted children on a tactual and performance test. *Exceptional Children,* Dec. 1970, Vol. 37, No. 4, pp. 269–73.

Forty blind and 40 sighted children compared on a Tactual Performance Test. No significant differences between the 2 groups.

2022. Elonen, Anna S. Assessment of the nontestable blind child. In Proceedings of the Conference on New Approaches to the Evaluation of Blind Persons. New York: AFB, 1970, pp. 104–11. Mimeo.

Too often inadequate assessment via surface manifestations is made of the nontestable blind child. Adequate assessment needs not only the skills of one individual, trained in a particular field, but the cooperation of many with breadth of knowledge, awareness, and point of view, to pick up significant and subtle elements from the general picture.

2023. Forman, Hortense. An experiment in group use of the Seashore Measures of Musical Talents. *International Journal for the Education of the Blind,* Dec. 1958, Vol. 8, No. 2, pp. 41–45.

Describes the SMMT and reasons for giving it. This project involved developing a special answer sheet and setting up details of administration. The answer sheets proved satisfactory, and scores for a test group of 16 appeared reasonably accurate.

2024. Foulke, Emerson. A multi-sensory test of conceptual ability. *New Outlook for the Blind,* Mar. 1964, Vol. 58, No. 3, pp. 75–77.

A test was developed using 14 blocks that could be divided into 2 groups based on 7 different types of sensory cues. Author thinks results with children show test could be useful as a research or clinical tool.

2025. Gardner, R. C. A language aptitude test for blind students. *Journal of Applied Psychology,* 1965, Vol. 49, No. 2, pp. 135–41.

Three studies are reported which assess the validity of subtests of the Modern Language Aptitude Test modified for use with blind students of a foreign language.

2026. Ga. Univ. *The development and application of intelligence tests for the blind: A research utilization conference. Final report.* Athens, Ga.: Author, 1972, 55 pp.

Reports proceedings and recommendations of conference on topic. Gives information on various tests for use with blind adults in social and vocational rehabilitation. Lists tests by name, purpose, description, etc.

2027. Gilbert, Jeanne G., & Rubin, Edmund J. Evaluating the intellect of blind children. *New Outlook for the Blind*, Sept. 1965, Vol. 59, No. 7, pp. 238–40.

Through analysis of test records of 30 chiefly residential school children, compares the Hayes-Binet and WISC in terms of usefulness in evaluation of blind children. Recommends development of a new test standardized on blind children.

2028. Gloeckler, Theodore L. The relationship of selected variables to changes in IQ scores in a group of visually handicapped adults. Lansing: Univ. of Mich., 1973, vi + 120 pp., app. Dissertation.

Studies changes in intelligence test performance of a group of 159 visually handicapped adults.

2029. Goldman, Herbert. Psychological testing of blind children. *American Foundation for the Blind Research Bulletin 21*, Aug. 1970, pp. 77–90.

Performance testing, verbal testing, prediction of academic achievement, and studies relating intellectual evaluation to academic achievement are discussed. Includes review of literature and research. Author concludes there is a dearth of studies explicitly concerned with prediction of academic achievement in blind children.

2030. Gore, George V., III. Retrolental fibroplasia and I.Q. *New Outlook for the Blind*, Dec. 1966, Vol. 60, No. 10, pp. 305–6.

Analysis of IQs of RLF population on a state agency register shows no difference between RLF and non-RLF populations. Bib.

2031. Hallenbeck, Phyllis N. Some issues concerning the use of standard personality tests with the blind. In Proceedings of the Conference on New Approaches to the Evaluation of Blind Persons. New York: AFB, 1970, pp. 70–82. Mimeo.

The paper suggests and discusses some of the problems involved with the use of standard personality tests with the blind. Examples cited and practical considerations included.

2032. Hammill, Donald D., et al. The Slosson Intelligence Test adapted for visually limited children. *Exceptional Children*, Mar. 1970, Vol. 36, No. 7, pp. 535–36.

Shortened version of SIT was adapted for visually handicapped and administered to 32 students. Test reliability on shortened version was .95; it appears that the SIT can be useful in testing visually impaired children.

2033. Hammill, Donald, & Crandell, John M., Jr. Implications of tactile-kinesthetic ability in visually handicapped children. *Education of the Visually Handicapped*, Oct. 1969, Vol. 1, No. 3, pp. 65–69.

Study of 50 randomly selected *S*s to examine reliability, validity, and relationship between the Tactile Kinesthetic Forms Discrimination Test and other characteristics.

2034. Hammill, Donald D., & Powell, Lafayette S. An abstraction test for visually handicapped children. *Exceptional Children*, May 1967, Vol. 33, No. 9, pp. 646–47.

To determine if Form X of Abstraction Test, originally designed for cerebral palsied, could be used with visually handicapped, it was administered to 94 children. Affirmative conclusion.

2035. Hardy, Richard E. *The Anxiety Scale for the Blind.* New York: AFB, 1968, 12 pp., $2.

Presents an instrument designed to measure manifest anxiety among totally blind and partially sighted persons. Includes suggestions for administration.

2036. Hayes, Samuel P. A new series of standard achievement tests adapted for use with blind and partially seeing pupils. *International Journal for the Education of the Blind,* Dec. 1955, Vol. 5, No. 2, pp. 44–45.

Stanford Achievement Tests series J-N can be used below 4th grade. Discussion of oral method, simplification of testing procedure, scoring keys, norms used, and comparison between blind and seeing in same grades. Mention of arithmetic computation and use of Taylor or Nemeth Codes.

2037. ———. Is achievement testing practical in the primary grades? *International Journal for the Education of the Blind,* Mar. 1956, Vol. 5, No. 3, pp. 51–54.

Reports on a trial use of the primary arithmetic tests (in the SAT series) offered for first time. Offers explanation of how administered and of problems involved. Tables showing 4th, 3rd and 2nd grades' results in arithmetic games and problems. Includes tables.

2038. Hecht, Patricia J., & Newland, T. Ernest. Learning potential and learning achievement of educationally blind third–eighth graders in a residential school. *International Journal for the Education of the Blind,* Dec. 1965, Vol. 15, No. 2, pp. 33–38.

For a total sample of 69 residential school pupils, divided into 3 age groups, correlations were done between Interim Hayes-Binet, Wechsler Intelligence Scale for Children, Blind Learning Aptitude Test (nonverbal), and 4 sections of the Stanford Achievement Test. Statistical results and interpretation are presented.

2039. Hepfinger, Lucy M. Psychological evaluation of young blind children. *New Outlook for the Blind,* Nov. 1962, Vol. 56, No. 9, pp. 309–15.

Discusses various approaches and procedures in evaluating blind children between ages of 4 and 6 years, such as testing vs. clinical approach; the psychologist's need for a background of work with blind people; parent interviews, and case conferences. Lists psychometric devices and information which should be included in the evaluator's report.

2040. Hoffman, Simon. Some predictors of the manual work success of blind persons. *Personnel and Guidance Journal,* 1958, Vol. 36, pp. 542–44.

Study of 36 blind adults showed performance on Purdue Pegboard and Minnesota Rate of Manipulation tests correlated with their earnings. A survey of hobbies and interests is also a significant predictor.

2041. Hopkins, Kenneth D., & McGuire, Lenore. Mental measurement of the blind: The validity of the Wechsler Intelligence Scale for Children. *International Journal for the Education of the Blind,* Mar. 1966, Vol. 15, No. 3, pp. 65–73.

To answer 7 questions regarding the WISC, 30 blind students, ranging in age from 9 to 15 years, were administered the Hayes-Binet and the WISC. Results are compared in statistical tables and graphs, with conclusion that the 2 tests are not interchangeable.

2042. ———. IQ constancy and the blind child. *International Journal for the Education of the Blind*, May 1967, Vol. 16, No. 4, pp. 113–14.

The 4-year constancy of the IQ was investigated for a group of 30 blind children. Initial Hayes-Binet IQ scores were more comparable to subsequent WISC IQ scores than to the re-test scores on the Hayes-Binet. Authors conclude that renorming for the Hayes-Binet is indicated.

2043. Huckabee, Malcolm H., & Ferrell, Jack G., Jr. The tactual Embedded Figures task as a measure of field dependence-independence in blind adolescents. *Education of the Visually Handicapped*, May 1971, Vol. 3, No. 2, pp. 37–40.

Six totally blind, 12 legally blind, and 30 sighted *S*s were tested. Study findings were felt to support previous research that blind children require significantly longer mean time to discover the embedded figure than do sighted. The legally blind showed better differentiation than the totally blind.

2044. Husni-Palacios, May, & Palacios, John R. Auditory perception and personality patterns of blind adults. *Journal of Projective Techniques and Personality Assessment*, 1964, Vol. 28, No. 3, pp. 284–92.

Two hundred twelve blind adults were given the Sound Test to study their perceptual style and relate it to their functioning employment criterion groups. Results discussed in terms of Witkin's principles of differentiation, field-dependency, and field-independence. Cross-validation study supports results.

2045. ———. The diagnostic interview. In Proceedings of the Conference on New Approaches to the Evaluation of Blind Persons. New York: AFB, 1970, pp. 38–54. Mimeo.

An interview of 68 open-ended questions constructed to probe certain areas of adjustment applicable to an adult blind population.

2046. ———. Personality dynamics and vocational success of blind adults. In Proceedings of the Conference on New Approaches to the Evaluation of Blind Persons. New York: AFB, 1970, pp. 19–37. Mimeo.

Discussion of the development and application of a psychological test battery for use with the blind. *S*s = 626 blind adults (legally) aged 20–50. The battery was designed to investigate the intellectual, attitudinal, developmental, and perceptual aspects, and then to relate the findings to vocational success.

2047. Joiner, Lee M., & Erickson, Edsel L. *Scales and procedures for assessing social psychological characteristics of visually impaired and hearing impaired students.* Kalamazoo: W. Mich. Univ., 1967, 111 pp.

Methodological study to evaluate scales related to self-concept.

2048. Jones, Reginald L., & McGhee, Paul E. Locus of control, reference group, and achievement in blind children. *Rehabilitation Psychology*, Spring 1972, Vol. 19, No. 1, pp. 18–26.

Group of 45 blind males stated expectancies and performed block-sorting. Bialer Locus of Control Scale and Crandall's Intellectual Achievement Responsibility Questionnaire were used.

2049. Kahn, T. C. Kahn Intelligence Tests: Experimental Form (KIT: EXP). *Perceptual and Motor Skills*, 1960, Vol. 10, pp. 123–53.

Includes: A Main Scale, Brief Placement Scale to determine level of entry into Main Scale, special shorter scales to estimate ability in areas of concept formation, recall, and motor coordination, and scales for administration by sign language and for testing the sight-handicapped and blind.

2050. Kephart, John G.; Kephart, Christine P.; & Schwarz, George C. A journey into the world of the blind child. *Exceptional Children*, Mar. 1974, Vol. 40, No. 6, pp. 421–27.

Comparison of responses of 49 blind and 37 sighted children, ages 5–7, on Kephart Scale suggested that blind children are deprived of information-gathering modes available to sighted children and that for them total sensory experiences are needed.

2051. Klimasinski, Krzysztof. An attempt to test the personality of the blind using the MMPI. *American Foundation for the Blind Research Bulletin 24*, Mar. 1972, pp. 65–74.

Minnesota Multiphasic Personality Inventory was found useful for testing the visually handicapped after changes in procedure and interpretation of some responses. Degree of loss of vision does not significantly influence emotional adjustment.

2052. Koestline, W. Charles; Dent, Oran B., & Giambra, Leonard M. Verbal mediation on a nonvisual formboard task with blind, partially sighted, and sighted subjects. *Journal of Consulting and Clinical Psychology*, Apr. 1972, Vol. 38, No. 2, pp. 169–73.

Compares 46 congenitally blind, partially sighted, and sighted adolescents. Facilitating effects of verbal mediation not confirmed.

2053. Komisar, David, & MacDonnell, Marian. Gains in IQ for students attending a school for the blind. *Exceptional Children*, Jan. 1955.

A study of the results of intelligence retests for 89 students. Some caution is necessary in prediction of achievement on basis of initial examinations.

2054. Kramer, Harvey J. *Stimulus variables in auditory projective testing.* New York: AFB, 1962, 81 pp.

The principal purpose of the study was to devise a method for measuring psychological ambiguity, and to examine the relationships between ambiguity, content, and projection using 3 varying levels of ambiguous auditory stimuli and 2 types of auditory stimulus content.

2055. ————. Stimulus variables in auditory projective testing. *American Foundation for the Blind Research Bulletin 1*, Jan. 1962, pp. 33–40. Chap. 3 of #2054 above.

Experiment comparing human and nonhuman projective content of varying ambiguity shows that human content produced significantly more projection than stimuli with nonhuman content. The projection curve for nonhuman content also increased between least and intermediate ambiguous sets of auditory stimuli.

2056. Land, Shirley L., & Vineberg, Shalom E. Locus of control in blind children. *Exceptional Children*, 1965, Vol. 31, No. 5, pp. 257–60.

The Bialer-Cromwell Children's Locus of Control Scale was administered to 54 blind children and sighted children matched for mental age.

Found to be a valid measure of a trait seemingly related to an individual's ability to perceive himself in control of events around him.

2057. Lebo, Dell. The development and employment of VTAT's or pictureless TAT's. *American Foundation for the Blind Research Bulletin 1*, Jan. 1962, pp. 58–63. Reprinted from *Journal of Psychology*, 1960.

Compares TAT descriptions provided by Murray and Rankin's adaptation for use with blind persons. Concludes that a pictureless TAT administered by means of card descriptions has proven diagnostically useful.

2058. Lebo, Dell, & Bruce, Roselyn S. Projective methods recommended for use with the blind. *American Foundation for the Blind Research Bulletin 1*, Jan. 1962, pp. 41–58. Reprinted from *Journal of Psychology*, 1960.

Projective stimuli recommended or used as suitable evaluative procedures with blind persons are presented, and many are discussed in detail. Ref.

2059. Lewis, Lena L. The relation of measured mental ability to school marks and academic survival in the Texas School for the Blind. *International Journal for the Education of the Blind*, Mar. 1957, Vol. 6, No. 3, pp. 56–60.

With detailed evidence of the statistics used, reports a study that there is (1) a positive relation between tests of intelligence adapted for the blind, (2) a positive relationship between mental ability and academic achievement, and (3) a positive relationship between mental ability and academic survival.

2060. Lowenfeld, Berthold. The visually handicapped. *Review of Educational Research*, 1963, Vol. 33, pp. 38–47.

Emphasizes need for supplementation of verbal intelligence tests by performance tests to measure the global intelligence of the blind. Bib.

2061. McCoy, George F. *The team approach in diagnosing and educating the visually impaired pupil.* Springfield: Ill. State Univ., 1972, 89 pp.

Gives each member of the interdisciplinary team (physician, optometrist, social worker, psychologist, teacher) a working knowledge of what each can do for the visually handicapped child.

2062. Malikin, David, & Freedman, Saul. Test construction or adaptation for use with blind persons. In Proceedings of the Conference on New Approaches to the Evaluation of Blind Persons. New York: AFB, 1970, pp. 7–18. Mimeo.

Discussion of basic concepts involved in diagnostic testing. Also, experience of using psychological tests with the blind and considering diagnostic needs for the future.

2063. Margach, Charles, & Kern, Kate C. Visual impairment, partial-sight and the school psychologist. *Journal of Learning Disabilities*, Aug. 1969, Vol. 2, No. 8, pp. 407–14.

Discusses special techniques in both administration and interpretation of the Wechsler Intelligence Scale for Children when used in testing of partially sighted children.

2064. Maxfield, Kathryn E., & Buchholz, Sandra. *A social maturity scale for blind preschool children: A guide to its use.* New York: AFB, 1957, 44 pp., $2.

Scale was developed to measure the social quotient of blind children from infancy through 6 years. Standardization based on 717 ratings of 484 children. Insufficient data for reliability and validity studies. Includes instructions for administration and scoring as well as a copy of the scale.

2065. Maxfield, Kathryn E., & Kenyon, Eunice L. *A guide to the use of the Maxfield-Fjeld tentative adaptation of the Vineland Social Maturity Scale for use with visually handicapped preschool children.* New York: AFB, 1953, 30 pp.

Directions for administering and scoring, and suggestions for interpretation are given.

2066. Maxfield, Kathryn E., & Perry, James D. Performance of blind vocational rehabilitation clients on the Purdue Pegboard. *Perceptual and Motor Skills*, 1960, Vol. 11, pp. 139–46.

Analysis of performance of 275 blind clients in terms of 3 vision groups (legally blind with usable vision, blind from birth or an early age, more recently blind), age, education, sex, and work experience. Comparison of results with similar data gathered in 1953 by Bigman.

2067. ————. The intelligence status of some vocational rehabilitation clients. *New Outlook for the Blind*, Jan. 1961, Vol. 55, No. 1, pp. 19–20.

IQ of blind clients as measured by Wechsler Verbal Scales compared in various ways. Conclusions are that men and women were sent for evaluation who seemed able to profit from vocational training; also, blind adults compared favorably with seeing adults on this measure.

2068. Mayer, Joseph. Difficulties in handling the "human element" in the psychological evaluation of blind children. *International Journal for the Education of the Blind*, May 1966, Vol. 15, No. 4, pp. 101. Also in *New Outlook for the Blind*, Nov. 1966, Vol. 60, No. 9.

Discusses feelings and attitudes of the primary individuals in a psychological evaluation, i.e., person evaluated, examiner, referring person, and parents. An open and honest approach is emphasized.

2069. Monbeck, Michael E., & Mulholland, Mary E. Introduction to assessment and the blind. *New Outlook for the Blind*, Oct. 1975, Vol. 69, No. 8, pp. 337–39.

Describes history of this special issue of *Outlook*, general aspects of assessment that must be considered, and questions about assessment that need to be resolved.

2070. Morris, June E. 1973 Stanford Achievement Test Series as adapted for use by the visually handicapped. *Education of the Visually Handicapped*, May 1974, Vol. 6, No. 2, pp. 33–40.

Adaptation, done by the American Printing House for the Blind, was necessary in 1973 because of significant curriculum changes and a need to update the norms. Among other things, adaptation involved removing items which could not be adapted. Testers are cautioned on various points.

2071. ————. *Stanford Achievement Test, Forms A and B: Directions for administering braille editions.* Also *Directions for administering large type editions.* Louisville, Ky.: American Printing House for the Blind, 1975.

Published as a series in separate volumes: 2 levels of primary, 2 levels of intermediate, and 1 advanced.

2072. ———. *Stanford TASK— Test of Academic Skills, Forms A and B: Directions for administering braille editions.* Also, *Directions for administering large type editions.* Louisville, Ky.: American Printing House for the Blind, 1975.

Manuals for a new achievement test.

2073. Morris, June E., & Nolan, Carson Y., Comps. Bibliography on tests and testing of the blind. Louisville, Ky.: American Printing House for the Blind, 1971, 31 pp. Mimeo.

Includes references on: Theoretical or practical aspects of testing, history, manuals, descriptions and evaluations of tests, adaptation for the blind, and various uses of tests. Testing and guidance programs not included.

2074. Morse, John L. The adaptation of a non-verbal abstract reasoning test for use with the blind. *Education of the Visually Handicapped,* Oct. 1970, Vol. 2, No. 3, pp. 79–80.

Twenty-eight blind 9th graders at Perkins School were tested. Predictive validity was determined by correlating the test performance with the grades the *S*s received in their academic subjects 3 mos. after test administration. Was concluded that the adapted test was reliable.

2075. ———. The adaptation of a non-verbal abstract reasoning test for use with the blind: Review of related research and bibliography. *American Foundation for the Blind Research Bulletin 23,* June 1971, pp. 39–46.

Research involving sighted and blind *S*s is reviewed to determine a means of adapting group-administered, visually perceived, abstract reasoning intelligence tests with the blind.

2076. ———. Answering the questions of the psychologist assessing the visually handicapped child. *New Outlook for the Blind,* Oct. 1975, Vol. 69, No. 8, pp. 350–53.

Questions include such areas as required information concerning visual condition, background of client, test conditions, role of parents, classroom observation, behaviors observed during testing, evaluation of results, expectations of parents and teachers, and modification of a child's inappropriate behaviors.

2077. Napier, Charles S. "What do you at Royer-Greaves do with testing?" *International Journal for the Education of the Blind,* Mar. 1954, Vol. 3, No. 3, pp. 240–41.

Discusses testing at school for retarded blind children. Compares different types of tests used. Many tests are not useful for this type child. Teacher's judgment with qualifying statement helpful.

2078. ———. Reliability of an orally presented interest measure. *Dissertation Abstracts International,* Sept. 1971, Vol. 32 (3-A), pp. 1340–41.

Comprehension of oral presentation of Kuder Preference Record, Occupational Form D, reliability, seeing vs. visually handicapped *S*s under 18 years.

2079. Nevil Interagency Referral Service. Use of work samples with blind clients. Philadelphia: Author, 1975, iii + 70 pp. Mimeo.

Papers and conference discussions relating various aspects of work samples to vocational problems of blind clients.

2080. Newland, T. Ernest. Prediction and evaluation of academic learning by blind children. Part 1: Problems and procedures in prediction. *International Journal for the Education of the Blind*, Oct. 1964, Vol. 14, No. 1, pp. 1–7. Part 2, Dec. 1964.

Teaching should be determined by the amount and nature of learning potential in each child. Predicting capacity to learn depends on good measures of the extent to which he has already learned and of basic capacity to acquire symbols.

2081. ———. Prediction and evaluation of academic learning by blind children. Part 2: Problems and procedures in evaluation. *International Journal for the Education of the Blind*, Dec. 1964, Vol. 14, No. 2, pp. 42–51. Part 1, Oct. 1964.

Differentiates between prediction and evaluation. Discusses verbal measures of mental ability and the need for a nonverbal measure less affected by achievement. Evaluation requires answering whether the child is performing as well as we have a right to expect him to perform, but measuring that is very complex.

2082. ———. *The Blind Learning Aptitude Test.* Urbana: Univ. of Ill., 1969, 103 pp., illus.

Final report, including review of tests for the blind, description of development of BLAT, statistical data, findings based on use, and suggestions for further research.

2083. Nolan, Carson Y. Achievement in arithmetic computation. *International Journal for the Education of the Blind*, May 1959, Vol. 8, No. 4, pp. 125–28.

Data resulting from experimental use of a new arithmetic achievement test made possible comparison of arithmetic skills in 9 schools. Without using school names, this comparison is reported and interpreted.

2084. ———. Roughness discrimination among blind children in the primary grades. *International Journal for the Education of the Blind*, May 1960, Vol. 9, No. 4, pp. 97–100.

Reports an exploratory study of differences in ability to discriminate degrees of roughness. Fourteen different grades of sandpaper were used to make 27 test items which were administered to 94 residential school students, ages 5 to 13.

2085. Nolan, Carson Y., & Ashcroft, Samuel C. The Stanford Achievement Arithmetic Computation Tests. *International Journal for the Education of the Blind*, Mar. 1959, Vol. 8, No. 3, pp. 89–92.

Following some years of omitting arithmetic from achievement tests for blind students, an adaptation of Form J of the Stanford was made. Results of its experimental use show adequate reliability and general usefulness.

2086. Nolan, Carson Y., & Morris, June E. Variability among young blind children in object recognition. *International Journal for the Education of the Blind*, Oct. 1960, Vol. 10, No. 1, pp. 23–25.

Reports a pilot study of object recognition using 78 young blind children as subjects. Test items were 30 objects commonly found in homes. Significant differences were found but did not correlate with chronological age. Items of this type might be used to estimate level of concept development.

2087. ———. Further results in the development of a test of roughness discrimination. *International Journal for the Education of the Blind*, Dec. 1960, Vol. 10, No. 2, pp. 48–50.

An earlier report on this test indicated that it showed promise of usefulness. Therefore, the test was refined and administered to 98 children in grades K–4. Grade means increased through grade 3, and low correlation was found with IQ and chronological age.

2088. ———. Roughness Discrimination Test manual. Louisville, Ky.: American Printing House for the Blind, 1965, 17 pp. Mimeo.

Designed as a readiness test for braille reading, this test consists of a set of cards upon each of which is mounted 4 pieces of sandpaper, 3 alike and 1 different. Manual provides instructions and interpretive data.

2089. ———. Development and validation of the Roughness Discrimination Test. *International Journal for the Education of the Blind*, Oct. 1965, Vol. 15, No. 1, pp. 1–6.

The final version of the RDT, a reading readiness test for braille, is composed of 69 cards upon each of which 4 pieces of sandpaper are mounted. The student is asked to find the 1 piece of sandpaper on each card which feels different from the others. Reliability and validity are presented.

2090. Ohwaki, Yoshikazu. *Manual of the Ohwaki-Kohs Tactile Block Design Intelligence Test for the Blind.* Japan: Ohwaki Institute of Child Psychology, n.d. (U.S. Distributor: Western Psychological Services, Los Angeles.)

2091. Ohwaki, Yoshikazu; Tanno, Yuji; Ohwaki, Mieko; et al. Construction of an intelligence test for the blind. *Tohoku Psychologica Folia*, 1960, Vol. 18, pp. 45–65.

The Kohs Block Design Test was translated into varying tactile surfaces using cloths of different textures, with blocks enlarged and time allowed increased. Three hundred forty-five totally blind *S*s aged 8–20 were tested. Conclusions are doubtful because of the small number of *S*s.

2092. Ozias, Douglas K. Achievement assessment of the visually handicapped. *Education of the Visually Handicapped*, Oct. 1975, Vol. 7, No. 3, pp. 76–84.

Following a brief history of achievement testing, discusses the following current issues: Problems with modification of tests, norm or criterion reference issues, problems regarding subject matter content such as maps, graphs, and mathematics, and identification of referent population. Suggests questions yet to be answered in relation to achievement assessment. Ref.

2093. Parker, James. Adapting school psychological evaluation to the blind child. *New Outlook for the Blind*, Dec. 1969, Vol. 63, No. 10, pp. 305–11.

Methods of testing individual intelligence and adaptation of current instruments. Mentions the ease of adapting the Wechsler for use with the blind. Points out need for test of neuro-motor components.

2094. Pearson, Margaret A. The establishment of School and College Ability Test norms for blind children in grades 4, 5, and 6. *International Journal for the Education of the Blind*, May 1963, Vol. 12, No. 4, pp. 110–12.

The SCAT was put into braille and large type, and norms, not presented in this article, have been established on 197 white students. Author concludes research is needed to develop a test of intelligence which requires no vision and measures both verbal and quantitative abilities.

2095. Rawls, Rachel. Objective tests and testing of blind children. *New Outlook for the Blind*, Feb. 1954, Vol. 48, No. 2, pp. 39–45.

Describes tests of intelligence, aptitude, personality, and interest as adapted for blind children. General and specific achievement tests are also described. Psychological tests have an important place in the guidance program, but certain cautions are important in interpreting results.

2096. Rich, Charles C., & Anderson, Robert P. A tactual form of the progressive matrices for use with blind children. *American Foundation for the Blind Research Bulletin 15*, Jan. 1968, pp. 49–60. Reprinted from *Personnel and Guidance Journal*, May 1965.

Used an experimental test, Children's Tactual Progressive Matrices, with 115 blind children, ages 6–15. Concluded test could be used successfully above age 8, had high reliability and moderate validity.

2097. Rogers, Floyd S. *Report of a Title VI, ESEA, summer screening clinic sponsored by El Paso County School Education.* Colorado Springs, Colo.: Public Schools, 1968, 35 pp.

Summer clinic established which screened 425 *S*s for visual and auditory disorders. Vision, hearing, and auditory discrimination problems did not seem to affect reading achievement or IQ scores on standardized tests.

2098. Romig, Dennis A., & Van Atta, Ralph E. A validity study of the Adolescent Emotional Factors Inventory. *Education of the Visually Handicapped*, May 1970, Vol. 2, No. 2, pp. 38–46.

One hundred fifty-five *S*s were given the AEFI and the scores were intercorrelated separately and in combination with 15 measures of adjustment and achievement. All but 1 subscale were statistically significant. Suggests that because the 9 other subscales had a high correlation, the test is probably not useful for differential diagnosis.

2099. Rothschild, Jacob. A battery of psychological tests in rehabilitation services. *New Outlook for the Blind*, Sept. 1959, Vol. 53, No. 7, pp. 249–51.

Reports on the test records of 275 clients of a division of the Industrial Home for the Blind. Wechsler, dexterity, and personality tests were used.

2100. Rowe, Raymond. Measuring capabilities of the visually limited. *New Outlook for the Blind*, Mar. 1963, Vol. 57, No. 3, pp. 94–96.

A general capacities scale covering 5 levels in each of 5 areas provides a client profile which makes important information easily available to the agency staff.

2101. Rusalem, Herbert. The assessment of blind persons. In Proceedings of the Conference on New Approaches to the Evaluation of Blind Persons. New York: AFB, 1970, pp. 1–5. Mimeo.

An introduction to the conference held in order to examine and take stock of the present state of testing and evaluation of blind and visually impaired persons.

2102. Sakellariou, Georgiou T. *An explorative study of the personality of the blind.* Athens: Hellenic Psychol. Assoc., 1964, 36 pp.

Fifteen blind *S*s were tested with the Sakellariou Personality Scale. Results indicate a marked difference in reaction and emotional response between those born blind and others who developed blindness later in life. Discussion of specific personality traits provided.

2103. Sargent, Helen D. Insight Test prognosis in successful and unsuccessful rehabilitation of the blind. *Journal of Projective Techniques,* 1956, Vol. 20, pp. 429–41.

Results of a study of 27 blind clients of a rehabilitation agency suggest that the Insight Test is a potentially useful clinical device for selecting those who are personally best equipped to benefit from rehabilitation.

2104. Scholl, Geraldine T. Intelligence tests for visually handicapped children. *Exceptional Children,* Dec. 1953, Vol. 20, No. 3, pp. 116–20.

Describes intelligence tests which have been adapted for use with visually handicapped children and, especially, use of the Wechsler Intelligence Scale for Children at Michigan School for the Blind. Data relates to 23 students, aged 7–14 years.

2105. ———. Some notes on the use of two personality tests with visually handicapped students. *New Outlook for the Blind,* Dec. 1953, Vol. 47, No. 10, pp. 287–95.

Details method of administering the Personality Inventory (Bernreuter) and the Adjustment Inventory (Bell) using tape recorder and response tickets. Gives scoring procedure, interpretation and results for 62 students at Michigan School for the Blind.

2106. Scholl, Geraldine, & Schnur, Ronald N. Measures of psychological, vocational, and educational functioning in the blind and visually handicapped: Introductory remarks. *New Outlook for the Blind,* Oct. 1975, Vol. 69, No. 8, pp. 365–70.

Based on introductory chapters of AFB's forthcoming *Measures of psychological, vocational and educational functioning in the blind and visually handicapped,* briefly discusses general factors of testing the visually impaired and describes the book.

2107. Shurrager, Harriett C., & Shurrager, Phil S. *HISAB manual: Haptic Intelligence Scale for Adult Blind.* Chicago: Psychology Research, Technology Center, 1964, 45 pp.

The HISAB is a performance scale for totally blind persons age 16+. Provides instructions, norms, and material necessary for interpretation.

2108. Spungin, Susan J., & Swallow, Rose-Marie. Psychoeducational assessment: Role of psychologist to teacher of the visually handicapped. *Education of the Visually Handicapped,* Oct. 1975, Vol. 7, No. 3, pp. 67–76.

Discusses relatively new role of teachers in assessment, importance of accurate and detailed observation. Detailed discussion of interpretation of WISC-R Verbal Scale. Psychoeducational assessment requires scores or observations in at least the following: Verbal, spatial, conceptual, sequential, attention/concentration, functional learning styles, and behavioral operatives. Ref.

2109. Stillman, Robert, Ed. *The Callier-Azusa Scale.* Dallas: Callier Center for Communication Disorders, 1974, 132 pp.

Presents Scale designed to aid assessment of deaf-blind and multihandicapped children in areas of motor development, perceptual abilities, daily living skills, socialization. Scale said to be useful for initial assessment, measuring progress over time, planning developmentally appropriate programs. Should be administered by individuals familiar with the child.

2110. Streitfeld, Julian W., & Avery, Constance D. The WAIS and HIS Tests as predictors of academic achievement in a residential school for the blind. *International Journal for the Education of the Blind,* Oct. 1968, Vol. 18, No. 3, pp. 73–77.

WAIS and HIS were administered to 31 students, ages 16–19, of whom 20 were partially sighted, 11 totally blind. Correlation with achievement ratings showed that for the totally blind WAIS and HIS predicted grades equally well, but for the partially sighted WAIS predicted better.

2111. Suinn, Richard M.; Dauterman, William; & Shapiro, Bernice. The Stanford Ohwaki-Kohs Tactile Block Design Intelligence Test for the Blind. *New Outlook for the Blind,* Mar. 1966, Vol. 60, No. 3, pp. 77–79.

Discusses test as instrument of measurement and prediction. Based on 1 yr. experience, suggests crucial issues in test studies with the blind, including 5 modifications of the Ohwaki-Kohs materials.

2112. ———. The WAIS as a predictor of educational and occupational achievement in the adult blind. *New Outlook for the Blind,* Feb. 1967, Vol. 61, No. 2, pp. 41–43.

With supporting statistical data, reports correlations of WAIS IQs and subtests with education, income, and occupational level for 135 blind adults. Reports significant correlations with educational and occupational information.

2113. Templer, D., & Hartlage, L. The reliability and utilization of the hand-face test with the retarded blind. *American Journal of Mental Deficiency,* 1965, Vol. 70, No. 1, pp. 139–41.

Hand-face test was administered to 24 Ss, 12 blind and 12 sighted, matched for MA, CA, and sex. The reliability of the test was demonstrated.

2114. Tiffin, Joseph, Proj. Dir. *An investigation of vocational success with the blind.* Final report, OVR Grantee Designation PRF 1588. Lafayette, Ind.: Purdue Research Foundation, Purdue Univ. Press, 1960, 142 pp.

Report of a 3-year project through which tests were developed and related to the vocational success of a large sample of blind clients. The resulting tests are: Tactual Reproduction Pegboard, Vocational Intelligence Scale for the Adult Blind, Asher-Frohman Maze, McDaniel Sentence Completion Test, and Sound Test.

2115. Tillman, Murray H. The performance of blind and sighted children on the Wechsler Intelligence Scale for Children: Study I. *International Journal for the Education of the Blind,* Mar. 1967, Vol. 16, No. 3, pp. 65–74. Study II, May 1967.

Results of WISC are compared for matched groups of blind and sighted children ranging in age from 7 to 12 years. Tables and graphs support the verbal analysis, by subtest. Blind children scored about the same as sighted children on Arithmetic, Information and Vocabulary, less well on Comprehension and Similarities.

2116. ———. The performance of blind and sighted children on the Wechsler Intelligence Scale for Children: Study II. *International Journal for the Education of the Blind*, May 1967, Vol. 16, No. 4, pp. 106–12. Study I, Mar. 1967.

A second article presenting data on 110 blind children and a matched sighted group. Application of factor analysis suggests that the blind lack integration among educational experiences with result that each bit of knowledge is isolated. Also, verbal abilities focus on basic vocabulary without much elaboration, and in conceptualization, blind lag behind sighted children.

2117. ———. Intelligence scales for the blind: A review with implications for research. *Journal of School Psychology*, Mar. 1973, Vol. 11, No. 1, pp. 80–87.

Focuses on reliability, validity, and research strategy, in studies using the verbal section of the WISC.

2118. Tillman, Murray H., & Bashaw, W. L. Multivariate analysis of the WISC scales for blind and sighted children. *Psychological Reports*, 1968, Vol. 23, No. 2, pp. 523–26.

Examined Verbal IQ in terms of subtest scores. Results indicated future studies of the predictive validity of the WISC with blind children should use individual subtests as variables rather than the single Verbal IQ measure.

2119. Tillman, Murray H., & Osborne, R. T. The performance of blind and sighted children on the Wechsler Intelligence Scale for Children: Interaction effects. *Education of the Visually Handicapped*, Mar. 1969, Vol. 1, No. 1, pp. 1–4.

Study of 167 WISC forms to determine whether blind and sighted children have similar WISC profiles when equated on total Verbal IQ.

2120. Tobin, M. J., & Hunter, B. Assessing the manual dexterity of the visually handicapped. *New Beacon*, July 1974, Vol. 58, No. 687, pp. 169–72.

Report on research conducted in England using the 1960 version of the Purdue Pegboard. The Ss were 100 visually handicapped boys (58) and girls (42), aged 16–19.

2121. Trisman, Donald A. Equating braille forms of the Sequential Tests of Educational Progress. *Exceptional Children*, Feb. 1967, Vol. 33, No. 6, pp. 419–24.

Tests of social studies, science, and mathematics were adapted and brailled, to compare achievement of blind and sighted students.

2122. U.S. Civil Service Commission, Standards Div., Test Development Section. *Tests for blind competitors for trades and industrial jobs in the Federal civil service.* Washington, D.C.: Author, 1956, vi + 72 pp.

Study to provide tests in which blind or sighted workers at the same level of efficiency would receive equivalent scores.

2123. Van der Merwe, S. W. Pictures of the intellectual orientation of partially-sighted children. *Educational Studies*, 1966, No. 48, 133 pp.

The Williams Intelligence Test for Children with Defective Vision, a reading test, a dictation test, Rorschach cards, and other specially constructed tests of visual and graphic expression were used in the study. Findings show a high incidence of emotional disturbance, inadequate attunement to spiritual values, poor to indifferent quantitative indices, and insufficient intellectual development.

2124. Vega, Manuel, & Powell, Arnold. Visual defects and performance on psychological tests. *Journal of Negro Education*, Winter 1974, Vol. 43, No. 1, pp. 127–30.

Sixty-eight children with visual defects such as astigmatism or substandard acuity, and 129 visually normal children tested twice. Lists tests used and implications, such as indication that a period of learning is required after optometric correction of defective vision which caused behavioral deficits.

2125. Wacks, Theodore D. Personality testing of the handicapped: A review. *Journal of Projective Techniques and Personality Assessment*, 1966, Vol. 30, No. 4, pp. 339–55.

The validity and utility of various projective and non-projective tests with handicapped populations are reviewed. Five areas of handicapping conditions are considered: Blindness, deafness, speech disorders, motor disorders, and intellectual retardation.

2126. Walls, Richard T.; MacDonald, A. P., Jr.; & Gulkus, Steven P. The disability seriousness scale: Rating the effects of blindness. *New Outlook for the Blind*, Apr. 1974, Vol. 68, No. 4, pp. 174–75, 177.

The test instrument developed for this study seeks to measure the extent to which the subject perceives his own or a named disability as debilitating in nine life areas or skills. It was administered to 46 visually handicapped persons and 50 sighted. Results indicate substantial agreement between the 2 groups regarding the seriousness of blindness in life activities.

2127. Wardell, Kent T. Assessment of blind students' conceptual understanding. *New Outlook for the Blind*, Dec. 1975, Vol. 69, No. 10, pp. 445–46.

Briefly discusses need for assessment and what it should encompass.

2128. Wattron, John B. A suggested performance test of intelligence. *New Outlook for the Blind*, Apr. 1956, Vol. 50, No. 4, pp. 115–21.

An early attempt to develop a performance test based on copying patterns with rough and smooth sides of blocks. Gives results for 20 student *S*s ranging in age from 7 to 17 years.

2129. Weiner, Bluma B. A new outlook on assessment. *New Outlook for the Blind*, Mar. 1967, Vol. 61, No. 3, pp. 73–78.

Assessment should relate to educability in terms of level, rate, range, efficiency, and autonomy. Curriculum should avoid limiting the child with complex disabilities. Describes tools for bringing these concepts of assessment and curriculum together.

2130. Weiner, Lawrence H. The performance of good and poor braille readers on certain tests involving tactual perception. *International Journal for the Education of the Blind*, Mar. 1963, Vol. 12, No. 3, pp. 72–77.

Two groups of 25 children each, good and poor braille readers, did 6 experimental tests of tactual perception. Complex tests of tactual perception showed a relationship to braille reading ability. Other intercorrelations are provided.

2131. Williams, Myfanwy. An intelligence test for blind and partially sighted children. *Bulletin of the British Psychological Society*, 1956, Vol. 30, p. 32.

2132. ———. *Williams Intelligence Test for children with defective vision.* Birmingham, England: Univ. of Birmingham, 1956.

An individually administered intelligence test on the general pattern of the Binet, specifically designed for blind children.

2133. Wilson, Edouard L. The use of psychological tests in diagnosing the vocational potential of visually handicapped persons who enter supportive and unskilled occupations. *New Outlook for the Blind*, Mar. 1971, Vol. 65, No. 3, pp. 79–88.

Discusses client-oriented psychological testing, the choice and interpretation of tests related to individual backgrounds and needs, and the importance of relating vocational testing to vocational goals. Ref.

2134. Winer, David. The relationships among intelligence, emotional stability and use of auditory cues by the blind. *American Foundation for the Blind Research Bulletin 2*, Dec. 1962, pp. 88–93.

For 22 totally blind Ss, WAIS and Emotional Factors Inventory were related to use of auditory cues in traveling. Information produced can be useful in selecting appropriate travel aid.

2135. Wisland, Milton V. *Psychoeducational diagnosis of exceptional children.* Springfield, Ill.: Charles C Thomas, 1974, 398 pp.

Collection of articles concerned with problems of diagnosis and assessment of different types of exceptional children. Ref. at end of each chapter.

22.　Personality, Adjustment, Psychosocial Studies

2136. Adams, George L., & Pearlman, Jerome T. Emotional response and management of visually handicapped patients. *Psychiatry in Medicine,* July 1970, Vol. 1, No. 3, pp. 233–40.

Patients react to visual loss as they do to other crises; 3 cases illustrate acceptance, denial, and depression.

2137. Altshuler, K. Z. Reaction to and management of sensory loss: Blindness and deafness. In Bernard Schoenberg, Arthur C. Carr, David Peretz, et al., Eds., *Loss and grief: Psychological management in medical practice.* New York: Columbia Univ. Press, 1970, pp. 140–55.

Reactions to and subsequent adjustments to sudden blindness. Effects of blindness from birth, especially psychological.

2138. American Assoc. of Workers for the Blind. *Contemporary papers, Volume III: The role of the psychiatrist in better service to blind persons.* Washington, D.C.: Author, 1968, 19 pp.

Papers on the psychiatrist in rehabilitation centers, W. Payton Kolb; psychiatrist and multi-handicapped, Edith M. Jurka; and rehabilitation of mentally retarded blind, Eugene A. Hargrove.

2139. Avery, Constance. Para-analytic group therapy with adolescent multi-handicapped blind. *New Outlook for the Blind,* Mar. 1968, Vol. 62, No. 3, pp. 65–72.

Illustrated by some case studies, describes group psychotherapy with 14–19 year olds in a residential school. Process, outcomes, and role of therapist are discussed.

2140. ———. Play therapy with the blind. *International Journal for the Education of the Blind,* May 1968, Vol. 18, No. 2, pp. 41–46.

Explains some unusual aspects of play therapy with a blind child, including need to orient the child to the playroom, and the originality with which the child may incorporate toys into his activity. Two case reports are given.

2141. Barker, Roger G., et al. Somatopsychological significance of impaired vision. In *Adjustment to physical handicap and illness: A survey of the social psychology of physique and disability,* rev., 2nd ed. New York: Social Science Research Council, 1953, pp. 269–308.

Significance of somatopsychological aspects reviewed. Includes social effects, personality development, behavioral characteristics, research summaries, attitudinal traits.

2142. Bauman, Mary K. *Adjustment to blindness: A study as reported by the Committee to Study Adjustment to Blindness.* Harrisburg, Pa.: State Council for the Blind, 1954, 198 pp.

Chosen by their counselors to represent 3 levels of employment and adjustment, 443 blind persons were tested and interviewed. Statistical analysis of the results provides some guidelines for rehabilitation.

2143. ———. A measure of personality change through adjustment training. *New Outlook for the Blind,* Feb. 1954, Vol. 48, No. 2, pp. 31–34.

Describes the Emotional Factors Inventory and the results of its use with 104 blind clients in an adjustment training center. All diagnostic categories showed some tendency to improve; several showed significant improvement.

2144. ———. The initial psychological reaction to blindness. *New Outlook for the Blind,* May 1959, Vol. 53, No. 5, pp. 165–69.

Describes some of the psychological reactions to adventitious blindness and suggests reasons for them.

2145. Bauman, Mary K., & Yoder, Norman M. *Adjustment to blindness— Re-viewed.* Springfield, Ill.: Charles C Thomas, 1966, 272 pp., $7.50.

A historical approach, the view of psychiatrists, the practical approach through training, and the contributions of research are considered in relation to adjustment to blindness. Includes summary of a study including the employment record of *S,* and discussion of prematurity and blindness, impact of the child on the family, early lack of mothering, parent-child relationships, rocking, early effects of development, reaction to loss, aging and blindness as well as the place of the counselor.

2146. Berger, Maria K. A threat of irreparable damage. In *Studies in child psychoanalysis: Pure and applied.* New Haven: Yale Univ. Press, 1975, 175 pp., $12.50.

Describes the problem of masculine identification of an 11-year-old boy whose development from infancy was affected by severely impaired sight and conflicts with his parents.

2147. Berkson, Gershon. Visual defect does not produce stereotyped movements. *American Journal of Mental Deficiency,* July 1973, Vol. 78, No. 1, pp. 89–94.

Monkeys with severe visual deficit were reared in social isolation to determine factors related to stereotyped movements also observed in visually handicapped persons. Results suggest that isolation, not visual deficit, relates to development of stereotyped acts.

2148. Blank, H. Robert. *Psychoanalytic considerations for professional workers in the prevention of blindness.* New York: National Society for the Prevention of Blindness, 1955, 11 pp. Also in *Social Case Work,* 1955, Vol. 36.

Gives author's observations and opinions in an attempt to answer the question, "What psychological factors sabotage the successful treatment of eye disorders and the prevention of blindness?"

2149. ———. Psychoanalysis and blindness. *Psychoanalytic Quarterly,* 1957, Vol. 26, pp. 1–24.

A presentation of the applications of psychoanalytic principles to the treatment of the problems of the blind. Implications of this study for the theory of ego development were suggested.

2150. ————. Psychiatric problems associated with congenital blindness due to retrolental fibroplasia. *New Outlook for the Blind*, Sept. 1959, Vol. 53, No. 7, pp. 237–44.

The greater incidence of psychiatric and educational problems in RLF children is largely related to the presence of other neurological problems, a very traumatic impact on the family, and the family's inability to cope. Recommends specific helps for parents and child.

2151. Bonaccorsi, M. T., & Caplan, Hyman. Psychotherapy with a blind child. *Canadian Psychiatric Association Journal*, 1965, Vol. 10, No. 5, pp. 393–98.

The 8-month, 1 session per week treatment of a 12-year-old boy elicited a significant change in symptomatology after 3 months. It also revealed the interrelationship between sensory deprivation, affect, and cognitive development.

2152. Boston Center for Blind Children. *Problems of adjustment of handicapped children.* Boston: Author, 1959, 115 pp.

Provides most of the papers presented at an institute in May 1958. Topics covered are: Procedures and problems in diagnosis, psychiatric consultation to the agency, medical problems associated with blindness, therapeutic implications of group living, parental problems associated with adjustment of the children and how such problems are met in a residential school.

2153. Bottrill, John H. Effectiveness of an adjustment course for those recently rendered blind. *Perceptual and Motor Skills*, 1968, Vol. 26, No. 2, p. 366.

Evaluation of course held for 4 males and 3 females recently blinded.

2154. Brooks, Karen, & Dunn, Susan. Dancers in darkness. *Journal of School Health*, Mar. 1974, Vol. 44, No. 3, pp. 147–51.

A 25-year-old woman discusses her reaction to recent blindness from diabetes, attitudes of friends and strangers, and her struggle to maintain her concept of self rather than of a blind person.

2155. Browne, Louise J.; Goldsberry, John H., Jr.; & Bull, Janet K. Rehabilitating blind psychiatric patients. *Hospital and Community Psychiatry*, 1968, Vol. 19, No. 4, pp. 116–17.

Analyzes a program in which patients were tested for legal blindness as a selective device for *S*s' participation in specific therapeutic sessions to improve integration in the hospital community. Improvement shown in independence and sociability after sessions.

2156. Bucknam, Frank G. Preventive child psychiatry at a residential school for the blind. *New Outlook for the Blind*, Sept. 1967, Vol. 61, No. 7, pp. 232–37.

Concludes that preventive work can be done in the areas of excessive dependency and adjustment to adolescence. A 5-step program is worked out.

2157. Burleson, Georgia. Modeling: An effective behavior change technique for teaching blind persons. *New Outlook for the Blind,* Dec. 1973, Vol. 67, No. 10, pp. 433–41, 469.

A description of Bandura's modeling—presented as one of the most effective behavior change techniques used. *S,* a 38-year-old male institutionalized since age 12, acquired self-confidence, self-respect, trust of others, motivation and socialization, concern for others, and a hope for the future. Description of how modeling works in various aspects of rehabilitation with a blind person.

2158. Burlingham, Dorothy. *Psychoanalytic studies of the sighted and the blind.* New York: International Univ. Press, 1972, vi + 396 pp., $15.

Six psychoanalytic studies concern blind children. Delves into the difficulties of the child building up ties to the mother when lacking vision. Focuses on such topics as the role of hearing as a substitute for vision, problems of ego development, and developmental considerations in the occupations of the blind.

2159. Caetano, Anthony P., & Kauffman, James M. Reduction of rocking mannerisms in two blind children. *Education of the Visually Handicapped,* Dec. 1975, Vol. 7, No. 4, pp. 101–5.

Study of use of Foxx and Azrin's Overcorrection procedure to reduce rocking mannerisms in 2 legally blind girls, ages 9 and 10. Analyzes the objectives and reasons for achieved success.

2160. Calek, Oldrich. Distressful life situations and the emotional strain felt by subjects with severe visual defects. *American Foundation for the Blind Research Bulletin 25,* Jan. 1973, pp. 59–67.

Problems noted by 11 young adults include inability to achieve success in activities at which visually normal people succeed, decreased range of free-time activities, selection of a profession, and relations with visually normal persons.

2161. Catena, Josephine. Symposium—Self-image: A guide to adjustment II. Emotional disturbance—Pre-adolescence: The caseworker and the family. *New Outlook for the Blind,* Nov. 1961, Vol. 55, No. 9, pp. 297–99.

Primarily talks of problems of children aged 7–12 with blindness plus another handicap. Discussion of parental problems and how caseworker can deal with them as well as own feelings.

2162. Cerulli, Frank, & Shugerman, Estelle E. Symposium—Self-image: A guide to adjustment II. Emotional disturbance—Infancy: Counseling the family. *New Outlook for the Blind,* Nov. 1961, Vol. 55, No. 9, pp. 294–97.

Importance of immediate counseling with the family of a child born blind is emphasized. The counseling must continue since authors think that learning not done at proper time is difficult to compensate for later. Brief mention of 3 cases worked with.

2163. Chess, Stella; Korn, Sam J.; & Fernandez, Paulina B. *Psychiatric disorders of children with congenital rubella.* New York: Brunner/Mazel, 1971, 178 pp., $7.50.

Reports results of a behavioral study done in collaboration with the

Rubella Birth Defect Evaluation Project. Two hundred forty-three children were assessed for physical impairments, psychiatric status, behavioral disturbance, intellectual development, levels of functioning, and temperamental dimensions. Book includes discussion of clinical issues surrounding neurological defects, autistic symptoms, and impact upon families. Case histories.

2164. Cholden, Louis. Group therapy with the blind. *Group Psychotherapy,* 1953, Vol. 6, pp. 21–29.

An evaluation of group therapy conducted over a 2–5 year period with an adult blind group.

2165. ———. Some psychiatric problems in the rehabilitation of the blind. *Bulletin of the Menniger Clinic,* 1954, Vol. 18, pp. 107–12.

Report on the emotional experience involved in loss of vision. Discussion of the "mourning period."

2166. ———. *A psychiatrist works with blindness.* New York: AFB, 1958, 119 pp.

A memorial edition of selected papers of this psychiatrist, who worked with the blind before his death in 1956.

2167. Cole, Nyla J., & Tarboroff, Leonard H. The psychological problems of the congenitally blind child. *American Journal of Orthopsychiatry,* 1955, Vol. 25, pp. 627–43.

Detailed study of the psychotherapy of a 16-year-old congenitally blind girl.

2168. Cruickshank, William M., Ed. *Psychology of exceptional children and youth.* Englewood Cliffs, N.J.: Prentice-Hall, rev. 1963, 623 pp.

Eleven authorities discuss the psychological characteristics of children with exceptionalities: A theoretical framework for understanding the behavior of persons with physical disability; psychological assessment of exceptional children; psychological problems of children with impaired vision; psychotherapy and play techniques with exceptional children. Ref.

2169. Cutsforth, Thomas D. Blindness as an adequate expression of anxiety. *American Foundation for the Blind Research Bulletin 12,* Jan. 1966, pp. 49–52.

Presents an interesting theory concerning personality responses to the condition of blindness and its social impact.

2170. ———. Personality and social adjustment among the blind. *American Foundation for the Blind Research Bulletin 12,* Jan. 1966, pp. 53–67.

A thoughtful analysis of the influences which affect the development of personality in blind persons. "The blind individual should be taught to assume full emotional responsibility for his physical condition, and should become aware of and refuse to employ his physical condition as either a negative or a positive factor in his social relations."

2171. ———. Role of emotion in a synaesthetic subject: Summary and discussion. *American Foundation for the Blind Research Bulletin 12,* Jan. 1966, pp. 19–22.

On evidence available concludes that in certain individuals synaesthetic phenomena pervade the entire mental life, often with rich emotional overtones.

2172. Davis, Carl J. Development of the self-concept. *New Outlook for the Blind*, Feb. 1964, Vol. 58, No. 2, pp. 49–51.

The self-concept and close relationship of this to body image. Problems in development of self-concept unique to blind people and differences caused by being born blind vs. becoming so later in life.

2173. Dean, Sidney I. Some experimental findings about blind adjustment. *New Outlook for the Blind*, May 1958, Vol. 52, No. 5, pp. 182–84.

Discusses method, measures of adjustment, results, characteristics of the blind, anxiety, defensiveness, and conclusions.

2174. Diamond, B. L., & Ross, Alice. Emotional adjustment of newly blind soldiers. *American Journal of Psychiatry*, 1945, Vol. 102, pp. 367–71.

Reports neurological and psychiatric examinations and hospital observations on 150 newly blinded soldiers, apparently an excellent sample of blinded soldiers in which the somatopsychological problem is represented in relatively pure form. Good adjustment is reported in 59%, borderline adjustment in 23%, and maladjustment in 18%.

2175. Dickinson, Frances H. *My eyes were opened by the blind.* New York: Vantage Press, 1967, 152 pp., illus.

The author, who lost and then recovered her sight, tells her own story and that of the Lydia Hayes Memorial Association Home for the Aging Blind in Kenvil, N.J.

2176. Dimitriou, Evangelos C. Neuroticism in blind children, adolescents, and young adults. *American Foundation for the Blind Research Bulletin 25*, Jan. 1973, p. 261.

Brief report of clinical examination of 100 students in school for the blind in Greece, of whom 27 had full neurotic clinical picture.

2177. Dover, Francis T. Readjusting to the onset of blindness. *Social Casework*, June 1959, Vol. 40, pp. 334–38.

Deals with the newly blinded adult and some of the dynamics of the adjustive process.

2178. Dryer, Jerome, & Dix, James. Reaching the blind child through music therapy. *Journal of Emotional Education*, 1968, Vol. 8, No. 4, pp. 202–11.

A music therapist describes his methods for establishing contact with the withdrawn, nonverbal, or hostile child.

2179. Eissler, Ruth S., et al., Eds. *The psychoanalytic study of the child. Volume XXIII.* New York: International Univ. Press, 1968, 479 pp.

Included among 27 papers are some about blind and visually handicapped.

2180. Elonen, Anna S., & Cain, Albert C. Diagnostic evaluation and treatment of deviant blind children. *American Journal of Orthopsychiatry*, 1964, Vol. 34, No. 4, pp. 625–33.

Approach includes child therapy, environmental manipulation, parent treatment, and eventual placement in special classes. Results discussed.

2181. Elonen, Anna S., & Polzien, Margaret. Experimental program for deviant blind children. *New Outlook for the Blind*, Apr. 1965, Vol. 59, No. 4, pp. 122–26.

Summary of efforts in Mich. to change attitudes and extend services for multiply handicapped and deviant blind children listing problems and proposals for the future.

2182. Elonen, Anna S., & Zwarensteyn, Sarah B. Sexual trauma in young blind children. *New Outlook for the Blind*, Dec. 1975, Vol. 69, No. 10, pp. 440–42.

Severely disturbed blind children referred to authors had suffered wide range of sexually traumatic experiences. Cites specific cases. Prevention of deviant incidents is stressed. Makes plea for innovative sex education.

2183. Fike, Norma. Social treatment of long-term dependency. *New Outlook for the Blind*, Feb. 1958, Vol. 52, No. 2, pp. 50–56.

Discusses chronic maladjustment at great length. Since it is impossible for existing agencies to provide intensive casework treatment to all people who need such service, it seems practical to concentrate attention on preventive measures.

2184. Fitting, Edward A. *Evaluation of adjustment to blindness.* New York: AFB, 1954, 84 pp.

Analysis of 155 case records (63 Negroes) from 9 state and private adjustment centers shows better adjustment for whites with work experience, single Negroes, and those who become blind before age 20. Ref.

2185. Fitzgerald, H. Kenneth. Symposium—Self-image: A guide to adjustment. A social worker speaks out. *New Outlook for the Blind*, Mar. 1961, Vol. 55, No. 3, pp. 90–97.

Overall picture of social worker's role as investigator and diagnostic evaluator, planner, and facilitator. During these activities he consults and works with other professionals, the client and the client's parents. Goals are adjustment, economic independence, and participation in community life.

2186. Fitzgerald, Roy G. Reactions to blindness: An exploratory study of adults with recent loss of sight. *Archives of General Psychiatry*, Apr. 1970, Vol. 22, No. 4, pp. 370–79. Also in *Rehabilitation Teacher*, May 1971.

Interviewed 66 recently blind adults (ages 21–65) from a large metropolitan area. Discusses their reactions and experiences in detail.

2187. ———. Visual phenomenology in recently blinded adults. *American Journal of Psychiatry*, May 1971, Vol. 127, No. 11, pp. 1533–39. Also in *Southern Regional Review Blind Welfare*, Mar. 1972.

A psychosocial investigation conducted in London of 66 recently blinded adults shows depressive reactions, visual residue, and behaviors irrelevant to blindness.

2188. ———. The newly blind: Mental distress, somatic illness, disability and management. *Eye, Ear, Nose and Throat Monthly*, Mar. 1973, Vol. 52, No. 3, pp. 99–102, & Apr. 1973, No. 4, pp. 127–32.

Two-part article on research in London. An investigation of psychiatric and medical effects of loss of sight of 66 recently blind adults, aged 21–65. The most common cause was diabetic retinopathy. The psychological reaction was initially overwhelming; depression, anxiety, and suicidal ideation were most prominent in a reaction that generally abated in 10–12 mos.

2189. Foulke, Emerson. The personality of the blind: A non-valid concept. *New Outlook for the Blind*, Feb. 1972, Vol. 66, No. 2, pp. 33–37, 42. Also in *New Beacon*, June 1972.

Refutes "personality of the blind" theory that adjustment to adventitious blindness entails a dying as a sighted person and a rebirth as a blind person. Describes human organism as an active system, seeking information. Different personalities result from different capacities interacting with different environments and experiences.

2190. Frank, Joseph J. Symposium—Self-image: A guide to adjustment. As seen by the ophthalmologist. *New Outlook for the Blind*, Mar. 1961, Vol. 55, No. 3, pp. 99–101.

Mentions important points in eye care and seeks to dispel some widely believed myths.

2191. Freedman, Saul. Reactions to blindness. *New Outlook for the Blind*, Dec. 1965, Vol. 59, No. 10, pp. 344–46.

Reviews some typical reactions of a newly blind person and of the public to blind people. Emphasis is on the multiple influences of blindness, the complexity of interacting reactions.

2192. ———. Personality growth. *New Outlook for the Blind*, June 1966, Vol. 60, No. 6, pp. 173–76.

Identifies some areas exerting critical influence upon personality growth, ways in which these areas may exert negative influence; positive conditioning of the environment; ways in which positive influence may be encouraged and implemented.

2193. Freedman, Sidney. Group workers in an institution. *New Outlook for the Blind*, Feb. 1964, Vol. 58, No. 2, pp. 47–48.

Somewhat unorthodox ways to get clients in an institution to participate in group activities which can also meet the needs of individuals.

2194. Freeman, Roger D. Emotional components in pediatric ophthalmology. In Robison D. Harley, Ed., *Pediatric Ophthalmology*. Philadelphia: W. B. Saunders, 1975, pp. 795–815, $50.

A psychiatrist presents a brief statement of those aspects of child development with which he thinks all ophthalmologists should be familiar, with some guidelines on handling children in office practice and in hospitalization. Describes the emotional effects of certain familiar eye problems and of severe visual impairment and blindness.

2195. Goldman, Herbert. The use of encounter microlabs with a group of visually handicapped rehabilitation clients. *New Outlook for the Blind*, Sept. 1970, Vol. 64, No. 7, pp. 219–26.

Attempts to define, illustrate, and clinically assess the use of group psychotherapeutic techniques with young visually handicapped clients.

2196. Greenberg, Herbert, & Jordan, Sidney. Differential effects of total blindness and partial sight on several personality traits. *Exceptional Children*, 1957, Vol. 24, pp. 123–24.

The Bernreuter Personality Inventory and the F scale were administered to 191 legally blind students. The totally blind group was found to be less authoritarian than the partially sighted. No differences found on Bernreuter scales.

2197. Grosz, Hanus J., & Zimmerman, Joseph. Experimental analysis of hysterical blindness. *Archives of General Psychiatry*, 1965, Vol. 13, No. 3, pp. 255–60.

Purpose of paper is to indicate that original report on this patient (Brady & Lind, *Archives of General Psychiatry*, 1961, Vol. 4) is being misused in the literature, to present follow-up data on present status of the patient, and to comment on diagnostic issue of hyseria vs. malingering and to present new experimental data.

2198. ————. A second detailed case study of functional blindness: Further demonstration of the contribution of objective psychological laboratory data. *Behavior Therapy*, Mar. 1970, Vol. 1, No. 1, pp. 115–23.

Case report of a 15-year-old girl in whom an acute attack of meningo-encephalitis coincided with development of functional blindness. Documented over 6-year period.

2199. Hallenbeck, Phyllis N. *Dogmatism and visual loss.* New York: AFB, 1967, 108 pp., $2.50.

A study of how open-minded and dogmatic attitudes affect rehabilitation following loss of vision.

2200. Hallenbeck, Phyllis N., & Lundstedt, Sven. Some relations between dogmatism, denial, and depression. *Journal of Social Psychology*, 1966, Vol. 70, No. 1, pp. 53–58.

Thirty-two *S*s studied. Findings: (1) inverse relationship between depression and dogmatism, (2) positive relationship between denial and dogmatism, (3) only in gradual onset cases was there a positive correlation of dogmatism and denial tendency.

2201. Hardy, Richard E. Prediction of manifest anxiety levels of blind persons through the use of a multiple regression technique. *International Journal for the Education of the Blind*, Dec. 1967, Vol. 17, No. 2, pp. 51–55.

Reports research to ascertain whether manifest anxiety levels of blind residential school students, as indicated by 2 anxiety tests, could be predicted through a short teacher-rating scale and biographical data. Lists positive relationships found.

2202. ————. A study of manifest anxiety among blind residential school students. *New Outlook for the Blind*, June 1968, Vol. 62, No. 6, pp. 173–80.

An anxiety scale of 78 items was used with 122 blind residential school students, ages 13–22. Statistical analysis of the results is provided, and it is concluded that the new scale and Taylor's Manifest Anxiety Scale measure essentially the same qualities.

2203. Harlow, Steven, et al., Eds. *The child who is special.* New York: MSS Information Corp., 1971, 244 pp.

Papers on blindisms and sensory impairments are included in this general volume of readings on various handicapping conditions.

2204. Harper, Mary L. Personality and the visually handicapped. *International Journal for the Education of the Visually Handicapped*, Oct. 1952, Vol. 2, No. 1, pp. 121–22.

Discusses aspects of a pleasing personality and its influence upon financial success and public relations.

2205. Harth, Robert. The emotional problems of people who are blind: A review. *International Journal for the Education of the Blind,* Dec. 1965, Vol. 15, No. 2, pp. 52–58.

The literature, 1960–65, is reviewed under 5 headings: (1) adjustment, (2) treatment, (3) education for children who are blind and emotionally disturbed, (4) attitudes, and (5) personality testing. Ref.

2206. Haspiel, George S. Communication breakdown in the blind emotionally disturbed child. *New Outlook for the Blind,* Mar. 1965, Vol. 59, No. 3, pp. 98–99.

Reports the results of giving 60 visually impaired emotionally disturbed children complete audiological, speech, and language evaluations, plus follow-up. This is the first step in an extended communications evaluation.

2207. Heyes, Anthony D. Blindness and yoga. *New Outlook for the Blind,* Nov. 1974, Vol. 68, No. 9, pp. 385–93.

Evidence is presented to show that physical fitness may be achieved by means of Hatha Yoga and that anxiety may be reduced and lasting effects of anxiety moderated by the practice of meditation. An attempt is made, on behalf of the blind population, to extract from Yogic knowledge those aspects which are likely to be beneficial.

2208. Hoshmand, Lisa T. "Blindisms": Some observations and propositions. *Education of the Visually Handicapped,* May 1975, Vol. 7, No. 2, pp. 56–60.

Discusses "blindism" problematically, etiologically, and propositionally. In her conclusion the author proposes the adaptation of an existing behavioral clinical procedure for the treatment of similar behavior problems to the management of the autisticlike behaviors in question.

2209. Jervis, Frederick M. The self in process of obtaining and maintaining self-esteem. *New Outlook for the Blind,* Feb. 1964, Vol. 58, No. 2, pp. 51–54.

Author sees process of obtaining self-esteem as interaction of self-concept and the environment. Need for adequacy and avoidance of anxiety are prime forces in developing beliefs about self. Discusses implications of blindness on development of positive self-esteem.

2210. Keegan, David L. Adaptation to visual handicap: Short-term group approach. *Psychosomatics,* 1974, Vol. 15, No. 2, pp. 76–78.

Presents short-term group therapy for visual disability as an approach to adjustment and rehabilitation during blindness.

2211. Keehn, J. D.; Kuechler, H. A.; & Wilkinson, S. A. Behavior therapy in a transactional context: The case of a blind drunk. *American Journal of Mental Deficiency,* Jan. 1973, Vol. 77, No. 4, pp. 147–49.

Case of 23-year-old blind man whose blindness is probably hysterical.

2212. Kinnane, John F., & Suziedelis, Antanas. Sources of interpersonal anxiety in the physically handicapped. Washington, D.C.: Catholic Univ. of America, Dec. 1974, 73 pp.

The Schedule of Interpersonal Concerns, based on Schultz's 3-dimensional model, was developed to measure the sources of interpersonal concerns among the physically handicapped. Two groups with sensory handicaps (including 56 deaf and 42 blind) were predicted to show concern over rejection. Data analysis showed significant support of the hypotheses.

2213. Kirtley, Donald D. *The psychology of blindness.* Chicago: Nelson-Hall, 1975, 312 pp., $15.

Book has 2 major sections: Part I, Attitudes toward Blindness, includes the place of the blind in history, symbolism of the eyes, blindness in the arts, and research on attitudes toward blindness; Part II, Blindness and Personality, includes discussion of some prominent sightless persons, adjustment in the visually handicapped, studies of dreaming and one detailed study of the personality of an adventitiously blinded man through his reported dreams.

2214. Kirtley, Donald D., & Cannistraci, Katherine. Dreams of the visually handicapped: Toward a normative approach. *American Foundation for the Blind Research Bulletin 27*, Apr. 1974, pp. 111–33.

Through analysis of the dream diaries of 7 visually handicapped *S*s, seeks to develop procedures to make reporting of this kind of data standard and comparable. Also provides detailed comparisons with norms.

2215. Knight, John J. Mannerisms in the congenitally blind child. *New Outlook for the Blind,* Nov. 1972, Vol. 66, No. 9, pp. 297–302.

Explains the change, at about 3 mos. of age, from noninstrumental gross motor activities to instrumental behaviors. The latter enable child to cope with problems in environment and reduce tension. States that mannerisms are behaviors blind child uses to cope with tension since he does not have strong instrumental coping behaviors because lack of vision impedes their development.

2216. Krause, Elliott A. Dependency and the blind: Family *vs.* therapeutic work setting. *New Outlook for the Blind,* Dec. 1962, Vol. 56, No. 10, pp. 353–57.

Reports on research investigating effect of temporarily breaking patterns of psychosocial dependency on the family setting, with blind clients having definite problems in the area of dependency. Includes description of facility, clients studied, experiment, results, theoretical and practical implications.

2217. La Sater, Hubert E. Flight from destruction: The newly blind. *Journal of Rehabilitation,* 1963, Vol. 29, No. 1, pp. 26–29.

Concludes that in the case of the flight-from-destruction syndrome, immediate cursory examination of client would possibly lead to assumptions which would not be entirely in keeping with recognizing his strengths and weaknesses. It is essential to see the client as a totality in which multiple factors interact and affect each other.

2218. Lehon, Lester. *Adjustment and blindness: A selected bibliography.* Working Paper, Vol. 1, No. 4. New York: Columbia Univ., 1969, 8 pp.

Selected bibliography including 110 articles and books concerning psychological problems and adjustment of the visually handicapped.

2219. Lester, David. Suicide after restoration of sight: II. *JAMA: Journal of the American Medical Association,* Feb. 1972, Vol. 219, No. 6, p. 757.

Discusses possibility of suicide when removal of blindness withdraws the cause on which patient can blame his unhappiness.

2220. London, Ivan D. A Russian report on the postoperative newly seeing. *American Journal of Psychology*, 1960, Vol. 73, pp. 478–82.

A 1953 report containing some unusual findings that form an interesting addition to the literature on the restoration of sight to congenitally blind individuals.

2221. Lukoff, Irving F. Psychosocial research and severe visual impairment. In M. D. Graham, Ed., *Science and blindness: Retrospective and prospective.* New York: AFB, 1972, $3.75.

Notes that most research on visual impairment tends to exclude the aged blind and those with multiple handicaps. Research is recommended on the family and kinship patterns of the aged blind, socialization of the atypical blind individual, stigma labeling theory in blindness, and the service structure of agencies serving the blind.

2222. McCoy, Marie B. *Journey out of darkness.* New York: David McKay, 1963, 205 pp.

Personal account of managing the emotional and physical adjustment to blindness.

2223. McGuire, Lenore L., & Meyers, C. E. Early personality in the congenitally blind child. *New Outlook for the Blind*, May 1971, Vol. 65, No. 5, pp. 137–43.

Study of 27 totally blind children who were followed for from 1 to 8 years shows no clear relationship between causes of blindness and behavior patterns. Behavior disturbances have a psychogenic base, are a high risk of, but not inevitable to, congenital blindness. Ref.

2224. Maire, Frederick W. Van Gogh's suicide. *JAMA: Journal of the American Medical Association*, Aug. 1971, Vol. 217, No. 7, pp. 938–39.

Speculates that Van Gogh had glaucoma and that realization of approaching blindness incited suicide.

2225. Mehr, Helen M.; Mehr, Edwin B.; & Auld, Carrol. Psychological aspects of low vision rehabilitation. *American Journal of Optometry and Archives of American Academy of Optometry*, Aug. 1970, Vol. 47, No. 8, pp. 605–12.

Discusses the formation of a group of partially sighted 15–16 year old *S*s and professional people of various disciplines to learn about the problems of being partially sighted. Observation revealed (1) denial reactions, (2) over–independent reactions, and (3) defensive reactions.

2226. Miller, E. A note on the visual performance of a subject with unilateral functional blindness. *Behaviour Research and Therapy*, 1968, Vol. 6, No. 1, pp. 115–16.

Reports the case of a 37-year-old woman whose lack of vision was diagnosed as "hysterical" blindness. After testing and reexamination a return of visual ability was noted.

2227. Morse, John L. Mannerisms, not blindisms: Causation and treatment. *International Journal for the Education of the Blind*, Oct. 1965, Vol. 15, No. 1, pp. 12–16.

Reviews literature on causation of mannerisms. In his role as guidance counselor, author is convinced that mannerisms are reactions to stress, most frequently appearing when the student feels pressure. Describes ways in which stress and mannerisms may be reduced.

2228. Rapaport, Irene. Symposium—Self-image: A guide to adjustment. A psychologist's view. *New Outlook for the Blind*, Mar. 1961, Vol. 55, No. 3, pp. 101–2.

Mentions general psychological considerations in dealing with visually handicapped children.

2229. Raskin, Nathaniel J. Play therapy with blind children. *New Outlook for the Blind*, Oct. 1954, Vol. 48, No. 8, pp. 290–92.

Describes procedures and results of play therapy, which the author describes as a chance for the child to discover himself.

2230. ———. Visual disability. In James F. Garrett & Edna S. Levine, Eds., *Psychological practices with the physically disabled.* New York: Columbia Univ. Press, 1962, pp. 341–75.

2231. Riddle, Irene L. Communicative behaviors of hospitalized school age children with binocular bandages. *Maternal-Child Nursing Journal*, Winter 1972, Vol. 1, No. 4, pp. 291–354.

Studied 5 school children who had adequate vision for activities of daily living prior to hospitalization. Four had sustained traumatic eye injuries; 1 had a retinal detachment. It is concluded that school-age children are vulnerable to feelings of interpersonal estrangement.

2232. Roberts, Alvin. *Psychosocial rehabilitation of the blind.* Springfield, Ill.: Charles C Thomas, 1973, xv + 83 pp., $8.95.

Using the terminology of Transactional Analysis, this text is a compilation of techniques which the author has found especially useful in helping newly blinded individuals.

2233. Ross, John R., Jr.; Braen, Bernard B., & Chaput, Ruth. Patterns of change in disturbed blind children in residential treatment. *New Outlook for the Blind*, Apr. 1969, Vol. 63, No. 4, pp. 106–13. Reprinted from *Children*, 1967, Vol. 14, No. 6.

Process and results of rehabilitation for 20 children, ages 6–12. Describes change from withdrawal and total rejection of external world to use of language, development of mobility, and evidences of normal functioning.

2234. Rothschild, Jacob. Play therapy with blind children. *New Outlook for the Blind*, Nov. 1960, Vol. 54, No. 9, pp. 329–33.

Discusses introduction to play, therapist's role, and aids for self-expression. Very nondirective methods are unsuitable; simultaneous therapy with mother is advantageous.

2235. Routh, Thomas A. A study of the use of group psychotherapy in rehabilitation centers for the blind. *Group Psychotherapy*, 1957, Vol. 10, pp. 38–50.

Evaluation of the usefulness of group psychotherapy in centers for the blind. Survey indicates that it is considered an important part of the rehabilitation program.

2236. ———. Psychotherapy as used in a rehabilitation centre for the blind. *Indian Journal of Social Work*, 1962, Vol. 23, No. 2, pp. 173–78.

Modified group psychotherapy is described. Topics include: Social life, courtship, marriage, heredity, and family.

2237. Saul, Sidney R. Group work with blind people. *New Outlook for the Blind*, May 1958, Vol. 52, No. 5, pp. 166–72.

Defines and illustrates functions of a group worker. Discusses how agency program is shaped to needs of group involved, how resulting problems are alleviated by group activity, how attitudes toward blindness complicate social adjustment.

2238. ————. Groupwork and integration. *New Outlook for the Blind*, Feb. 1959, Vol. 53, No. 2, pp. 58–60.

Describes a variety of programs resulting in integration in the sighted community, including basic social and emotional rehabilitation for the blind prior to integration.

2239. ————. The evolution of a social group work service. *New Outlook for the Blind*, Feb. 1963, Vol. 57, No. 2, pp. 44–51.

Discusses purposes of group work program, methods employed in developing group work services, and future planning.

2240. ————. New uses of social group work. *New Outlook for the Blind*, Feb. 1965, Vol. 59, No. 2, pp. 66–68.

Describes social group work based on experience at the Jewish Guild for the Blind, lists its values for the individual, and suggests program content.

2241. Saul, Sidney R.; Eisman, Nadine; & Saul, Shura. The use of the small group in the helping process. *New Outlook for the Blind*, Apr. 1964, Vol. 58, No. 4, pp. 122–25.

Analysis of use of small group to assess social behavior of clients and to aid in planning for placement. Groups also helped with preparation for and adjustment to new situations.

2242. Schneiders, Alexander. Blindness: A psychologist's view of handicap. *New Outlook for the Blind*, Feb. 1965, Vol. 59, No. 2, pp. 69–72.

With the Adlerian theory of inferiority as the pattern, develops a theory of the psychology of disability. Reviews writing on the psychological impact of blindness and theorizes on the adjustment process.

2243. Scholl, Geraldine T. Understanding the behavior of the non-adjusted visually handicapped client. *Rehabilitation Teacher*, Mar. 1973, Vol. 5, No. 3, pp. 3–16.

Guidelines suggested include the identification of appropriate goals and client involvement in goal definitions, objectives, and decision-making.

2244. Scott, Robert A., Comp. *Adjustment to blindness and severe visual impairment: A selected bibliography.* New York: AFB, 1967, 35 pp., $2.

The books, articles, and essays cited were extracted from 3 primary sources: (1) reference documents of the social sciences for 1955–66, (2) literature from work for the blind, and (3) standard bib. on adjustment to blindness.

2245. Sennet, Edith L. A negative learning force becomes a positive teaching tool. *TEACHING Exceptional Children*, Winter 1970, Vol. 2, No. 2, pp. 54–61, illus. (Commentary on article by Virginia L. Brown pp. 61–62.)

Describes program to overcome hostility in a blind 8-year-old boy with resulting improvement in reading, writing, listening, speaking, and mobility.

2246. Severson, Alfred L. Adjustment to blindness. *New Outlook for the Blind*, Mar. 1953, Vol. 47, No. 3, pp. 81–82.

Three areas of adjustment: Acceptance of loss, acquiring specialized skills, and learning to deal with the attitudes and actions of the sighted toward the blind. Defines a well-adjusted blind person and argues that the phrase "adjustment to blindness" should replace the phrase "adjustment of the blind."

2247. Smith, Honor R. Hysterical blindness. *Nursing Mirror*, Jan. 16, 1970, Vol. 130, No. 3, pp. 22–23.

Case history of case of hysterical blindness referred to psychiatrist. Patient's living conditions were such that her symptoms were a way to escape from intolerable surroundings.

2248. Smith, Marguerite A.; Chethik, Morton; & Adelson, Edna. Differential assessments of "blindisms." *American Journal of Orthopsychiatry*, Oct. 1969, Vol. 39, No. 5, pp. 807–17.

Etiology and psychological significance of "blindisms" in a longitudinal study of 3 congenitally blind infants. Etiology compared with related behaviors in sighted children.

2249. Tate, B. G., & Baroff, George S. Aversive control of self-injurious behavior in a psychotic boy. *Behavior Research and Therapy*, 1966, Vol. 4, No. 4, pp. 281–87.

Reports 2 studies showing how chronic self-injurious behavior was controlled in a 9-year-old blind psychotic boy.

2250. Thomson, Solveig H. Insight for the sightless: A TA group for the blind. *Transactional Analysis Journal*, 1974, Vol. 4, No. 1, pp. 13–17.

Conducted Transactional Analysis group therapy for 9 legally blind *S*s with favorable results.

2251. Thomson, Solveig H., & Mosher, John R. An eye to change: Transactional analysis in rehabilitation. *New Outlook for the Blind*, Feb. 1975, Vol. 69, No. 2, pp. 64–72.

Transactional analysis differs from other approaches in its emphasis on educating clients; concentrating on present behaviors; the active, action approach of counselor and client; the therapeutic contract; and having fun. Examples relating to blindness and a sampling of some of the techniques of analysis are given.

2252. Thurrell, Richard J., & Rice, David G. Eye rubbing in blind children: Application of a sensory deprivation model. *Exceptional Children*, Jan. 1970, Vol. 36, No. 5, pp. 325–30.

Examines eye-rubbing as one of the stereotyped behaviors occurring in blind children and its relevance to child development, sensory deprivation, and critical periods.

2253. Tinkham, Wilma N. Symposium—Self-image: A guide to adjustment. Thoughts on the resource room. *New Outlook for the Blind*, Mar. 1961, Vol. 55, No. 3, p. 85.

Presents goals and techniques used in the resource room.

2254. Turbyfill, Kelly. Focus on self help. *Performance*, Oct. 1972, Vol. 23, No. 4, pp. 5–9.

FOCUS (Family Oriented Counseling for Understanding Sight Loss) is a project started in Milwaukee to help the newly blind and their families adjust to the problems occasioned by blindness.

2255. Unkefer, Robert K. *Music therapy in the rehabilitation of the adult blind.* Topeka: State Dept. of Social Welfare of Kans., 1956?, 80 pp., app.

Results of study conducted to evaluate effectiveness of music therapy as part of an overall program for rehabilitation of the blind.

2256. Upshaw, McAllister. Blindness as a factor of disability. *New Outlook for the Blind*, Nov. 1965, Vol. 59, No. 9, pp. 301–8.

With explanatory introduction, uses a fairly detailed case report to show the significance of a client's acceptance of blindness and its impact in his life before true rehabilitation can occur. "It's hard to solve problems that you pretend you don't have."

2257. Valvo, Alberto. Behavior patterns and visual rehabilitation after early and long-lasting blindness. *American Journal of Ophthalmology*, Jan. 1968, Vol. 65, No. 1, pp. 19–24.

Problems of visual rehabilitation illustrated by case report of 33-year-old man who regained vision through surgery after 27 years of blindness. Problems discussed include psychic depression and conversion from tactile to visual patterns.

2258. Verma, Parshotam L. Probe into the adjustment problems of the blind. *Indian Journal of Social Work*, Apr. 1971, Vol. 32, No. 1, pp. 53–62.

General discussion of factors related to maladjustment in blindness.

2259. Wagner, Georgiana. Symposium—Self-image: A guide to adjustment II. Emotional disturbance—The caseworker faces the adolescent. *New Outlook for the Blind*, Nov. 1961, Vol. 55, No. 9, pp. 299–302.

Information relating to blind, emotionally disturbed adolescents. Two case histories are given.

2260. Weiner, Lawrence H. Educating the emotionally disturbed blind child. *International Journal for the Education of the Blind*, Mar. 1962, Vol. 11, No. 3, pp. 77–79.

After describing some typical behaviors of emotionally disturbed blind children, the author suggests 5 steps toward improving that behavior.

2261. Williams, Cyril E. The Mary Sheridan Unit. *Nursing Mirror*, Oct. 23, 1970, Vol. 130, No. 17, pp. 57–58.

Describes unit for blind children with psychiatric disorders. Studies problems, tries to modify behavior and give children a better chance.

2262. Willma, Irene R. As a blind nurse sees. *American Journal of Nursing*, 1955, Vol. 55, pp. 205–8.

The author discusses in detail the psychological impact of losing and then, after 5 years, gradually regaining her vision.

2263. Wilson, Edouard L. Group therapy in a rehabilitation program. *New Outlook for the Blind*, Sept. 1970, Vol. 64, No. 7, pp. 237–39.

Describes the use of group therapy sessions in a rehabilitation program for blind high school students. Concludes that such therapy is a valuable adjunctive therapeutic technique in prevocational and personal adjustment programs.

2264. Winkler, Doreen W. Some needs created by blindness. *Rehabilitation Teacher*, Oct. 1972, Vol. 4, No. 10, pp. 3–20.

Discusses the psychological needs of blind people and their families.

2265. Wintermantel, Ann C. A rebirth in the family. *New Outlook for the Blind*, Sept. 1964, Vol. 58, No. 7, pp. 209–11.

Description of program for families of newly blinded trainees to help them deal with the effects of the blindness on the family. Also shows families how they can be of most help to the trainee.

2266. Winton, Chester A. On the realization of blindness. *New Outlook for the Blind*, Jan. 1970, Vol. 64, No. 1, pp. 16–24.

Discusses the relation of George H. Mead's theories to the legally blind including man's concept of himself, self-reflection, self-communication, and the use of language in its indications (meanings) for orderly behavior. Discussion of need for early detection, school's responsibility, need for parent education and visual examinations.

2267. ———. The beautiful blind. *American Foundation for the Blind Research Bulletin 23*, June 1971, pp. 9–38.

Examines research findings on work roles as they affect self-concepts of legally blind young adults. Five adaptive factors are cited, all of which are shown to bolster ego of the blind in spite of social rejection and enable him to maintain a basically positive self-concept.

2268. Wolf, Sanford R. Psychiatric reaction to threatened blindness: A personal account. *Psychosomatics*, Sept. 1971, Vol. 12, No. 5, pp. 316–20.

Reviews literature on postoperative reactions to surgery for organic eye disease; then describes the author's personal experience.

2269. Zaladup, Emma. On the psychology of the newly blind. *International Journal for the Education of the Blind*, June 1952, Vol. 1, No. 4, pp. 97–100.

Discusses initial attitude and adjustment, relationship to remaining senses, rehabilitation, training, and work. States that other countries offer greater opportunities for the blind. It is hoped Israel will be able to offer wider vocational training.

2270. Zarlock, Stanley P. Magical thinking and associated psychological reactions to blindness. *Journal of Consulting Psychology*, 1961, Vol. 25, pp. 155–59.

Fifty-two blind *S*s were rated on Social Adjustment Scale and tested for ego strength, anxiety, attitudes toward blindness, medicine and religion, and degrees of antidemocratic personality.

2271. Zimmerman, Joseph, & Grosz, Hanus J. "Visual" performance of a functionally blind person. *Behaviour Research and Therapy*, 1966, Vol. 4, No. 2, pp. 119–34.

Describes in detail the application of an operant-reinforcement procedure to the objective description and assessment of visual behavior in a functionally blind patient.

2272. Zunich, M., & Ledwith, B. E. Self-concepts of visually handicapped and sighted children. *Perceptual and Motor Skills*, 1965, Vol. 21, No. 3, pp. 771–74.

Fifty-eight students, 29 visually handicapped and 29 sighted, were *S*s. The self-concept scale designed by Lipsitt was utilized. Only 4 significant differences among 22 comparisons were indicated.

23. Psychology of Blindness

2273. Ahmad, Shahab. The difference between the haptic perception of sighted and blind persons. *American Foundation for the Blind Research Bulletin 23*, June 1971, pp. 103–4.

Brief report of 4 experiments in tactile recognition.

2274. Amadeo, Marco, & Gomez, Evaristo. Eye movements, attention and dreaming in subjects with lifelong blindness. *Canadian Psychiatric Association Journal*, 1966, Vol. 11, No. 6, pp. 501–7.

Study to determine increases in REM rate during states of heightened attention; and to investigate patterns of eye movements in the sleep of congenitally blind *S*s.

2275. Axelrod, Seymour. *Effects of early blindness: Performance of blind and sighted children on tactile and auditory tasks.* New York: AFB, 1959, 83 pp.

Study investigated effects of blindness on functioning in the remaining sense modalities—82 blind *S*s of school age matched with 82 sighted. Results indicate that early-blind *S*s had lower 2-point limens than sighted on the index finger and performed significantly less well. Late-blind *S*s did not differ significantly from sighted.

2276. ———. Severe visual handicap and kinesthetic figural aftereffects. *American Foundation for the Blind Research Bulletin 17*, July 1968, pp. 1–4. Reprinted from *Perceptual and Motor Skills*, 1961.

Amount of kinesthetic figural aftereffect was compared for 37 blind and 33 sighted high school students. KFAE for the blind were significantly smaller than for the controls. Insignificant differences were found for degree of residual vision, age at onset of visual loss, and sex.

2277. Baird, Richard M. Haptic and visual perception of shapes that vary in three dimensions. *American Foundation for the Blind Research Bulletin 28*, Oct. 1974, pp. 219–22.

Report of 2 experiments. One assessed abilities of haptic and visual systems to discriminate shapes varying in 3 dimensions. The other assessed relative efficiencies of intramodal and intermodal transfer of identification learning.

2278. Baker, Larry D. Blindness and social behavior: A need for research. *New Outlook for the Blind*, Sept. 1973, Vol. 67, No. 7, pp. 315–18.

Regrets lack of theory development and research related to psychology of blind persons and suggests possible areas: Attitudes toward blind, behavior of sighted interacting with blind, self-concepts, and behavior of blind interacting with others.

2279. Bartholomeus, Bonnie. Naming of meaningful nonverbal sounds by blind childern. *Perceptual and Motor Skills*, Dec. 1971, Vol. 33, No. 3, pp. 1289–90.

Compared 34 6–15 year-old blind *S*s and 34 matched seeing controls on auditory naming test. Lower scores by blind *S*s suggest that previously acquired visual naming responses facilitate acquisition of names for sounds.

2280. Benedetti, Lois H., & Loeb, Michel. A comparison of auditory monitoring performances in blind subjects with that of sighted subjects in light and dark. *Perception and Psychophysics*, Jan. 1972, Vol. 11 (1-A), pp. 10–16.

Two experiments compare 20 blind with sighted on auditory watchkeeping task. Blind *S*s show superior detection efficiency.

2281. Berger, R. J.; Olley, P.; & Oswald, I. The EEG, eye-movements and dreams of the blind. *Quarterly Journal of Experimental Psychology*, 1962, Vol. 14, No. 3, pp. 183–86.

Rapid eye movements were absent during dream periods of 3 men with life-long blindness, and of 2 men, 30 and 40 years blind, but were present in 3 men blind only 3, 10, and 15 years, respectively.

2282. Berlá, Edward P. Effects of physical size and complexity on tactual discrimination of blind children. *Exceptional Children*, Oct. 1972, Vol. 39, No. 2, pp. 120–24.

Metric figures varying on 3 levels of complexity were combined factorially with 3 physical sizes. Speed and accuracy of recognition were investigated for 36 blind children in grades 1 and 2.

2283. ————. Tactual orientation performance of blind children in different grade levels. *American Foundation for the Blind Research Bulletin 27*, Apr. 1974, pp. 1–10.

Effects of stimulus complexity and degree of rotation on tactual figural orientation performance were investigated with 72 blind children in grades 2, 4, 6, and 8. Differences in tactual search patterns seem responsible for differences in accuracy.

2284. Berlá, Edward P., & Murr, Marvin J. Psycho-physical functions for active tactual discrimination of line width by blind children. *Perception and Psychophysics*, June 1975, Vol. 17, No. 6, pp. 607–12.

Results of 2 psycho-physical experiments using the method of constant stimuli. Found no differences in accuracy of discrimination between sex groupings, age groupings, or grade groupings.

2285. Bitterman, M. E., & Worchel, Philip. The phenomenal vertical and horizontal in blind and sighted subjects. *American Journal of Psychology*, Nov. 1953, Vol. 66, pp. 598–602.

Tests showed that when body was tilted, greater disorientation was shown by sighted *S*s. Interpreted as evidence for dominance of vision in orientation of normal individuals.

2286. Blank, H. Robert. Dreams of the blind. *Psychoanalytic Quarterly*, 1958, Vol. 27, pp. 158–74.

Concludes that the phenomenological differences between the dreams of the blind and the sighted require no revision of the psychoanalytic theory of dreams.

2287. Blass, Thomas; Freedman, Norbert; & Steingart, Irving. Body movement and verbal encoding in the congenitally blind. *Perceptual and Motor Skills*, Aug. 1974, Vol. 39, No. 1, pp. 279–93.

Report on part of a study which examined the prevalence of object- and body-focused hand movements of 10 congenitally blind individuals (aged 17–21) engaged in a 5-minute monologue task. The hand movements were analyzed to determine their relationship to verbal performance.

2288. Bottrill, John H. Difference in curiosity levels of blind and sighted subjects. *Perceptual and Motor Skills*, 1968, Vol. 26, No. 1, pp. 189–90.

A test of perceptual curiosity showed sighted to be more curious than blind, although a locomotor test showed no such significant difference. No significant variation was found among Ss divided as to source of blindness.

2289. ———. Locomotor learning by the blind and sighted. *Perceptual and Motor Skills*, 1968, Vol. 26, No. 1, p. 282.

Studied location learning and spatial cognition in 33 blind and 33 blindfolded sighted students by means of a semilinear U-finger maze. Concluded that both groups have equal ability in this area, or that the measuring instrument was inappropriate.

2290. Brekke, Beverly; Williams, John D.; & Tait, Perla. The acquisition of conservation of weight by visually impaired children. *Journal of Genetic Psychology*, 1974, Vol. 125, No. 1, pp. 89–97.

Studied 72 legally blind Ss 6–14 years of age to determine whether cognitive development of visually impaired children follows stages of development similar to sighted children.

2291. Cohen, Jerome. The effects of blindness on children's development. *New Outlook for the Blind*, May 1966, Vol. 60, No. 5, pp. 150–54. Also in *Children*, 1966, Vol. 13, No. 1.

Factors in quality of adjustment of 57 Ss include intellectual functioning, psychological impairment resulting from blindness or familial reactions, effects of oxygenation, effects of visual deprivation, and adjustment differences between congenitally and adventitiously blind.

2292. ———. Brain waves and blindness. In Proceedings of the Conference on New Approaches to the Evaluation of Blind Persons. New York: AFB, 1970, pp. 112–32. Mimeo .

Reported findings on 42 cases of RLF, 15 children with blindness due to other causes, and 24 adults. Also included as a control were 32 matched sighted prematures.

2293. Cohn, L. Substitute functions of the blind and the deaf and blind. *British Journal of Ophthalmology*, 1954, Vol. 38, pp. 680–84.

2294. Connor, Gordon B., & Muldoon, John F. A statement of the needs of blind and visually impaired individuals. *New Outlook for the Blind*, Oct. 1973, Vol. 67, No. 8, pp. 352–62.

Descriptions of blind and visually impaired should include 3 levels: Physiological, personal, and social. Discusses needs shared by all individuals plus detailed discussion of special needs of congenitally and adventitiously blind.

2295. Cornwell, Christine. The development of depth perception in blind children: A theory of the development of creative ability. *Education of the Visually Handicapped,* Dec. 1969, Vol. 1, No. 4, pp. 97–100.

Development of creativity is discussed as it is related to visual experience and depth perception.

2296. Cotzin, Milton, & Dallenbach, Karl M. "Facial Vision": The role of pitch and loudness in the perception of obstacles by the blind. *American Foundation for the Blind Research Bulletin 13,* July 1966, pp. 113–52, illus. Reprinted from *American Journal of Psychology,* Oct. 1950.

Detailed description of experiments with 2 blind and 2 sighted Ss. Changes in pitch, rather than loudness of stimulus sounds, provide the basic cues for perception of obstacles.

2297. Cowan, Mary K. Sex role typing in the blind child as measured by play activity choices. *American Journal of Occupational Therapy,* Mar. 1972, Vol. 26, No. 2, pp. 85–87.

Compared male–female choices in play activities of 21 blind Ss and 21 matched controls in 2–8 grades. Found no differences between blind and sighted.

2298. Craig, Ellis M. Role of mental imagery in free recall of deaf, blind, and normal subjects. *Journal of Experimental Psychology,* Feb. 1973, Vol. 97, No. 2, pp. 249–53.

Tested A. Paivio's dual coding hypothesis in an experiment with 40 undergraduates, 40 deaf adolescents, and 40 blind adolescents. It was hypothesized that the deaf store information almost exclusively in a nonverbal code while the blind primarily use an auditory-motor (verbal) code. Serial position effects support the dual coding hypothesis.

2299. Crandell, John M., Jr.; Hammill, Donald D.; Witkowski, Casimar; et al. Measuring form-discrimination in blind individuals. *International Journal for the Education of the Blind,* Oct. 1968, Vol. 18, No. 3, pp. 65–68.

Preliminary work to develop a measure of form discrimination which utilizes tactual and kinesthetic modalities used 51 residential school subjects, aged 12–21. Concluded the test holds promise as a simple, efficient measure of tactile-kinesthetic form discrimination.

2300. Cull, John G., & Hardy, Richard E. Language meaning (gender shaping) among blind and sighted students. *American Foundation for the Blind Research Bulletin 27,* Apr. 1974, pp. 275–76. Reprinted from *Journal of Psychology,* 1973, Vol. 83, No. 2.

Blind students differed from sighted in assigning gender to 17 commonly used words out of 50. Authors conclude that blind persons have different interpretations of meaning of the words.

2301. Curtis, Jack F., & Winer, David M. The auditory abilities of the blind as compared with the sighted. *Journal of Auditory Research,* 1969, Vol. 9, No. 1, pp. 57–59.

Tests of primary auditory abilities were presented to 3 groups of listeners: Normal sighted, expert blind travelers, and homebound blind Ss. Results indicate that the expert blind travelers exhibited an increased sensitivity to differences in intensity as compared with either homebound blind or normal sighted. Latter performed better on a test of loudness discrimination of a broad band noise.

2302. Cutsforth, Thomas D. An analysis of the relationship between tactual and visual perception. *American Foundation for the Blind Research Bulletin 12*, Jan. 1966, pp. 23–47.

Reports experiments to determine whether a perception, supposedly originating and developing in one sense modality (touch), could be reproduced or duplicated in another (vision).

2303. Cutsforth, Thomas D., & Wheeler, R. T. The synaesthesia of a blind subject with comparative data from an asynaesthetic blind subject. *American Foundation for the Blind Research Bulletin 12*, Jan. 1966, pp. 1–17.

Intensive study of 2 subjects leads authors to posit a theoretical framework for synaesthesia and its place in the total thought process. No evidence that mental processes of blind differed from those of seeing.

2304. Dauterman, William L. A study of imagery in the sighted and the blind. *American Foundation for the Blind Research Bulletin 25*, Jan. 1973, pp. 95–167.

Compares many kinds of imagery to develop and standardize an objective measure of imagery ability of blind persons. Considers congenitally and adventitiously blind. Includes 44 summaries of experiments and reports of 17 subjective tests.

2305. Davidson, Philip W. The role of exploratory activity in haptic perception: Some issues, data, and hypotheses. *American Foundation for the Blind Research Bulletin 24*, Mar. 1972, pp. 21–27.

Chiefly a review of the relevant literature, including studies with blind *S*s.

2306. ——. Haptic judgments of curvature by blind and sighted humans. *Journal of Experimental Psychology*, Apr. 1972, Vol. 93, No. 1, pp. 43–55.

Report on 3 experiments investigating the relationship between active handling and the haptic perception of curves. Sixteen blind and 16 sighted *S*s. Blind used more effective scanning technique.

2307. Davidson, Philip W.; Barnes, Judith K.; & Mullen, Gina. Differential effects of task memory demand on haptic matching of shape by blind and sighted humans. *Neuropsychologia*, 1974, Vol. 12, No. 3, pp. 395–97.

Study of the role of prior perception experience in retention of haptic information by comparing 22 blind and 23 sighted adolescents (matched for IQ) in a matching task that systematically varied task memory demand.

2308. Dean, Sidney I. Some notes on research problems with the blind. *New Outlook for the Blind*, June 1956, Vol. 50, No. 6, pp. 200–204.

In doing research the author found the relevant literature in many out-of-the-way publications and not indexed in an accessible way, references sometimes inaccurate, terminology of the field inexact, and overall quality of research lacking.

2309. DeMott, Richard M. Verbalism and affective meaning for blind, severely visually impaired, and normally sighted children. *New Outlook for the Blind*, Jan. 1972, Vol. 66, No. 1, pp. 1–9, 25.

Purpose of study "was to determine the degree to which concrete words having visual connotations share similar meanings for individuals differing in visual experience." Forty-one congenitally blind, 41 severely impaired, 61 normally sighted *S*s. "There appear to be no significant differences in the meaning of general concepts as a function of visual experience."

2310. DeRenzi, Ennio; Scotti, Giuseppe; & Spinnler, Hans. Perceptual and associative disorders of visual recognition. *Neurology*, July 1969, Vol. 19, No. 7, pp. 634–41.

Two hemispheric groups were given 4 visual-perceptual tests: Overlapping figures, face identification, the Farnsworth 100 Hue, and objective-figure matching. The findings are suggestive of a differential specialization between the 2 hemispheres in the process of visual impairment.

2311. Dimmick, Kenneth. *Psychoacoustics—A selected bibliography.* New York: AFB, 1966, 24 pp., $2.

The 346 bibliographic entries include material in books, journals, and monographs in fields related to sensory impairment, especially the blind and partially sighted. The dates range from 1934–65.

2312. Dokecki, Paul. Verbalism and the blind: A critical review of the concept and the literature. *Exceptional Children*, Apr. 1966, Vol. 32, No. 8, pp. 525–30.

Summarizes current theory in psycholinguistics and argues that some concepts are inadequate explanations for blind children. Suggests research.

2313. Drever, James. Early learning and the perception of space. *American Journal of Psychology*, Dec. 1955, Vol. 68, No. 4, pp. 605–14.

Research project in which early blind, late blind, and sighted *S*s were given 3 spatial tests.

2314. Duran, Peter, & Tufenkjian, Sylvia. Tactile-kinesthetic methods for measuring length used by congenitally blind children. *Perceptual and Motor Skills*, 1969, Vol. 28, No. 2, pp. 395–400.

Analyzes and describes the use of the haptic sense as it bears on the blind child's measurement of length.

2315. ———. The measurement of length by congenitally blind children and a quasiformal approach for spatial concepts. *American Foundation for the Blind Research Bulletin 22*, Dec. 1970, pp. 47–70.

An analysis and description of use of haptic sense as it relates to the congenitally blind child's perception of length. Concluded that physical size of objects will determine the technique used for measurement and that as the physical length increases the corresponding difference threshold increases independently of the technique used.

2316. Edelheit, Henry. The relationship of language development to problem-solving ability. *Journal of the American Psychoanalytic Association.* Jan. 1972, Vol. 20, No. 1, pp. 145–55.

Reports a panel discussion in which some case histories (including blind) are cited. No strong concensus was reached in the discussion.

2317. Eldridge, Roswell; O'Meara, Kathy; & Kitchin, David. Superior intelligence in sighted retinoblastoma patients and their families. *Journal of Medical Genetics*, 1972, Vol. 9, No. 3, pp. 331–35.

Average overall IQ of the patients and (family) controls were significantly above U.S. average. It is unlikely that high intelligence in the retinoblastoma survivor is due to the gene for retinoblastoma. Suggests more feasible possibilities.

2318. Elonen, Anna S.; Polzien, Margaret; & Zwarensteyn, Sarah B. The "uncommitted" blind child: Results of intensive training of children formerly committed to institutions for the retarded. *Exceptional Children*, Jan. 1967, Vol. 33, No. 5, pp. 301–7.

Six blind children who spent varying periods of time in institutions for the mentally defective were placed in a residential school for the blind and given intensive care and special attention. Advances in IQ, progress in behavior, and educational achievement are described.

2319. Ewart, Anne G., & Carp, Frances M. Recognition of tactual form by sighted and blind subjects. *American Journal of Psychology*, 1963, Vol. 76, No. 3, pp. 488–91.

Ss were 30 blind and 30 sighted children. Results indicated that visual imagery is not a critical factor in this kind of form-recognition.

2320. Fay, Warren H. On the echolalia of the blind and of the autistic child. *Journal of Speech and Hearing Disorders*, Nov. 1973, Vol. 38, No. 4, pp. 478–89.

Author theorizes that the similarities in echolalic blind and echolalic autistic children stem from sensory deprivation in the one and perceptual restriction in the other acting in a like manner to delay or preclude language acquisition.

2321. Ferrell, William R. A study of the effect of motion size on performance for a task involving kinesthetic feedback. *American Foundation for the Blind Research Bulletin 1*, Jan. 1962, pp. 10–42 + app., illus.

Describes an experiment to determine whether a change in size of task might enable a manipulator to make better use of his kinesthetic senses and so result in improved performance. Concluded that a fairly clear maximum in performance might be expected if proper motion size were used but, for a given task, this would need to be experimentally determined.

2322. Fisher, Gerald H. Spatial localization by the blind. *American Foundation for the Blind Research Bulletin 15*, Jan. 1968, pp. 147–57. Reprinted from *American Journal of Psychology*, 1964, No. 1.

Using 5 blind Ss, investigated ability to localize by sound and by touch. Warns of possible sources of error in such experiments.

2323. Flax, Nathan. The contribution of visual problems to learning disability. *Journal of the American Optometric Association*, Oct. 1970, Vol. 41, No. 10, pp. 841–45.

Asserts that the control and integrative functions of the visual system influence learning more than the refractive state of the eye.

2324. Flynn, W. R. Visual hallucinations in sensory deprivation. *Psychiatric Quarterly*, 1963, Vol. 36, No. 1, pp. 55–65.

Case of a 72-year-old blind woman with visual hallucinations of unusually long duration was reported. Discussed in light of the psychoanalytic theory of hallucinations.

2325. Foulke, Emerson. The role of experience in the formation of concepts. *International Journal for the Education of the Blind*, Oct. 1962, Vol. 12, No. 1, pp. 1–6.

Defines concepts and how they relate to information from the senses. Examines the kind of experience peculiar to each of the senses. The blind child must be encouraged to seek as much and as many kinds of sensory experiences as possible, to be attentive to all aspects of his environment.

2326. ———. Transfer of a complex perceptual skill. *Perceptual and Motor Skills*, 1964, Vol. 18, No. 3, pp. 733–40.

To explore the problem, braille readers served as Ss in an experiment. They were required to read with each of 8 fingers. Performance best when forefingers were used and fell off sharply as the little fingers were approached.

2327. Foulke, Emerson, & Warm, Joel S. Effects of complexity and redundancy on the tactual recognition of metric figures. *Perceptual and Motor Skills*, 1967, Vol. 25, No. 1, pp. 177–87.

As result of study of 24 sighted and 24 blind Ss the following overall trends were noted: (1) efficiency of performance was greater in the blind, (2) speed and accuracy of recognition tended to decrease with increments in stimulus complexity.

2328. Freedman, David A. On hearing, oral language, and psychic structure. *Psychoanalysis & Contemporary Science*, 1972, Vol. 1, pp. 57–69.

Reviews studies on the effects of some organismic factors (e.g., normal development of sight and hearing vs. blindness and deafness) and related environmental factors on the development of personality, behavior, and cognitive processes.

2329. Friedman, Judith, & Pasnak, Robert. Attainment of classification and seriation concepts by blind and sighted children. *Education of the Visually Handicapped*, May 1973, Vol. 5, No. 2, pp. 55–62.

Testing of Piagetian concepts on 21 blind and 30 sighted children found the children approximately equal in seriation and classification skills until 8 years of age, after which the blind fell behind, particularly on verbal tasks.

2330. Garry, Ralph, & Ascarelli, Anna. *An experiment in teaching topographical orientation and spatial organization to congenitally blind children.* Boston: Boston Univ., 1959, 87 pp.

Through a special training program attempted to establish better understanding of the problems of totally blind children in general orientation and space perception. Statistically significant gains over the control group were shown by the experimental group. Further study recommended.

2331. Gibbs, Sally H., & Rice, James A. The psycholinguistic characteristics of visually impaired children: An ITPA pattern analyses [sic]. *Education of the Visually Handicapped*, Oct. 1974, Vol. 6, No. 3, pp. 80–88.

Sighted and nonsighted children compared. Latter performed less well because of weakness on 4 primarily visual subtests. Degree of vision impairment did not have significant effect. Ref.

2332. Gottesman, Milton. A comparative study of Piaget's developmental schema of sighted children with that of a group of blind children. *Child Development*, June 1971, Vol. 42, No. 2, pp. 573–80.

Compared performance of 15 congenitally blind children with 30 sighted children, 15 of whom were not permitted use of vision. Developmental stages of blind and sighted similar.

2333. ———. Conservation development in blind children. *Child Development*, Dec. 1973, Vol. 44, No. 4, pp. 824–27.

In a study based on work of Piaget and Inhelder, conservation tasks were given 45 congenitally blind and 90 sighted Ss, half of whom were blindfolded. Study indicated that developmental stages of 2 groups are similar.

2334. Gross, Joseph; Byrne, Joseph; & Fisher, Charles. Eye movements during emergent stage 1 EEG in subjects with lifelong blindness. *Journal of Nervous and Mental Disease*, 1965, Vol. 141, No. 3, pp. 365–70.

Employing a movement transducer for recording eye movements together with direct observation, 5 Ss, blind since birth, showed recurring rapid eye movement periods during emergent stage 1, similar to normals. Corneofundal potentials as measured by EEG were absent or greatly diminished.

2335. Guess, Doug. The influence of visual and ambulation restrictions on stereotyped behavior. *American Journal of Mental Deficiency*, 1966, Vol. 70, No. 4, pp. 542–47.

Sample for the study included 32 Ss equally divided into blind ambulatory, blind non-ambulatory, sighted ambulatory, and sighted non-ambulatory groups. A reciprocal relationship between environmental manipulation and stereotyped behavior was demonstrated.

2336. Halpin, Gerald; Halpin, Glennelle; & Tillman, Murray H. Relationships between creative thinking, intelligence, and teacher-rated characteristics of blind children. *Education of the Visually Handicapped*, May 1973, Vol. 5, No. 2, pp. 33–38.

Four activities of the Torrance Tests of Creative Thinking were administered to 63 blind children. No conclusive data was found on relationships between creative thinking and mobility, adjustment to blindness, social acceptance, etc., but otherwise unobtainable information on individual differences was gathered.

2337. Halpin, Gerald; Halpin, Glennelle; & Torrance, E. Paul. Comparison of creative thinking abilities of blind and deaf children. *Perceptual and Motor Skills*, Aug. 1973, Vol. 37, No. 1, p. 154.

Brief report on a study comparing 34 blind and 34 deaf children matched for sex, race, and age.

2338. ———. Effects of sex, race, and age on creative thinking abilities of blind children. *Perceptual and Motor Skills*, Oct. 1973, Vol. 37, No. 2, pp. 389–90.

Report on a study of 61 functionally blind children, aged 6–12, in residential schools for the blind in Ala., Ga., and S.C.

2339. Hanninen, Kenneth A. The effect of texture on tactual perception of length. *Exceptional Children*, May 1970, Vol. 36, No. 9, pp. 655–59.

Study of 107 blind and sighted *S*s to prove that children would underestimate coarse and overestimate fine textures in judging lengths of abrasive paper presented individually. Negative findings; however, analysis of errors to criterion in training supported the idea that texture facilitated or interfered with making judgments of length.

2340. ———. Review of the educational potential of texture and tactually discriminable patterns. *Journal of Special Education*, Summer 1971, Vol. 5, No. 2, pp. 133–41.

Reviews tactile perception research; relationship to education of blind is obvious but may be useful in education of nonblind, as well.

2341. Hans, Michael A. Imagery and modality in paired associate learning in the blind. *Bulletin of the Psychonomic Society*, 1974, Vol. 4, No. 1, pp. 22–24.

Thirteen congenitally blind *S*s learned lists of 12 noun-noun word pairs in a paired-associates task, where the visual and auditory image-producing qualities of the stimulus and response terms of the pairs were varied. Data are interpreted as a rejection of a modality-specific imagery hypothesis.

2342. Hare, Betty A.; Hammill, Donald D.; & Crandell, John M., Jr. Auditory discrimination ability of visually limited children. *New Outlook for the Blind*, Nov. 1970, Vol. 64, No. 9, pp. 287–92.

Study made to examine selected characteristics of auditory discrimination in visually limited and sighted children. No significant differences were detected in the overall performances of the visually handicapped and sighted children.

2343. Harley, Randall K., Jr. *Verbalism among blind children: An investigation and analysis.* New York: AFB, 1963, 61 pp., $2.

Relationship of verbalism among blind children to age, intelligence, experience, and personal adjustment was studied by giving 40 blind *S*s tasks to perform.

2344. Harris, Charles S. The effect of *S*'s interpretation of "straight ahead" upon measures of prism adaptation. In Robert B. Welch & Charles Hallenbeck, Ed., Recombination and visual perception. *American Foundation for the Blind Research Bulletin 29*, June 1975, pp. 114–15.

A warning that *E* and *S* may interpret "straight ahead" differently. Article is summary of a conference presentation.

2345. Hartlage, Lawrence C. Verbal tests of spatial conceptualization. *Journal of Experimental Psychology*, 1969, Vol. 80, No. 1, pp. 181–82.

Measured spatial conceptualization in blind and sighted 7–18 year-old *S*s. Blind *S*s without other impairment matched with sighted for age, sex, estimated intellectual ability. Concluded that vision may be crucial in development of spatial ability.

2346. Hay, John C. Motor transformation learning. In Robert B. Welch & Charles Hallenbeck, Ed., Recombination and visual perception. *American Foundation for the Blind Research Bulletin 29*, June 1975, pp. 109–11.

Research on vision related to the theory that organisms learn not the particular stimuli associated with motor activity, but the transformations imposed on stimuli by the motor activity. Article is summary of a conference presentation.

2347. Hermelin, Beate. Locating events in space and time: Experiments with autistic, blind, and deaf children. *Journal of Autism and Childhood Schizophrenia*, July 1972, Vol. 2, No. 3, pp. 288–89.

Compaired autistic, blind, deaf (10 each) and 20 normal children in 2 experiments focused on responses to stimuli in situations allowing for alternative strategies and coding processes.

2348. Hermelin, Beate, & O'Connor, N. Spatial coding in normal, autistic and blind children. *Perceptual and Motor Skills*, Aug. 1971, Vol. 33, No. 1, pp. 127–32.

Report on an experiment testing spatial location using tactile stimulation. *S*s were 10 blind, 10 blindfolded, 10 sighted normal, 10 sighted autistic children, and 10 blindfolded adults.

2349. ————. Location and distance estimates by blind and sighted children. *Quarterly Journal of Experimental Psychology*, 1975, Vol. 27, No. 2, pp. 295–301.

Discussion of results of an experiment in which 3 groups of 24 blindfolded normal, blindfolded autistic, and congenitally blind children (average age 13) made reproduction location and distance estimates of an arm movement. Results discussed in terms of role of visual reference system for different aspects of motor movements.

2350. Higgins, Leslie C. *Classification in congenitally blind children: An examination of Inhelder and Piaget's theory.* New York: AFB, 1973, 52 pp., $2.

Children examined to determine relationship between total congenital blindness and development of mental structure underlying classification, and to test validity of central aspects of J. Piaget's theory of intelligence. Data supported some hypotheses, raised questions on others. 39 *S*s, in Australian schools for the blind. Three control groups of sighted children.

2351. Hill, Everett. The formation of concepts involved in body position in space. *Education of the Visually Handicapped*, Dec. 1970, Vol. 2, No. 4, pp. 112–15. 2nd in 4-part series. (1st, Mills, Oct. 1970; 3rd, Hill, Mar. 1971; last, Mills, May 1971.)

A study to explore the possibility of teaching selected terms in a formalized manner to congenitally blind children between the ages of 7 and 9.

2352. ————. The formation of concepts involved in body position in space. *Education of the Visually Handicapped*, Mar. 1971, Vol. 3, No. 1, pp. 22–25. 3rd in 4-part series (1st, Mills, Oct. 1970; 2nd, Hill, Dec. 1970; last, Mills, May 1971.)

This article has 3 purposes: (1) discuss the performance test given and implications for the classroom teacher, (2) provide information about selected games and activities used in developmental phases, and (3) answer the question "How can these be incorporated into the classroom?"

2353. Hill, John W., & Bliss, James C. Modeling a tactile sensory register. *American Foundation for the Blind Research Bulletin 17*, July 1968, pp. 91–130, app., illus.

Data from 2 blind and 3 sighted Ss results in reporting techniques for tactile short-term memory.

2354. Hintz, J. M. & Nelson, T. M. Haptic aesthetic value of the golden section. *British Journal of Psychology*, May 1971, Vol. 62, No. 2, pp. 217–23.

Presented rectangles for preference to Ss: Congenitally vs. late blind vs. blindfolded vs. unblindfolded normally sighted. Results indicate that the haptic perception of the golden rectangle as aesthetically pleasing is contingent on contact with the visual world.

2355. Hochstim, Joseph R. Comparison of three information-gathering strategies in a population study of socio-medical variables. *American Foundation for the Blind Research Bulletin 3*, Aug. 1963, pp. 72–83.

Compares 3 strategies of information-gathering: Mail, telephone, and personal interviewing, used in certain combinations, in terms of rate of return, the completeness of the returns, and cost. Data in processing stage, and so no results given.

2356. Howard, Ian P. Proposals for the study of adaptation to anomalous causal schemata. In Robert B. Welch & Charles Hallenbeck, Ed., Recombination and visual perception. *American Foundation for the Blind Research Bulletin 29*, June 1975, pp. 111–13.

A brief discussion of author's recent research on prism adaptation and a number of research ideas in area of perceptual-motor schemata which he plans to implement. Article is summary of a conference presentation.

2357. Hunter, Ian M. Tactile-kinaesthetic perception of straightness in blind and sighted humans. *Quarterly Journal of Experimental Psychology*, 1954, Vol. 6, pp. 149–54.

The tactile-kinaesthetic perception of the straightness of a "plus-curved" edge in 20 blind and 20 sighted Ss were compared. In this area, the blind's perception is more highly developed.

2358. Hunter, William F. An analysis of space perception in congenitally blind and sighted individuals. *Perceptual and Motor Skills*, 1962, Vol. 15, No. 3, p. 754.

Blind Ss were not as efficient in manipulating a curved surface into a flat one or in orienting objects in space. The blind habitually underestimated space.

2359. ———. The role of space perception in the education of the congenitally blind. *International Journal for the Education of the Blind*, May 1962, Vol. 11, No. 4, pp. 125–30.

Reviews the relevant literature and describes educational and rehabilitation procedures which contribute to good orientation in space. This includes all types of moving the body through space, and use of hands in eating, dressing, working, and playing.

2360. ———. An analysis of space perception in congenitally blind and in sighted individuals. *Journal of General Psychology*, 1964, Vol. 70, No. 2, pp. 325–29.

Sample consisted of 12 congenitally blind adolescents matched with sighted children as to age, sex, and IQ. Results indicated a lack of ability in blind to utilize various types of stimuli to the degree accomplished by sighted.

2361. Huntly, C. W., & Yarus, Gary J. Horizontal-vertical illusion in haptic space. *Catalog of Selected Documents in Psychology,* Winter 1973, No. 3. Blind vs. sighted subjects.

2362. Inoue, Katsuya. A study on interaction among sense modalities in memory: 1. *Journal of Child Development,* 1968, Vol. 4, pp. 28–37.

Sixty-six normal and 46 blind students were presented with nonsense syllables in a retroactive inhibition paradigm. *S*s were divided into visual, auditory, and cutaneous learning groups. Results suggest benefit of poly-sensory learning and use of cutaneous material in all learning programs.

2363. Jeavons, P. M.; Harding, G. F. A.; Ferries, G. W.; et al. Alpha rhythm in totally blind children. *British Journal of Ophthalmology,* Dec. 1970, Vol. 54, No. 12, pp. 786–93.

Study conducted in England with 32 totally blind children. Results failed to support previous findings that the presence of some vision in early life is related to amount of alpha rhythm in the electroencephalo-gram of the totally blind child later in life.

2364. Jones, Bill. Development of cutaneous and kinesthetic localization by blind and sighted children. *Developmental Psychology,* Mar. 1972, Vol. 6, No. 2, pp. 349–52.

Compared 78 blind and 160 sighted 5–12 year olds in cutaneous and kinesthetic localization under 2 conditions. Blind found superior to sighted without visual cues.

2365. Jones, Reginald L. Learning and association in the presence of the blind. *New Outlook for the Blind,* Dec. 1970, Vol. 64, No. 10, pp. 317–24.

Two studies conducted to explore the feelings of nonhandicapped students toward the handicapped. Sighted *S* did not perform more poorly when learning in the presence of a blind person, but there was a tendency for them to believe that their performance was impaired.

2366. Jonides, John; Kahn, Robert; & Rozin, Paul. Imagery instructions improve memory in blind subjects. *Bulletin of the Psychonomic Society,* 1975, Vol. 5, No. 5, pp. 424–26.

Data from 16 congenitally and totally blind and 16 sighted *S*s show that the typical improvement in memory with imagery instructions that occurs in normal *S*s also occurs in the blind.

2367. Jordan, John E., & Felty, John. Factors associated with intellectual variation among visually impaired children. *American Foundation for the Blind Research Bulletin 15,* Jan. 1968, pp. 61–70.

Using 253 records of residential school students, tested two hypotheses: (1) intelligence varies directly with variations in blindness, and (2) intelligence varies according to social-psychological influences. Only (2) is supported by the results. Ref.

2368. Juurmaa, Jyrki. *Ability structure and loss of vision.* Helsinki, Finland: Institute of Occupational Health, 1967, 128 pp. (Avail.: AFB, New York, $3.)

In the analysis of ability structure and loss of vision a battery of tests, followed by factor analysis, were given 228 heterogenous blind *S*s, and sighted controls. Included were tests for verbal comprehension, arithmetic reasoning, spatial ability, kinesthetic memory, discrimination sensitivities. Results given.

2369. ————. The ability structure of the blind and the deaf: Final report. *American Foundation for the Blind Research Bulletin 14*, Mar. 1967, pp. 109–21.

Briefly reports results of a complex study of the mental abilities of blind persons. Eight major results relate to general mental makeup of the blind, memory, arithmetic, musical aptitude, tactual discrimination, kinesthetic mastery of hand positions, and dexterity.

2370. ————. A comparative analysis of the effects of blindness and deafness on psychic functions. *Eye, Ear, Nose and Throat Monthly*, Nov. 1968, Vol. 47, No. 11, pp. 553–61.

Finnish *S*s were tested on verbal comprehension, numerical ability, spatiality, and memory to determine in what specific traits the blind and deaf differ from those with no sensory defects, and how to account for the differences.

2371. ————. "A reanalysis and critique of 'sensory discrimination' as an ability component of the blind": A reply. *Perceptual and Motor Skills*, 1969, Vol. 29, No. 1, pp. 289–90.

A reply to the criticism presented by M. H. Tillman, W. L. Bashaw, & M. Bradley, concerning the author's study "Ability Structure and Loss of Vision." A reanalysis of former data is presented supporting the author's views.

2372. ————. On the accuracy of obstacle detection by the blind—Part 1. *New Outlook for the Blind*, Mar. 1970, Vol. 64, No. 3, pp. 64–72. Part 2, Apr. 1970.

Discusses the perception of obstacles through hearing and tactile or skin sensations. Research reviewed including work with bats, discrimination levels, sound shadow studies, and echo acuity. Potential for guidance devices discussed.

2373. ————. The spatial sense of the blind: A plan for research. *American Foundation for the Blind Research Bulletin 24*, Mar. 1972, pp. 57–64.

Reviews theoretical background and outlines a planned study of several aspects of the spatial sense in blind *S*s.

2374. ————. Transposition in mental spatial manipulation: A theoretical analysis. *American Foundation for the Blind Research Bulletin 26*, June 1973, pp. 87–134.

Technical analysis of evidence from a variety of sources leads to conclusion that previous visual experience helps in tactual recognition and in mobility, i.e., that there is association in the central nervous system of relationships familiar from prior experience.

2375. Juurmaa, Jyrki, & Suonio, Kyosti. *Optification tendency in tactual spatial manipulation: An experimental study.* Helsinki, Finland: 1969, 22 pp.

These reports from the Institute of Occupational Health compared ability to identify tactually in 20 congenitally blind, 20 adventitiously blind, and 20 sighted 13–46 year olds. Concluded role of visual imagery depends on method employed.

2376. Kanno, Yasuo, & Ohwaki, Yoshikazu. Formation of the Charpentier weight illusion in the blind. *American Foundation for the Blind Research Bulletin 24*, Mar. 1972, pp. 37–56.

Describes experiments in which the Charpentier illusion is related to various characteristics of blindness. No significant relationships found.

2377. Karp, S. An experiment using revised stimulus presentation. *American Foundation for the Blind Research Bulletin 2*, Dec. 1962, pp. 12–14.

This paper records an experiment to check on the methodology of earlier experiments. Three stimulus conditions for discriminating braille type material were evaluated in order of effectiveness.

2378. ————. Experiments in tactual perception. *American Foundation for the Blind Research Bulletin 2*, Dec. 1962, pp. 14–20.

Evaluates the results of 4 experiments in tactile discrimination, especially with regard to the role of motor activity in tactile sensing.

2379. Kellogg, Winthrop N. Sonar systems of the blind. *American Foundation for the Blind Research Bulletin 4*, Jan. 1964, pp. 55–69, illus. Reprinted from *Science*, Aug. 1962.

With 2 blind and 2 blindfolded sighted college students as Ss, experiments showed blind Ss better able to perceive small differences in size and distance of objects.

2380. Kent, Allen; Stevens, Godfrey D.; & Clark, Leslie L., Eds. *Proceedings of the conference on documentation and information retrieval in human sensory processes.* New York: AFB, 1972, 66 pp., $2.50.

Includes 11 papers and a discussion summary of conference held June 1968.

2381. Kirk, Samuel A., & Weiner, Bluma B. *Behavioral research on exceptional children.* Washington, D.C.: Council for Exceptional Children, 1963, 377 pp.

Reviews behavioral research studies, giving author, title, purpose, subjects, methods and procedures, and results. Includes studies on visually impaired.

2382. Klich, Beatriz De M., & Wierig, George J. Social interaction and emotional adjustment among the blind. *Perceptual and Motor Skills*, Apr. 1971, Vol. 32, No. 2, pp. 516–18.

Study based on 41 blinded veterans, VA Hospital, Hines, Ill.

2383. Kohler, Ivo. Past, present, and future of the recombination procedure. In Robert B. Welch & Charles Hallenbeck, Ed., Recombination and visual perception. *American Foundation for the Blind Research Bulletin 29*, June 1975, pp. 118–22.

A brief review of the origins of the use of recombination procedures, comments on the 9 other papers in the section, and suggestions for future research. Article is summary of a conference presentation.

2384. Lairy, Gabrielle C., & Netchine, S. The electroencephalogram in par-

tially sighted children related to clinical and psychological data. *American Foundation for the Blind Research Bulletin* 2, Dec. 1962, pp. 38–56.
Discusses comparison of EEG records of blind, partially sighted, and normally sighted.

2385. Levitt, Eugene A.; Rosenbaum, Arthur L.; Willerman, Lee; et al. Intelligence of retinoblastoma patients and their siblings. *Child Development*, Sept. 1972, Vol. 43, No. 3, pp. 939–48.
Compared 25 sighted and 19 blind retinoblastoma patients with their normal siblings (N=59) on WAIS, WISC, Stanford-Binet, or Williams Intelligence Scale. Concluded retinoblastoma associated with blindness may result in selective cognitive superiority.

2386. Lindley, Sondra. Kinesthetic perception in early blind adults. *American Foundation for the Blind Research Bulletin 25*, Jan. 1973, pp. 175–91.
Experiments to investigate the role of vision in organizing body sensations show that a large number of variables play a role. An adequate model of personal space can be developed without vision but mere repetition, without feedback, will not improve functioning. Ref.

2387. McFadden, Dennis. Detection and lateralization of interaural differences of time and level by the blind. *Perceptual and Motor Skills*, Feb. 1974, Vol. 38, No. 1, pp. 211–15.
Comparison of performance by blind and sighted subjects on auditory tasks involving binaural cues.

2388. McReynolds, Jane, & Worchel, Philip. Geographic orientation in the blind. *Journal of General Psychology*, 1954, Vol. 51, pp. 221–36.
Study to test the hypothesis that visual imagery is fundamental to geographic orientation. Under the conditions of this study, the hypothesis was disproved.

2389. Magary, James F., et al. *Piagetian theory and its implications for the helping professions: Invitational interdisciplinary seminar. (Third).* Los Angeles: Univ. of S. Calif., School of Education, 1973, 109 pp.
Presents 25 papers given at the conference. Topics include the implications of Piaget for the development of moral judgment in children, Piaget and the early education of handicapped children, Piaget and psychometric assessment. Example of included titles: "Spatial education for blind children."

2390. Martin, Clessen J. *Associative learning strategies employed by deaf, blind, retarded and normal children. Final report.* Washington, D.C.: Bureau of Research, 1967, 219 pp.
Detailed studies discuss verbalization by blind children and include 4 app., 31 tables, 18 figures presenting data and a bib. listing 38 items.

2391. Martin, Clessen J., & Herndon, Mary A. Facilitation of associative learning among blind children. *Proceedings of the Annual Convention of the American Psychological Association*, 1971, Vol. 6 (Part 2), pp. 629–30.
Examined the associative strategies reported by blind children, and attempted to determine whether syntactical strategy aids facilitate the storage of verbal associations in memory for these *S*s.

2392. Miller, Charles K. Conservation in blind children. *Education of the Visually Handicapped*, Dec. 1969, Vol. 1, No. 4, pp. 101–5.

Explanation of Piagetian framework of conservation. Results of a study indicated that a partially sighted group did significantly better than a low vision group in their ability to conserve.

2393. Moreno, Zerka T. Note on spontaneous learning "in situ" versus learning the academic way. *Group Psychotherapy*, 1958, Vol. 11, pp. 50–51.

Suggested that psychodrama would be a profitable teaching technique for deaf-dumb and blind children.

2394. Morin, Stephen F., & Jones, Reginald L. Social comparison of opinions among blind children and adolescents. In *Proceedings, 80th Annual Convention, 1972.* Washington, D.C.: American Psychological Assoc., 1972, pp. 721–22.

Structured interviews with 45 institutionalized blind school-age subjects were used to verify Festinger's theory that "given a range of possible persons for comparison, someone close to one's own ability or opinion will be chosen for comparison."

2395. Morris, June E., & Nolan, Carson Y. Discriminability of tactual patterns. *International Journal for the Education of the Blind*, Dec. 1961, Vol. 11, No. 2, pp. 50–54.

The discriminability of 12 tactual patterns was judged by 96 legally blind students. Ability to discriminate was not related to sex, grade, or chronological age, but did appear slightly related to intelligence.

2396. Mostofsky, David I. Anchor referral: A new technique. *Neuropsychologia*, Sept. 1972, Vol. 10, No. 3, pp. 321–25.

Describes a modification of the standard category judgment technique which permits an analysis of predicision behavior. *S*s included 54 blind, 33 normal, and 10 hemiplegic males.

2397. Naddeo, Candice L., & Curtis, W. Scott. Some effects of the disorientation of tactical-kinesthesia. *International Journal for the Education of the Blind*, Oct. 1968, Vol. 18, No. 3, pp. 69–73.

Two groups of sighted blindfolded *S*s identified missing parts of objects, one group receiving the objects while their hands were held normally in front of them, other group receiving the objects while their hands were in distorted position. Differences in recognition time and errors have implications for testing procedures.

2398. Neisworth, John R., & Smith, Robert M. *Congenital blindness as an instance of sensory deprivation, implications for rehabilitation.* Newark, Del.: Del. Univ., 1965, 15 pp.

Research concerning sensory deprivation and its relationship to personality, behavior, and cognitive changes is reviewed. Three limitations of congenitally blind are: restriction in experience, deficits in mobility, and deficits in control of environment and self in relation to it.

2399. Nelson, Thomas M., & Haney, R. R. Force perception by blind and blindfolded subjects. *International Journal for the Education of the Blind*, Dec. 1968, Vol. 18, No. 4, pp. 116–19.

Early blind, later blind, and blindfolded sighted *S*s judged the force with which an object struck them. Results suggest blind over-react to impinging physical forces as compared with blindfolded sighted.

2400. Nelson, Thomas M., & MacDonald, Brian H. Experience of cause in sighted and blind samples. *Perceptual and Motor Skills*, Dec. 1973, Vol. 37, No. 3, pp. 903–10.

Report on testing of perceptual causality by means of fixed sequences of haptic stimulation. Comparisons are made of the reactions of subjects who were early blinded, late blinded, and blindfolded sighted.

2401. Nolan, Carson Y. On the unreality of words to the blind. *New Outlook for the Blind*, Mar. 1960, Vol. 54, No. 3, pp. 100–102.

Thirty-nine stimulus words given 39 blind *S*s to compare the number of visual responses they made against the number of visual responses reportedly made by a similar group tested by Cutsforth. Concluded that verbal unreality was not a significant problem for the group studied by Nolan.

2402. Norton, Fay-Tyler M. Training normal hearing to greater usefulness. *New Outlook for the Blind*, Dec. 1959, Vol. 53, No. 10, pp. 357–60.

Hearing is the only sense the blind person can use to get information about the more distant environment, therefore emphasis on training of hearing is important. Describes binaural tape recordings used to train hearing at Cleveland Society for the Blind and early results of training.

2403. ————. *Improving and accelerating the process of raising the hearing of blinded persons to a greater degree of usefulness: A final report.* Cleveland, Ohio: Cleveland Society for the Blind, 1960, 34 pp., app.

Results of 3-year project to determine whether the hearing of blinded persons can be improved/accelerated by new teaching techniques. Research efforts concentrated on testing effectiveness of the use of binaural tape recordings. Bib.

2404. ————. Training normal hearing to greater usefulness: A progress report. *New Outlook for the Blind*, June 1960, Vol. 54, No. 6, pp. 199–205.

Binaural tape recordings prove useful in training for localization and identification of sounds. Presents procedures, lists types of recordings, description of *S*s, and conclusions.

2405. Novikova, L. A. The role of visual afferentation in forming the electrical activity of the cortex of the human brain. *American Foundation for the Blind Research Bulletin 24*, Mar. 1972, pp. 75–94.

Study of visual characteristics and electroencepholography.

2406. ————. *Blindness and the electrical activity of the brain: Electroencephalographic studies of the effects of sensory impairment.* Zofja S. Jastrzembska, Ed. Eng. lang. edition. B. Sznycer & L. Zielinski, Trans. New York: AFB, 1974, 341 pp., $9.

Part one covers electrical activity of human brain when basic distance receptors are impaired; Part two describes use of electroencephalographic method in diagnosis of central nervous system damage in visually impaired; Part three examines electrical activity of brain of rabbit when distance receptors are excluded. Illus. include 144 EEG tracings.

2407. O'Connor, N., & Hermelin, B. Inter- & intra-modal transfer in children with modality specific and general handicaps. *British Journal of Social and Clinical Psychology*, Dec. 1971, Vol. 10, No. 4, pp. 346–54.

Compared 10 blind with groups of normal, subnormal, and deaf *S*s on touch discrimination. Transfer to other modalities was difficult.

2408. ———. Seeing and hearing and space and time. *Perception and Psychophysics*, Jan. 1972, Vol. 11 (1-A), pp. 46–48.

Sought to determine central digit in sequences of digits presented auditorally or visually to deaf, blind, and normal 12–14 year olds. Mode of presentation does affect choice.

2409. ———. The reordering of three-term series problems by blind and sighted children. *British Journal of Psychology*, Aug. 1972, Vol. 63, No. 3, pp. 381–86.

Compared the strategies used by 10 blind and 10 sighted 7–9 year olds in attempts to solve 2 forms of the 3-term series problem. Results show that both groups used a sequential rather than a logical order as a guide in answering questions. There was no indication that sighted *S*s used a strategy of spatial coding.

2410. ———. Modality-specific spatial coordinates. *Perception and Psychophysics*, 1975, Vol. 17, No. 2, pp. 213–16.

Results of 2 experiments conducted to determine whether the development of spatial coordinates depends on the integration of information from different modalities or is based on modality-specific coding.

2411. Paivio, Allan, & Okavita, Hymie W. Word imagery modalities and associative learning in blind and sighted subjects. *Journal of Verbal Learning and Verbal Behavior*, Oct. 1971, Vol. 10, No. 5, pp. 506–10.

Paired-associate lists of nouns were learned by blind and sighted *S*s in 2 experiments in Canada. Blind *S*s were affected by auditory but not visual word imagery, while reverse occurred for sighted *S*s.

2412. Parmelee, Arthur H., Jr., & Wolff, Peter. Developmental studies of blind children: Parts I and II. *New Outlook for the Blind*, June 1966, Vol. 60, No. 6, pp. 177–79, 179–81.

Part I—behavioral studies can be of importance to understanding vision vs. other perceptual processes in cognitive/personality development. Discusses pseudo-retardation. Part II—accounts of early cognitive development stressing hand-eye-mouth coordination, and visually guided manipulation of objects raise questions for investigation of concept of space, causality, and object permanence. Ref.

2413. Parrish, John L., & Chassen, Larry R. Variables in tactual perception. *Education of the Visually Handicapped*, Oct. 1972, Vol. 4, No. 3, pp. 76–79.

Review of selected research on tactual perception including performance of good and poor braille readers and recognition of tactual form by sighted and blind subjects.

2414. Pasnak, Robert, & Ahr, Paul. Tactual poggendorff illusion in blind and blindfolded subjects. *Perceptual and Motor Skills*, Aug. 1970, Vol. 31, No. 1, pp. 151–54.

Presented tactual poggendorff illusions to blind and blindfolded Ss according to the method of constant stimuli. Results show no significant difference between the two.

2415. Patterson, James, & Deffenbacher, Kenneth. Haptic perception of the Mueller-Lyer illusion by the blind. *Perceptual and Motor Skills*, Dec. 1972, Vol. 35, No. 3, pp. 819–24.

Presented haptic versions of the Mueller-Lyer illusion to 4 groups of 10 Ss each: Congenital blind, blinded in adulthood, sighted blindfolded, and sighted visual. Implications for theories of visual illusions and the blind Ss' presumably better utilization of short-term memory for retaining haptic relationships are discussed.

2416. Pick, Anne D., & Pick, Herbert L., Jr. A developmental study of tactual discrimination in blind and sighted children and adults. *Psychonomic Science*, 1966, Vol. 6, No. 8, pp. 367–68.

Normally sighted, partially sighted, and totally blind Ss from 6 years to adults performed tactual discrimination task. Number of errors made depended on age of S, amount of vision present, and nature of the differences between pairs of presented stimuli.

2417. Pick, Herbert L., Jr.; Klein, Robert E.; & Pick, Anne D. Visual and tactual identification of form orientation. *Journal of Experimental Child Psychology*, Dec. 1966, Vol. 4, No. 4, pp. 391–97.

Orientation identification was used as a tool for investigating the relationship between the development of visual and tactual form perception; 208 normal Ss, 39 partially sighted Ss, and 33 total blind Ss (ages 6–adult).

2418. Raskin, Nathaniel J., & Weller, Marian F. *Current research in work for the blind: A survey.* New York: AFB, 1953, 34 pp.

Describes in detail 17 studies and relates them to past research, including studies on intelligence, achievement, and aptitude.

2419. Rice, Charles E. Perceptual enhancement in the early blind? *Psychological Record*, 1969, Vol. 19, No. 1, pp. 1–14.

Six Ss blind from birth were significantly superior to 8 adventitiously blind and 8 sighted Ss in tests of auditory localization ability, and evidence from a tactile immediate memory test similarly favored the early blind.

2420. ———. Early blindness, early experience and perceptual enhancement. *American Foundation for the Blind Research Bulletin 22*, Dec. 1970, pp. 1–22.

Two experiments conducted using individuals blind from infancy, blinded later in life, and sighted, to determine perceptual enhancement. Early blindness was seen as a correlate which could affect perceptual enhancement.

2421. Rice, Charles E., & Feinstein, Stephen H. Sonar system of the blind: Size discrimination. *Science*, 1965, Vol. 148, No. 3673, pp. 1107–8.

Measurements were made of the ability of 4 blind Ss to use echoes to discriminate between objects of different sizes placed in front of them. Threshold estimates indicate that objects with area ratios as low as 1.07/1 could be discriminated.

2422. Rice, Charles E.; Feinstein, Stephen H.; & Schusterman, Ronald J. Echo-detection ability of the blind: Size and distance factors. *Journal of Experimental Psychology*, 1965, Vol. 70, No. 3, pp. 246–51.

The ability of 5 blind *S*s to detect metal discs placed in front of them by use of echoes was measured. Compares performance using a vocal echo signal with performance using signal characteristics as independent variables.

2423. Rivenes, Richard S., & Cordellos, Harry C. Kinesthetic performance by blind and sighted. *Perceptual and Motor Skills*, Feb. 1970, Vol. 30, No. 1, p. 76.

Studied relative performance of 10 blind and 10 blindfolded/sighted *S*s on a kinesthetic task involving space perception. Results support J. H. Bottrill's findings that blind *S*s do not develop a special ability to perform kinesthetic tasks.

2424. Rogow, Sally. Perceptual organization in blind children. *New Outlook for the Blind*, May 1975, Vol. 69, No. 5, pp. 226–29, 231, 233.

On the basis of review of literature, especially on form and spatial relationships by blind persons, suggests that differences between tactual and visual information result in differences in perceptual organization but that blind children reach developmental milestones (e.g., conservation) at approximately the same ages as sighted children.

2425. Rosenstein, Joseph. Tactile perception of rhythmic patterns by normal, blind, deaf, and aphasic children. *American Annals of the Deaf*, 1957, Vol. 102, pp. 399–403.

Ten *S*s in each group (ages 11–13) were tested on trials of Series "A" of the rhythm test of the Seashore Measures of Musical Talents, adapted for tactile use. The blind performed best on each trial.

2426. Rubin, Edmund J. *Abstract functioning in the blind.* New York: AFB, 1964, 64 pp.

Hypothesized that congenitally blind adults would score lower on tests of abstraction than adventitiously blind or sighted adults. Total of 75 *S*s were used (25 in each category). Tests used were: Similarities Test, Proverbs Test, Kohn Test of Symbol Arrangement, and the Number Series Completion Test. Hypothesis supported.

2427. Sato, Yasumasa. Comparison of group judgments made by blind and sighted subjects. *Perceptual and Motor Skills*, 1963, Vol. 17, No. 3, p. 654.

*S*s were 38 blind pupils (13–15 yrs.) and 40 sighted *S*s of the same age range. Concluded that essentially no difference is observed on the judgments made by the blind and sighted *S*s as a result of their participating in a group situation.

2428. Schlaegel, T. F., Jr. The dominant method of imagery in blind as compared to sighted adolescents. *Journal of Genetic Psychology*, 1953, Vol. 83, pp. 265–77.

Study showed the imagery of the blind to be significantly affected by (1) present visual acuity (2) age of onset of incapacitating loss of vision.

2429. Schwartz, Ralph J., & Steer, M. D. Vocal responses to delayed auditory feedback in congenitally blind adults. *Journal of Speech and Hearing Research*, 1962, Vol. 5, No. 3, pp. 228–36.

Results of a test done with 7 young blind adults and 10 adults with normal vision, all normal speakers.

2430. Singer, Jerome L., & Streiner, Bella F. Imaginative content in the dreams and fantasy play of blind and sighted children. *Perceptual and Motor Skills,* 1966, Vol. 22, No. 2, pp. 475–82.

The role of vision in the development of a differentiated capacity for imagination was tested with 20 pairs of matched blind and sighted children (ages 8–12). Results indicated that sighted children proved more imaginative.

2431. Stellwagen, William T., & Culbert, Sidney S. Comparison of blind and sighted subjects in the discrimination of texture. *Perceptual and Motor Skills,* 1963, Vol. 17, No. 1, pp. 61–62.

Ability of 50 blind and 50 sighted Ss to discriminate among all combinations of pairs of 10 embossed textural patterns was compared.

2432. Stephens, Beth. Cognitive processes in the visually impaired. *Education of the Visually Handicapped,* Dec. 1972, Vol. 4, No. 4, pp. 106–11.

Piaget's stages of intellectual development reviewed. Behavior of normally sighted and visually handicapped infants at each stage, and the effect on the equilibrium between assimilation and accommodation are discussed. There is great need with visually handicapped for tactual knowledge of objects to counterbalance the negative effects of sensory privation.

2433. Stephens, Beth, & Simpkins, Katherine. *The reasoning, moral judgment, and moral conduct of the congenitally blind.* Washington, D.C.: Dept. of HEW, 1974, v + 117 pp.

Report of research project to probe specific effects blindness has on development of reasoning, moral judgment, and moral conduct in persons 6–18. Sample was 75 sighted and 75 congenitally blind persons.

2434. Suinn, Richard M. The theory of cognitive style: A partial replication. *Journal of General Psychology,* 1967, Vol. 77, No. 1, pp. 11–15.

Articulation scores on 108 adventitiously and congenitally blind Ss confirm that cognitive style measures are needed in addition to traditional verbal IQ tests.

2435. Supa, Michael; Cotzin, Milton; & Dallenbach, Karl M. "Facial vision": The perception of obstacles by the blind. *American Foundation for the Blind Research Bulletin 13,* July 1966, pp. 1–53, illus. Reprinted from *American Journal of Psychology,* Apr. 1944.

Detailed account of experiments with 2 sources of sensation—exposed areas of skin and ears—and 2 kinds of stimuli—air currents and "air waves" outside the auditory range. Findings are corroborated by studies on bats.

2436. Suppes, Patrick. *A survey of cognition in handicapped children. Technical report no. 197.* Palo Alto, Calif.: Stanford Univ., Calif. Institute for Mathematical Studies in Social Science, 1972, 77 pp.

Reviews research on the development of cognitive skills of language, concept formation, and arithmetic in blind, mentally retarded, or deaf children.

2437. ———. A survey of cognition in handicapped children. *Review of Educational Research,* Spring 1974, Vol. 44, No. 2, pp. 145–76.

Literature survey divided into 3 main parts: (1) problems of language and language development, (2) concept formation and abstraction, (3) elementary mathematical skills. The 3 handicaps concerned are blindness, mental retardation, and deafness.

2438. Swallow, Rose-Marie, & Poulsen, Marie K. An exploratory study of Piagetian space concepts in secondary low-vision girls. *American Foundation for the Blind Research Bulletin 26,* June 1973, pp. 139–49.

Assessed relevant concept development in 10 Ss, whose age indicated they should have mastered concepts involved on a concrete level, using tasks developed by Piaget. Includes considerations of oscillation between intuitive ideas and concrete operational thinking.

2439. Tillman, Murray H.; Bashaw, W. L.; & Bradley, Michael. Reanalysis and critique of "sensory discrimination" as an ability component of the blind. *Perceptual and Motor Skills,* 1969, Vol. 29, No. 1, pp. 283–88.

Explores the interpretation of Juurmaa's findings on ability structure and loss of vision and raises methodological issues about his analyses. Considers makeup of blind sample, choice of factor analytic tools, and arbitrariness of decision concerning dimensionality.

2440. Tillman, Murray H., & Williams, Charlotte. Associative characteristics of blind and sighted children to selected form classes. *International Journal for the Education of the Blind,* May 1968, Vol. 18, No. 2, pp. 33–40.

A study, across age, of effect of severe visual impairment on word associations to selected grammatical form classes. Subjects were 35 blind children from 3 southeastern residential schools and 35 sighted children of similar backgrounds. With supporting statistical data, rather complex findings are reported.

2441. Tisdall, William J., et al. *Divergent thinking in blind children.* Lexington: Ky. Univ., 1967, 93 pp.

Compared divergent thinking in blind and sighted children to determine relationship with onset of blindness, mobility, achievement, and sex.

2442. Tisdall, William J.; Blackhurst, A. Edward; & Marks, Claude H. Divergent thinking in blind children. *Journal of Educational Psychology,* Dec. 1971, Vol. 62, No. 6, pp. 468–73.

Studied influence of visual deprivation upon divergent thinking aspects of intelligence in 10–12 year olds. Compared 76 seeing children, 76 blind children in residential schools, and 76 blind children in day school programs. Differences found to be small.

2443. Tobin, Michael J. Conservation of substance in the blind and partially sighted. *British Journal of Educational Psychology,* June 1972, Vol. 42, No. 2, pp. 192–97.

Experiments suggest that while the best of blind or partially sighted 5–15 year olds perform on a par with the best of their sighted peers, the age range in which conservation is obtained is more extended for the visually handicapped.

2444. Toonen, Bonita L., & Wilson, Jere P. Learning eye fixation without visual feedback. *American Foundation for the Blind Research Bulletin 19,* June 1969, pp. 123–28.

Detailed report of experiment to determine if a blind person can learn to direct his gaze at a sound source.

2445. Tsai, Loh S. Mueller-Lyer illusion by the blind. *Perceptual and Motor Skills*, 1967, Vol. 25, No. 2, pp. 641–44.

Nine blind *S*s (3 born blind, 3 blinded in childhood, 3 blinded as adults) all exhibited the haptic illusion to an extent comparable to the optical illusion of 4 normal controls. The author's theory emphasizes the total impression in explaining optical and haptic Mueller-Lyer illusions.

2446. Uhlarik, John J. Some effects of exposure to optical disarrangement on adaptation to optical rearrangement. In Robert B. Welch & Charles Hallenbeck, Ed., Recombination and visual perception. *American Foundation for the Blind Research Bulletin 29*, June 1975, pp. 97–100.

Two studies on adaptation to prism-displaced vision are described. Article is summary of a conference presentation.

2447. Walker, Don L. Body image and blindness: A review of related theory and research. *American Foundation for the Blind Research Bulletin 25*, Jan. 1973, pp. 211–31.

Reviews the Freudian subconscious theory and a more physical sensory motor theory. Hypothesizes that in visually handicapped children differentiation may proceed from specific to general, whereas in normal children the process is from general to specific.

2448. Warren, David H. Early vs. late vision: The role of early vision in spatial reference systems. *New Outlook for the Blind*, Apr. 1974, Vol. 68, No. 4, pp. 157–62.

Studies of tactual form discrimination and finger maze learning and experiments involving extended space to test the hypothesis that the early visual experience of adventitiously blind persons gives them a visual frame of reference after the onset of blindness. The length of early visual experience was found to be important.

2449. Warren, David H.; Anooshian, Linda J.; & Bollinger, Janet G. Early vs. late blindness: The role of early vision in spatial behavior. *American Foundation for the Blind Research Bulletin 26*, June 1973, pp. 151–70.

Reviews literature comparing spatial behavior of blind with sighted and congenitally with adventitiously blind *S*s. Suggests that early visual experiences produce frame of reference with enduring effects. Implications for mobility training.

2450. Warren, David H., & Pick, Herbert L. Intermodality relations in localization in blind and sighted people. *Perception and Psychophysics*, Dec. 1970, Vol. 8, No. 6, pp. 430–32.

Comparing with a sighted group, tested 116 blind children in 3 age groups under auditory-proprioceptive conflict conditions. No age changes found. Also a second study of congenitally blind.

2451. Whitcraft, Carol J. Motoric engramming for sensory deprivation or disability. *Exceptional Children*, Feb. 1972, Vol. 38, No. 6, pp. 475–78.

Relationships of motoric involvement, perceptual-motor theories, and neurophysiological evidence are examined for support of a motoric engramming approach to learning.

2452. Williams, M. Superior intelligence of children blinded from retinoblastoma. *Archives of Disease in Childhood*, 1968, Vol. 43, No. 228, pp. 214–20.

A group of 50 children blinded by retinoblastoma is shown to have significantly higher intelligence than children blind from other causes, and sighted children. No satisfactory explanation found.

2453. Witkin, Herman A., et al. Cognitive patterning in congenitally totally blind children. *Child Development*, Sept. 1968, Vol. 39, No. 3, pp. 767–86.

Using a special battery of perceptual and problem-solving tests and models of the human figure to assess articulation of body concept, hypothesis that lack of vision hampers development of articulation and fosters dependence on others confirmed.

2454. Witkin, Herman A.; Oltman, Philip K.; Chase, Joan B., et al. Cognitive patterning in the blind. In Jerome Hellmuth, Ed., *Cognitive studies, Vol. 2: Deficits in cognition.* New York: Brunner/Mazel, 1971, pp. 16–46, $15.

The 1st section of the chapter is adapted from a paper in *Child Development* (Sept. 1968) entitled "Cognitive patterning in congenitally totally blind children." The 2nd section adds information re adventitiously totally blind retinoblastoma children.

2455. Yates, J. T.; Johnson, R. M.; & Starz, W. J. Loudness perception of the blind. *Audiology*, Sept. 1972, Vol. 11, Nos. 5–6, pp. 368–76.

Constructed equal-loudness contours from the results of loudness judgments by 20 blind and 20 sighted adults. Results indicate that very little difference existed between data for blind and sighted Ss for the overall equal-loudness contours or within any single frequency or across any of the phone contours.

2456. Zemtzova, M. I.; Kulagin, J. A.; & Novikova, L. A. The use of the remaining sensory channels (safe analyzers) in compensation of visual function in blindness. *American Foundation for the Blind Research Bulletin 2*, Dec. 1962, pp. 72–87, illus.

Reviews then-current Russian research on perception. Discusses electroencephalographic and tactile tests, records and results, and briefly, hearing and spatial perception. Compares blind and sighted test results in some cases. Some EEG profiles included.

2457. Zweibelson, I., & Barg, C. Fisher. Concept development of blind children. *New Outlook for the Blind*, Sept. 1967, Vol. 61, No. 7, pp. 218–22.

Comparison of 8 blind with 8 sighted children, ages 11–13, suggests less use of abstract concepts by blind.

24.   Partially Sighted

2458. Allan, Dennis. Yet another minority. *Education of the Visually Handi-capped*, Mar. 1972. Vol. 4, No. 1, pp. 30–32.

World of the partially sighted is described as that of a rejected minor-ity. Discusses problems of personal adjustment for the partially sighted person who tries to act like a seeing person.

2459. Bateman, Barbara D. *Reading and psycholinguistic processes of partially seeing children. CEC Research Monograph, Series A, Number 5.* Washington, D.C.: Council for Exceptional Children, 1963, 51 pp.

Investigates the effects of visual defect on the reading and psycholin-guistic processes through results obtained for partially seeing children on various reading and aptitude tests. Provides 8 figures, 12 tables, 4 case histories. Ref.

2460. ———. Reading and psycholinguistic processes of partially seeing children. *American Foundation for the Blind Research Bulletin 8,* Jan. 1965, pp. 29–44.

Compares performance of 93 partially seeing children in Illinois Test of Psycholinguistic Abilities (ITPA) to norms assumed to be based on chil-dren with normal sight. Gives analysis of results and 3 case histories.

2461. Brazelton, Frank A.; Stamper, Bruce; & Stern, Victor. Vocational re-habilitation of the partially sighted. *American Journal of Optometry and Archives of American Academy of Optometry*, Aug. 1970, Vol. 47, No. 8, pp. 612–18.

Reports of 55 patients who were evaluated to determine whether any type of visual appliance would be helpful in obtaining or maintaining em-ployment or education.

2462. Christner, Florence. A partially seeing child learns to read. *Opto-metric Weekly*, 1954, Vol. 45, pp. 736–39.

General application of principles of teaching reading were applied to a child whose acuity was 20/300 in each eye.

2463. Cunliffe, W. Partially sighted or blind? *New Beacon*, Sept. 1973, Vol. 57, No. 677, pp. 231–34.

Suggests ways for England's special teachers to help partially sighted students develop skills independent of vision use; discusses scale compar-ing blind, partially sighted, and normal students, indicating partially sighted at least proficient in social initiative.

2464. Froistad, Wilmer M. The partially seeing are not blind. *New Outlook for the Blind*, Oct. 1966, Vol. 60, No. 8, pp. 239–42.

Partial sight presents psychological and physical problems different from those of blindness; illustrated by history of a child. Questions appropriate recognition of partially sighted by agencies.

2465. Genensky, Samuel M. *Binoculars: A long ignored aid for the partially sighted.* Santa Monica, Calif.: Rand Corp., 1973, 59 pp., $3.

Defines the visually handicapped population that could benefit from use of binoculars, and describes the use of binoculars and additional equipment.

2466. Hoffman, Simon. Counseling the client with useful vision. *New Outlook for the Blind*, Feb. 1955, Vol. 49, No. 2, pp. 49–53.

Discusses the importance of effective use of remaining vision and the relationship of that use to personality. Case histories.

2467. Horn, Thomas D., & Ebert, Dorothy J. *Books for the partially sighted child.* Champaign, Ill.: National Council of Teachers of English, 1965, 81 pp.

Annotated bibliography of books selected according to typography, type of illustration, and literary worth. Divided into 3 sections: Non-fiction, fiction, and easy books. Includes information about price, type size, type face, and approximate grade level.

2468. Jose, Randall T., & Butler, James H., Jr. Driver's training for partially sighted persons: An interdisciplinary approach. *New Outlook for the Blind*, Sept. 1975, Vol. 69, No. 7, pp. 305–7, 311.

Through a program involving optometric and special education professionals, partially sighted persons can be trained to use bioptic telescopes for driving. Special performance tests, given by Dept. of Motor Vehicles, insure that a safe and dependable driver will be placed on our highways.

2469. Karnes, Merle B., & Wollersheim, Janet P. *An intensive differential diagnosis of partially seeing children to determine the implications for education.* Champaign, Ill.: Champaign Community Unit 4 Schools, Dept. of Special Services, 1963, 83 pp.

A battery of tests given 16 partially sighted children grades 1–8, characteristics as a group and as individuals delineated, hypotheses regarding partially seeing tested. Areas tested include intelligence, psycholinguistic abilities, visual retention, social maturity, actual achievement. Three case studies provided.

2470. ———. An intensive differential diagnosis of partially seeing children to determine the implications of education. *Exceptional Children*, 1963, Vol. 30, No. 1, pp. 17–25.

A study of 16 such children concludes that "psycholingualistic processes involving visual and motor abilities . . . are significantly inferior to their auditory and vocal abilities." Hypothesis that these childern are not achieving at a level commensurate with their potential was strongly but not fully confirmed.

2471. Kirk, Edith C. The future of reading for partially seeing children. *Reading Teacher*, Dec. 1970, Vol. 24, No. 3, pp. 195–202.

Considers the future reading of partially seeing children in the light of new developments in improving vision and improving reading instruction. Discusses definition of the partially seeing child, necessity for early identification, role of parents, and optimum physical conditions for reading in school. Considers mechanical aids, class organization, comprehension, study skills, and materials.

2472. Parmenter, Trevor R. Self-concept development of the partially seeing. *Slow Learning Child: The Australian Journal on the Education of Backward Children*, Nov. 1970, Vol. 17, No. 3, pp. 178–85.

Self-concept inventories were administered to adolescent partially seeing *S*s. Results indicate that there are no significant differences in self-concept development between 2 groups.

2473. Putnam, W. D. *On becoming partially sighted: A personal account of loss of sight.* Santa Monica, Calif.: Rand Corp., 1974, 26 pp.

Author relates his experiences and describes his adjustment to the problem.

2474. Soll, David M. Vision care for the partially sighted child. *New England Journal of Optometry*, Sept. 1973, Vol. 24, No. 7, pp. 202–5.

2475. Stone, Patricia. The peculiar problems of partial sight. *New Outlook for the Blind*, June 1965, Vol. 59, No. 6, pp. 211–12.

Describes special problems of the partially sighted, especially related to mobility, eating in public, and interpersonal relationships.

2476. Warren, R. L. What constitutes blindness? II Psychology. *Journal of the American Optometric Association*, Nov. 1969, Vol. 40, No. 11, pp. 1116–20.

Provides practical suggestions for understanding the low-vision patient.

2477. Wolf, Benjamin. Visual impairment is not blindness. *New Outlook for the Blind*, Dec. 1971, Vol. 65, No. 10, pp. 334–36.

Visual impairment is differentiated from blindness in degree and educational needs. Blind persons rely on other senses for normal functioning, while partially sighted persons need help to use and coordinate their limited vision with their other senses.

2478. Zimmerman, A. Alfred. An appraisal of partial vision: Its dual nature and problems. *New Outlook for the Blind*, May 1965, Vol. 59, No. 5, pp. 153–56.

Describes the special and highly individual problems of partially sighted and suggests ways in which counselors may help.

25.   The Older Blind

2479. American Foundation for the Blind. *The aging person who is visually handicapped: A handbook.* New York: Author, 1971.

This manual, which contains both practical and theoretical information of use to social workers, nurses, therapists, families who are in regular contact with older visually handicapped persons grew out of recommendations made by AFB's Task Force on Geriatric Blindness.

2480. ———. *How to integrate aging persons who are visually handicapped into community senior programs.* New York: Author, 1972, 35 pp.

Documentation of experiences of a number of different agencies which were able to join forces and collaborate successfully within a community to meet the needs of the older blind person.

2481. ———. *An introduction to working with the aging person who is visually handicapped.* New York: Author, 1972, 51 pp., illus., $3.

A resource guide for persons with little or no previous experience with aging blind persons. Includes sections on the medical and psychological aspects of aging and blindness, personal contact, available services, solving other problems, and further reading.

2482. ———. *First National Conference on Aging and Blindness. Theme: Meeting the challenges of elderly persons with sight difficulties—Action 76.* New York: Author, 1975, 104 pp., app.

Proceedings of conference to identify needs and gaps in service, to recommend solutions, and to outline a concrete plan of action for 1976.

2483. ———. *Conference on aging and blindness, College of Physicians, Philadelphia, Pa., April, 1975.* New York: Author, 1975, 102 pp.

Papers and summaries of discussions on aging and blindness in the general areas of: Demography, health, economic and social factors, and psychological-psychiatric factors. Local sources of help are stressed.

2484. Barnett, M. Robert. Blindness among the aging—A growing dual problem. *New Outlook for the Blind,* Feb. 1956, Vol. 50, No. 2, pp. 65–68.

Analyzes the needs of the growing population of older blind and makes detailed recommendations regarding income maintenance, public assistance, health maintenance, recreation, and housing.

2485. Berg, Murray, & Durchslag, Betty. Observations on visually handicapped residents in a geriatrics setting. *New Outlook for the Blind,* Oct. 1964, Vol. 58, No. 8, pp. 243–45.

Description of a home for the aged's endeavor to deal more positively with their visually handicapped residents. Suggestions for carrying out such a program successfully.

2486. Bledsoe, C. W. Blind patients as domiciliary members. *New Outlook for the Blind*, Apr. 1957, Vol. 51, No. 4, pp. 140–44.

Combination of philosophy and practical suggestions related to the older blind in institutional settings.

2487. ———. Rehabilitation of the blind geriatric patient. *Geriatrics*, 1958, Vol. 13, pp. 91–96.

Specific emotional problems typically found with onset of blindness of the aged are discussed.

2488. ———. Geriatrics and the venerable. *New Outlook for the Blind*, Dec. 1958, Vol. 52, No. 10, pp. 371–76.

Discusses 3 problems which merge in efforts to assist the geriatric blind: Dependency of patient on doctor; relationships between doctors and workers for the blind; learning/knowing the actual needs and wants of the blind geriatric patient.

2489. Boninger, Walter B. Aging and blindness. *New Outlook for the Blind*, June 1969, Vol. 63, No. 60, pp. 178–84.

Guidelines and philosophy through which a program for aged blind can be developed: Look at each person individually, believe in the person's right to quality service, believe the older person can learn, and workers must involve themselves actively in the overall problems of the aged.

2490. Burnside, Irene M. A nurse's perspective: Blindness in long-term care facilities. *New Outlook for the Blind*, Apr. 1974, Vol. 68, No. 4, pp. 145–50.

More intensive in-service staff education programs are needed to improve care of blind elderly residents of long-term care facilities. Many specific suggestions for improving care are given.

2491. Carolan, Robert H. Sensory stimulation in the nursing home. *New Outlook for the Blind*, Mar. 1973, Vol. 67, No. 3, pp. 126–30.

As stimulation is often neglected in the nursing home environment, specific suggestions are provided for improving this situation. Orientation and mobility specialists can be invaluable catalysts. Specialists and regular staff can, by analyzing the person's entire daily routine, provide many opportunities for additional sensory stimulation.

2492. Carroll, Thomas J. A look at aging. *New Outlook for the Blind*, Apr. 1972, Vol. 66, No. 4, pp. 97–103, 118–19. Also in *New Beacon*, July 1972.

Published posthumously, this address reviews problems of aging in modern society and stresses the value of providing even minimal gains in vision.

2493. Clark, Leslie L., Ed. *Proceedings of the Research Conference on Geriatric Blindness and Severe Visual Impairment, September 7–8, 1967.* New York: AFB, 1968, 83 pp., $2.50.

Presented are the proceedings of a research-related conference on aging discussing current knowledge about the status and welfare of aged blind persons. Includes presentations by Hyman Goldstein, Robert A. Scott, Jeanne G. Gilbert, and D. C. MacFarland.

2494. Cohen, Ruth G. Casework with older persons. *New Outlook for the Blind*, Oct. 1957, Vol. 51, No. 8, pp. 363–69.

Staff must like older people, perceive aging as a normal phase of life, and balance between "doing for" and "doing with." Social work should provide the milieu in which activity and creativity can survive for the older person.

2495. Colligan, J. C. Special problems of aging blind persons in the modern world. *New Outlook for the Blind*, Feb. 1965, Vol. 59, No. 2, pp. 45–49.

Discusses needs in the general areas of friendly visiting, communication skills, housing, companionship, radio, and a holiday change in environment.

2496. Copeland, Arthur E. Recreation for the aging blind. *New Outlook for the Blind*, Feb. 1961, Vol. 55, No. 2, pp. 44–49.

Comprehensive discussion of reasons for recreation programs for older people and the blind, especially. Leadership, how to set up program and what to include are all discussed.

2497. Coughlin, Barbara C. Future directions of government programs. *New Outlook for the Blind*, Sept. 1971, Vol. 65, No. 7, pp. 215–17.

Explores progress in government programs serving aged blind persons which can be anticipated during the next decade.

2498. Dickey, Thomas W. Meeting the vocational needs of the older blind person. *New Outlook for the Blind*, May 1975, Vol. 69, No. 5, pp. 218–25.

Experienced placement specialist reviews the special challenges of placing older blind, reviewing vision and employment characteristics of that population, and suggesting some responses to employers' objections.

2499. Faye, Eleanor E. Visual function in geriatric eye disease. *New Outlook for the Blind*, Sept. 1971, Vol. 65, No. 7, pp. 204–9.

Identifies 4 major eye diseases of the elderly (cataracts, macular degeneration, glaucoma, diabetic retinopathy) and discusses treatment available. Suggests most older persons can enjoy at least partial restoration of vision.

2500. Fisch, Mayer. Organic and psychiatric disorders of the aged blind. *New Outlook for the Blind*, May 1958, Vol. 52, No. 5, pp. 161–65.

Discusses nature of changes of the brain in aging, and blindness compounding problem on 2 levels: Orientation affect and treatment.

2501. Franke, Eleanor D. A study of the over 65's. *New Outlook for the Blind*, Oct. 1960, Vol. 54, No. 8, pp. 285–88.

A very general discussion of conditions which caused study to be made, how it was made, and what was found as a result.

2502. Freedman, Saul. The assessment of older visually impaired adults by a psychologist. *New Outlook for the Blind*, Oct. 1975, Vol. 69, No. 8, pp. 361–64.

Describes psychologist's role in a specific rehab. facility. Specific tests that have been used with this older population effectively are mentioned.

2503. Gilbert, Jeanne G. Aging among sighted and blind persons. *New Outlook for the Blind*, Sept. 1964, Vol. 58, No. 7, pp. 197–201.

General consideration of aging process. Discussion of differences between those who have always been blind and those who become so through the aging process.

2504. ———. Old age and blindness—Research needs. *New Outlook for the Blind,* Feb. 1965, Vol. 59, No. 2, pp. 49–51.

Outlines areas of research related to physical, intellectual, and emotional changes in aging and as narrowed by blindness. Decline can be retarded and research should be directed toward this. Contributions of work and psychotherapy should be evaluated.

2505. Gobetz, Giles E.; Drane, Harold W.; & Underwood, Eleanor L. *Home teaching of the geriatric blind.* Cleveland, Ohio: Cleveland Society for the Blind, 1969, 103 pp., app., illus.

Comprehensive study and evaluation of a home teaching demonstration project with the geriatric blind.

2506. Griffis, Gretta. The aging—The home teacher's challenge. *New Outlook for the Blind,* Dec. 1954, Vol. 48, No. 10, pp. 360–64.

Describes 4 levels of potential in older blind clients, their special needs, the problem of role reversal, and the need to make services individual.

2507. Heeren, Ethel. The blind person in the home for the aged. *New Outlook for the Blind,* Oct. 1960, Vol. 54, No. 8, pp. 280–84.

Examines ways to reassure the elderly blind person, to provide a sense of importance and identity, to reestablish his independence and feeling of equality. Discusses denial, manifestations of dependency, transference from childhood in dependent situations, attitudes toward blindness and aging, balance problems, staff assistance in orientation, social intercourse, optical aids.

2508. Held, Marian, & Wartenberg, Stanley. Blind people fifty and over. *New Outlook for the Blind,* May 1961, Vol. 55, No. 5, pp. 165–68.

Discusses the services most useful to blind clients over 50 years of age.

2509. Hellinger, George. Vision rehabilitation for aged blind persons. *New Outlook for the Blind,* June 1969, Vol. 63, No. 6, pp. 175–77.

Details practical steps in providing optical aids to older people and supporting services so they make optimum use of the aids. Older persons present special problems: Lack of motivation, resignation to limitations of old age, disbelief in desirability of using the eyes, decreased attention span, limited energy, and some mild mental confusion.

2510. ———. Providing ophthalmological and optometric diagnostic examinations and optical aids for legally blind aged persons under Medicare. *New Outlook for the Blind,* Jan. 1971, Vol. 65, No. 1, pp. 18–20.

Survey of over 5,400 institutionalized aged persons found over 16% of them legally blind. Guidelines given for guarding against possible abuse of Medicare regulations to provide ophthalmological and optometric examinations and aids to the aged.

2511. Hoffman, Simon. Employment for the older blind worker. *New Outlook for the Blind,* Dec. 1954, Vol. 48, No. 10, pp. 354–59.

Discusses the older worker in general and how blindness augments the problems. Case histories of several successful older blind workers.

2512. Jolicoeur, Roger M., Sr. *Caring for the visually impaired older person.* Minneapolis: Minneapolis Society for the Blind, 1970, 47 pp.

Especially designed for staff of nursing homes, details the characteristics of dependent older blind persons and suggestions for their care.

2513. Kornzweig, Abraham L. Progress in the prevention of blindness among the aged. *New Outlook for the Blind*, Sept. 1971, Vol. 65, No. 7, pp. 209–13.

Discusses progress in methods of preventing injuries to the eye and of treating cataract, glaucoma, diabetic retinopathy, and macular degeneration. Stresses early detection and treatment of eye diseases by the ophthalmologist.

2514. Lockerbie, Cleda, & Rodenberg, L. W. The need for homes for aged and dependent blind persons. *New Outlook for the Blind*, Oct. 1964, Vol. 58, No. 8, pp. 252–53.

Authors feel there is definite need for homes for aged blind. Examples are given of type of person who will be most content in a home of this kind.

2515. Lokshin, Helen. Psychological factors in casework with blind older persons. *New Outlook for the Blind*, Jan. 1957, Vol. 51, No. 1, pp. 1–8.

On the basis of review of records of the Social Service Dept. of the New York Guild for the Jewish Blind, and with a number of brief case histories, discusses the reactions of older people to blindness and the highly individual nature of solutions to their problems.

2516. Maloney, Elizabeth. Social service implications of the Community Aging Project. *New Outlook for the Blind*, June 1969, Vol. 63, No. 6, pp. 165–67.

Services must be individualized, prevention and remedial care are important, and specialized project staff are usually welcomed by the institutions in which older blind people are living.

2517. Mercer, Alonzo V. A recreational survey of blind persons who are 60 years of age and older. *New Outlook for the Blind*, Feb. 1971, Vol. 65, No. 2, pp. 63–71.

Survey of 137 persons included questions re knowledge of recreational facilities, size of groups preferred, hobbies before and after loss of sight, and reasons for not using known facilities. Survey indicated gap between need and services for elderly blind persons.

2518. Merrill, Toni. *Activities for the aged and infirm: A handbook for the untrained worker.* Springfield, Ill.: Charles C Thomas, 1967, 372 pp.

Describes games and activities, some of which are suitable for the elderly visually handicapped. Discusses role of leader, program planning, etc.

2519. Miller, David, & Stern, Rachel. Vision screening and hearing in the elderly. *Eye, Ear, Nose and Throat Monthly*, Apr. 1974, Vol. 53, No. 4, pp. 128–33.

Report on the audiometric and ophthalmologic results of a screening survey of 115 persons living in a housing project for the elderly.

2520. Minkoff, Harry. An approach to providing services to aged blind persons. *New Outlook for the Blind*, Apr. 1972, Vol. 66, No. 4, pp. 104–8, 119.

Discussion of centers in the community which serve as bridges "by which aged blind persons may enter and enjoy community programs and services otherwise limited to the sighted." Primary object is to help blind adults make use of neighborhood centers and to move from this to the use of other agencies and resources. Cites problems, including recruitment of volunteers and transportation, which the project encountered.

2521. ————. Integrating the aging visually handicapped into community groups in New York City. *New Outlook for the Blind*, Nov. 1975, Vol. 69, No. 9, pp. 396–98.

Reports results of 3-year funded project. Describes project's structure, how groups are organized, site selection, orientation of host center staff and members, activities, and transportation. A special program in an area nursing home is also described.

2522. **Morris, Robert.** Realizing a comprehensive national policy on aging and blindness. *New Outlook for the Blind*, Sept. 1972, Vol. 66, No. 7, pp. 233–35.

Author expresses the need for a national policy that gives as much attention to day-to-day living of the handicapped as is now given medical treatment and rehabilitation. Feels that "a personal care benefit paid for a condition . . . promises to bring into being the requisite range of personal care services now lacking."

2523. **Morrison, A. Marie.** Some guidelines for providing in-service training to the staff of nursing homes and homes for the aged. *New Outlook for the Blind*, Mar. 1970, Vol. 64, No. 3, pp. 81–85, 91.

Results of a workshop held to familiarize staff personnel caring for aged blind. Recommendations were: In-service training valuable, information should be on practical rather than technical level, follow-up questionnaire should be used. Information is provided for development of a workshop.

2524. **Mummah, Hazel R.** Group work with the aged blind Japanese in the nursing home and in the community. *New Outlook for the Blind*, Apr. 1975, Vol. 69, No. 4, pp. 160–67.

A nurse views the multiple losses complicated by cultural differences affecting aged blind Japanese and discusses the program in the nursing home in which she is employed.

2525. **National Society for the Prevention of Blindness.** Presby . . . . what, Doctor? *Sight-Saving Review*, Spring 1974, Vol. 44, No. 1, pp. 31–39.

Description of a program on cataracts and eye care taken to older people attending senior centers throughout New York City. Includes questions most frequently asked at the centers and the types of responses that seem most useful and supportive to the older population.

2526. **N.J. State Commission for the Blind and Visually Impaired.** *Blindness and the vintage years.* Newark, N.J.: Author, 1972, 42 pp., app.

An assessment of the needs of the aged blind in N.J.

2527. **Pastalan, Leon A.** The simulation of age-related sensory losses: A new approach to the study of environmental barriers. *New Outlook for the Blind*, Oct. 1974, Vol. 68, No. 8, pp. 356–62.

Through use of mechanical appliances to simulate the usual sensory losses of the aged, demonstrated such losses can constrain a person from freely using buildings, facilities, and other environments as presently designed.

2528. Pattison, Claudia C. The blind nursing home patient: A question of real kindness—A discussion of sighted guide, room familiarization, and independent travel for the geriatric blind person. *Rehabilitation Teacher,* Fall 1975, Vol. 7, No. 5, pp. 7–15.

Nursing home personnel need training in work with the blind; otherwise, they do too much or too little.

2529. Randall, Ollie A. The aging blind in an aging population. *New Outlook for the Blind,* June 1956, Vol. 50, No. 6, pp. 210–15.

The problems of the aging blind in a generally aging population call for emphasis upon the person, not the handicap. Criticizes the frequently negative attitudes toward the blind in homes for the aged and calls for new methods and new facilities. Must treat all as individuals.

2530. Range, M. Conrad. An outline of project objectives and procedures. *New Outlook for the Blind,* June 1969, Vol. 63, No. 6, pp. 163–64.

Objectives of the Community Aging Project are: (1) to identify aging blind persons in institutions; (2) increase their self-reliance and reduce their need for protective care; and (3) utilize the IHB residence as a rehabilitation center. Reports progress to date.

2531. Riffenburgh, Ralph S. The psychology of blindness. *Geriatrics,* 1967, Vol. 22, No. 10, pp. 127–33.

Discusses the behavioral effects of blindness with emphasis on adjustment at the onset and the management of the newly blinded geriatric patient.

2532. Roberts, Harold G. White House Conference on the Aging—Implications for blind persons. *New Outlook for the Blind,* Apr. 1961, Vol. 55, No. 4, pp. 132–34.

Results of White House Conference on Aging in general with particular emphasis on policy statement relating to blindness.

2533. Rogot, Eugene. Survivorship among the aged blind. *New Outlook for the Blind,* Dec. 1965, Vol. 59, No. 10, pp. 333–38.

Analysis of the records of the Massachusetts register of the blind for 5,976 persons who were 65 years of age or older at time of registration. Analysis shows survivorship by sex, age, cause of blindness, and cause of death. Statistical tables.

2534. Rosenbloom, Alfred A., Jr. Prognostic factors in the visual rehabilitation of aging patients. *New Outlook for the Blind,* Mar. 1974, Vol. 68, No. 3, pp. 124–27.

Follow-up study of 150 patients to analyze physical, psychological, social-emotional, and occupational factors and their relationship to predicting success in the use of low vision aids. Revealed the importance of residual vision, the patient's life situation, and the extent of the training in the use of the aid.

2535. Rusalem, Herbert. A study of the incidence of blindness in homes for the aged and nursing homes. *New Outlook for the Blind,* June 1969, Vol. 63, No. 6, pp. 168–74.

Vision screening was provided for 5,376 individuals in 56 institutions, median age 82. Of these, 19% failed the screening and were presumed blind, an incidence far greater than previously supposed. Unless blindness is recognized early, suitable prevention and treatment are delayed.

2536. Rusalem, Herbert; Bettica, Louis; & Urguhart, John. An experiment in improving communication between blind and deaf-blind persons in a residence for older blind persons. *New Outlook for the Blind*, Oct. 1966, Vol. 60, No. 8, pp. 255–56.

Reports on a 10-session course in printing in the palm, given 5 volunteer blind Ss. No significant changes in attitude and behavior in either experimental or control group were observed.

2537. Salmon, Peter J. The community aging project. Introduction: Geriatric rehabilitation for the aging blind. *New Outlook for the Blind*, June 1969, Vol. 63, No. 6, p. 162.

A brief introduction to the following papers which report various aspects of a federally funded project at Industrial Home for the Blind, Brooklyn.

2538. Saterbak, Melvin; Sineps, John; & Relaford, Raymond. *The relocation of blind persons from a residential home for the blind and the development of specialized community services for the older visually handicapped population.* Minneapolis: Minneapolis Society for the Blind, Nov. 1, 1970, 78+ pp., $1.

Final report on study begun in 1966 when the planned closing of the Home for the Blind necessitated relocation of 65 residents. Study continued for 2½ years following the relocation to obtain information re the factors leading to successful community integration and adjustment.

2539. Solomon, Aaron. Recreation and the aged blind. *New Outlook for the Blind*, Feb. 1955, Vol. 49, No. 2, pp. 55–61.

Universal basic needs for self-expression, approval, security, and belonging may be satisfied in the aged blind through recreation programs. Discusses the varied program offered by the New York Guild.

2540. Stern, Mildred F. Activity or idleness: Restoration of social contacts among the elderly blind. *New Outlook for the Blind*, June 1969, Vol. 63, No. 6, pp. 185–89.

Project of Metropolitan Society for the Blind, Detroit, to reintegrate older blind persons in the community through instruction for residence and nursing home staff, a camping experience, day center programs, and providing transportation for recreation.

2541. ———. The aging blind and leisure time activities. *New Outlook for the Blind*, Feb. 1970, Vol. 64, No. 2, pp. 46–50.

Includes discussion of camping sessions, volunteer work at Christmas, Project Restore (providing activities such as sewing, crafts, games, and group singing), and mobility instruction. Reactions of participants cited and considerations for the future noted.

2542. Stevens, F. J. Social rehabilitation. *New Outlook for the Blind*, Feb. 1963, Vol. 57, No. 2, pp. 62–63.

A glimpse into the problems of training older persons to live satisfactorily in their local communities, as seen by a worker in England.

26. Mobility, Posture, Guidance Devices, and Dog Guides

2543. Airasian, Peter W. Evaluation of the binaural sensory aid. *American Foundation for the Blind Research Bulletin 26*, June 1973, pp. 51–71.

Summarizes data from questionnaire responses of trainers and trainees in a Sonic Glasses training project. Reports characteristics of respondents, training practices and experiences, mobility before and after training, adequacy of device, and attitudes toward training and device.

2544. Alameda County [Calif.] School Dept. *Orientation and mobility for blind adolescents in public schools.* Washington, D.C.: Rehabilitation Services Admin., HEW, 1969, 72 pp.

Description of a project which provided instruction to 50 visually handicapped students. Students instructed in long cane usage. Tactual maps used for orientation. Evaluation showed 21 of 27 students improved. Case records included.

2545. Alameda County Public Schools. *Itinerant instruction in orientation and mobility for blind adolescents in public schools.* Hayward, Calif.: Supt. of Schools of Alameda Co., 1966, 69 pp.

Description of a program begun in 1963 in 2 Calif. counties. The program showed that orientation-mobility on an itinerant basis was feasible administratively and financially and was successful with the students.

2546. Alonso, Lou. The educator's vital role in mobility and orientation. *New Outlook for the Blind*, Sept. 1965, Vol. 59, No. 7, pp. 249–51.

Although the teacher's role in developing basic mobility skills has been recognized, only recently has the teacher preparation curriculum included training for this. Urges better developed teacher preparation for stimulating and developing mobility-relevant attitudes and skills.

2547. Altmann, John, & Hatlen, Philip H. New dimensions in sound for the blind. *American Foundation for the Blind Research Bulletin 25*, Jan. 1973, pp. 249–52.

Describes a sound laboratory to encourage creative expression and aid mobility training.

2548. American Foundation for the Blind. *Bibliography of mobility research and mobility instrumentation research: A provisional bibliography.* New York: Author, 1964, 30 pp.

Cites 355 research and development reports from 1927 to 1964. Among areas treated are mobility training, sensory devices, travel aids, perception and echo location, guide dogs, orientation.

2549. ———. *Dog guides for the blind.* New York: Author, 1969, 6 pp., free.

Describes briefly the history of dog guides and the selection and training of both user and dog.

2550. Ammons, Carol H.; Worchel, Philip; & Dallenbach, Karl M. "Facial vision": The perception of obstacles out of doors by blindfolded and blindfolded-deafened subjects. *American Foundation for the Blind Research Bulletin 13*, July 1966, pp. 153–92. Reprinted from *American Journal of Psychology*, Oct. 1953.

Study had 2 purposes: (1) determine whether results of indoor experiments could be duplicated outdoors, and (2) discover whether every person with normal hearing could learn to perceive obstacles. Blindfolded *S*s quickly learned to perceive obstacles; blindfolded-deafened *S*s did not.

2551. Angus, Herbert D.; Howell, Bob; & Lynch, Jacqueline. Twenty questions about mobility. *New Outlook for the Blind,* Sept. 1969, Vol. 63, No. 7, pp. 214–18.

Questions parents are likely to ask about mobility and encouraging answers. There is no substitute for independent travel.

2552. Apple, Loyal E., & May, Marianne. *Distance vision and perceptual training: A concept for use in the mobility training of low vision clients.* New York: AFB, 1971, 23 pp., $2.25.

2553. Ark. Enterprises for the Blind. *Final report: The mobility and orientation instruction of blind people.* Little Rock: Author, 1966, 38 pp.

Purpose was to demonstrate value of systematic teaching of mobility skills to blind and to measure results of training. Materials and lesson plans described. Results positive, especially in increasing independence of clients. Various mobility techniques evaluated.

2554. Armstrong, John D. A head-mounted version of the sonic aid. *New Beacon,* Sept. 1970, Vol. 54, No. 641, pp. 227–30.

Aid is discussed in terms of its development, use, advantages, and user training. Reports on the use by 9 blind persons who reported it to be of some assistance to them.

2555. ———. Blind mobility current research program. *American Foundation for the Blind Research Bulletin 29*, June 1975, pp. 145–48.

Overview of research being done at the Univ. of Nottingham, England. Includes evaluation of mobility performance and aids, mobility of deaf-blind, mobility maps, adjustment to blindness, and problems of low-vision blind.

2556. Auzenne, George R. Some observations on peripatology. *New Outlook for the Blind,* Nov. 1965, Vol. 59, No. 9, pp. 313–15.

At once justifies and answers some criticisms of peripatology, using a team approach with the peripatologist's responsibility in perspective.

2557. Baecker, Ronald M. Computer simulation of mobility aids: A feasibility study. *American Foundation for the Blind Research Bulletin 16*, May 1968, pp. 141–206, illus.

Details the methods and problems in computer simulation and concludes that a multichannel system would be superior.

2558. Bann, Win. The case for the partially sighted syndrome. *Chronicle,* Dec. 1973, Vol. 11, No. 13, pp. 7–10.

The head of the Adult Rehabilitation Unit of the Royal New Zealand

Foundation for the Blind discusses the special problems that occur in mobility and orientation programs for the partially sighted.

2559. Barnett, M. Robert, Ed. Mobility and orientation—A symposium. I. National Conference on Mobility and Orientation. *New Outlook for the Blind*, Mar. 1960, Vol. 54, No. 3, pp. 77–81.

Presents findings relative to establishing criteria for selection of O & M personnel, curriculum, and recommended length of training and sponsorship.

2560. Baumann, D. M.; Gerstley, L. A.; Neuman, L. A., et al. The collapsible cane project. *American Foundation for the Blind Research Bulletin 3*, Aug. 1963, pp. 1–12, illus.

Detailed report of efforts to develop an improved cane.

2561. Benham, Thomas A. A guidance device for the blind. *Physics Today*, Dec. 1954, Vol. 7, No. 12, pp. 11–14.

Gives the technical operation of an electronic guidance device and results of tests with 67 *S*s.

2562. Bishop, Alexander R. Independence for the blind. *International Journal for the Education of the Blind*, Feb. 1953, Vol. 2, No. 2, pp. 147–48.

Describes a mandatory course in travel at the Alabama School for the Blind, and course objectives. The techniques used were developed by branches of the U.S. military. The course is said to be successful and as important to the blind individual's well-being as any academic or vocational course.

2563. Blackhurst, A. Edward; Marks, Claude H.; & Tisdall, William J. Relationship between mobility and divergent thinking in blind children. *Education of the Visually Handicapped*, May 1969, Vol. 1, No. 2, pp. 33–36.

One hundred fifty-two students from day and residential schools were scored on 6 tests to determine if a relationship exists between mobility and divergent thinking. Conclusion was that if a relationship exists in day school students, it is a slight one. No significant correlation was found in the residential group.

2564. Blasch, Bruce B.; Welsh, Richard L.; & Davidson, Terry. Auditory maps: An orientation aid for visually handicapped persons. *New Outlook for the Blind*, Apr. 1973, Vol. 67, No. 4, pp. 145–58.

Auditory maps (cassette tapes) can successfully orient a skilled blind traveler to a specific area or guide him to a particular objective. Discusses types of maps, portability, and hardware.

2565. Bohman, Richard V.; Bryan, William H.; & Tapp, Kenneth L. The Auditory Quiz Board: An orientation and mobility game for visually handicapped elementary school children. *New Outlook for the Blind*, Dec. 1972, Vol. 66, No. 10, pp. 371–73.

The Board utilizes multiple-choice questions printed or brailled on a specially wired form which is clipped to the surface of a battery-operated box; when the "right" choice is made, the box buzzes. Authors explain how the system is used in orientation and mobility training and list 9 advantages they have found in working with this learning aid.

2566. Boughton, Douglass. Teaching compass directions to the visually handicapped. *Pointer*, Winter 1974, Vol. 19, No. 2, p. 134.

Compass directions can provide student with independent means of orientation and are taught on basis of knowledge of angles and clock positions.

2567. Brambring, Michael. Technical and practical utilization of electronic mobility aids for the blind. *American Foundation for the Blind Research Bulletin 25,* Jan. 1973, p. 257.

Brief report of field tests of Kay Sonic Aid and Laser Cane, using 24 blind *S*s, aged 14–22. Reports 8 conclusions and urges further improvements in design.

2568. Brothers, Roy J. Stimulating learning through physical activity. In *Association for Education of the Visually Handicapped—Forty-ninth Biennial Conference, June 1968, Toronto, Canada.* Philadelphia: AEVH, 1969, pp. 49–60.

Discussion of research on physical education and the movement theory programs of Kephart and Barsch.

2569. Brothers, Roy J., & Huff, Roger A. *Sound localization; suggested activities for the development of sound localization skills.* Louisville, Ky.: American Printing House for the Blind, Aug. 1972, 18 pp., $1.

Manual of activities and learning situations based on data supplied by participants in the Sound Localization Institute held Apr. 1972 in Louisville.

2570. Brown, G. D., & Jessen, W. E. Evaluation of an orientation, mobility, and living skills workshop for blind children. *Exceptional Children,* 1968, Vol. 35, No. 3, pp. 239–40.

Developed the Orientation and Mobility Test Battery to evaluate a 3-week workshop.

2571. ———. Preliminary performance test battery of orientation, mobility and living skills. *American Foundation for the Blind Research Bulletin 24,* Mar. 1972, pp. 1–20.

Administration of 21 preliminary tests to blind children shows feasibility of battery of orientation, mobility, and living skills measures.

2572. Busbridge, John. Mobility and the almost blind. *New Beacon,* Apr. 1973, Vol. 57, No. 672, pp. 92–93.

Partially sighted author describes mobility problems specific to that group, ways in which he tries to cope with problems, mobility instructors' seeming neglect of partially sighted.

2573. Carney, James R. An orientation and mobility program for the geriatric blind adult. *New Outlook for the Blind,* Nov. 1970, Vol. 64, No. 9, pp. 285–86.

Makes suggestions for planning a program including concepts of environment and travel training, the significance of correct timing in presenting the lessons, and the value of the long cane.

2574. Clark, Leslie L., Ed. *Proceedings of the Rotterdam mobility research conference.* New York: AFB, 1965, 294 pp.

Five sections entitled respectively: State of the art reports on the utilization of the electromagnetic spectrum for mobility implementation; special problems of mobility training; social and demographic research; research and development of mobility aids; evaluations in field laboratory for performance parameters of objects using mobility aids.

2575. Clarke, N. V.; Pick, G. F.; & Wilson, J. P. Obstacle detection with and without the aid of a directional noise generator. *American Foundation for the Blind Research Bulletin 29*, June 1975, pp. 67–85, illus.

Investigation shows use of aid approximately doubled both number of detections and distance at which detection occurred.

2576. Coon, Nelson. Guide dogs for the blind—Whose idea was it? *New Outlook for the Blind*, Apr. 1956, Vol. 50, No. 4, pp. 132–33.

Ancient art of more than one country shows dogs in guiding positions, but it was Johann Wilhelm Klein who set down in print the procedure for training the guide dog.

2577. ———. *A brief history of dog guides for the blind.* Morristown, N.J.: Seeing Eye, 1959.

A concise and informative history of dog guides with many illustrations showing the use of dogs throughout the centuries.

2578. Corbett, Michael. Professionalism in mobility. *New Outlook for the Blind*, Mar. 1974, Vol. 68, No. 3, pp. 104–7, 123.

Discussion of ways in which the professionalism of mobility instructors can be increased. Some of the items mentioned are a forum for dialogue and dissemination of information, a central resource for information, public relations materials, greater attention to individual differences in clients, and emphasis on the interpersonal aspects of mobility.

2579. Couchell, Peter, Jr., et al. *The value of mobility instruction as a technique to motivate blind individuals.* Charlotte, N.C.: Mecklenberg Assoc. for Blind, Aug. 1966, 62 pp.

Reports 3-year demonstration project involving 73 Ss, ages 14–70. Success in mobility seemed to improve motivation in other areas of social functioning.

2580. Cratty, Bryant J. Perception of inclined plane while walking without vision. *Perceptual and Motor Skills*, 1966, Vol. 22, No. 2, pp. 547–56.

One hundred sixty-four blind Ss and 30 blindfolded sighted controls walked and reported their perceptions of a pathway whose surface contained grades of 1, 2, 4 and 6° of incline and decline from the horizontal. Results are described and discussed.

2581. ———. The perception of gradient and the veering tendency while walking without vision. *American Foundation for the Blind Research Bulletin 14*, Mar. 1967, pp. 31–51, illus.

Studies 164 blind Ss and 30 sighted controls to investigate tendency to veer and perception of gradient. Influence of leg length, posture, and stride length was measured.

2582. ———. *Perceptual-motor behavior and educational processes.* Springfield, Ill.: Charles C Thomas, 1969, 265 pp., app.

This text for elementary school and special class teachers presents research-based information and research guidelines. In considering special education, perceptual-motor abilities are discussed with reference to the blind, among others. App. includes a mobility orientation test for the blind.

2583. Cratty, Bryant J., & Williams, Harriet G. *Perceptual thresholds of* *non-visual locomotion.* Los Angeles: Dept. of Physical Education, Univ. of Calif., 1966, 100 pp.

With blindfolded and blind *S*s, studied effects of practice upon veer, facing movements, and position relocation; also lateral tilt in pathways and curvature of curbs.

2584. Crouse, Robert V. The long cane in Great Britain. *New Outlook for the Blind,* Jan. 1969, Vol. 63, No. 1, pp. 20–22.

History of gradual acceptance, after initial opposition, and current status of long cane use in Great Britain.

2585. Curtin, George T. Mobility: Social and psychological implications. *New Outlook for the Blind,* Jan. 1962, Vol. 56, No. 1, pp. 14–18.

Describes mobility as psychological movement involving attitudes, ideas, aspirations, and emotions. Discusses casework services in detail.

2586. Curtis, Jack F., & Winer, David M. A comparison of the efficacy of two methods of mobility training for the blind, using blindfolded sighted subjects. *American Foundation for the Blind Research Bulletin 22,* Dec. 1970, pp. 119–29, app.

Two methods of mobility training were evaluated by measuring travel of 7 groups of blindfolded sighted *S*s.

2587. DeFazio, T. L., & Sheridan, T. B. Vibration analysis of the cane. *American Foundation for the Blind Research Bulletin 3,* Aug. 1963, pp. 13–18.

An example of how one would consider a cane according to classical vibration theory. The proposed analysis was not completed because impracticable in this context.

2588. de Silva, Anthony. Guide dog or long cane? *New Beacon,* Dec. 1974, Vol. 58, No. 692, pp. 320–22.

The author, who is blind, discusses the advantages and disadvantages of both guide dog and long cane and gives his reasons for using both.

2589. Dickinson, Raymond M. *Mobility training for the visually handicapped: A guide for teachers.* Springfield, Ill.: Office of Public Instruction, 1968, 43 pp.

Discusses terminology, home learning processes, introduction to the outside world, fears and anxieties, parent-teacher cooperation. Also includes information on posture and gait, learning space relationships, using sensory clues, orientation and mobility skills, and formal training.

2590. ――――. *Orientation and mobility for the visually handicapped: A guide for parents.* Springfield, Ill.: Office of Public Instruction, 1968, 33 pp.

Discusses available services, recognition of infant's needs, adventitious loss, encouraging exploration, social adjustment, school preparation, and training at elementary, junior, and senior high school levels.

2591. Dupress, J. K., & Wright, H. N. Identifying and teaching auditory cues for traveling in the blind. *American Foundation for the Blind Research Bulletin 1,* Jan. 1962, pp. 3–9.

Project goals are: (1) to study differences between good and poor travelers especially in auditory task performance; (2) to provide measures of mobility capability which can be used in rehabilitation centers; and (3) to develop training tapes for use in mobility programs.

2592. Eichorn, John R., & Vigaroso, Hugo R. Orientation and mobility for pre-school blind children. *International Journal for the Education of the Blind*, Dec. 1967, Vol. 17, No. 2, pp. 48–50.

Suggestions for parents on helping the young child to experience and find meaning in his environment. Features of his home and neighborhood, streets and sidewalks, how cars travel, and safety rules, can be understood at an early age. Even a beginning understanding of direction is possible at this age.

2593. Enzinna, A. James. Orientation and mobility for a totally blind, bilateral hand amputee. *New Outlook for the Blind*, Mar. 1975, Vol. 69, No. 3, pp. 103–8, illus.

This program for a severely injured veteran involved the use of the long cane method and also included self-care skills and recreational activities.

2594. Farmer, Leicester W. Travel in adverse weather using electronic mobility guidance devices. *New Outlook for the Blind*, Dec. 1975, Vol. 69, No. 10, pp. 433–39, 451, illus.

Discusses characteristics of ideal aid and describes 4 devices in detail: Mowat Sonar Sensor; Russell E Model Pathsounder; Bionic C-5 Laser Cane; and Mark II Binaural Sensory Aid. Feels intensive training is necessary for effective use. Experiences of 2 users in snowy weather are reported.

2595. Finestone, Samuel; Lukoff, Irving F.; & Whiteman, Martin. *The demand for dog guides and the travel adjustment of blind persons.* New York: Equity Press, 1960, 131 pp.

Study undertaken to determine qualifications for potential users of dog guides, amount and nature of demand for dog guide training, volume of existing services, factors which influence choice of the dog guide as a mode of travel, and the travel adjustment of blind persons. Bib.

2596. Flannagan, Clara H. *A concentrated mobility and orientation approach for the improvement of education for partially seeing and blind children in day school settings. Final report.* Washington, D.C.: Office of Education, HEW, 1969, 79 pp.

Results of program in which training was given to 36 children were positive and demonstrated the need for mobility and orientation instruction beginning in infancy and continuing throughout the school years.

2597. Fla. Council for the Blind. *Preparation of blind students for vocational rehabilitation through early training in mobility and orientation: A final report.* Tallahassee: Author, 1968, 37 pp., app., illus.

Results of project to develop a well-organized orientation and mobility program as an addition to public school educational programs, thus better preparing the blind student to function self-sufficiently to succeed in rehabilitation efforts.

2598. Foulke, Emerson. The development and testing of the Caster Cane. *New Outlook for the Blind*, Oct. 1969, Vol. 63, No. 8, pp. 247–50.

Three reported evaluation procedures show some promise in a wheel-tipped cane.

2599. ———. The perceptual basis for mobility. *American Foundation for the Blind Research Bulletin 23*, June 1971, pp. 1–8. [Corrections appear in *Bulletin 24*, pp. 143–44.]

Detailed analysis of the perceptual experience in mobility.

2600. Freiberger, Howard. Mobility aids for the blind. *Bulletin of Prosthetics Research*, Fall 1974, BPR-10-22, pp. 73–78.

Pinpoints areas in need of improvement and more technological research in the mobility services for the blind provided by the VA. Discusses Laser Typhlocane, Binaural Sensory Aid, Lindsay Russell Pathsounder, Mowat Sonar Sensor, and Mims Seeing Aid.

2601. Friedman, Robert M. Patterns of travel for blind travelers. *Long Cane News*, May 1972, Vol. 5, No. 1, pp. 12–22.

A scheme, presented in outline form, designed to develop a blind person's ability to conceptualize trips as an aid to orientation.

2602. Gallagher, Patricia. A correlation study of Haptic subtest scores and travel rating skills of blind adolescents. *New Outlook for the Blind*, Oct. 1968, Vol. 62, No. 8, pp. 240–46.

After discussing the need for a readiness test for mobility training, reports the relationship between mobility skills and the Pattern Board subtest of the Haptic Intelligence Scale for 33 adolescents in 2 residential schools.

2603. Gissoni, Fred. My "cane" is twenty feet long. *New Outlook for the Blind*, Feb. 1966, Vol. 60, No. 2, pp. 33–38.

The author, a satisfied user of the Ultra-Sonic Travel Aid for the Blind, discusses uses for, benefits of, components of this device.

2604. Gobetz, Giles E. *Learning mobility in blind children and the geriatric blind: Final research report.* Cleveland, Ohio: Cleveland Society for the Blind, 1967, 140 pp., app., illus.

Summary of project developed to provide comprehensive orientation and mobility training to juvenile and geriatric clients, and to compare learning potential, achievement, and adjustment of the 2 groups and various subgroups. Bib.

2605. Gockman, Robert. *Independent travel training for blind children.* Chicago: Catholic Charities of the Archdiocese of Chicago, 1967, 143 pp., illus.

Positive findings related to introduction of mobility instruction at grade school level. Psychological factors affecting success. Importance of parent-teacher cooperation. Lesson planning and timing.

2606. Goodman, William. Is mobility education a one-man job? *New Outlook for the Blind*, Jan. 1964, Vol. 58, No. 1, pp. 16–18.

Description of mobility workshops held for teachers. Considered important because teacher in classroom can then reinforce indoor techniques and have proper attitude about mobility to pass on to students.

2607. ———. Peer group influences on mobility education. *New Outlook for the Blind*, Sept. 1965, Vol. 59, No. 7, pp. 251–54.

Describes program of mobility stimulation, motivation, and training with 8 junior high students in a day school program.

2608. ———. The making of a traveler. *Education of the Visually Handicapped*, Mar. 1969, Vol. 1, No. 1, pp. 11–14.

Theoretical case history of a blind child learning mobility. Importance of mobility on overall attitude toward life.

2609. Graham, Milton D. Wanted: A readiness test for mobility training. *New Outlook for the Blind*, May 1965, Vol. 59, No. 5, pp. 157–62.

Based on evaluation records of 100 blind male adults suggests characteristics which might be used to predict mobility patterns. Indicates need for a better predictor. Ref.

2610. Hamilton-Wilkes, Monty. *Guide dogs in Australia.* Melbourne: Royal Guide Dogs for the Blind Assoc. of Australia, 1970, 86 pp., illus.

Describes Australia's systematic training program of guide dogs as mobility aids for the blind.

2611. Hapeman, Lawrence. The Ultra Sonic Aid for the blind. *New Outlook for the Blind*, May 1967, Vol. 61, No. 5, pp. 142–45.

A mobility specialist evaluates the Aid and poses questions about its usefulness.

2612. ———. Developmental concepts of blind children between the ages of three and six as they relate to orientation and mobility. *International Journal for the Education of the Blind*, Dec. 1967, Vol. 17, No. 2, pp. 41–48.

Presents basic concepts needed by a blind traveler and shows how these concepts can be developed early in childhood. The parent or teacher can find opportunities for the child to experience and, through repetition, learn these concepts. Ref.

2613. Harris, Janet C. Veering tendency as a function of anxiety in the blind. *American Foundation for the Blind Research Bulletin 14*, Mar. 1967, pp. 53–63, illus.

Relates veering tendency to anxiety level through a study of 44 blind *Ss*. Suggests that personality evaluation should precede mobility training.

2614. Hartong, Jack R. A special orientation and mobility project at a residential school. *New Outlook for the Blind*, Apr. 1968, Vol. 62, No. 4, pp. 118–21.

A 5-unit mobility program covers all levels of travel needs including summer follow-up contact and travel in student's home community.

2615. Hatchley, Eric. The Kay binaural ultrasonic sensory aid: A personal evaluation. *Rehabilitation Teacher*, Nov. 1972, Vol. 4, No. 11, pp. 3–24.

Describes aid and training course for use in mobility by blind persons.

2616. ———. More instructors for sonic glasses. *Guide Dog Magazine*, Sept. 1974, Vol. 9, No. 3, p. 13.

Eight sighted O & M and guide dog instructors attended a 4-week course in Australia on use of sonic spectacles to complement travel with dog or cane. Instructors used the Binaural Sensory Aid MK II in suburban and city travel.

2617. Hetherington, Francis. Travel at the Michigan School for the Blind. *International Journal for the Education of the Blind*, June 1952, Vol. 1, No. 4, pp. 93–95.

Gives details of the course in travel, indicating schools which feel the course had beneficial results economically, socially, etc. States belief that course in travel should be compulsory.

2618. ———. Elementary school travel program. *International Journal for the Education of the Blind*, Oct. 1955, Vol. 5, No. 1, pp. 15–17.

Describes foot travel instruction in 4th, 5th and 6th grades in 1952: Techniques, areas covered, obstacle perception training. Travel begins at home in preschool years. Mention of gratifying results from Parent Institute and Play School for parent instruction.

2619. Holdsworth, J. K. Research may give a new breed. *Faithfully Theirs*, Mar. 1972, Vol. 7, No. 1, p. 9.

Discusses a new breeding plan for guide dogs in Australia which is hoped to lead to development of an entirely new breed.

2620. ———. New approaches to mobility training. *New Beacon*, May 1975, Vol. 59, No. 697, pp. 116–22.

Using both dog guides and canes, a multi-aid mobility service has been established in Australia, including assessment of mobility needs on an individual basis and use of many community resources.

2621. Hubbard, James A. A program of orientation and mobility for the aged blind in the community. *New Outlook for the Blind*, Sept. 1969, Vol. 63, No. 7, pp. 211–13.

A 3-year project in mobility for older blind persons differed from mobility training in a rehabilitation center in being home-based, adjusted to individual needs, and including in-service training for medical and institutional personnel.

2622. Hughes, Robert K. Orientation and mobility for the partially sighted. *International Journal for the Education of the Blind*, May 1967, Vol. 16, No. 4, pp. 119–20.

Lists reasons why some partially sighted persons have mobility problems. Reports a program at the Western Pennsylvania School for Blind Children to meet needs of partially sighted travelers.

2623. Ill. Office of Education. *A curriculum guide for the development of body and sensory awareness for the visually impaired.* Springfield: Author, 1974, 312 pp., illus.

Guide for educators to develop pre-cane skills, listing materials, activities and references, charts and worksheets.

2624. Ill. State Dept. of Children and Family Services. *Orientation and mobility for the visually handicapped: A guide for parents.* Springfield: Author, 1968, 33 pp., illus.

2625. Ill. State Office of the Supt. of Public Instruction. *Mobility training for the visually handicapped: A guide for teachers.* Springfield: Author, 1968, 43 pp., illus.

2626. Industrial Home for the Blind. *Instruction in physical orientation and independent mobility: A lesson plan outline.* Brooklyn: Author, 1973, 51 pp., $2.50.

Revised edition of an instruction manual (1960) based on the techniques developed by Dr. Richard E. Hoover during his work with blinded servicemen of W.W. II.

2627. Jackson, Ned T. Some problems encountered in a summer orientation and mobility follow-up program for blind students of a residential school.

International Journal for the Education of the Blind, May 1967, Vol. 16, No. 4, pp. 121–22.

In a federally funded program at the Illinois Braille and Sight Saving School a mobility instructor provided a week of follow-up training in the home community of each mobility student. Difficulties encountered are listed, including changed motivation on part of some students.

2628. Jackson, Ned T., & Hartong, Jack R. Orientation and mobility instruction and sequential school for the blind. Unpublished final report. Jacksonville: Ill. Braille and Sight Saving School, 1968.

2629. James, Grahame, & Armstrong, John. An evaluation of the Silva braille compass: 1—Static tests. *New Beacon*, Sept. 1974, Vol. 58, No. 689, pp. 225–29, illus. Part 2 in Oct. 1974.

Study report and evaluation of this new mobility device—5 Ss, 1 male, aged 11.5 to 15.9 years, tested compass. Conclusion that compass is only useful in determining gross directions. Future study indicated.

2630. James, Grahame; Armstrong, John; & Campbell, Dennys. Verbal instructions used by mobility teachers to give navigational directions to their clients. *New Beacon*, Apr. 1973, Vol. 57, No. 672, pp. 86–91.

Analysis of questionnaire replies from 21 mobility instructors surveyed for the purpose of assessing methods commonly used in presenting directions to clients.

2631. ———. An evaluation of the Silva braille compass: 2—Field trials. *New Beacon*, Oct. 1974, Vol. 58, No. 690, pp. 253–55, illus. Part 1 in Sept. 1974.

Study did not confirm usefulness of compass used in conjunction with tactual map, did confirm usefulness in reorientation when used by deliberately disoriented blind person. Implications for use as navigational aid.

2632. Juurmaa, Jyrki. On the accuracy of obstacle detection by the blind— Part 2. *New Outlook for the Blind*, Apr. 1970, Vol. 64, No. 4, pp. 104–18. Part 1, Mar. 1970, pp. 65–72.

Tests of 7 blind Ss showed Kay mobility aid effective in some areas. Mobility trainers should investigate the natural auditory capabilities of the blind.

2633. Juurmaa, Jyrki; Suonio, Kyösti; & Moilanen, Aatu. The effect of training in the perception of obstacles without vision. *Reports from the Institute of Occupational Health*, June 1968, No. 55, 37 pp.

Three visually handicapped males with no obstacle sense were trained to perceive obstacles. Rapid learning occurred.

2634. Kallman, Heinz E. Optar, a method of optical automatic ranging, as applied to a guidance device for the blind. *Proceedings of the Institute of Radio Engineers*, Sept. 1954.

A small hand-held guidance device operates on ambient light when that exceeds 1 foot-candle. Image space is explored several times per second.

2635. Kay, Leslie. A preliminary report on ultrasonic spectacles for the blind. *American Foundation for the Blind Research Bulletin 21*, Aug. 1970, pp. 91–100.

Described the device, its performance, and initial training of blind people in its use.

2636. ———. The sonic glasses evaluated. *New Outlook for the Blind*, Jan. 1973, Vol. 67, No. 1, pp. 7–11.

Précis of findings from 2 questionnaires to evaluate the ultrasonic Binaural Sensory Aid, a mobility and orientation device invented by the author. The results, although influenced by inadequacies, show that the aid achieved a high level of acceptance by both teachers and students. Only 7% of the users indicated that they did not want to keep the aid.

2637. ———. Sonic glasses for the blind: A progress report. *American Foundation for the Blind Research Bulletin 25*, Jan. 1973, pp. 25–58.

Evaluates preliminary use of the Binaural Sensory Aid for the blind. Describes and illustrates the device.

2638. ———. Sonic glasses for the blind: Presentation of evaluation data. *American Foundation for the Blind Research Bulletin 26*, June 1973, pp. 35–50.

Presents data collected from questionnaires sent to 94 blind users and 25 teachers in sensory aid training program. Notes differences between trainer and trainee responses. App. includes 88 item trainer and 169 trainee questionnaires with number of *S*s responding to each alternative given.

2639. ———. Toward objective mobility evaluation: Some thoughts on a theory. New York: AFB, 1974, 55 pp. Mimeo.

An effort to isolate and define some of the factors that might form the basis for a viable theory of mobility. The author, a professor of electrical engineering at the Univ. of Christchurch, New Zealand, developed the binaural sensor, a mobility device.

2640. ———. Orientation for blind persons: Clear path indicator or environmental sensor. *New Outlook for the Blind*, Sept. 1974, Vol. 68, No. 7, pp. 289–96.

The aim of sensory aids for blind persons that indicate the presence or absence of obstructions in the travel path is compared with the aim of possible devices that would provide more detailed information about various aspects of the environment.

2641. ———. A sonar aid to enhance spatial perception of the blind: Engineering design and evaluation. *Radio and Electronic Engineer*, Nov. 1974, Vol. 44, No. 11, pp. 605–27, illus.

Explains use and design of Binaural Sensory Aid. Includes detailed report of evaluation conducted using O & M specialists and blind and sighted *S*s in U.S., New Zealand, and Australia.

2642. Keating, William P. Mobility and orientation seminars for parents and teachers of blind children. *New Outlook for the Blind*, June 1964, Vol. 58, No. 6, pp. 183–84.

Discussion of development and content of seminars in a N.C. county. A booklet developed as a result of the meetings.

2643. ———. Peripatology in practice. *New Outlook for the Blind*, Dec. 1965, Vol. 59, No. 10, pp. 346–48.

A brief history of the evolution of the formal mobility training program.

2644. Keller, George W. *A mobility project with blind public school stu-*

dents and other selected rehabilitation clients. Final report. Baltimore: Div. of Vocational Rehab., July 1970, 20 pp.

Designed to demonstrate the value of teaching modern mobility techniques to legally blind public school students and other vocational clients beyond school age. While no new or significant results emerged, the recognition and acceptance of mobility as an area needing special attention constitutes a worthwhile achievement.

2645. Kimbrough, James A. Concerning certification of orientation and mobility specialists. *New Outlook for the Blind,* Nov. 1969, Vol. 63, No. 9, pp. 275–79.

Specialty of orientation and mobility is based on (1) a method, (2) someone to teach the method, and (3) someone to teach the teacher. Ability to teach O & M is not determined by place of training. Describes Pittsburgh Guild program and urges a graduate degree should not be a requirement for certification.

2646. Kirk, Edith C. A Mobility Evaluation Report for parents. *Exceptional Children,* 1968, Vol. 35, No. 1, pp. 57–62.

Describes report developed to aid in recognition of strengths and weaknesses in mobility of blind children.

2647. Klee, K. E. The long cane and the guide dog as mobility aids. *New Beacon,* June 1975, Vol. 59, No. 698, pp. 141–47.

Basic differences between cane and dog, advantages and disadvantages of each, differences in teaching and learning processes with each, and specific guidelines for instructors with each.

2648. Klein, Karl K.; Budd, Otis; Welch, Patti, et al. A preliminary report of a pilot study on postural balancing on tracking efficiency of blind subjects, school year 1969–70. *American Foundation for the Blind Research Bulletin 23,* June 1971, pp. 93–99.

With 39 totally blind boys, ages 9–18, as subjects, tested the heel lift procedure to balance the pelvis and spine to increase tracking efficiency in straight line walking.

2649. ———. The effect of lateral postural balancing on gait patterns of blind subjects. *American Foundation for the Blind Research Bulletin 25,* Jan. 1973, pp. 241–48.

Data suggests that lateral postural correction can increase efficiency.

2650. Kohler, Ivo. Orientation by aural clues. *American Foundation for the Blind Research Bulletin 4,* Jan. 1964, pp. 14–53, illus.

Research on the mechanisms of obstacle detection without the use of sight, especially through orientation by hearing, is summarized. Methods of training in orientation by sound are discussed. Ref.

2651. LaDuke, Robert O. An analysis of current issues and trends in orientation and mobility. *Education of the Visually Handicapped,* Mar. 1973, Vol. 5, No. 1, pp. 20–27.

Among issues are the recommendation that certification of instructors be based on competency rather than on graduation from an approved program and that many needs of the blind population are not being met.

2652. Langan, Paul J. Orientation and travel programs at residential schools.

International Journal for the Education of the Blind, Dec. 1953, Vol. 3, No. 2, pp. 218–19.

Discusses recent recognition of importance of orientation, adjustment, and travel training, student incentive, helpfulness of public school attendance. Some information on course of training at Kentucky School.

2653. Lefkowitz, Leon J. A role for the physical educator in the education of the blind. *International Journal for the Education of the Blind,* Oct. 1962, Vol. 12, No. 1, pp. 6–7.

Proposes that mobility training lies naturally within the province of the physical education dept. in residential schools.

2654. Lehon, Lester H. The relationship between intelligence and the mastery of mobility skills among blind persons. *New Outlook for the Blind,* Apr. 1972, Vol. 66, No. 4, pp. 115–18. Also in *New Beacon,* Sept. 1972.

After brief review of the literature, reports relationship between intelligence of 90 mobility students and their acquisition of mobility skills. Age range for *S*s was 17–60. Less intelligent *S*s learned more slowly, but final achievement was not a function of intelligence.

2655. Kruger, Irving J. Mobility and orientation—A symposium. III. Orientation and mobility in the vocational area. *New Outlook for the Blind,* Mar. 1960, Vol. 54, No. 3, pp. 87–90.

Discusses both orientation and reorientation, the latter in terms of both the adventitiously blind and of any blind person entering a truly new area of physical endeavor. Lists 6 O & M program goals specifically related to vocational goals, and 7 examples of program activities specifically related to reorientation.

2656. Leonard, J. Alfred. Mobility and the blind—A survey. *American Foundation for the Blind Research Bulletin 7,* Dec. 1964, pp. 1–25. Reprinted from *Medical Electronics and Biological Engineering,* 1963, Vol. 1.

A British summary of various mobility aids including recent sophisticated instrumentation. Ref.

2657. ———. Towards a unified approach to the mobility of blind people. *American Foundation for the Blind Research Bulletin 18,* Dec. 1968, pp. 1–21.

Since integration with sighted requires independent mobility, standards for mobility are suggested and the necessary cooperation of others described.

2658. ———. Modern trends in mobility. *American Foundation for the Blind Research Bulletin 19,* June 1969, pp. 73–89.

Reports survey of mobility habits and needs of about 1,500 blind in England and Wales. Describes various guidance devices and their potential usefulness to that population.

2659. ———. Studies in blind mobility. *Applied Ergonomics,* Mar. 1972, Vol. 3, No. 1, pp. 37–46.

Reviews the work of the Nottingham (England) Blind Mobility Research Unit in assessing the general situation of the blind population, analyzing the skills involved in blind mobility, insuring the availability of information about existing best method, and providing new methods to close the gap between levels of sighted and blind mobility. Several new devices and aids for the blind are described, including hand-held and head-worn ultrasonic detectors and tactual route maps with braille directions.

2660. ————. The evaluation of blind mobility. *American Foundation for the Blind Research Bulletin 26*, June 1973, pp. 73–76.

Takes position that blind mobility should be a matter of scientific and professional concern, a subject matter in its own right, achieved by collaboration between users, practitioners, inventors, designers, and researchers.

2661. Leonard, J. Alfred, & Carpenter, A. Trial of an acoustic blind aid. *American Foundation for the Blind Research Bulletin 4*, Jan. 1964, pp. 70–119, illus.

In one study, results of evaluation indicated that the aid appeared more useful in detecting obstacles than in negotiating them. A second study indicated that poor acceptance of the aid may have been due to inadequate training procedure, instruments insufficiently reliable, and low motivation.

2662. Leonard, J. Alfred, & Newman, R. C. Spatial orientation in the blind. *Nature*, 1967, Vol. 215, No. 5108, pp. 1413–14.

Concludes that whatever "difficulties congenitally blind *S*s may experience in problems of spatial orientation are more likely to be caused by lack of experience than by blindness as such."

2663. Lessard, Kevin. Orientation and mobility program. *Lantern*, June 1975, Vol. 4, No. 3, pp. 5–10.

Describes program at Perkins School for the Blind which now includes even the youngest students. Concentrates on such areas as body image, posture, gait, motor coordination, position, directionality, and spatial awareness.

2664. Levine, Helen G. *Planning to meet peripatology needs of visually handicapped pupils in a public school program.* Cincinnati: Cincinnati Public Schools, 1968, 41 pp.

An evaluation of information about and attitudes toward orientation and mobility training as they pertain to the Cincinnati Public School program for visually handicapped.

2665. Liddle, D. Cane travel: Techniques and difficulties. *American Foundation for the Blind Research Bulletin 11*, Oct. 1965, pp. 1–62.

Analyzes the answers of 100 blind individuals to a questionnaire on the problems of mobility. Results indicated that most of the blind persons relied heavily on auditory clues and all but a few always used a cane.

2666. ————. The effect of signal strength on reaction times to auditory signals in noise. *American Foundation for the Blind Research Bulletin 19*, June 1969, pp. 129–90, illus.

Differs from earlier studies of reaction time in use of background noise. Includes blind *S*s and relates findings to travel devices. Statistics and graphs.

2667. LoGuidice, Donald D. Research on a comprehensive follow-up program for mobility service. *New Outlook for the Blind*, May 1969, Vol. 63, No. 5, pp. 137–41.

With supporting statistical data, describes the procedures and results of programmed follow-up of mobility training for 91 clients.

2668. LoGuidice, Donald D., & Patton, William E. *A state-wide community-oriented mobility and orientation program in New Hampshire.* Concord: Assoc. for the Blind, 1968, 64 pp., app., illus.

Significant results in areas of designing and implementing a meaningful follow-up program. Client readiness, rural mobility, casework service, and use of a community program were found as consequence of this study. Project forms and questionnaires are included. Bib.

2669. Lord, Francis E. *Preliminary standardization of a scale of orientation and mobility skills of young blind children. Final report.* Los Angeles: Calif. State Col., 1967, 161 pp.

Mobility rating scales were developed, reliability established, and norms provided on 173 *S*s, ages 3–12.

2670. ————. Development of scales for the measurement of orientation and mobility of young blind children. *Exceptional Children*, Oct. 1969, Vol. 36, No. 2, pp. 77–81.

The construction of the scales is described, and results with 173 blind children are presented.

2671. Lord, Francis E., & Blaha, Lawrence E. *Demonstration of home and community support needed to facilitate mobility instruction for blind youth. Final report.* Los Angeles: Calif. State Col., Special Education Center, 1968, 101 pp.

In a project involving 101 blind adolescents, training in mobility was supported by parental cooperation and results analyzed.

2672. Luini, Eugene, & Ryder, James. *Mobility and orientation instruction of blind persons.* Rochester, N.Y.: Assoc. for the Blind of Rochester and Monroe Co., 1967, 78 pp.

A project description and evaluation involving blind and partially sighted individuals taught mobility and orientation by a peripatologist. Illustrates construction of the sliding cane and outlines subjects' lesson plans.

2673. McCarty, Bruce, & Worchel, Philip. Rate of motion and object perception in the blind. *New Outlook for the Blind*, Nov. 1954, Vol. 48, No. 9, pp. 316–22.

Study was undertaken to investigate the relationship between rate of motion and blind person's ability to perceive obstacles. Subject was a totally blind 11-year-old boy. For this boy, higher speeds did not impair object perception.

2674. McDonald, Edward H. Mobility-Occlusion versus low vision aids. *New Outlook for the Blind*, May 1966, Vol. 60, No. 5, pp. 157–58.

Lists and refutes most common arguments for use of occluders. Presents 3 case examples illustrating that with expert instruction residual vision is a mobility asset rather than a negative factor.

2675. Manley, Jesse. Orientation and foot travel for the blind child. *International Journal for the Education of the Blind*, Oct. 1962, Vol. 12, No. 1, pp. 8–13.

For the totally blind child, orientation requires very complete knowledge and awareness of his environment. Details what cues the child can use and how to teach him to use them. Briefly discusses leading the blind child, trailing, training for travel off-campus, and motivation.

2676. Mann, Robert W. The evaluation and simulation of mobility aids for the blind. *American Foundation for the Blind Research Bulletin 11*, Oct. 1965, pp. 93–98.

Mobility devices for the blind are considered in the light of problems faced by the user in display and assimilation of the information acquired by the instrument.

2677. Mass. Institute of Technology. *Conference for Mobility Trainers and Technologists: Proceedings.* New York: Hartford Foundation, 1968, 76 pp.

Conference held at M.I.T. in Dec. 1967 discusses specific developments in mobility aids and training for the blind. Reports action in implementation of a committee on orientation and mobility as well as on other projects.

2678. Menzel, Rudolphina. Mobility and orientation in Israel. *New Outlook for the Blind*, May 1964, Vol. 58, No. 5, pp. 157–58.

Problems relating to mobility and ways in which they are solved in Israel.

2679. Menzel, Rudolphina; Shapira, G.; & Dreifuss, E. A proposed test for mobility-training readiness. *New Outlook for the Blind*, Feb. 1967, Vol. 61, No. 2, pp. 33–40.

Presents in complete detail a form on which factors related to mobility readiness can be recorded for evaluation, as developed in Israel. Data included: Personal, medical, remaining senses, outdoor mobility as reported by client, educational, occupational, temperament, and motivation.

2680. Mich. School for the Blind. *Pre-cane mobility and orientation skills for the blind.* Lansing, Mich.: State Dept. of Education, 1965, 58 pp.

Units, activities, lesson plans, and resource materials to help elementary teachers reinforce instruction in pre-cane mobility and orientation. Bib.

2681. Mickunas, J., Jr., & Sheridan, T. B. Use of an obstacle course in evaluating mobility of the blind. *American Foundation for the Blind Research Bulletin 3*, Aug. 1963, pp. 35–54, illus.

Study to design an obstacle course with the most salient features of the real environment, and to develop techniques to evaluate the behavior of blind persons in traversing such an experimental obstacle course.

2682. Miller, Josephine. Mobility training for blind children. *New Outlook for the Blind*, Dec. 1964, Vol. 58, No. 10, pp. 305–7.

Emphasizes need for early training in mobility. Discussion of use of long cane with Hoover technique.

2683. Mills, Robert J. Orientation and mobility for teachers. *Education of the Visually Handicapped*, Oct. 1970, Vol. 2, No. 3, pp. 80–82. 1st in 4-part series. (2nd, Hill, Dec. 1970; 3rd, Hill, Mar. 1971; last, Mills, May 1971.)

This article discusses 3 areas: Body image, walking gait and stride, and posture. Also included is information on material development for classroom use in the given instances.

2684. ————. Orientation and mobility for teachers. *Education of the Visually Handicapped*, May 1971, Vol. 3, No. 2, pp. 58–59. Last in 4-part series. (1st, Mills, Oct. 1970; 2nd, Hill, Dec. 1970; 3rd, Hill, Mar. 1971.)

This article deals with environmental awareness. Three methods with values other than establishing an individual awareness activity within the classroom are included.

2685. Mills, Robert J., & Adamshick, Donald R. The effectiveness of structured sensory training experiences prior to formal orientation and mobility instruction. *Education of the Visually Handicapped*, Mar. 1969, Vol. 1, No. 1, pp. 14–21.

Forty-four blind students were given a sensory training program to develop nonvisual perceptions in small group settings to accelerate ability to learn travel skills. Comparison with a control group showed that the pretrained group had more skills and higher proficiency ratings and performance ratings after a 5-week orientation program.

2686. Mims, Forrest. Eyeglass mobility aid for the blind. *Journal of the American Optometric Association*, June 1972, Vol. 43, No. 6, pp. 673–76.

Describes an infrared mobility aid that is mounted on spectacle frames. Objects intersecting a beam of radiant energy reflect enough energy back to the receiver to trigger a threshold circuit and cause an audio tone to be transmitted to one of the blind user's ears.

2687. ———. Energy radiating mobility aids for the blind: Design considerations and a progress report on an eyeglass mounted infrared aid. *American Foundation for the Blind Research Bulletin 27*, Apr. 1974, pp. 135–58.

Reviews current research on ultrasonic and electro-optical mobility aids. Gives detailed description of development of an infrared mobility aid. Describes some technological spinoffs from the research.

2688. Miyagawa, Stephen H. My experiences with the laser cane. *New Outlook for the Blind*, Nov. 1974, Vol. 68, No. 9, pp. 404–7.

The VA conducted a 5-week training program and subsequent evaluation of the C-4 Laser Cane. Account of 1 participant's experiences in the project.

2689. Morris, Robert H. Evaluation of a play environment for blind children. *Therapeutic Recreation Journal*, 4th Quarter 1974, Vol. 8, No. 4, pp. 151–55.

An investigation to determine the effectiveness of a series of specially designed play courts in helping blind children improve their orientation and mobility skills.

2690. Murphy, Jo Anne. *How does a blind person get around?* New York: AFB, 1973, 20 pp.

Discusses orientation and mobility skills, including a brief history, ramifications of good skills, travel aids, use of other senses by blind travelers, mobility readiness for children.

2691. Murphy, Thomas J. Motivation for mobility. *New Outlook for the Blind*, May 1965, Vol. 59, No. 5, pp. 178–80.

Discusses client needs as a necessary motivation for mobility. In many, only rewarding employment can motivate independent travel.

2692. ———. Reflections on a readiness test for mobility training. *New Outlook for the Blind*, Feb. 1966, Vol. 60, No. 2, pp. 47–48.

Response to 5/65 *Outlook* article by M. Graham questions finding client sample to serve as valid basis for readiness test. Discusses problem factors: Degree of blindness, motivation, conceptual differences, age at onset.

2693. Nichos, R. H., Jr. Ultrasonic spectacles for the blind. *Journal of the Acoustical Society of America*, 1966, Vol. 40, No. 6, p. 1564.

Describes 2 recently developed sensory devices: The binaural aid, and a "small personal radar set" allowing the wearer to hear objects in his environment.

2694. O'Neill, John J.; Oyer, Herbert J.; & Baker, Donald J. Auditory skills of blinded individuals with pilot dogs. *Journal of Speech and Hearing Research*, Sept. 1958, Vol. 1, No. 3, pp. 262–67.

Study of the hearing acuity, hearing discrimination, and sound localization ability of 53 guide dog users. Those above average in their use of the dog had better hearing.

2695. Patton, William E. Research on criteria for measuring mobility readiness of adventitiously blind adults. *New Outlook for the Blind*, Mar. 1970, Vol. 64, No. 3, pp. 73–79.

In preparation of an instrument to measure mobility readiness the following were found to have a positive correlation with performance: Willingness to leave home area with a guide, realistic acceptance of visual problems, need for training, intelligence, motivation, willingness for community knowledge of blindness, acceptance of white cane, and adjustment to blindness.

2696. Peel, Jennifer C. Psychological aspects of long cane orientation training: Parts 1–4. *American Foundation for the Blind Research Bulletin 27*, Apr. 1974, pp. 159–86. Part 5 in *Bulletin 28.*

Critique of "standard training method" for mobility in Great Britain which is derived from American long cane training. On the basis of observation and several small experiments, analyzes difficulties encountered by trainees and suggests changes in methodology.

2697. ————. Psychological aspects of long cane orientation training: Part 5. *American Foundation for the Blind Research Bulletin 28*, Oct. 1974, pp. 111–24. Parts 1–4 in *Bulletin 27.*

The evaluation in a real life setting of the experimental training techniques discussed in Parts 1–4. Includes summary of entire study.

2698. Potash, Leonard. Correlates of the tactual and kinesthetic stimuli in the blind man's cane. *American Foundation for the Blind Research Bulletin 1*, Jan. 1962, pp. 117–29, illus.

Experiment to study the mechanical interactions between a blind man and his environment through the medium of the cane. Force discrimination thresholds and displacement discrimination level were measured.

2699. Randolph, Leo G. The classroom teacher speaks: Don't rearrange the classroom. Why not? A proposal for meaningful classroom mobility. *Education of the Visually Handicapped*, Oct. 1970, Vol. 2, No. 3, pp. 83–86.

Encourages rearrangement of furniture in a classroom for the blind with suggested techniques for teaching mobility skills. Four techniques for room familiarization (perimeter, door object, criss cross, object object) are provided.

2700. R.I. Assoc. for the Blind. *Final report: Mobility and orientation instruction for the blind. Project No. RD-1539.* Providence: Author, 1968, 16 pp., app.

Describes the initiation and development of mobility training for the blind residents of R.I.

2701. Richardson, Clarence V. Aids for good mobility in the blind. *International Journal for the Education of the Blind,* Oct. 1958, Vol. 8, No. 1, pp. 1–11.

Detailed discussion of cane and electronic guidance devices and of the psychological factors needed for good mobility. Ref.

2702. Richterman, Harold. Mobility instruction for the partially seeing. *New Outlook for the Blind,* Oct. 1966, Vol. 60, No. 8, pp. 236–38.

Compares mobility problems of the partially sighted client and his instructor with those of the blind client and his instructor. Negative opinion on use of occluders.

2703. Riley, Leo H.; Luterman, David M., & Cohen, Marion F. Relationship between hearing ability and mobility in a blinded adult population. *New Outlook for the Blind,* May 1964, Vol. 58, No. 5, pp. 139–41.

Study dealing with hearing and mobility concludes that there is a significant relationship between pure tone thresholds as well as speech reception thresholds and mobility. Interaural differences were also studied.

2704. Rintelmann, William; Harford, Earl; & Burchfield, Samuel. A special case of auditory localization: CROS for blind persons with unilateral hearing loss. *Archives of Otolaryngology,* Mar. 1970, Vol. 91, No. 3, pp. 284–88.

Observation of 2 clinical cases leads the authors to believe that the contralateral routing of signals (CROS) by a hearing aid provides sufficient clues to the direction of sounds to be of significant value in the mobility training of blind individuals with good hearing in only 1 ear.

2705. Robson, Howard. The dog as a mobility aid. *New Beacon,* Jan. 1973, Vol. 57, No. 669, pp. 3–6.

Discusses factors in selection of trainees to receive guide dogs, factors influencing successful dog use, figures on characteristics of the British blind population and dog users.

2706. ———. The practice of guide dog mobility in the United Kingdom. *New Outlook for the Blind,* Feb. 1974, Vol. 68, No. 2, pp. 72–78.

The Guide Dogs for the Blind Assoc. is fully described as well as the services and concessions available to guide dog owners. Standards both for applicants for dogs and for the dogs themselves are described.

2707. ———. The mobility aid that happens to suit. *New Beacon,* Dec. 1975, Vol. 59, No. 704, pp. 309–11.

General discussion of a variety of aids to mobility including long and short canes, dogs, use of the senses of smell and taste, with some evaluative comments.

2708. Rodgers, Carl T., & Voorhees, Arthur L. Some thoughts on white cane philosophy and problems. *New Outlook for the Blind,* May 1961, Vol. 55, No. 5, pp. 173–77.

History of laws governing and philosophy behind the use of the white cane.

2709. Ronayne, C. Edward. *The teacher and the orientor: The teacher's role in helping the visually handicapped student develop mobility skills.* Denver: State Dept. of Education, 1963, 10 pp.

Describes 3 modes of travel: Guide dog, sighted guide, cane. College courses in mobility training are mentioned and skills which the classroom teacher can help develop are listed.

2710. Rossi, Peter. A bibliography of orientation and mobility articles since 1964 (A provisional bibliography). New York: AFB, 1971, 49 pp. Mimeo.

Lists 570 references on above topic.

2711. Rouse, Dudley L., & Worchel, Philip. Veering tendency in the blind. *New Outlook for the Blind,* Apr. 1955, Vol. 49, No. 4, pp. 115–19.

After reviewing the literature which shows that blindfolded sighted *S*s tend to veer, describes an experiment to determine whether veering would occur in *S*s who had been blind from birth. Results from 18 *S*s show veering is present, consistent in direction for each subject, and not increased by removal of auditory or facial tactile cues.

2712. Royster, Preston M. Peripatology and the development of the blind child. *New Outlook for the Blind,* May 1964, Vol. 58, No. 5, pp. 136–38.

Outlines special needs of blind child from birth to adulthood. Emphasizes need for peripatologist at many stages of development.

2713. Rudkin, S. W. Cane travel in winter. *New Outlook for the Blind,* Jan. 1971, Vol. 65, No. 1, pp. 8–11.

Difficulties presented by winter conditions, especially the variability of conditions, are noted, and modifications in travel technique suggested.

2714. Rupf, John A., Jr. Time expansion of ultrasonic echoes as a display method in echolocation. *American Foundation for the Blind Research Bulletin 15,* Jan. 1968, pp. 1–33.

A useful mobility device should indicate presence of obstacles, locate them, and identify them. Describes experiments to investigate whether object identity information can be obtained by listening to the time expansion of the ultrasonic echoes produced by a sound source.

2715. Rusalem, Herbert. Mobility and orientation—A symposium. II. The dilemma in training mobility instructors. *New Outlook for the Blind,* Mar. 1960, Vol. 54, No. 3, pp. 82–87.

Presents critique on low standards and lack of defined qualifications for employing O & M personnel. Presents and analyzes proposals on curriculum and standards for training instructors, mobility instruction as a profession, the possibility of retaining instructors with master's degrees. Recommendations for research.

2716. Schulz, Paul J. Psychological factors in orientation and mobility training. *New Outlook for the Blind,* May 1972, Vol. 66, No. 5, pp. 129–34.

A psychologist discusses the emotional interaction between O & M instructors and students which may interfere with or facilitate learning process. Uses a Q & A format to report on an in-service training program with mobility instructors. Deals with discontinuing a student, lack of carryover from lesson to independent travel, preventing overprotectiveness, avoiding overdependence, severing a strong attachment, setting meaningful goals, and dealing with fear and anxiety.

2717. Seelye, Wilma S., & Thomas, John E. Is mobility feasible with multiply handicapped blind children? *Exceptional Children*, 1966, Vol. 32, No. 9, pp. 613–17.

Discusses the relationship of parents and teachers as well as that of self-image and independence to mobility instruction.

2718. ————. Is mobility feasible with: A blind girl with leg braces and crutches? A deaf-blind girl with a tested I.Q. of 50? A blind boy with an I.Q. of 51? *New Outlook for the Blind*, June 1966, Vol. 60, No. 6, pp. 187–90.

An additional handicap does not invariably disqualify a child from mobility training. Three case reviews, each including description of relevant technique modifications, instruction location and objectives, results.

2719. Sensory Aids Evaluation and Development Center. *Proceedings: Conference for mobility trainers and technologists.* Cambridge, Mass.: Author, 1967, 69 pp.

Conference action, suggested projects, and 10 papers. Topics include: Mobility training for children and the aged, the long cane and laser cane, the pathsounder, travel skill performance measurement.

2720. Siegel, Irwin M. The expression of posture in the blind. *International Journal for the Education of the Blind*, Oct. 1965, Vol. 15, No. 1, pp. 23–24.

To achieve fluid movement the individual requires: (1) adequate spatial orientation including a valid concept of the vertical; (2) well-conditioned postural reflex mechanisms; and (3) appropriate and accurate body awareness against which stance and motion can be patterned.

2721. ————. *Posture in the blind: The use of its determinants in the diagnosis and treatment of its problems.* New York: AFB, 1966, 39 pp.

Concludes that effective mobility in the blind is predicted upon proper dynamic posture, which is conditioned primarily by 3 influences: (1) proprioceptive spacial orientation, (2) postural reflex, (3) body image. These determinants must be considered in a program of postural education.

2722. ————. Selected athletics in a posture training program for the blind. *New Outlook for the Blind*, Oct. 1966, Vol. 60, No. 8, pp. 248–49.

Workers in the field should be concerned with the blind person's development of good dynamic posture. Ice skating, fencing, and skiing are discussed, benefits cited, and general account of method of procedure in instruction.

2723. ————. Postural compensation in the motor-handicapped blind. *New Outlook for the Blind*, Dec. 1967, Vol. 61, No. 10, pp. 328–32.

With case reports and pictures, describes posture training. Causes of malposture must be determined on an individual basis and appropriate treatment undertaken.

2724. Siegel, Irwin M., & Murphy, Thomas J. *Postural determinants in the blind. Final report.* Chicago: Ill. Visually Handicapped Institute, Aug. 1970, 113 pp.

Explores problem of malposture in the blind and its effect on orientation and travel skills. Hypothesis tested was that improvement in posture contributed to improvement in mobility. Results indicated that such a correlation exists.

2725. Silver, Frederick A. Peripatology—A new profession. *New Outlook for the Blind*, June 1962, Vol. 56, No. 6, pp. 200–02.

Discusses emergence of profession and why author thinks mobility instructors should be called peripatologists.

2726. ———. How the home teacher can help the mobility instructor. *New Outlook for the Blind*, May 1965, Vol. 59, No. 5, pp. 173–74.

Lists information needed by and goals to be attained by a mobility instructor with general implications about how home teachers can be helpful.

2727. Spittler, Margaret. Games for the development of pre-orientation and mobility skills. *New Outlook for the Blind*, Dec. 1975, Vol. 69, No. 10, pp. 453–56.

Twelve games for nursery school to junior high are described.

2728. Thomas, John E. Detroit school students evaluate mobility education program. *New Outlook for the Blind*, June 1970, Vol. 64, No. 6, pp. 182–85.

Twenty-one children were surveyed indicating favorable results in confidence and skill. Areas of concern are the basic ideas behind the program and its aims, in addition to the student reactions.

2729. Thornton, Walter. The binaural sensor as a mobility aid. *New Outlook for the Blind*, Dec. 1971, Vol. 65, No. 10, pp. 324–26.

Describes the binaural sensor, an electromechanical mobility aid for the visually handicapped. Sensor is shown to be easy to learn and use; speculates that with practice the wearer may be able to interpret the signals to the extent that he can identify objects reflected.

2730. ———. What's in a cane? *New Beacon*, June 1974, Vol. 58, No. 686, pp. 141–43.

Discusses the Typhlocane, folding canes. Gives brief history cane development and use, U.S. and United Kingdom.

2731. ———. Four years' use of the binaural sensory aid. *New Outlook for the Blind*, Jan. 1975, Vol. 69, No. 1, pp. 7–10.

Having used the aid in conjunction with the long cane, the author feels it is a successful mobility aid and environmental sensor. Various models of Mark I as well as the new Mark II were used.

2732. Thume, L., & Murphree, O. D. Acceptance of the white cane and hope for the restoration of sight in blind persons as an indicator of adjustment. *Journal of Clinical Psychology*, 1961, Vol. 17, No. 2, pp. 208–9.

Seventy-seven blind Ss were studied. The detrimental effect of hope for return of sight with its accompanying non-use of cane and poor vocational adjustment is the most significant finding of the study.

2733. Trevena, Thomas M. *The role of the resource teacher in mobility instruction.* Hayward, Calif.: Alameda Co. School Dept., 1971, 18 pp., $1.

Suggests activities a resource teacher can use to ready students for the orientation and mobility specialist. Includes suggestions of books and articles for the teacher and devices and equipment useful for the student.

2734. Twersky, V. Auxiliary mechanical sound sources for obstacle perception by audition. *Journal of the Acoustical Society of America*, 1953, Vol. 25, pp. 156–57.

Several auditory devices for obstacle avoidance by the blind are described. Preliminary results suggest that a simple high-frequency whistle yields satisfactory results.

2735. Uslan, Mark M., & Manning, Paul. A graphic analysis of touch technique safety. *American Foundation for the Blind Research Bulletin 28*, Oct. 1974, pp. 175–89.

Existing long cane techniques and their execution were analyzed by graph methods. Suggestions for improvement are given.

2736. Voorhees, Arthur. Professional trends in mobility training. *New Outlook for the Blind*, Jan. 1962, Vol. 56, No. 1, pp. 4–9.

Discusses who should teach mobility, choice of a dog or a cane, length and material for a cane, white canes. Lists minimum realistic standards for the selection of training personnel, and areas of study to be included in the curriculum.

2737. Vopata, Alvin E. Making mobility meaningful. *New Outlook for the Blind*, Apr. 1973, Vol. 67, No. 4, pp. 161–67.

Explanation of a sequential orientation and mobility curriculum at the Iowa Braille and Sight Saving School consisting of 127 lessons divided into 5 units (shown in the app.). Motivation techniques discussed. While lesson plans are quite specific, authors conclude that the plans are most effective when used flexibly and creatively in relation to individual students.

2738. Walker, Don L. Practices in teaching orientation, mobility, and travel. *International Journal for the Education of the Blind*, Dec. 1961, Vol. 11, No. 2, pp. 56–58.

In cooperation with the AAIB Mobility Workshop, the Iowa Braille and Sight Saving School conducted a questionnaire survey of mobility teaching practices in 41 residential schools and 17 day schools. Results suggest the need for better standards.

2739. Wallace, Bruce. Aberrations from improper touch techniques. *Long Cane News*, May 1972, Vol. 5, No. 1, pp. 6–11.

An outline of the various problems that arise from improper handling of the cane.

2740. Ward, Rex. Diabetics in orientation and mobility: A discussion guide concerning blind diabetics with special emphasis regarding the role of orientation and mobility specialist. *Education of the Visually Handicapped*, Mar. 1972, Vol. 4, No. 1, pp. 26–29.

Successful rehabilitation of a blind diabetic depends upon a nonprofessional orientation and mobility specialist who understands the nature and symptoms of diabetes, the emergency treatment concerning reactions, the aftereffects of a reaction, and the individual blind diabetic's physical and mental capabilities.

2741. Wardell, Kent T. Preparatory concepts of orientation and mobility training. *Education of the Visually Handicapped*, Oct. 1972, Vol. 4, No. 3, pp. 86–87.

Intended as a springboard for teachers who attempt to overcome faulty concept development in congenitally blind or partially sighted students.

Provides 120 general concepts in directionality, motion, time-distance in addition to orientation.

2742. ———. The blind walk faster. *Journal of Rehabilitation,* Mar.–Apr. 1973, Vol. 39, No. 2, pp. 23–24, 40.

Brief sample program of orientation and mobility instruction for the long cane traveler.

2743. Warren, David H., & Kocon, Joe A. Factors in the successful mobility of the blind: A review. *American Foundation for the Blind Research Bulletin 28,* Oct. 1974, pp. 191–218.

The major part of the review consists of 3 sections: Perceptual factors in mobility, with sections on body image and spatial relations; IQ and cognitive factors; and personality, social, and environmental factors. Ref.

2744. Welsh, Richard L., & Blasch, Bruce B. Manpower needs in orientation and mobility. *New Outlook for the Blind,* Dec. 1974, Vol. 68, No. 10, pp. 433–43.

Based on survey of administrators of agencies and schools serving blind persons, day-school programs, hospitals, and residential schools for other handicapped persons, the authors conclude that university-level training of orientation and mobility specialists should be expanded.

2745. Whitstock, Robert H. Mobility and orientation—A symposium. IV. Orientation and mobility for blind children. *New Outlook for the Blind,* Mar. 1960, Vol. 54, No. 3, pp. 90–94.

Includes suggestions relevant to mobility readiness, a list of 13 nonvisual cues, and discussion of the selection of travel "technique" (in this article, largely a discussion of The Seeing Eye).

2746. ———. A dog guide user speaks on mobility. *New Outlook for the Blind,* Jan. 1962, No. 56, No. 1, pp. 19–23.

Discusses some of the factors involved in preparing and referring a blind person for dog guide training. Covers some of the qualifications, techniques, and implications involved in dog guide use.

2747. Williams, Joan. Clear path our way. *St. Dunstan's Review,* Feb. 1972, No. 627, pp. 3–9.

Personal experiences in using Kay's binaural sensor and other types of mobility aids.

2748. Williamson, Donald R. Cane travel techniques. *Rehabilitation Teacher,* May 1972, Vol. 4, No. 5, pp. 3–23, & June 1972, No. 6, pp. 3–23.

A 2-part article based on personal experiences of the author, who is blind. Material is divided into 15 lessons covering simple as well as complex problems encountered in the course of daily 3-mile walks which he takes for pleasure and exercise.

2749. Wilson, Edouard L. A developmental approach to psychological factors which may inhibit mobility in the visually handicapped person. *New Outlook for the Blind,* Nov. 1967, Vol. 61, No. 9, pp. 283–89, 308.

Illustrated by 2 case reports, discusses influences inhibiting mobility in blind children, how to encourage maturation and overcome immobility; also forces inhibiting mobility in the aged blind whose integration in the community often depends upon it.

2750. Witcher, Clifford M. Electronic travel aids. *New Outlook for the Blind*, May 1955, Vol. 49, No. 5, pp. 161–65.

Describes standards of performance a travel aid should meet and several experimental forms of electronic aids matched against these standards. Predicts that a travel aid which meets those standards should be ready for testing in about 2 years.

2751. ⸻. General consideration on guidance devices. *American Foundation for the Blind Research Bulletin 7*, Dec. 1964, pp. 53–61.

Summary of the statements by a group of blind persons about problems with guidance devices. Important factors are: Maintenance, production cost, acceptable performance characteristics, and power consumption.

2752. Worchel, Philip; Byrne, Donn; & Young, Robert K. Evaluation of an obstacle detector for the blind. *Journal of Applied Psychology*, 1966, Vol. 50, No. 3, pp. 225–28.

Three series of training sessions were conducted to evaluate an obstacle detector, using 26 totally blind subjects. Results of the test are described and discussed in relation to the value of the instrument.

2753. Wycherley, R. J., & Nicklin, B. H. The heart rate of blind and sighted pedestrians on a town route. *Ergonomics*, 1970, Vol. 13, No. 2, pp. 181–92.

The heart rate of 6 matched pairs of blind and sighted *S*s were telemetered as they walked over an unfamiliar town route on 5 consecutive occasions. Results are discussed in detail in terms of the degree to which blind mobility aids reduce user stress.

2754. Yamanashi, Masao. Cane technique for the blind with hemiplegia. *Bulletin of the Tokyo Metropolitan Rehabilitation Center for the Physically and Mentally Handicapped*, 1973, pp. 9–16.

Full case report of the mobility training of a blind hemiplegic.

2755. Zetsche, Laura, & Woodcock, Charles C. Orientation-mobility and living skills workshop: An evaluative resumé. *New Outlook for the Blind*, Nov. 1964, Vol. 58, No. 9, pp. 290–92.

Discussion of a summer workshop in orientation-mobility and living skills for blind students from 11–17 who had average or better academic ability.

27. Communications: Braille, Listening, Nonverbal Communication, and Related Devices of All Types

2756. Abel, Georgie Lee, et al. *Learning through listening: Applying listening skills to the curriculum.* Sacramento: State Dept. of Education, Div. of Special Education, 1973, 68 pp., app.

Presents 4 papers and brief reports of 6 demonstrations. Topics include use of technology, reading by listening, compressed speech, listening related to classroom performance.

2757. American Foundation for the Blind. *Report of proceedings of Conference on Research Needs in Braille.* New York: Author, 1961, 100 pp.

Detailed papers on a variety of technical problems in braille, especially problems in discrimination and reading.

2758. ———. *Report of the proceedings of the Conference on Nine-Dot Braille (New York, New York, June 19, 1964).* New York: Author, 1964, 126 pp.

Includes resumé of the nine-dot braille code development, readability of the first nine-dot proposal, readability of nine-dot cell characters, and the orthographic efficiency and space saving of nine-dot braille. Also includes presentation of the mathematics of six-dot braille and expanded punctographic codes for touch reading and writing.

2759. ———. *Understanding braille.* New York: Author, 1968, 12 pp.

The raised dot system of braille—how it works, how it started, how it is read and written, and the different grades—is described, as are the other raised dot systems.

2760. American Printing House for the Blind. *Suggested activities for the development of sound localization skills.* Louisville, Ky.: Author, n.d., 18 pp.

A manual for use with the American Printing House goal indicator.

2761. ———. *Proceedings, Conference on New Processes for Braille Manufacture.* New York: Hartford Foundation, 1968, 86 pp.

Papers on new braille translation program and research at APH, math translation program, and plans for computerized braille.

2762. ———. *Key braille contraction contexts.* Louisville, Ky.: Author, 1969, 110 pp.

Lists occurrences of braille contraction sequences. Attention focused on occurrences in which syllabification, pronunciation, and meaning determine the use or nonuse of the contraction.

2763. Anderson, Gary B., & Rogers, David W. An inexpensive braille terminal device. *American Foundation for the Blind Research Bulletin 22*, Dec. 1970, pp. 111–17.

Gives details for construction of a brailler from a Model 33 teletype and of the programming needed.

2764. Apple, Marianne M. Kinesic training for blind persons: A vital means of communication. *New Outlook for the Blind*, Sept. 1972, Vol. 66, No. 7, pp. 201–8.

Defines problems in use of nonverbal communication (kinesics) by blind persons, reviews the literature, and proposes a set of gestures which might be taught. Suggests that further effort be made to explore some of the areas outlined and to create an effective training program in nonverbal communication techniques for blind persons.

2765. Ark. Enterprises for the Blind. *Syllabus and its development for instruction of communicative skills in a rehabilitation center for the blind: Final report.* Little Rock: Author, 1969, 90 pp., illus.

Project to determine what syllabus existed for teaching communicative skills in rehabilitation center for blind and to develop appropriate syllabi for these skills. Helpful to instructors in evaluating client, setting reasonable goals, interpreting progress. Syllabi included.

2766. Ashcroft, Samuel C. Programmed instruction in braille. *International Journal for the Education of the Blind*, Dec. 1961, Vol. 11, No. 2, pp. 46–50.

To reduce the stress and increase the efficiency of the braille course in a teacher preparation center, a teaching-machine-type program for learning braille was developed and a specialized text prepared. This should be useful to all who need to acquire braille skills quickly.

2767. Ball, Jay H. Synthesis of original vocal pitch in accelerated playback speech. *American Foundation for the Blind Research Bulletin 9*, Apr. 1965, pp. 23–69.

Very technical discussion of why tape recordings of speech become essentially unintelligible when greatly speeded in playback. Several schemes for improving intelligibility are suggested. Many diagrams, charts, graphs, tables. Ref.

2768. Barr, Ruth L. Developing and evaluating a simplified braille writing device. *New Outlook for the Blind*, May 1968, Vol. 62, No. 5, pp. 148–52.

To eliminate the need to write braille from right to left, a new slate and stylus were developed. Reports in detail the development and trial of this slate.

2769. Bassler, Harry. The Optacon: A personal report. *Rehabilitation Teacher*, Oct. 1973, Vol. 5, No. 10, pp. 13–16.

Description of the electronic reading device and the author's experiences in learning and using it.

2770. Beddoes, M. P. Simple reading machines for the blind. *American Foundation for the Blind Research Bulletin 9*, Apr. 1965, pp. 1–11, illus. Reprinted from *Engineering Journal*, May 1963.

Classifies reading machines as 2 types: Direct translation and letter recognition. Optophone and Argyle's Reading Machine are direct translation machines. Experimental studies are reported and limitations discussed.

2771. Berger, Allen, & Kautz, Constance. Diagnostic reading test for the blind. *Perceptual and Motor Skills,* 1967, Vol. 24, No. 3, p. 850.

Describes the first Braille Informal Reading Inventory and its value in diagnosing reading abilities of blind children.

2772. ――――. The Braille Informal Reading Inventory. *Reading Teacher,* Nov. 1967, Vol. 21, No. 2, pp. 149–52.

Presents an instrument to measure reading level, rate, and comprehension, describing it in terms of its development, research possibilities, population sample, and procedures.

2773. ――――. The Braille Informal Reading Inventory: Implications for the teacher. *New Outlook for the Blind,* May 1968, Vol. 62, No. 5, pp. 153–58.

Detailed description of a new inventory which allows the teacher to observe how far ahead of his oral reading the child's fingers are and reaction to increasingly difficult passages.

2774. Bieber, James C. Visual sensory-motor considerations in reading. *Optometric Weekly,* Dec. 1970, Vol. 61, No. 52, pp. 1153–55.

Deals with vision problems of a sensory-motor nature which should be considered in relation to reading.

2775. Bixler, Ray H., et al. *Comprehension of rapid speech by the blind, Part I.* Washington, D.C.: Office of Education, HEW, 1961, 46 pp.

Reading comprehension of blind children reading braille selections compared with comprehension of blind children who heard same selections at varied rates. Results showed that the children who listened to the recorded materials suffered no significant loss of literary comprehension through 225 wpm at the .01 level and no significant loss of scientific through 275 wpm.

2776. Bixler, Ray H., & Foulke, Emerson. Current status of research in rapid speech. *International Journal for the Education of the Blind,* Dec. 1963, Vol. 13, No. 2, pp. 57–59.

Reviews studies which show the feasibility of rapid speech from the technical point of view and user comprehension and acceptance. Outlines further needed research.

2777. Bliss, James C. Communication via the kinesthetic and tactile senses. *American Foundation for the Blind Research Bulletin 1,* Jan. 1962, pp. 89–116 + illus.

A general model for a sensory aid communication system is proposed which contains a source, sensor, processor, display, sensor channels, and user. The coding, display, and control aspects of this model are discussed in relation to communication via the tactile and kinesthetic senses.

2778. ――――. Comments on the Tobin and James paper, "Evaluating the Optacon: General reflections on reading machines for the blind." *American Foundation for the Blind Research Bulletin 28,* Oct. 1974, pp. 159–64.

Asserts that the Tobin-James evaluation was severely limited in terms of duration, amount of available equipment, number of subjects, choice of dependent variables, and motivation of the subjects.

2779. ――――, Ed. *Optacon training - teaching guidelines.* Palo Alto, Calif.: Telesensory Systems, 1973, 137 pp.

A manual aid to the training of blind persons in the use of the Optacon, a device which converts normal print into tactile form. Describes Optacon concept. Summarizes learning process. Includes sample 9-day teacher training program, sections on student factors, equipment, teaching techniques, class organization and administration, follow-up training.

2780. Bliss, James C., & Crane, Hewitt D. Tactile perception. *American Foundation for the Blind Research Bulletin 19*, June 1969, pp. 205–30, illus.

Reviews tactile neurology and initial experiments in tactile reading which led to the Optacon.

2781. Bliss, James C.; Katcher, Michael H.; Rogers, Charles H., et al. Optical-to-tactile image conversion for the blind. *IEEE Transactions on Man-Machine Systems*, 1970, MMS-11, No. 1, pp. 58–65.

Describes 2 conversion systems being developed for the blind; in one, area of printed page is translated into vibratory tactile image, while in the other information is acquired from the environment. Ultimately, 1 system with 2 sets of optics might be used.

2782. Bliss, James C., & Moore, Mary W. The Optacon reading system. *Education of the Visually Handicapped*, Dec. 1974, Vol. 6, No. 4, pp. 98–102. 1st in 3-part series. (2nd, Moore, Mar. 1975; last, Moore, May 1975.)

Describes development and mechanical and electrical aspects of Optacon; lists independent evaluations of Optacon.

2783. Bouma, H. The Philips television enlarger. *American Foundation for the Blind Research Bulletin 27*, Apr. 1974, p. 266.

Very brief report of adaptation of CCTV reading device in the Netherlands.

2784. Boyle, J.; Jacobs, W.; & Loeber, N. A Braille code for interactive terminal use. *American Foundation for the Blind Research Bulletin 27*, Apr. 1974, pp. 267–72.

Presents in chart form a proposed single-celled braille code for interactive computer terminal use. Chart also provides comparison of literary grades 1 and 2, programmer's code, and terminal Braille.

2785. Britz, Karl. The German system of contracted braille: Some critical points of view. *American Foundation for the Blind Research Bulletin 14*, Mar. 1967, pp. 95–97.

Suggests that simplification, resulting in fewer and less complex rules, would be desirable.

2786. Brodlie, James F., & Burke, John. Perceptual learning disabilities in blind children. *Perceptual and Motor Skills*, Feb. 1971, Vol. 32, No. 1, pp. 313–14.

Two hundred legally and totally blind children were observed for perceptual problems in learning to read and write.

2787. Brothers, Roy J. Learning through listening: A review of the relevant factors. *New Outlook for the Blind*, Sept. 1971, Vol. 65, No. 7, pp. 224–31.

Reviews research focused upon aural study and learning, particularly as it relates to the visually handicapped.

2788. ———. Aural study systems for the visually handicapped: Effects of message length. *Education of the Visually Handicapped*, Oct. 1971, Vol. 3, No. 3, pp. 65–70.

Segmenting stimulus materials in varied message lengths did not significantly affect comprehension or recall when Ss had equal time to complete the material.

2789. Brown, William H. Harmonic compression: Double-tempo recordings with no rise in pitch. *New Outlook for the Blind,* Oct. 1969, Vol. 63, No. 8, pp. 245–46.

Brief report of desirable results of harmonic compressor in speeding speech.

2790. Brugler, J. S., & Young, W. T. Reading aid for the blind. *Rehabilitation Teacher,* May 1970, Vol. 2, No. 5, pp. 21–27.

Considers development of reading machines for the blind focusing on a direct-translation machine with tactile output. Describes the way the machine operates.

2791. Burns, Jim. Braille: A birthday look at its past, present, and future. *Braille Monitor,* Mar. 1975, pp. 117–20.

Briefly discusses the beginning of the system 150 years ago, the present use of braille and its advantages over other systems. Author feels that braille will continue to be used and is important for a blind person's independence.

2792. Calhoun, C. Robert, et al. *San Diego Optacon project, 1971–1972, teacher's manual and student's manual.* San Diego: San Diego Unified School District, 1973, 260 pp.

Goals, objectives, procedures, and explanations are given for the 36 student lesson plans included.

2793. Cardinale, John F. Methods and procedures of braille reading. *American Foundation for the Blind Research Bulletin 26,* June 1973, pp. 171–83.

Surveyed 39 residential schools for the blind to determine braille teaching methods used with elementary school children and the children's characteristics. Report findings. Suggests many methods used are outdated.

2794. Centrum Obliczeniowe PAN. Electromechanical perforated tape reader for the blind. *American Foundation for the Blind Research Bulletin 27,* Apr. 1974, pp. 273–74.

Brief account of the first device built in Poland to enable blind persons to work as programmers.

2795. Cheadle, Geoffrey. Sensory reading aid for the blind. *American Foundation for the Blind Research Bulletin 5,* July 1964, pp. 1–30, app., illus.

An experiment to determine whether a Stenotype machine, with its activity sequence reversed, could be used as a reading machine. A number of additional modifications were shown to be necessary.

2796. Clewett, R. W.; Genensky, S. M.; & Petersen, H. E. *An X-Y platform for Randsight-Type instruments.* Santa Monica, Calif.: Rand Corp., 1971, 30 pp., illus.

Describes hand-operated mechanical device which, when used in conjunction with CCTV system, permits the partially sighted to read printed and handwritten material and to write with a pen or pencil.

2797. Cline, Carol A., & Cardinale, John F. Braille reading: A review of research. *Education of the Visually Handicapped,* Mar. 1971, Vol. 3, No. 1, pp. 7–10.

Through an historical perspective of trends, a reevaluation of present approaches to braille reading is emphasized. Cites training students to read with both hands, stressing concept and vocabulary development, and reexamining content in braille reading with emphasis on tactual and other experiences.

2798. Cooper, Franklin S. Review and summary of reading machines. *American Foundation for the Blind Research Bulletin 3*, Aug. 1963, pp. 84–93.
Reports experiments with various types of reading machines as of 1962.

2799. Council for Exceptional Children (CEC) Information Center. *Reading —aurally handicapped and visually impaired: A selective bibliography.* Exceptional Child Bibliography Series No. 666. Reston, Va.: CEC, 1974, 7 pp.
Bibliography of 38 references, with descriptors and abstracts, for the visually impaired.

2800. Craig, Ruth H. A personal approach to teaching braille reading to youths and adults. *New Outlook for the Blind*, Jan. 1975, Vol. 69, No. 1, pp. 11–19.
A 4-phase approach with emphasis on good reading skills is described in detail.

2801. Crandell, John M., Jr., & Wallace, David H. Speed reading in braille: An empirical study. *New Outlook for the Blind*, Jan. 1974, Vol. 68, No. 1, pp. 13–19.
Study of the effects of 6 days of rapid reading training and rapid reading plus recognition training on the reading rates and comprehension of blind braille-reading adults. Speeds of up to 225 wpm are feasible without significant loss of comprehension.

2802. Critchley, MacDonald. Tactile thought, with special reference to the blind. *Proceedings of the Royal Society of Medicine*, Jan. 1953, Vol. 46. Also in *Brain*, 1953, Vol. 76.
Observations on the neurological aspects of braille reading. An interpretation of observed behavior, not a research study.

2803. Cronin, Bob. A new technique using braille to teach print reading to dyslexic children. *New Outlook for the Blind*, Mar. 1972, Vol. 66, No. 3, pp. 71–74.
Suggests that braille can serve as a useful medium to teach reading to dyslexics who have impaired ability to understand and interpret visual symbols. Describes experiment with one child, where transference from the tactile to visual mode of reading started to take place in less than 4 weeks.

2804. Crowley, Francis J., et al. *A comparison of the listening ability of blind students and the listening ability of sighted students in the intermediate grades.* Bronx, N.Y.: Fordham Univ., 1965, 131 pp.
Studies conducted with 152 blind braille-reading and 152 sighted children in the intermediate grades. Makes recommendations for education and research. Cites 83 items in bib. and presents 32 tables.

2805. Dalrymple, George F. *Transcription of "In Darkness" via DOTSYS III and the BRAILLEMBOSS.* Cambridge: M.I.T., Sensory Aids Evaluation & Development Center, 1972, 23 pp.
Describes the use of DOTSYS III (a braille computer translation pro-

gram) and the BRAILLEMBOSS (a braille page printer designed to emboss braille at similar or faster rates than teletypes).

2806. ———. *Development and demonstration of communication systems for the blind and deaf/blind. Braille communication terminal and tactile paging systems. Final report.* Cambridge: M.I.T., Sensory Aids Evaluation & Development Center, 1973, 91 pp.

Describes the BRAILLEMBOSS (a braille page printer), the TACCOM (a wireless signaling device for the deaf-blind), and the PATHSOUNDER (ultrasonic mobility aid for the blind). Examples of applications are given.

2807. Daugherty, Kathryn M. Listening skills: A review of the literature. *New Outlook for the Blind,* Oct. 1974, Vol. 68, No. 8, pp. 363–69; Nov. 1974, No. 9, pp. 415–19, 21; & Dec. 1974, No. 10, pp. 460–69.

Includes 106-item annotated bibliography, annotated list of 8 tests, and list of problems that need further research.

2808. Davis, Finis E. APH announces new braille printing process: Marks 100th anniversary. *New Outlook for the Blind,* Mar. 1958, Vol. 52, No. 3, pp. 92–93.

Discusses the purpose of this process: To take advantage of the work of volunteer transcribers who make the original single, hand-transcribed paper copies.

2809. Davis, Flora. *Inside intuition: What we know about nonverbal communication.* New York: McGraw-Hill, 1973, xi + 245 pp., $7.95.

The implicit effects of blindness on communicational behavior are contained in a chapter devoted to eye behavior.

2810. Davis, Philip; Asarkof, John; & Tallman, Carter B. A closed-circuit television system as a reading aid for visually handicapped persons. *New Outlook for the Blind,* Mar. 1973, Vol. 67, No. 3, pp. 97–101, illus.

Gives brief history of CCTV. In this study, 6 of 17 patients tested with such a system could benefit from it. CCTV seems most appropriate for patients with vision of less than 10/200 and as low as 2/200, and for patients whose reading rate with their best other optical aid is less than 70 wpm.

2811. Dorf, Maxine B., & Scharry, Earl R. *Instruction manual for braille transcribing.* Washington, D.C.: Div. for the Blind, Library of Congress, 1961, xv + 125 pp.

With initial orientation to braille system, presents 19 detailed lessons on reading and writing braille.

2812. Downing, Winifred. More about rapid reading for the blind. *Braille Monitor,* June 1975, pp. 226–29.

Letter in response to Feb. 1975 article. Author's experience in course on rapid reading. While did note improvement, feels that work needs to be done to determine just what improvements can be made and how they can be brought about.

2813. Dupress, John K. Braille research and development: Progress and predictions. *International Journal for the Education of the Blind,* Mar. 1966, Vol. 15, No. 3, pp. 74–78.

Projects are described under the following headings: Computer translation of braille, special braille displays, generating embossed pictures and other graphic forms, grade 2 braille from publishing tapes, and special braille codes. Implications of research are listed. Ref.

2814. Dupress, John K., et al. *Towards making braille as accessible as print.* Cambridge: M.I.T., 1968, 20 pp.

Present state of effort to make braille available with index to more detailed material.

2815. Elms, Hazel. Short cuts in learning braille. *International Journal for the Education of the Blind,* Oct. 1959, Vol. 9, No. 1, pp. 4–9.

Describes a series of teaching methods and materials which may represent short cuts to mastering braille. Memory clues are helpful.

2816. Enc, Mitat E., & Stolurow, Lawrence M. A comparison of the effects of two recording speeds on learning and retention. *New Outlook for the Blind,* Feb. 1960, Vol. 54, No. 2, pp. 39–48.

A study of the ability to learn from listening, or the temporal contiguity factor, had implications for the preparation of recordings for the blind. Includes tables, graphs, results.

2817. Feuk, Tore. A new closed circuit television system for the visually impaired. *American Foundation for the Blind Research Bulletin 26,* June 1973, pp. 1–3.

Describes a CCTV system to scan text, providing magnification up to 50 times, and allowing for contrast reversal.

2818. Fisher, Harvey. Braille rapid reading workshop. *Rehabilitation Teacher,* Jan. 1974, Vol. 6, No. 1, pp. 31–35.

Braille instructors participated in the workshop 3 hours daily for 10 days. Resulting increase in reading speed has implications for teaching braille.

2819. Flanigan, Patrick J. Automated training and braille reading. *New Outlook for the Blind,* May 1966, Vol. 60, No. 5, pp. 141–46.

Positive results. Tables included.

2820. Flanigan, Patrick J., & Joslin, Elizabeth S. Patterns of response in the perception of braille configurations. *New Outlook for the Blind,* Oct. 1969, Vol. 63, No. 8, pp. 232–44.

With 27 residential school subjects, aged 9–17, discrimination of braille stimuli and remediation of related slow reading were studied. Extensive statistical data reports traditional and machine presentation, gains resulting from training, and potential usefulness of an automated learning device. Ref.

2821. Flowers, David M. Expansion of the intelligibility of speech by blind and sighted, nonretarded and retarded individuals. *American Journal of Mental Deficiency,* Mar. 1974, Vol. 78, No. 5, pp. 619–24.

Intelligibility of words was measured for 10 blind non-retarded, 10 blind retarded, 10 sighted non-retarded, and 10 sighted retarded *S*s in a control condition and 2 conditions of expanded speech (30 and 50%). Under the conditions of expansion, blind subjects performed significantly better than their respective sighted group.

2822. Fonda, Gerald E.; Thomas, Henry; & Schnur, Ronald N. Evaluation of closed-circuit television as an optical aid for the low-vision patient.

Transactions of American Academy of Ophthalmology and Otolaryngology, May–June 1975, pp. 468–80, illus.

Evaluation was of reading speed, endurance, comfort, and subjective reactions of client.

2823. For the blind reader—New braille machine from U.S.A. *Nursing Mirror*, Feb. 12, 1971, Vol. 132, No. 7, p. 19.

Describes braille machine using magnetic tape which raises dots on plastic belt which is then touched by blind person.

2824. Foulke, Emerson. The retention of information presented at an accelerated word rate. *International Journal for the Education of the Blind*, Oct. 1966, Vol. 16, No. 1, pp. 11–15.

To explore retention of materials presented at an accelerated word rate, a 2-factor experiment was performed in which word rate and retention interval were varied; 315 junior high school students served as Ss. No difference was found in retention of material presented at an accelerated rate and that presented at a normal rate.

2825. ———. A survey of the acceptability of rapid speech. *New Outlook for the Blind*, Nov. 1966, Vol. 60, No. 9, pp. 261–65.

Discusses and evaluates 3 methods of increasing the spoken word rate on recordings.

2826. ———. The influence of a reader's voice and style of reading on comprehension of time-compressed speech. *New Outlook for the Blind*, Mar. 1967, Vol. 61, No. 3, pp. 65–68.

To evaluate characteristics of a reader's voice which affect comprehension of accelerated speech, a 2-factor experiment varied word rate in 2 ways and oral reading factor in 3 ways. Results were negative.

2827. ———. *The comprehension of rapid speech by the blind: Part III. Final report.* Washington, D.C.: Office of Education, HEW, Sept. 1969, 168 pp.

Accounts of completed and ongoing research conducted 1964–68 on accelerated speech as substitute for the written word. Includes a review of the research methods for controlling the word rate of recorded speech, and comparison of types of speech compression.

2828. ———. Non-visual communication. A series in *International Journal for the Education of the Blind* and *Education of the Visually Handicapped*.

1. Introduction. *IJEB*, Oct. 1968, Vol. 18, No. 3, pp. 77–78.

2 & 3. The visual reading system. *IJEB*, Dec. 1968, Vol. 18, No. 4, p. 122; and *EVH*, Mar. 1969, Vol. 1, No. 1, pp. 25–26.

4, 5, 6 & 7. Reading by listening. *EVH*, Oct. 1969, Vol. 1, No. 3, pp. 79–81; Dec. 1969, Vol. 1, No. 4, pp. 120–21; Mar. 1970, Vol. 2, No. 1, pp. 23–24; May 1970, Vol. 2, No. 2, pp. 57–59.

8, 9, 10 & 11. Reading by touch. *EVH*, Oct. 1970, Vol. 2, No. 3, pp. 87–88; Dec. 1970, Vol. 2, No. 4, pp. 122–24; Mar. 1971, Vol. 3, No. 1, pp. 25–28; May 1971, Vol. 3, No. 2, pp. 55–58.

2829. ———. A comparison of harmonic compression and compression by the sampling method. *American Foundation for the Blind Research Bulletin 23*, June 1971, pp. 100–102.

Two methods of speech compression were studied with college students. Comprehension scores and supporting statistics are shown.

2830. Foulke, Emerson; Amster, Clarence H.; Nolan, Carson Y., et al. The comprehension of rapid speech by the blind. *Exceptional Children*, 1962, Vol. 29, No. 3, pp. 134–41.

"It was felt that those losses in comprehension that were statistically significant were not at all educationally important, especially when time saved in presenting material was considered."

2831. Foulke, Emerson, & Robinson, Jacques. *The development of accelerated speech as a useful communication tool in the education of blind and other handicapped children: Progress report.* Washington, D.C.: Office of Education, HEW, Feb. 1970, 42 pp.

Research institute and laboratory established as part of the compressed speech project. Reports on completed research on aural tests and the use, methods, and variables of compressed speech. In addition, a new speech compressor was utilized.

2832. Foulke, Emerson, & Warm, Joel. *The development of an expanded reading code for the blind: Interim technical report.* Louisville, Ky.: Louisville Univ., May 1967, 16 pp.

Suggests revision of braille code based on tactual identification experiment with matched groups of 24 blind and 24 sighted college students.

2833. Freiberger, Howard. Deployment of reading machines for the blind. *Bulletin of Prosthetics Research*, Spring 1971, BPR 10–15, pp. 144–156.

History of reading machines over the past 50 years with emphasis on the portable machines, prototypes of which have been developed under contracts from the VA.

2834. ———. Reading machines for the blind, the Veterans Administration, and the non-veteran blind. *American Foundation for the Blind Research Bulletin 24*, Mar. 1972, pp. 29–35.

After sketching the history of reading machine development, author indicates why there is now a great need for independent reading by some blind persons. Suggests devices which could make this a reality.

2835. Friedman, Gerald R. The closed-circuit television reading system: Fact or fiasco? *New Outlook for the Blind*, Oct. 1973, Vol. 67, No. 8, pp. 346–51.

After describing the basic principles of CCTV and its uses in low vision rehabilitation, the author provides a general critique of the system. It is concluded that the current devices do not meet the needs of low vision patients. Modifications in design are suggested.

2836. Gaitenby, Jane H. The machine conversion of print to speech: Two papers. *New Outlook for the Blind*, Apr. 1969, Vol. 63, No. 4, pp. 114–26.

Two technical papers describing (1) problems in machine conversion of print to "speech," and (2) rules for word stress analysis for conversion. Numerous charts.

2837. Garland, C. W. Methods of producing embossed material. *New Beacon*, Feb. 1972, Vol. 56, No. 658, pp. 33–35.

Brief survey of methods used at Royal National Institute for the Blind for the production of braille, Moon type, and diagrams.

2838. Garland, Harry. An experimental one-hand Optacon. *American Foundation for the Blind Research Bulletin 28*, Oct. 1974, pp. 165–68.

As the 2 hemispheres of the brain can act independently, it was felt that a 1-hand Optacon would be more effective. Three Ss, experienced in the use of the "2-hand" Optacon participated in the evaluation of the experimental model.

2839. Genensky, Samuel M. *Some comments on a closed circuit TV system for the visually handicapped.* Santa Monica, Calif.: Rand Corp., 1968, 16 pp.

Description, discussion, and evaluation.

2840. Genensky, Samuel M., et al. *An interactive CCTV system for educating partially sighted and some other types of handicapped children.* Santa Monica, Calif.: Rand Corp., 1974, 37 pp., app.

Describes use and benefits (on basis of short-term evaluation) of a highly interactive multicamera-multimonitor system permitting a resource teacher and her handicapped elementary school students to be in continuous visual communication with one another.

2841. Genensky, Samuel M.; Barak, P.; Moshin, Hubert L.; et al. *A closed circuit TV system for the visually handicapped.* Santa Monica, Calif.: Rand Corp., 1968, 22 pp., illus.

Describes an experimental system to help the visually handicapped read, write, and perform precise manual operations.

2842. ———. A closed circuit TV system for the visually handicapped. *American Foundation for the Blind Research Bulletin 19,* June 1969, pp. 191–204.

Reports experiments with early prototypes of TV reading devices. Many illus.

2843. Genensky, Samuel M.; Moshin, Hubert L.; & Petersen, Harold E. *Performance of partially sighted with Randsight I equipped with an X-Y Platform.* Santa Monica, Calif.: Rand Corp., 1973, 32 pp., illus.

Describes test used to determine how well a partially sighted subject can read and write with the help of CCTV system, Randsight I. Results for 81 Ss provided.

2844. Genensky, Samuel M.; Petersen, Harold E.; Clewett, R.W.; et al. *A double X-Y Platform for Randsight-Type instruments.* Santa Monica, Calif.: Rand Corp., 1974, 43 pp., illus.

Detailed description of double X-Y Platform to be used in conjunction with a CCTV system and substituted for the single X-Y Platform. Permits partially sighted to read printed and handwritten material and take notes on what has been read.

2845. ———. *Information transfer problems of the partially sighted: Recent results and project summary.* Santa Monica, Calif.: Rand Corp., 1975, 62 pp., illus.

Description of an experimental secretarial CCTV system that permits the partially sighted to type from printed or handwritten manuscript and a pseudocolor system. Discusses experiment concerning reading speed of normally sighted using CCTV system. Four methods for detecting visual color deficiencies.

2846. Genensky, Samuel M.; Petersen, Harold E.; Moshin, Hubert L.; et al. *Advances in Closed Circuit TV systems for the partially sighted.* Santa Monica, Calif.: Rand Corp., 1972, 88 pp., app., illus.

Reports accomplishments of Rand in CCTV systems from May 1, 1970, to Apr. 30, 1972.

2847. Germanov, M. M. Apparatus for the blind to be used in reading ordinary typographic texts (Polyphonic and tactile). *American Foundation for the Blind Research Bulletin 3*, Aug. 1963, pp. 94–104, illus.

Translated from the Russian. Techno-philosophical discussion of need for reading machines and some general principles on which they might be developed.

2848. Goldish, Louis H. *Braille in the United States: Its production, distribution, and use.* New York: AFB, 1968, 106 pp.

Outlines an approach to braille system development including the marketing approach, marketing, braille research philosophy, and the future. Cites references for each area and provides 70 exhibits.

2849. ———. The braille embosser terminal: Creating new jobs for the blind. *Rehabilitation Record*, July–Aug. 1973, Vol. 14, No. 4, pp. 4–6.

Description of the braille embosser terminal as "the braille equivalent of the tele-typewriter, computer terminal and stock ticker." Author feels that as they become available commercially they will open many additional employment fields to the blind.

2850. Goldish, Louis H., & Taylor, Harry E. The Optacon: A valuable device for blind persons. *New Outlook for the Blind*, Feb. 1974, Vol. 68, No. 2, pp. 49–56.

Results of survey of more than 100 blind users by AFB. Questions about characteristics of the user, the uses being made of the Optacon, advantages and disadvantages, reliability and training were included.

2851. Gore, George V., III. *An analysis of the effects three modes of oral presentation have on certain cognitive skills as measured by scores obtained by blind senior high school students.* Washington, D.C.: Office of Education, HEW, 1969, 8 pp.

Analyzed the results of testing blind students on normal, compressed and accelerated (57% increase) materials to determine the effect on comprehension and recall of speeding up recorded material. Conclusion that compressed form better of 2 accelerated forms and that normal speed presentation is best.

2852. ———. A comparison of two methods of speeded speech. *Education of the Visually Handicapped*, Oct. 1969, Vol. 1, No. 3, pp. 69–76.

Thirty-two blind Ss were tested to examine comprehension and recall of speeded speech. Ss divided into 2 groups—accelerated vs. compressed methods and normal vs. speeded methods, accelerated and compressed. Results indicated Ss achieved higher comprehension by listening to compressed rather than accelerated material, and all Ss will achieve higher recall scores on compressed material rather than accelerated material.

2853. ———. The effects modes of oral presentation have on certain cognitive skills. *New Outlook for the Blind*, Mar. 1970, Vol. 64, No. 3, pp. 86–88.

Study to determine if listening time of recorded material could be reduced. Accelerated and compressed speech compared to normal. Normal and compressed more effective. Further studies necessary.

2854. Graham, Milton D. *Psychological research and braille: The need for a program of research and development.* New York: AFB, 1962, 23 pp.

Suggests studies to determine effects of braille's physical properties on legibility. Discusses current technical developments and suggests needed research.

2855. ————. Psychosocial research and braille: The need for a program of research and development. *American Foundation for the Blind Research Bulletin 2,* Dec. 1962, pp. 94–114.

Describes characteristics, uses, and potential uses of braille. Suggests how its value might be enhanced by technological developments, improved instructional methods, and proposed research.

2856. Grannis, Florence. Radio reading for the blind: Open channel broadcasting. *Braille Monitor,* Apr. 1975, pp. 150–53.

Suggestions for carrying newspaper content on the air. Open channel broadcasting vs. sub-channel.

2857. Greenwood, E. The braille reading scheme: Supplementary material for the reading scheme. *Teacher of the Blind,* Winter 1974–75, Vol. 63, No. 2, pp. 32–35.

Description of the supplementary material for the new braille reading scheme developed by the Reading Scheme Sub-Committee, teachers in some schools for blind children, and Mrs. Greenwood and her Student Workshop at Doncaster College of Education in England.

2858. Grumpelt, Howard R., & Rubin, Ellen. Speed listening skills by the blind as a function of training. *Journal of Educational Research,* July–Aug. 1972, Vol. 65, No. 10, pp. 467–71.

Tests were conducted with 66 blind high school students using both the time-compressed speech method and the rapid speech method. While training improved comprehension, the degree of improvement was not great.

2859. Grunwald, Arnold P. A braille-reading machine. *American Foundation for the Blind Research Bulletin 16,* May 1968, pp. 73–78. Reprinted from *Science,* Oct. 1966.

Summary of studies of certain basic qualities of a braille reading device.

2860. Hack, Walter A. Would this method help with your transcribing problems? *International Journal for the Education of the Blind,* May 1955, Vol. 4, No. 4, pp. 72–73.

Explanation of use of prison inmates in help in transcribing braille. Growth of project. Psychological lift for inmates.

2861. Hampshire, Barry E. Tactile and visual reading. *New Outlook for the Blind,* Apr. 1975, Vol. 69, No. 4, pp. 145–54.

Based on a review of the literature on reading, concludes that both visual and tactile reading involve the same basic processes. Simplifications in the braille code and changes in the mode of presentation are suggested to improve the efficiency of braille reading.

2862. ————. Braille, language and reading: 1. Some aspects of braille and reading. *Teacher of the Blind,* Spring 1975, Vol. 63, No. 3, pp. 60–63.

Discusses possible changes in braille code, including 2 levels of difficulty.

2863. ————. Braille, language and reading: 2. Some aspects of language and reading. *Teacher of the Blind,* Oct. 1975, Vol. 63, No. 4, pp. 100–105.

Discusses relationship of psycholinguistic research to braille reading materials for beginning school years.

2864. Hanley, Leo F. A brief review of the research on braille reading. *International Journal for the Education of the Blind*, Mar. 1961, Vol. 10, No. 3, pp. 65–70.

Following brief discussion of the need for research about braille, gives current status of the field and research on composition of braille, mechanics of braille reading, instruction in braille, and tests of braille reading achievement. Suggests future areas of research needed.

2865. Harley, Randall K. *Comparison of several approaches for teaching braille reading to blind children. Final report.* Nashville: George Peabody Col. for Teachers, Sept. 1969, 35 pp.

Thirty-nine *S*s from 6 residential schools evaluated to develop and test materials to be used in a study to compare 6 approaches in teaching braille. Results indicated that phonemic braille could be used with beginning braille readers; the analytic approach appeared to function more effectively for the phonemic materials than the synthetic approach.

2866. Harley, Randall K., & Rawls, Rachel. Comparison of several approaches for teaching braille reading to blind children. *Education of the Visually Handicapped*, May 1970, Vol. 2, No. 2, pp. 47–51.

Comparison of grade 1, grade 2, and phonemic braille media in synthetic and analytical approaches.

2867. ———. Comparison of several approaches for teaching braille reading to blind children. *American Foundation for the Blind Research Bulletin 23*, June 1971, pp. 63–85, app.

Reports the field testing of materials in two braille media—grade 1 and phonemic—with 39 students in residential schools.

2868. Harris, Theodore L. Summary of investigations relating to reading. *American Foundation for the Blind Research Bulletin 6*, Oct. 1964, pp. 1–88.

Covers entire field of reading: Sociology of reading, psychology of reading, physiology of reading and the teaching of reading. Includes the very small number of studies related to reading by the blind. Ref.

2869. Hartlage, Lawrence C. Differences in listening comprehension of the blind and the sighted. *International Journal for the Education of the Blind*, Oct. 1963, Vol. 13, No. 1, pp. 1–6.

Fifty blind high school students were paired with 50 sighted students on basis of age, sex, and test scores of mental ability. Listening comprehension was tested by a prose selection presented on tape recorder. No significant differences in listening comprehension were found.

2870. Hatchley, Eric. With the Optacon—The blind can read ordinary print. *Faithfully Theirs*, Mar. 1972, Vol. 7, No. 1, pp. 12–13.

Describes the Optacon, an electromechanical aid that enables the blind to read ordinary print.

2871. Haynes, Robert L. Processing optical character recognition (OCR) output into input for braille translation. *American Foundation for the Blind Research Bulletin 24*, Mar. 1972, pp. 145–48.

Detailed procedure for converting scanner output to translation input.

2872. Heinrichs, R. W., & Moorhouse, J. A. Touch-perception thresholds in blind diabetic subjects in relation to the reading of braille type. *New England Journal of Medicine*, 1969, Vol. 280, No. 2, pp. 72–75.

There were no differences in the thresholds for light touch, light contact vibration, and 2-point discrimination between 10 sighted Ss and 10 diabetic blind Ss. Nondiabetic blind Ss showed a mean threshold for 2-point discrimination of 1.6 mm. whereas in 10 diabetic blind Ss it was 2.5.

2873. Hellinger, George O., & Berger, Arthur W. The Optiscope Enlarger: A report of initial field trials. *New Outlook for the Blind*, Nov. 1972, Vol. 66, No. 9, pp. 320–22.

Evaluation of a projection device as an optical aid.

2874. Hendrickson, Walter B. The beginnings of the braille writer. *New Outlook for the Blind*, Oct. 1955, Vol. 49, No. 8, pp. 299–304.

The early history of the braillewriter, contributions of Hall and Sieber, and ultimate production of numbers of machines by larger organizations. Ref.

2875. Hermelin, Beate, & O'Connor, N. Right and left handed reading of braille. *Nature*, June 18, 1971, Vol. 231, p. 470.

Brief description of tests of 14 blind children aged 8–10. Speed and accuracy were scored for both right and left hands in reading braille using index or center fingers.

2876. ————. Functional asymmetry in the reading of braille. *Neuropsychologia*, Dec. 1971, Vol. 9, No. 4, pp. 431–35.

Findings in tests of differences between right- and left-handed reading of braille are discussed in relation to training effects and cortical asymmetry.

2877. Hoff, Paul W. Hoff writing aid to mathematics. *International Journal for the Education of the Blind*, Dec. 1954, Vol. 4, No. 2, pp. 34–35.

New type pocket braille slate with single movement cell to make it possible to write braille characters on observed side of paper. Advantages listed.

2878. House, Roger. *A survey of braille production devices with emphasis on the planned Zoltan Braille Embosser. Interim report number 18.* Stockholm: Research Group for Quantitative Linguistics, 1970, 12 pp.

Braille production techniques including low, moderate, and high volume production are surveyed. Zoltan described as filling the need for a high speed embosser.

2879. ————. *A tentative approach to braille translation by machine. Interim report number 16.* Stockholm: Research Group for Quantitative Linguistics, 1970, 30 pp.

Goals of project to develop a braille translator to translate text into braille presented. Discussion of a new Swedish braille using a changed abbreviation scheme is described.

2880. Huckins, Arline P. Teaching handwriting to the blind student. *New Outlook for the Blind*, Feb. 1965, Vol. 59, No. 2, pp. 63–65.

Describes equipment and provides rather detailed guides for teaching handwriting as gleaned from 18 years of experience and many sources in the literature.

2881. Illinois braille reading and writing manual: Part 1—A supplementary manual for rehabilitation teachers working with the adult blind. *Rehabilitation Teacher*, Aug. 1970, Vol. 2, No. 8, pp. 3–16.

Suggestions on motivation and preparation of students, introduction to first assignments, and problems often encountered.

2882. Ingham, Kenneth R. Braille, the language, its machine translation and display. *IEEE Transactions on Man-Machine Systems*, 1969, MMS-10, No. 4, Part 1, pp. 96–100.

Outlines the trend toward automatic braille production and describes the development of a low-cost braille translation and embossing system.

2883. Irwin, Robert B. *The war of the dots.* New York: AFB, 195–, 56 pp., $2.

An excerpt from Irwin's book, *As I Saw It*, this pamphlet details the struggle to achieve a uniform braille type in the U.S.

2884. Israel, Larry. CCTV reading machines for visually handicapped persons: A guide for selection. *New Outlook for the Blind*, Mar. 1973, Vol. 67, No. 3, pp. 102–10.

The following criteria are suggested as being vitally important: Magnification, focus, reversed image, sharpness (brightness), clarity (contrast), movable viewing table, adjustable monitor (distance, height, tilt), portability, accessories, monitor selections, aesthetics, warranty and service, long-term support, and user's manual and instructions.

2885. Iverson, Lee. Time compression: Can it help the blind, or should it be left to science fiction. *International Journal for the Education of the Blind*, May 1956, Vol. 5, No. 4, pp. 78–79.

"Time compression" (compressed speech) was demonstrated to 45 older blind students who were then asked 5 questions relevant to its advantages, disadvantages, and their acceptance of it. Questionnaires and responses (generally favorable) included.

2886. Jiggetts, Hattie. When should braille be taught? *International Journal for the Education of the Blind*, Mar. 1956, Vol. 5, No. 3, pp. 70–72.

Discusses child's readiness and extent of blindness, social and personal adjustment, preschool period. Specific suggestions. Suggests that prereadiness reading material now available is helpful. Considers braille in relationship to the partially sighted.

2887. Jogues, M. Francis. Chinese braille. *International Journal for the Education of the Blind*, Oct. 1960, Vol. 10, No. 1, pp. 1–5.

Following the story of the historical development of Chinese braille, describes the complexity of the Chinese language and how this complicates use of braille. The system for adaptation of braille to Mandarin and Cantonese now seems satisfactory.

2888. Kederis, Cleves J., et al. *Training for increasing braille reading rates: Final report.* Louisville, Ky.: American Printing House for the Blind, 1964, 15 pp.

Two studies using controlled exposure devices attempted to improve braille reading in visually handicapped elementary students.

2889. ———. *Bibliography of research on braille.* Louisville, Ky.: American Printing House for the Blind, 1968, 11 pp.

A 90-item bibliography including journal articles, theses, dissertations, unpublished reports, and manuals.

2890. Kederis, Cleves J., & Nolan, Carson Y. *Braille codes pilot project 1 December 1970–31 January 1972. Final report.* Louisville, Ky.: American Printing House for the Blind, 1972, 141 pp.

A feasibility and planning study was conducted on braille code problems. A large number of problems were found which could be resolved within 3–4 years. An application for a grant to study the problems was prepared.

2891. Kederis, Cleves J.; Nolan, Carson Y.; & Morris, June E. The use of controlled exposure devices to increase braille reading rates. *International Journal for the Education of the Blind,* May 1967, Vol. 16, No. 4, pp. 97–105.

Using an experimental and control group of 15 matched Ss 2 studies were made of effects of varied pacing of reading. Such reductions in reading time as occurred were evidently effect of motivation only.

2892. Kederis, Cleves J.; Siems, John R.; & Haynes, Robert L. A frequency count of the symbology of English braille Grade 2, American usage. *International Journal for the Education of the Blind,* Dec. 1965, Vol. 15, No. 2, pp. 38–46.

A count was done of the frequency of occurrence of elements of the braille code in randomly chosen volumes at 3 grade levels. A lengthy table shows frequency of braille elements and the ink print letters saved by the contracted forms. Other findings are noted.

2893. Keeping, Don. Computer braille system. *American Foundation for the Blind Research Bulletin 29,* June 1975, pp. 213–15.

Description of the Computer Braille Service at Univ. of Manitoba which prepares texts in braille for the Manitoba Dept. of Education.

2894. Kerney, Ellen. First tidings of literary braille in North America. *International Journal for the Education of the Blind,* Oct. 1952, Vol. 2, No. 1, pp. 112–18.

In commemoration of the 100th anniversary of Louis Braille's death, article reviews the arrival of braille and circumstances and discussions leading to its use in a number of locations, including the Halifax School in Canada, the New York Institute, and the Missouri School. Bib.

2895. Krebs, Bernard. A braillist talks with resource teachers. *New Outlook for the Blind,* Apr. 1959, Vol. 53, No. 4, pp. 132–36.

Discusses attitudes and responsibilities of the resource room teacher in the day school setting, supplying books, guiding volunteers, and the importance of braille.

2896. ———. Reviewing the new braille code. *New Outlook for the Blind,* Nov. 1959, Vol. 53, No. 9, pp. 328–29.

Discussion of significant changes in the braille system.

2897. ———. *Braille in brief.* Louisville, Ky.: American Printing House, 1968, 53 pp.

Accelerated course in braille reading.

2898. ————. *Teacher's guide to braille in brief.* Louisville, Ky.: American Printing House, 1968, 9 pp.

Suggests teaching techniques to *Braille in brief.*

2899. Kuck, John H. How to build a closed-circuit television reading aid. *American Foundation for the Blind Research Bulletin 21*, Aug. 1970, pp. 49–76.

Detailed description of CCTV. Discusses equipment and design, provides dimensional drawings. Possible improvements in TV reading aids discussed.

2900. Kurzhals, Ina W., & Caton, Hilda R. *A tactual road to reading.* Louisville, Ky.: American Printing House for the Blind, 1975.

2901. Kusajima, T. *Visual reading and braille reading: An experimental investigation of the physiology and psychology of visual and tactual reading.* New York: AFB, 1974, ix + 60 pp., illus., $3.50.

Presents experiments in visual and tactile reading based on 164 students of Tokyo School for the Blind 10–23 years of age. Classical theories of visual and tactile reading are compared with experimental results and found wanting. Develops an alternative derived from Gestalt theory. Bib.

2902. Langan, Paul J. The atomic dot. *International Journal for the Education of the Blind*, Mar. 1956, Vol. 5, No. 3, pp. 49–50.

Standard English Braille Code for 25 years, but inconsistencies, irregular practices, and confusion in books and magazines. Discusses efforts of joint Uniform Braille Committee and public reaction to idea of eliminating the Capitol dot: 10 to 1 against elimination.

2903. Lauer, Harvey. Personal reading machines: How they work, what they can do. *New Outlook for the Blind*, Nov. 1969, Vol. 63, No. 9, pp. 257–61.

Describes and compares Visotoner, Visotactor, and Cognodictor with predictions of future needs and reading systems.

2904. ————. Reading aids for the blind: Information for consumers and teachers. *Braille Monitor*, Jan. 1975, pp. 1–8.

Concerns inkprint reading aids for people who cannot use optical aids or CCTV systems. Available reading devices (including the Optacon) and some current research are described and discussed.

2905. Leach, Fay. *Commercially available recorded instructional materials for the development of communication skills.* Louisville, Ky.: American Printing House for the Blind, 1970, 48 pp.

A reference aid for teachers of the visually handicapped. Materials are grouped in categories: Communication programs, listening skills, phonics, speech, language concepts, spelling, teacher training, evaluated materials. Price, name of producer, and brief description of each item are given.

2906. Leavitt, Glenn S. *Oral-aural communications (OAC): A teacher's manual.* Springfield, Ill.: Charles C Thomas, 1974, 125 pp., app., $8/cloth, $5.95/paper.

Part One is an introduction to the subject; Part Two deals specifically with teaching OAC skills to visually impaired individuals, including listening and reading skills and working with blind persons using various kinds of equipment.

2907. Library of Congress, Div. for the Blind and Physically Handicapped. *Aids for handicapped readers.* Washington, D.C.: Author, Div. for the Blind and Physically Handicapped, Sept. 1972, 18 pp.

Provides information on approximately 50 reading and writing aids such as low vision aids, aids for holding a book, and sound reproducers. Listings usually include item name, brief nonevaluative description, manufacturing company, order number, and prices.

2908. ———. *Closed circuit television systems for the visually handicapped.* Washington, D.C.: Author, Dec. 1974, 4 pp. Reference circular.

Lists systems currently available including name and address of manufacturer and price. Also short list of articles about CCTV.

2909. Liechty, Howard M. New York Point: 1868–1963. *New Outlook for the Blind,* Mar. 1964, Vol. 58, No. 3, pp. 78–80.

History of a now defunct system of touch reading.

2910. Longini, Richard L. Spelltalk: A new approach to reading machine output for the blind. *American Foundation for the Blind Research Bulletin 24,* Mar. 1972, pp. 153–57.

Progress report on a reading device which produces 1 sound for each printed letter.

2911. Lorimer, John. A progress report on research on reading tests for the blind. *International Journal for the Education of the Blind,* May 1961, Vol. 10, No. 4, p. 116.

British research with Schonell's Silent Reading Test R3 used 333 blind children to provide standards.

2912. Lowenfeld, Berthold, & Abel, Georgie Lee. *Methods of teaching braille reading.* San Francisco: San Francisco St. Col., 1967, 113 pp.

To determine the status of braille reading instruction in 1965, 382 questionnaires were sent to residential schools and local classes for blind children, and 200 blind students from 4th and 8th grades with the sole handicap of visual acuity of 5/200 or less were administered the STEP and SAT tests and otherwise studied. Results include significant difference in reading rate between 8th-grade blind children, favoring those in public schools.

2913. Lowenfeld, Berthold; Abel, Georgie Lee; & Hatlen, Philip H. *Blind children learn to read.* Springfield, Ill.: Charles C Thomas, 1968, 185 pp. (rev. 1974.)

Discusses results of questionnaires on braille instruction and of questioning 200 students on personal characteristics. Compares comprehension of blind and sighted children. Includes history of Louis Braille and his system, discussion of reading readiness, teacher's role, special problems. Ref.

2914. Lucas, Jerrine M. Teaching machine in braille. *International Journal for the Education of the Blind,* May 1961, Vol. 10, No. 4, pp. 125–26.

Exact instructions for making a "Scrambled Book" which represents both fun and learning material in reading.

2915. McBride, Vearl G. Explorations in rapid reading in braille. *New Outlook for the Blind,* Jan. 1974, Vol. 68, No. 1, pp. 8–12.

Report of a July 1972 workshop in which techniques were developed through a series of exercises involving the rapid scanning of each page, using 1 or both hands and from 1 to 6 fingers. Speed increased from an average of 138 wpm to 710.

2916. MacKenzie, Clutha. *World Braille usage.* Paris: UNESCO, 1953, 172 pp. (Distributed by Columbia Univ. Press, New York).

Uses a very complete history of the development of braille as the universal script for the blind as framework for advancement of the philosophy of "World Braille." A book by an expert braillist for other expert braillists, but not a practical guide for writing braille.

2917. McLain, Julie R. A comparison of two methods of producing rapid speech. *International Journal for the Education of the Blind,* Dec. 1962, Vol. 12, No. 2, pp. 40–42.

Reports an experiment to compare comprehension by 7th grade pupils of speech that was compressed 46% by each of 2 methods, 1 a pitch-altering method and the other a sampling technique. The sampling group scored 6% higher than did the pitch-altering group.

2918. McLaughlin, W. J. Reading attainment of blind and partially-sighted children. A comparative study. *Teacher of the Blind,* Spring 1974, Vol. 62, No. 3, pp. 98–106.

Two tests were used in a school in the United Kingdom. 12 blind students (age 7–11 to 12–10) were given the same tests in braille as were given in inkprint to 31 partially sighted students (age 6–10 to 12–7). No significant differences were found between test scores of blind and partially sighted suggesting that the 2 could be educated in the same class without detriment.

2919. Margach, Charles B.; Reynolds, Robert A.; & Wallace, Dennis J. Some characteristics of electronic magnification systems. *Optical Journal and Review of Optometry,* Aug. 1975, Vol. 112, No. 15, pp. 16–21.

Report of study of use of CCTV by 6 low-vision patients. Use evaluated in terms of total magnification achieved, developed product of the electronic magnification, and the optical magnification used.

2920. Maris, Jeanette. *Learning to use braille.* Louisville, Ky.: American Printing House for the Blind, 1953.

Twenty lessons providing a logical sequence for teaching braille grade 2.

2921. Mass. Institute of Technology. *Conference on new processes for braille manufacture.* New York: Hartford Foundation, 1967, 25 pp.

Summarizes conference on braille production and services, primarily equipment ready for use; discusses specific production methods, problems, and cost of distribution and future projects.

2922. Mehr, Edwin B.; Frost, Alan B.; & Apple, Loyal E. Experience with closed-circuit television in blind rehabilitation program of the Veterans Administration. *Bulletin of Prosthetics Research,* Spring 1974, BPR 10-21, pp. 54–68. Reprinted from *American Journal of Optometry* and *Archives of American Academy of Optometry,* June 1973.

Report on study of 40 Ss, 28 of which were recommended for loan of a CCTV reading and writing system. VA program included screening, examination, evaluation, comparison with optical aids, training and subsequent follow-up of the 40 veterans.

2923. Melen, Roger D., & Meindl, James D. Electrocutaneous stimulation in a reading aid for the blind. *IEEE Transactions on Bio-Medical Engineering*, Jan. 1971, Vol. BME-18, No. 1, pp. 1–3.

Investigations conducted at Stanford Univ. indicate that electrocutaneous stimulation is not practical as a replacement for the tactile stimulation now used in the Optacon reading aid.

2924. Mich. Dept. of Education. *An exploration in braille speed reading: Report and evaluation of the McBride Institute in Michigan.* Lansing: Special Education Services, 1975.

Analyzes the Fourth Braille Speed Reading Institute, held July 1973.

2925. Mich. State Univ. Automated braille system (Autobraille). *American Foundation for the Blind Research Bulletin 19*, June 1969, pp. 231–33.

Describes a system with 2 aspects: (1) generation of tapes for storage of braille-transducing signals and (2) conversion of tape signals to tactile-reading display.

2926. Mick, David E., & Hittinger, Gerard N. An inexpensive, universal braille (UNIBRL) output device. *American Foundation for the Blind Research Bulletin 24*, Mar. 1972, pp. 158–60.

Detailed description of device for computer programmers.

2927. Millar, Susanna. Effects of tactual and phonological similarity on the recall of Braille letters by blind children. *British Journal of Psychology*, 1975, Vol. 66, No. 2, pp. 193–201.

Results of a study of 48 severely blind children show that tactual similarity produced recall decrements by Ss able to be tested under set sizes of up to 5 items, while phonological similarity produced recall decrements by Ss testable under set sizes of 5 and 6 items.

2928. Miller, Geraldine. The teaching of Braille reading. *International Journal for the Education of the Blind*, May 1955, Vol. 4, No. 4, pp. 69–71.

With emphasis on the importance of the teacher and the methods, discusses and suggests solutions for problems in the first few months of teaching braille.

2929. Miller, William H., & Porter, Jeffrey E. "Read it. Say it fast." The use of Distar Instructional Systems with visually impaired children. *Education of the Visually Handicapped*, Mar. 1973, Vol. 5, No. 1, pp. 1–8.

Describes instructional program for language and reading skills with precise behavioral objectives. Useful for large print and braille readers with possible benefits, through transfer of training, in other areas.

2930. Minn. State Services for the Blind and Visually Handicapped. The Radio Talking Book Network. *Rehabilitation Teacher*, June 1971, Vol. 3, No. 6, pp. 23–30.

Describes a program which uses the second sub-carrier of an FM radio station to broadcast reading materials to blind persons. Procedures for loaning receivers, copyright concerns, costs and operation of equipment are summarized.

2931. Misbach, Dorothy L. A reading program for little blind children. *New Outlook for the Blind*, Sept. 1954, Vol. 48, No. 7, pp. 218–22.

Know the child and his background well, adapt with imagination, evaluate reading readiness, train the other senses, and make books as attractive as possible. As reading develops, keep the child working at his own ability level.

2932. Moore, Mary W., et al. *Professional preparation of teachers of reading with the Optacon.* Pittsburgh, Pa.: Pittsburgh Univ., Dept. of Special Education and Rehabilitation, 1973, 70 pp., app.

Presents a guide used in a series of 2-week summer institutes on teaching Optacon use. Includes discussion of Optacon development, operation, and course outline, detailed instructions to teachers.

2933. Moore, Mary W., & Bliss, James C. The Optacon reading system. *Education of the Visually Handicapped*, Mar. 1975, Vol. 7, No. 1, pp. 15–21. 2nd in 3-part series. (1st, Bliss, Dec. 1974; last, Moore, May 1975.)

Describes the individual's use of the Optacon.

2934. ———. The Optacon reading system. *Education of the Visually Handicapped*, May 1975, Vol. 7, No. 2, pp. 33–39. 3rd in 3-part series. (1st, Bliss, Dec. 1974; 2nd, Moore, Mar. 1975.)

Theoretical analysis of the cognitive process involved in reading with the Optacon.

2935. Morris, June E., et al. *Aural study systems for the visually handicapped. Interim progress reports: No. 9 description of the aural study system; No. 10 field trial of the aural study system.* Louisville, Ky.: American Printing House for the Blind, 1973, 81 pp.

Describes system devised to help students learn more efficiently through listening rather than reading. Concludes that students could use the system after receiving more instruction and after refinements were incorporated in the system.

2936. Morrison, Ray E. Braille embossing and transmission equipment. *American Foundation for the Blind Research Bulletin 22*, Dec. 1970, pp. 71–82.

Very technical discussion of systems for distant transmission of coded braille, page embossers, tape embossers, and semiautomatic translation of grade 1 to grade 2. Many illus. and diagrams.

2937. Muranaka, Yoshio. A closed-circuit television reading aid for the visually handicapped (trans.) *Bulletin of the Tokyo Metropolitan Rehabilitation Center for the Physically and Mentally Handicapped*, 1974, pp. 19–26, illus.

Discusses appropriate magnification and comfortable viewing distance, sharp, clear, and flickerless screen image, and ease of operation as problems to be solved and their solutions in developing CCTV for the Japanese visually handicapped.

2938. Muratov, R. C.; Alekseev, O. L.; Verbuk, M. A.; et al. Typhological systems for the use of the blind and the visually impaired in education. In Leslie L. Clark, Ed., *Proceedings of the International Congress on Technology and Blindness.* New York: AFB, 1963, pp. 189–99, illus.

Describes a variety of equipment and techniques used for conveying information, including reading printed text.

2939. Murnane, James I. Aspects of some problems relating to the transliteration of the Hausa language into braille. *American Foundation for the Blind Research Bulletin 29*, June 1975, pp. 221–25.

Brief description of Hausa-speaking population and implied extent of need for braille transliteration, current very limited use and possible problems in achieving the goal.

2940. Napier, Grace D. A writing vocabulary study relative to braille contractions to be mastered by primary level children. *Colorado Journal of Educational Research,* Feb. 1973, Vol. 13, No. 1, pp. 2–5. Also in *Education of the Visually Handicapped,* Oct. 1973.

Evaluated Dolch, Fitzgerald, Ginn, Hildreth, and Rinsland vocabularies through 3rd grade level to determine which braille contractions occur most frequently. Composite vocabulary of part-word signs and whole-word contractions developed.

2941. Nelson, Calvin C. *An exploratory study of the development and utilization of a Grade Two Braille Translator for the Honeywell 222 High Speed Braille Printer. Final report.* Los Angeles: Univ. of S. Calif., Aug. 1967, 20 pp.

Description of 3 objectives to bring the Model 222 Modified Braille Printer to full utilization: Exploration of the problems related to the development of a translator system, exploration of a system for direct input of grade 2 braille, and exploration of the needs of teachers of the visually handicapped for brailled materials.

2942. Neou, I. M., & Erwin, W. F., Jr. Electromechanical braille copier. *American Foundation for the Blind Research Bulletin 27,* Apr. 1974, pp. 305–9, illus.

Describes and provides diagrams for a machine to copy braille without heat, vacuum, special paper, master plates, etc.

2943. Newman, J. D., & Lax, Bernard. Evaluation of closed circuit TV reading systems for the partially sighted. *Journal of the American Optometric Association,* Dec. 1972, Vol. 43, No. 13, pp. 1362–66.

Four models of closed-circuit TV reading systems were evaluated for 93 partially sighted individuals. In some, reading speed improved, but patients seemed to prefer simpler aids.

2944. Nolan, Carson Y. A program of research in braille reading. *International Journal for the Education of the Blind,* Oct. 1958, Vol. 8, No. 1, pp. 18–20.

A planned research program will have 2 sections, 1 related to the processes in learning to read, the other to reading itself.

2945. ———. Audio materials for the blind. *Audiovisual Instruction,* 1966, Vol. 11, No. 9, pp. 724–26.

Study results demonstrated that blind students learned as much listening to materials communicated at word rates of 275–325 wpm as they did reading it in braille at 57–70 wpm.

2946. ———. *Reading and listening in learning by the blind: Terminal progress report.* Lousville, Ky.: American Printing House for the Blind, 1968.

Final report of several years of research on this comparison.

2947. Nolan, Carson Y., & Kederis, Cleves J. *Perceptual factors in braille word recognition.* New York: AFB, 1969, 178 pp., $3.

Description of braille and review of research including 9 research studies in full and in summary. Research topics include effects of word length, braille word recognition by normal- and low-intelligence readers, influence of contractions. App. includes stimulus words used in studies.

2948. Nolan, Carson Y., & Morris, June E. Learning by blind students through active and passive listening. *Exceptional Children*, Nov. 1969, Vol. 36, No. 3, pp. 173–81.

Compares learning achieved by blind students at different grade levels for 3 types of material presented at normal and compressed rates under conditions of active and passive listening.

2949. ———. *Aural study systems for the visually handicapped. Final report.* Louisville, Ky.: American Printing House for the Blind, 1973, 29 pp.

Reports on study and identification of behavioral and procedural factors related to efficient study through listening and development of study system using recorded texts and playback recording device. Involved 1000 visually handicapped student *S*s. Includes results, recommendations.

2950. ———. *Program for facilitating the education of the visually handicapped through research in communications: The American Printing House Aural Study System as a reference source: Interim progress report no. 1* (Project No. 23 3492; Grant No. OEG-O-73-0642). Louisville, Ky.: American Printing House for the Blind, 1974.

2951. Nolan, Carson Y.; Morris, June E.; & Kederis, Cleves J., Comps. Bibliography of research on braille. Louisville, Ky.: American Printing House for the Blind, 1971, 12 pp. Mimeo.

Approximately 130 entries including journal articles, conference reports, doctoral dissertations, masters' theses, German publications, Japanese publications, and unpublished reports. Publication dates range from 1907 to the present.

2952. Nold, Don O. Optacon reader "explores" the printed page. *Dialogue*, Winter 1973, Vol. 12, No. 4, pp. 60–62.

Description for the congenitally blind of various sizes and faces of printing types as well as numerous decorative printing devices which can be quite puzzling when discovered by an Optacon probe.

2953. Norwegian Blind Organization. *European braille conference: Papers and recommendations.* Oslo, Norway: Author, 1973, 45 pp.

Presents 7 papers given at a 1973 conference on European braille by the World Council for the Welfare of the Blind. Includes papers on uniform international technical braille notation, modern transcription and printing methods, improved international lending arrangements. Gives recommendations.

2954. Nye, P. W. An investigation of audio outputs for a reading machine. *American Foundation for the Blind Research Bulletin 10*, July 1965, pp. 1–70.

Three experiments compared a data compression to a speech-like output in a reading machine for the blind. The Multidimensional Optaphone and Parametric Artificial Talking Device were superior to the optaphone and Variable Volume Optaphone.

2955. Olson, Myrna; Harlow, Steven D.; & Williams, John. Rapid reading in braille and large print: An examination of McBride's procedures. *New Outlook for the Blind*, Nov. 1975, Vol. 69, No. 9, pp. 392–95.

Three groups (2 braille, 1 large print) significantly increased their reading rates on both formal and informal tests; no corresponding loss in comprehension as measured by formal test. Younger *S*s appeared to make greatest gains.

2956. Ondricek, Robert C.; Meehan, Frank P.; & Love, James C. A new braille medium. *American Foundation for the Blind Research Bulletin 25,* Jan. 1973, pp. 69–94.

Describes a braille production system utilizing an inkprint medium.

2957. Paske, V., & Vinding, J. The "Perfect" braille system. *American Foundation for the Blind Research Bulletin 26,* June 1973, pp. 135–38.

Discusses and compares Danish braille system developed by computer evaluation and American English braille symbology in terms of ease in use, contractions, character saving, etc.

2958. Pick, Anne D.; Thomas, Margaret L.; & Pick, Herbert L., Jr. The role of grapheme-phoneme correspondences in the perception of braille. *Journal of Verbal Learning and Verbal Behavior,* 1966, Vol. 5, No. 3, pp. 298–300.

The results of tests with 26 braille readers suggest that grapheme-phoneme correspondences function as grouping principles in the perception of braille in the same manner as has been demonstrated for the perception of print by the sighted.

2959. Potter, C. Stanley. "Tuned-in" blind people. *Rehabilitation Record,* Mar.–Apr. 1973, Vol. 14, No. 2, pp. 1–5.

Description of Minn.'s Radio Talking Book program, inaugurated in Jan. 1969.

2960. Puckett, Russell E. *Enhancement of grade 2 braille translation.* Lexington: Univ. of Ky., Col. of Engineering, Feb. 28, 1971, 15 pp.

Final report on planning study re the use of computers to translate inkprint into grade 2 braille. Brief outlines on similar work being done by others are included.

2961. Rawls, Rachel F. Use of braille and print reading materials in schools for the blind. *International Journal for the Education of the Blind,* Oct. 1961, Vol. 11, No. 1, pp. 10–14.

Presents the analysis of questionnaire responses from 41 schools concerning relationship of visual acuity to use of print, how teaching of braille and large print is handled, and visual aids available. General agreement that choice of braille or ink print is an individual problem.

2962. Rawls, Rachel F., & Lewis, Ethel E. Braille writing in schools and day classes for the blind in the United States. *International Journal for the Education of the Blind,* Dec. 1961, Vol. 11, No. 2, pp. 42–46.

Tabular data resulting from questionnaires to 71 schools and day classes show the grade level at which braille writing is introduced, apparatus used, when that equipment is introduced, and when reading is introduced. Interpretation is provided.

2963. Reading through the medium of radio. *Seer,* Summer 1975, Vol. 46, No. 2, pp. 14–16.

Briefly describes Radio Talking Library in Erie, Pa., which provides reading of daily newspaper, books, magazines, and other types of entertainment.

2964. Rex, Evelyn J. A study of basal readers and experimental supplementary instructional materials for teaching primary reading in braille. Part I: An analysis of braille features in basal readers. *Education of the*

Visually Handicapped, Dec. 1970, Vol. 2, No. 4, pp. 97–107. Part II in Mar. 1971.

Braille features in 4 basal reader series were analyzed as to use of contractions in new vocabulary. Vocabulary lists at 7 reading levels were analyzed for appearance of contractions. Tables present data. Implications of the study for teachers of the blind are discussed.

2965. ————. A study of basal readers and experimental supplementary instructional materials for teaching primary reading in braille. Part II: Instructional materials for teaching reading in braille. *Education of the Visually Handicapped*, Mar. 1971, Vol. 3, No. 1, pp. 1–7. Part I in Dec. 1970.

Describes development of experimental materials which could become basis of more extensive set of materials for blind children. Reports on pilot study to test effectiveness of materials. Suggestions are made for further use of results of analysis.

2966. Robinson, D. P. The use of closed circuit television for partially-sighted pupils. *Teacher of the Blind*, Winter 1974–75, Vol. 63, No. 2, pp. 43–46.

Description and diagram of use of closed circuit television for partially-sighted children in England.

2967. Rodabaugh, Barbara J. *Optacon: Ink print reading for the blind.* Palo Alto, Calif.: American Institutes for Research, 1974, 44 pp., free.

Reports some of the results of a study of more than 85 Optacon users across the country. Briefly describes research in other countries.

2968. Schack, Ann, et al. *Computer-translation: Grade 2 Braille from print. Final report.* Louisville, Ky.: American Printing House for the Blind, June 1969, 98 pp.

Two studies demonstrated automation to be feasible, including mathematics and scientific notation. A program abstract and discussion of the potential of the IBM 360 series are included.

2969. Schoof, Loren T., II. An analysis of Optacon usage. *American Foundation for the Blind Research Bulletin 29*, June 1975, pp. 33–50.

Categorization of users by occupation, statistical analysis of factors which affect the performance levels attained by the end of the course, and a description of how 17 people are using their Optacons on the job.

2970. Schopper, Hans. The electro-brailler: A communications device and teaching aid for the blind and visually impaired at work and in school. *American Foundation for the Blind Research Bulletin 23*, June 1971, pp. 47–49.

Describes a braille transcribing aid consisting of a transmitting braille transcriber and receiving braillewriter.

2971. Schubert, Leland. *Handbook for learning to read braille by sight.* Louisville, Ky.: American Printing House, 1968, 170 pp.

To teach sighted to read braille by sight, not touch.

2972. Scruggs, B. Q. Improving listening. *International Journal for the Education of the Blind*, Oct. 1960, Vol. 10, No. 1, pp. 31–32.

A program to test, and then improve, listening in high school seniors showed beneficial results when they went on to college.

2973. Selfridge, Oliver G. Visual pattern recognition: The problems and promise. *American Foundation for the Blind Research Bulletin 3*, Aug. 1963, pp. 105–10.

General technological discussion of principles upon which reading machines might be developed.

2974. Sensory Aids Evaluation and Development Center. *Proceedings: Braille research and development conference.* Cambridge, Mass.: Author, 1966, 82 pp.

Highly technical discussions of braille production, especially computer functions.

2975. ———. *Proceedings: Conference on new processes for braille manufacture.* Cambridge, Mass.: Author, 1968, 76 pp.

Technical papers chiefly related to computer-translated braille.

2976. Siems, John R. *A program abstract for translating inkprint into braille by computer.* Louisville, Ky.: American Printing House for the Blind, 1969, 104 pp.

Presents an approach to computer processing of inkprint into braille including input, output, storage areas, and processing steps.

2977. Silberberg, Norman E., & Silberberg, Margaret C. Reading problems in two cases of persons who are legally blind. *Slow learning child: The Australian Journal on the Education of Backward Children*, Mar. 1972, Vol. 19, No. 1, pp. 17–21.

Presents 2 cases of (1) a 15-year-old blind boy who had a possible reading problem, and (2) a 26-year-old blind man who could not learn braille but later regained enough eyesight to see print but not to read well. Implications include the altering of school assignments and expectations for a child with reading problems.

2978. Silver, Sidney L. How speech can be compressed and expanded. *DB, The Sound Engineering Magazine*, Apr. 1975, Vol. 9, No. 4, pp. 32–35.

Discusses techniques (sample-and-discard, electromagnetic, electronic) of speeding or slowing speech reproduction without distorting nuance or intelligibility.

2979. Slamecka, Vladimir; Jensen, Alton P.; Valach, Miroslav; et al. A computer-aided multisensory instruction system for the blind. *IEEE Transactions on Bio-Medical Engineering*, Mar. 1972, Vol. 19, No. 2, pp. 157–60.

Describes a multisensory conversational learning facility which permits blind to share instructions of sighted persons. In classroom he perceives blackboard graphics, while in the self-instruction mode he connects to a remote bank of materials.

2980. Sloan, Louise L. Evaluation of closed-circuit television magnifiers. *Sight-Saving Review*, Fall–Winter 1974, Vol. 44, No. 3, pp. 123–33.

This study presents information to those interested in identifying patients likely to benefit from the use of electronic real-image magnification as a supplement to, or a substitute for, virtual image magnification by an optical device. Case histories are included.

2981. Smith, Glendon C., & Mauch, Hans A. Abstract of summary report on the development of a reading machine for the blind. *Bulletin of Prosthetics Research*, Fall 1972, pp. 195–96.

Describes the development of the Cognodictor (a personal type reading machine), Visotactor A and B, Digitactor, Visotoner, and the Stereotoner (an aural direct translation reading aid).

2982. Sprung, Minnie B. *Braille book of tests.* Philadelphia: Overbrook School for the Blind, 1961, 82 pp.

Designed to provide standardization in braille testing, this manual contains a regular, graded system of presenting tests for proficiency in braille.

2983. Staack, Gerald F. A study of braille code revisions. *American Foundation for the Blind Research Bulletin 2*, Dec. 1962, pp. 21–37.

Evaluates 199 contractions of grade 2 braille according to space saved, readability, translatability. Explores mathematical theory of communications relevant to described computer program for finding contractions. Gives tables of contractions, copy and evaluation of reading test to determine receptivity to braille changes, specific recommendations. Bib.

2984. Stilwell, Robert. The Optacon, a boon to visually handicapped? *West Virginia Tablet*, Feb. 1973, Vol. 96, No. 4, pp. 18–20.

Dr. Stilwell, who is blind, relates his experiences in using the Optacon himself and in teaching others to use it.

2985. Stocker, Claudell S. Restoration of communication skills. *New Outlook for the Blind*, Dec. 1964, Vol. 58, No. 10, pp. 327–28.

Author believes all communication skills should be taught in one department and coordinated by one person. Remedial help, as necessary, should be given as well as skills to restore former level of functioning in blinded person.

2986. ———. *Methods for improvement of listening efficiency in individuals with visual impairment: Final report of project 83–R025.6, July 1, 1967–June 30, 1970.* Topeka: Div. of Services for the Blind and Visually Handicapped, 1970, 43 pp.

Presents description and evaluation of a 3-year project to develop a listening curriculum. Instructional material in 3 listening comprehension skills, and recall and retention through techniques of review.

2987. ———. Listening education: From the Kansas project. *New Outlook for the Blind*, Oct. 1971, Vol. 65, No. 8, pp. 265–70.

Summarizes program of study resulting from a 3-year project on listening education. Covers the 3 phases of instruction in the program: Preskills or listening readiness, development of listening skills, and development of recall and retention.

2988. ———. *Listening for the visually impaired: A teaching manual.* Springfield, Ill.: Charles C Thomas, 1973, 167 pp. (rev. 1974).

Presents 47 exercises, 5 story texts accompanied by 14 tests to develop listening readiness, recall, skills, and retention. Designed in 3 phases for use in classes 3 hours per week over a 17 week period.

2989. Stocker, Claudell S., & Walton, Mary J. Exploring a more efficient method of teaching braille. *New Outlook for the Blind*, May 1967, Vol. 61, No. 5, pp. 151–54.

Some reasons why older blind people have difficulty learning braille and how working immediately with grade 2 braille may help.

2990. Stromer, Walter F. Listening for learning and living. *New Outlook for the Blind*, June 1954, Vol. 48, No. 6, pp. 171–78.

Words as symbols and how attention to these symbols can enrich listening.

2991. Suen, Ching Y., & Beddoes, Michael P. Spelled speech as an output for the Lexiphone reading machine and the Spellex talking typewriter. *American Foundation for the Blind Research Bulletin 29*, June 1975, pp. 51–66.

A series of experiments were conducted to test the feasibility of using a synthesized spelled speech code as an output for both machines. All 26 synthesized letter sounds were recognizable after training. Effects of presentation speed, bandwidth, word length, and pause between words on intelligibility of spelled sentences were also investigated.

2992. Thornhill, Daniel E. Translation from monotype tape to grade 2 braille. *American Foundation for the Blind Research Bulletin 5*, July 1964, pp. 63–85, app.

A computer system has been developed for producing grade 2 braille directly from the printer's monotype tape. Provision is made for inserting additional material and correcting errors.

2993. Tobin, Michael J., et al. *Print reading by the blind: An evaluation of the Optacon and an investigation of some learner variables and teaching methods.* Birmingham, England: Univ. of Birmingham, Research Centre for the Education of the Visually Handicapped, 1973, 2 vols., 131 pp. total, illus.

2994. Tobin, Michael J., & James, W. R. Evaluating the Optacon: General reflections on reading machines for the blind. *American Foundation for the Blind Research Bulletin 28*, Oct. 1974, pp. 145–57.

An evaluation, based on 30 Ss, conducted in the United Kingdom.

2995. Tooze, F. H. *The Tooze Braille Speed Test.* Bristol, England: Col. of Teachers of the Blind, 1962.

2996. Truquet, Monique. The automatic transcription of French ink print into braille. *American Foundation for the Blind Research Bulletin 28*, Oct. 1974, pp. 169–74.

A transcription program was devised, using an IBM 7044, with programming in FORTRAN and MAP language.

2997. Turner, Michael F. Audio-tactual braille: Some lines of research. *Focus*, Dec. 1972, pp. 51–52.

Brief report on efforts in New Zealand to develop a correspondence course suitable for blind adults to use in teaching themselves braille.

2998. ———. Teaching braille to adults. *Focus*, Mar. 1973, pp. 55–61.

Summary of a report based on survey of agencies and institutions in the U.S. and Britain re current policies and practices in the teaching of braille to newly-blinded adults.

2999. Tuttle, Dean W. A comparison of three reading media for the blind: Braille, normal recording, and compressed speech. *Education of the Visually Handicapped*, May 1972, Vol. 4, No. 2, pp. 40–44.

Reading comprehension and speed studied in 104 visually handicapped students who were given a reading test in braille, by listening to normal recording and by listening to compressed speech. No difference in comprehension among the 3. Compressed speech and normal recording faster than braille.

3000. ————. A comparison of three reading media for the blind: Braille, normal recording, and compressed speech. *American Foundation for the Blind Research Bulletin 27*, Apr. 1974, pp. 217–30.

Results from 104 blind students indicated that there was no difference in comprehension among the 3 media and that braille took almost twice as long as reading by listening to normal recording and almost 3 times as long as compressed speech.

3001. Umsted, Richard G. Improvement of braille reading through code recognition training: Review of the literature and bibliography. *American Foundation for the Blind Research Bulletin 23*, June 1971, pp. 50–62.

Discusses various influences on braille legibility and possible sources of improvement.

3002. ————. Improving braille reading. *New Outlook for the Blind*, June 1972, Vol. 66, No. 6, pp. 169–77.

Evaluation of an experimental instructional procedure yields favorable results.

3003. Ward, Ted. *Automated Braille System. (Autobraille). Dissemination document no. 3.* East Lansing: Mich. St. Univ. Regional Instructional Materials Center for Handicapped Children and Youth, 1967, 5 pp.

Describes a tactile communication mode employing a tabletop instrument. Gives advantages over standard braille books in areas such as storage and production costs, telephone transmission, and the potential for library-to-user transmission.

3004. Waterhouse, Edward J. Current status of the Perkins Brailler. *New Outlook for the Blind*, Apr. 1958, Vol. 52, No. 4, pp. 139–42.

Answers some of the many questions asked, such as: Why the long delays in obtaining these machines? Could we increase capacity? Do we lack technical knowledge? Are the Braillers handmade? What of future deliveries? What about other machines? Is Howe Press sabotaging our educational program?

3005. Weihl, Carolyn. The Optacon reading program at the Monroe Public School. *New Outlook for the Blind*, May 1971, Vol. 65, No. 5, pp. 155–62.

With some supporting tabular data, details the progress of 6 totally blind students of Optacon in a day school program.

3006. Weisgerber, Robert A., et al. *Educational evaluation of the Optacon (optical-to-tactile converter) as a reading aid to blind elementary and secdary students.* Palo Alto, Calif.: American Institutes for Research, 1974, 178 pp.

Summarizes research and demonstration activities of a 2-year national study which included 112 blind students. Instructional materials were developed and empirically tested, student selection procedures were established, and the extent to which ink print reading with the Optacon can be accomplished by elementary and secondary school students was explored.

3007. Werner, Helmut; Dost, Winfried; & Seibt, Peter. Automatic translation of inkprint to braille by electronic data processing systems. *American Foundation for the Blind Research Bulletin 14*, Mar. 1967, pp. 99–108.

Reports experiments over some 2 years on automatic braille translation and closes with proposals to reform German braille.

3008. Whitby, R. Writing braille by tape. *Teacher of the Blind*, Spring 1975, Vol. 63, No. 3, pp. 64–65.

Describes experimental taping of course in grade 2 braille to "automate" teaching.

3009. Williams, M. Braille reading. *Teacher of the Blind*, Apr. 1971, Vol. 59, No. 3, pp. 103–16.

Report on a survey (in England and Wales) of reading rates at the secondary school level, comparing braille readers to sighted readers.

3010. Williams, Marcelina I. Braille vs. spelling. *International Journal for the Education of the Blind*, Dec. 1955, Vol. 5, No. 2, pp. 45–48.

Discusses effect of braille contractions on student's ability to spell properly. Discusses and explains philosophies for teaching spelling to blind: Word method, phonic method, letter by letter. Suggests combination of word method and phonic method. Examines reasons for general difficulty in spelling for blind children and offers suggestions to remedy the problem.

3011. Wise, Janet. *Touch reading—A manual for adults who want to read braille.* New York: McKay Assoc., 1954. Inkprint supplementary manual, 124 pp. Braille, 2 vols., 85 pp. ea. (rev. 1959).

Manual for the blind adult who can and will study by himself with initial aid and intermittent assistance from a sighted person who need not know braille.

3012. Woodcock, Richard W. An electromechanical brailling system. *American Foundation for the Blind Research Bulletin 21*, Aug. 1970, pp. 101–7.

Development of the Tyco-brailler, an electric braillewriter, and early instructions for its use.

3013. Woodcock, Richard W., & Bourgeault, Stanley E. The Colorado Battery of Braille Skill Tests. *New Outlook for the Blind*, Oct. 1962, Vol. 56, No. 8, pp. 283–84.

Cites need for standardized braille test. Describes two sets of tests (battery of 12) to be standardized in a project by C.S.C. and HEW, and discusses standardization procedure.

3014. ———. *Construction and standardization of a battery of braille skill tests.* Greeley: Colo. State Col., 1964, 118 pp.

Development and standardization of 2 tests of braille mastery for grade 2 literary code and Nemeth code for mathematical notation.

3015. Zickel, Virgil E., & Hooper, Marjorie S. The program of braille research. *International Journal for the Education of the Blind*, May 1957, Vol. 6, No. 4, pp. 79–86.

Interest in the technical and mechanical aspects of braille production led to a project to improve the quality of braille printing, standardize production methods, and reduce costs. Reports on 6 separate but coordinated projects in U.S. and Great Britain.

3016. Ziegel, Helen, & Ostendorff, Margaret E. Why make braille more difficult for beginners? *International Journal for the Education of the Blind*, June 1953, Vol. 2, No. 4, pp. 182–83.

Presents reasons for preferring grade 1½ braille over grade 2 as a medium for teaching beginning reading, despite the fact that this practice is contrary to the trend.

28. Other Technology and General Reviews of Technology

3017. American Academy of Ophthalmology and Otolaryngology. Symposium: Prosthetic aids for the blind. *Transactions*, Sept.–Oct. 1974, Vol. 78, No. 5, pp. 711–46.

The 78th Annual Meeting of the AAOO, held Sept. 1973, discusses the use of prosthetic aids, instead of visual methods, in performing visual tasks.

3018. Ashcroft, Samuel C., & Harley, Randall K. The visually handicapped. *Review of Educational Research*, 1966, Vol. 36, No. 1, pp. 75–92.

A review of the space age and related technological advances as reflected in research and development contributions to the area of the visually handicapped, particularly those related to mobility and communication.

3019. Bach-y-Rita, Paul. Neurophysiological basis of a tactile vision-substitution system. *IEEE Transactions on Man-Machine Systems*, 1970, MMS-11, No. 1, pp. 108–10.

Describes instrumentation produced and results obtained with the tactile vision-substitution system (TVSS). Some of the neural mechanisms underlying the system's design are noted.

3020. Bach-y-Rita, Paul, et al. A tactile vision substitution system. *American Journal of Optometry and Archives of American Academy of Optometry*, 1969, Vol. 46, No. 2, pp. 109–11.

Developed a prototype of a tactile television system in which a television camera image is projected onto the skin of the back by means of vibrating electromechanical stimulators.

3021. Bach-y-Rita, Paul; Scadden, Lawrence A.; & Carter, Collins C. *Tactile Television System*. San Francisco: Smith-Kettlewell Institute of Visual Sciences, 1975, 81 pp., app.

Development of TVSS: Neurophysical basis, training techniques for blind subjects, and findings from perceptual and psychophysical investigations. Educational and employment field tests; usefulness to rehabilitation and social service workers.

3022. Beurle, R. L. Electronic aids for blind people. *American Foundation for the Blind Research Bulletin 14*, Mar. 1967, pp. 123–32. Reprinted from *British Journal of Psychology*, 1951.

Reports British research on guidance devices and reading aids, comparisons, field tests, and recommendations.

3023. Bisbee, Margaret K. Binaural sensory aid: Editor's report. *Rehabilitation Teacher*, Oct. 1973, Vol. 5, No. 10, pp. 17–21.

Description of the evaluation and testing of "Ultronic spectacles." About 100 blind persons in the U.S. have taken part in training sessions although the device is still in the preproduction stage.

3024. Black, William L. An acoustic pattern presentation. *American Foundation for the Blind Research Bulletin 16*, May 1968, pp. 93–132, app., illus.

Design and evaluation of a device to display acoustically the motion of a point in a plane. Experiments investigated *S*'s ability to follow small motions, fast motions, make judgments of position, and read letters.

3025. The blind in the age of technology: A public discussion. *New Outlook for the Blind*, Sept. 1970, Vol. 64, No. 7, pp. 201–18.

Discusses computer translation of braille, communication systems, mobility devices, compressed speech and reading devices. Detailed comments are presented.

3026. Bliss, J. C., Comp. *A bibliography on tactile displays.* New York: AFB, Nov. 1969, 24 pp., $2.

Bibliography covering interrelations among bioengineering, psychophysiology, and neurophysiology when attention is directed to the processes involved in information transfer across the skin.

3027. Budinger, Thomas F. Electrical stimulation of the visual apparatus. *American Foundation for the Blind Research Bulletin 16*, May 1968, pp. 133–40, illus.

Presents a survey of pertinent facts and progress in indirect electrical stimulation of the visual cortex in hope this phosphene approach might aid the visually impaired.

3028. Clark, Leslie L. The International Congress on Technology and Blindness: Summary report. *New Outlook for the Blind*, Mar. 1963, Vol. 57, No. 3, pp. 83–90.

General discussion of usefulness of an international congress. General areas considered, such as, sound recording and reproduction, adapted and special purpose devices.

3029. ———. The International Research Information Service. *New Outlook for the Blind*, Mar. 1964, Vol. 58, No. 3, pp. 85–89.

Tells of International Survey of technical devices and research techniques still in progress. Some developed hardware was not practical. Some basic research was never translated into something that could be used practically. Vast increase in amount of data is seen. Found areas in which more work is necessary.

3030. ———. Seminar Report: Information services for the visual sciences and related areas. *American Foundation for the Blind Research Bulletin 28*, Oct. 1974, pp. 1–18.

Report on a 2-day meeting which discussed problems with existing information services, needs and possible solutions, although setting only modest goals for the immediate future.

3031. ———. Research resource needs for the future. *New Beacon*, Jan. 1975, Vol. 59, No. 693, pp. 1–5. 1st of 2-part series.

Following introduction reviewing research accomplishments of the past decade, provides a combination of philosophical and practical comments which could become guidelines for research of the next decade; different consumers prefer different aids so there is no single solution, technologists and consumers need to understand each other better, and a central source of funding is needed.

3032. ————. Research resource needs for the future. *New Beacon,* Feb. 1975, Vol. 59, No. 694, pp. 29–33. 2nd of 2-part series.

Reviews technology gains, such as the difficulty in producing at reasonable cost devices for which demand is small, suggests possible allocation of resources for developing and providing devices, and makes a number of hopeful guesses about future technological developments.

3033. ————. Research resource needs for the future. *New Outlook for the Blind,* Feb. 1975, Vol. 69, No. 2, pp. 49–61.

Overview of the past, present, and future of research and development related to severely visually impaired persons. Ref.

3034. ————, **Ed.** *Proceedings of the International Congress on Technology and Blindness: Volume I: Man machine systems and Plinary session.* New York: AFB, 1963, 513 pp., $4.

Papers by various authors on man-machine systems including those dealing with: Mobility and mobility devices, direct translation and recognition reading machines, and indirect access to the printed page through braille, braille modifications, talking books and tapes.

3035. ————. *Proceedings of the International Congress on Technology and Blindness: Volume II: Living systems.* New York: AFB, 1963, 316 pp., $4.

Deals primarily with the nature of visual impairment and with the compensatory use of the remaining sensory channels. Includes papers on the mechanisms of seeing and the characterization of sight, the utilization of remaining sensory channels, theories and models of visual repair, and electroencephalograms of visually handicapped children.

3036. ————. *Proceedings of the International Congress on Technology and Blindness: Volume III: Sound recording and reproduction and Adapted and special purpose devices.* New York: AFB, 1963, 384 pp., illus., $4.

Presents 12 papers dealing with present status and future development of the talking book, booth disc recordings, and other tape recordings in the U.S. and other countries. Emphasis is primarily practical, but a few experimental devices are included.

3037. ————. *Proceedings of the International Congress on Technology and Blindness: Volume IV: Catalog appendix.* New York: AFB, 1963, 152 pp., $4.

International annotated catalog lists special purpose and adapted devices for the visually handicapped in the following areas: Braille duplication, education, household, personal, recreational, and· vocational.

3038. ————. *Proceedings of the Symposium on Research in Blindness and Severe Visual Impairment.* New York: AFB, 1964, 113 pp.

Account of proceedings of symposium held to stimulate further coordination of effort and dissemination of information between ophthalmologists and those from other disciplines who are engaged in research on visual impairment.

3039. ————. *International catalog of aids and appliances for blind and visually impaired persons.* New York: AFB, 1973, 224 pp., $2.

This 1st international compilation of aids and appliances in serial production from all over the world contains more than 1100 items. Listings for each item include name, manufacturer's or distributor's complete address, price, availability, and description. Will be revised and expanded periodically.

3040. Clark, Leslie L., & Holopigian, N. Charles. International survey of technical devices. *New Outlook for the Blind,* June 1961, Vol. 55, No. 6, pp. 216–19.

Authors, planning a report to an international conference in 1962 on technical devices, discuss source of problems in development of devices and request information.

3041. ————. European technology in problems of blindness. *New Outlook for the Blind,* Dec. 1961, Vol. 55, No. 10, pp. 340–46.

Overview of European technology in field of blindness focussing on (1) adapted devices, (2) sound recording and reproduction, (3) complex man-machine systems, and (4) living systems. Small amount of information relating to other areas of the world.

3042. Collins, Carter C. Tactile television: Mechanical and electrical image projection. *IEEE Transactions on Man-Machine Systems,* 1970, MMS-11, No. 1, pp. 65–71.

The system which is described in detail demonstrates the feasibility of communicating pictorial information through the skin. A tactile television system permitted blind *S*s to determine the position, size, shape, and orientation of visible objects and to track moving targets.

3043. Corp, Stephanie P., & Elliott, Richard R., Jr., Eds. Braille terminals. *Time-Sharing Today,* Oct. 1972, Vol. 3, No. 7, pp. 1–2.

Describes 3 terminal systems which enable blind persons to participate in interactive time-sharing computer activities. Comments by users emphasize the job opportunities opened by the systems.

3044. Cozman, Latif M. On the possibility of an entirely extracranial visual prosthesis. *American Foundation for the Blind Research Bulletin 29,* June 1975, pp. 1–7.

The stimulation of the visual cortex via extracranial electrodes is possible, at least in theory. Suggests that through appropriate correlation of the functions of alpha rhythms and the characteristics of brain cells it would be possible to build a visual prosthesis.

3045. Dalrymple, George F. Sensory aids at the Massachusetts Institute of Technology (MIT) Sensory Aids Evaluation and Development Center. *American Foundation for the Blind Research Bulletin 27,* Apr. 1974, pp. 11–32.

Describes development and application of the Braillemboss, TAC-COM, and the Pathsounder, 3 sensory aids for deaf and deaf-blind persons.

3046. ————. The braille computer terminal: Its applications in employment. *New Outlook for the Blind,* Jan. 1975, Vol. 69, No. 1, pp. 1–6, 10.

The production of braille simultaneously with print from a Teletype opens more jobs to appropriately trained blind persons. Explains use by a mathematician, a systems programmer, a taxpayer service rep., and a newscaster. Glossary.

3047. ————. An electromechanical numeric braille display: A familiar tactile representation of electrically encoded digital signals. *American Foundation for the Blind Research Bulletin 29*, June 1975, pp. 149–52, illus.

Description of the system. Enables blind person to meet restrictions placed on first-class radio telephone license by FCC and can be interfaced with almost any electronic instrument with digital binary coded decimal outputs.

3048. Davall, P. W., & Gill, J. M. A method for the comparative evaluation of visual and auditory displays. *American Foundation for the Blind Research Bulletin 29*, June 1975, pp. 9–21, illus.

Describes a method for comparing various displays and illustrates its use.

3049. Diespecker, D. D. Vibrotactile learning. *Psychonomic Science*, 1967, Vol. 9, No. 2, pp. 107–8.

An experiment was conducted with a group of sighted and a group of blind *S*s. Vibrators, Sherrick type, were placed at 5 body loci. A modification of the Howell system was used for encoding signals. No significant differences were found between the amounts of information transmitted in the 2 groups.

3050. Downey, Gregg. What a piece of work is Man. Restoring function to the disabled. *Modern Healthcare*, Aug. 1974, Vol. 2, No. 2, pp. 47–50.

Discusses prosthetics in general and bionic eye and laser canes for blind specifically.

3051. Dufton, Richard, Ed. *Proceedings of the International Conference on Sensory Devices for the Blind.* London: St. Dunstan's, 1967, 477 pp.

Conference held in 1966 includes papers on international evaluation and research of sensory aids for visually handicapped mobility and reading.

3052. Dupress, John K. Research, development and evaluation of sensory aids for the blind, *New Outlook for the Blind*, Mar. 1967, Vol. 61, No. 3, pp. 79–84. Also in Proceedings of the American Optometric Assoc. Conference on Aid to the Visually Limited, 1966.

Describes a number of past and current efforts to develop a useful direct translation (reading) machine. Alternatives are more effective production of braille, sound recording and compressed speech. Describes other instrumentation research and the importance of evaluation of sensory aids.

3053. Edwards, John L. An experimental investigation to determine whether the reading of color by transforming hues into audiofrequencies will affect the anxiety level of the visually handicapped. *American Foundation for the Blind Research Bulletin 17*, July 1968, pp. 5–81, app.

It was possible to teach a sample of blind students to distinguish colors with a colorscope, an electronic instrument designed for this study; however, anxiety was heightened.

3054. Fish, Raymond M. Visual substitution systems: Control and information processing considerations. *New Outlook for the Blind*, Sept. 1975, Vol. 69, No. 7, pp. 300–304.

Examines some functions of human and animal visual systems in order to define qualitatively and quantitatively the characteristics of an ideal sensory aid. Three types of substitution systems are discussed: Tactual display systems, audio display systems, and those involving direct stimulation of the brain. Ref.

3055. Fish, Raymond M., & Beschle, Richard G. An auditory display capable of presenting two-dimensional shapes to the blind. *American Foundation for the Blind Research Bulletin 26*, June 1973, pp. 5–18.

Describes tests on method of using sound to present 2-dimensional pictures of patterns to blind *S*s from 9 to 56 years of age.

3056. Fonda, Gerald. Bioptic telescopic spectacles for driving a motor vehicle. *Archives of Ophthalmology*, Oct. 1974, Vol. 92, pp. 348–49.

Brief report on an optical aid which has enabled persons with impaired vision to obtain licenses in some states—Mass., N.H., Calif., Maine, N.C.; and Fla.

3057. Foulke, Emerson. A language of the skin. *New Outlook for the Blind*, Jan. 1963, Vol. 57, No. 1, pp. 1–3.

Discusses communication by means of electrical stimulation of the skin and the task of providing suitable hardware. Promising research is underway.

3058. ———. Communication by electrical stimulation of the skin. *American Foundation for the Blind Research Bulletin 17*, July 1968, pp. 131–40.

A communication system using as signals simultaneously stimulated locations of the skin shows some promise.

3059. ———. Computer services for the blind. *Braille Monitor*, May 1972, pp. 207–10.

Description of the ARTS (Audio Response Time-Sharing) System developed at M.I.T. System utilizes a time-sharing computer to perform a wide variety of services for blind users.

3060. ———. Report of the Perceptual Alternatives Laboratory for the period July 1, 1972–June 30, 1973. *American Foundation for the Blind Research Bulletin 27*, Apr. 1974, pp. 277–301.

Reports activities and plans for developing perceptual alternatives for the blind. Discussion of such developments as the talking dictionary, print-to-speech transducers, a multisensory test of conceptual ability, tangible displays, computer services, etc.

3061. ———. Report of the Perceptual Alternatives Laboratory for the period July 1973–June 1974. *American Foundation for the Blind Research Bulletin 29*, June 1975, pp. 157–86.

Account of research projects of the laboratory which has its major concerns in acquiring information by listening and acquiring information by touch. Research also being done on the perceptual basis for mobility.

3062. Freiberger, Howard. Problems and accomplishments in sensory aids for the blind. *Transactions of the New York Academy of Sciences*, 1965, Vol. 27, No. 4, pp. 414–21.

Current problems in prosthetic development are delineated and some new mobility aids and reading machines are described.

3063. Geldard, Frank A. Body English. *Psychology Today*, Dec. 1968, Vol. 2, No. 7, pp. 43–47.

The skin is a relatively good organ for the reception of communicative signals. Perhaps the blind will be able to use their skin to "read."

3064. George, Faye. Verbatim reporting by means of oral stenography. *New Outlook for the Blind*, Mar. 1953, Vol. 47, No. 3, pp. 78–80.

Describes Dictavox (sometimes called Stenomask) and how it is used for court reporting.

3065. Gibson, Robert H., Comp. *Electrical stimulation of the skin—A selected bibliography.* New York: AFB, 1967, 23 pp., $2.

Lists 284 selected works—primarily journal articles but including some books and several theses. Items date from 1891 through 1967.

3066. Gill, J. M. Auditory and tactual displays for sensory aids for the visually impaired. *American Foundation for the Blind Research Bulletin 29*, June 1975, pp. 187–96.

Survey of nonvisual digital displays based on questionnaires circulated in Aug. 1973. Main features of 27 items, from foreign as well as U.S. sources, are given.

3067. ———. Non-visual computer peripherals. *American Foundation for the Blind Research Bulletin 29*, June 1975, pp. 197–212.

Survey of devices in production, or under development, based on questionnaires circulated in May 1974. Thirty-three items from foreign as well as U.S. sources. Selected bib. on use of computers by visually impaired included.

3068. Goldish, Louis H. The severely visually impaired population as a market for sensory aids and services: Part one. *New Outlook for the Blind*, June 1972, Vol. 66, No. 6, pp. 183–90, illus. Part two in Sept. 1973.

Presents the findings of the 1st stage of an intensive review of sensory aids conducted by AFB. Gives estimates of the visually impaired population in specific categories such as number of persons, age, visual ability, and major activity.

3069. Goldish, Louis H., & Marx, Michael H. The visually impaired as a market for sensory aids and services: Part two—Aids and services for partially sighted persons. *New Outlook for the Blind*, Sept. 1973, Vol. 67, No. 7, pp. 289–96, illus. Part one in June 1972.

Description of partially sighted population, low vision care, and range of low vision aids, optical (lens systems and electro-optical systems) and nonoptical (large print and misc.). Includes discussion of the need for aids and service, low vision care, and large print books. Encourages effort to increase public awareness of the partially sighted.

3070. Goldstein, Hyman. The need for sensory devices market research. *American Foundation for the Blind Research Bulletin 3*, Aug. 1963, pp. 66–71.

Argues that, in relation to the need for sensory devices, there is also need for (1) data on the size and demographic characteristics of the consumer population, (2) information on the minimum sensitivity required for effective use of devices utilizing specific modalities, and (3) controlled studies of the use of the selected devices by a panel of the blind.

3071. Guarniero, G. Experience of tactile vision. *Perception*, 1974, Vol. 3, No. 1, pp. 101–4.

The author, who is a doctoral candidate in philosophy and who is congenitally blind, describes his experiences during a 3-week training course with the Tactile Vision Substitution System, undertaken to give him some access to the concept of visual space.

3072. Hambrecht, F. T. The current status of visual prostheses. *American Journal of Ophthalmology*, July 1973, Vol. 76, No. 1, pp. 161–63.

Brief report on continuing experiments concerning electrical stimulation of the visual cortex.

3073. Jackson, John S., Ed. *Proceedings: 1973 Carnahan Conference on Electronic Prosthetics*. Lexington: Univ. of Ky., 1973, 133 pp., illus.

Prosthetics in general. Sections on reading and mobility aids for the blind: Transicon, sterotoner, C-5 laser cane, and tape recording retrieval techniques.

3074. Lauer, Harvey. Sensory aids for the blind: Are they automatic bonus or needed tools? *Education of the Visually Handicapped*, Dec. 1971, Vol. 3, No. 4, pp. 111–15.

Discusses need, availability, and development of sensory aids for the blind. Suggestions made concerning what blind persons and professionals can do to stimulate the development, production, and adoption of sensory aids.

3075. Lindberg, Bengt, & Hook, Olle. Telephone number dialing device for severely handicapped persons. *Scandinavian Journal of Rehabilitation Medicine*, 1973, Vol. 5, No. 4, pp. 183–85.

Describes device for physically, visually, or aurally handicapped persons, and use of same.

3076. Magill, Arthur N. The blind in the age of science. *New Outlook for the Blind*, Mar. 1970, Vol. 64, No. 3, pp. 89–91.

Discusses the impact of modern technological advances on the blind. Mention of research on a visual prosthesis and computer work with braille printing.

3077. Mann, Robert W. Sensory aids for the handicapped. *American Foundation for the Blind Research Bulletin 25*, Jan. 1973, pp. 193–204.

Proposed by the Subcommittee on Sensory Aids of the U.S. National Academy of Engineering is a long-term plan for the development and provision of sensory aids for the blind and deaf.

3078. ⸺. *Technology and human rehabilitation: Prostheses for sensory rehabilitation and/or sensory substitution*. New York: Academic Press, 1974, 144 pp., illus. Reprinted from *Advances in Biomedical Engineering*, 1974, Vol. 4.

Demography of sensory loss. Organization of literature on sensory aids. Details latest development in braille, Optacon, computer speech, mobility aids, sense substitution, psychophysical research, and practical application of results. Ref.

3079. Mass. Institute of Technology. *Accomplishments, administrative structure, and activities of the Sensory Aids Evaluation and Development Center. Annual report*. Washington, D.C.: Social Rehabilitation Admin., 1967, 30 pp.

Review of activities of the Center including work on: Compiled speech output for the DOTSYS Information System, monotype reader, braille embosser, folding canes, pathsounder, Perkins brailler, evaluation of braille, speeded hearing and experimental demonstration, the development of length concept of blind children.

3080. ————. *Final report to Social Rehabilitation Administration, Department of Health, Education, and Welfare.* Cambridge, Mass.: Author, 1970, 89 pp.

Technical report on braille codes, brailling devices, automated braille, mobility and orientation devices, and communication devices for deaf-blind.

3081. ————. *Harvard-MIT Rehabilitation Engineering Center: Progress and activities, February 1, 1973 to April 30, 1974.* Cambridge, Mass.: Author, 1974, 51 pp.

Reports of ongoing research in stimulation of afferent pathway for communication and control, development of creative technological aids. Advancements in employment opportunities for blind.

3082. Mims, Forrest. Sensory aids for blind persons. *New Outlook for the Blind,* Nov. 1973, Vol. 67, No. 9, pp. 407–14.

Reviews travel aids, electronic reading machines, and vision substitution systems. Discusses the future prospects for sensory aids in light of marketing problems, interest (and disinterest) of large companies in such research, and present levels of funding.

3083. National Academy of Sciences. *Sensory aids for the blind.* Washington, D.C.: VA, 1967, 57 pp.

Problems of providing sensory aids discussed as well as report of the status of direct translation and recognition reading machines and mobility aids. Evaluation of reading machines and mobility devices, introduction or deployment of new devices or techniques, and recommendations for a long-range program also considered.

3084. ————. *Evaluation of sensory aids for the visually handicapped.* Washington, D.C.: National Academy of Sciences—National Research Council, 1972, 194 pp.

Presents 11 papers evaluating mobility and reading aids beginning to be tested and distributed. Aids include the VA-Bionic Laser Cane, Optacon, and the Kay Binaural Sensor.

3085. New hope for the blind . . . substitute vision system. *Nursing Mirror,* Mar. 2, 1973, Vol. 136, No. 9, p. 40.

Describes Tactile Vision Substitution System. Translates TV images into tactile stimulation of abdomen. Progress correlates with manual dexterity not intelligence.

3086. Philips, John A., & Seligman, Peter M. Two instruments for the blind engineer. Part I: A braille-reading digital multimeter. *American Foundation for the Blind Research Bulletin 27,* Apr. 1974, pp. 187–203.

New model includes both a tactile digital output and an auditory continuous output device. Presents evaluative comments by a user.

3087. ————. Two instruments for the blind engineer. Part II: An auditory oscilloscope. *American Foundation for the Blind Research Bulletin 27,* Apr. 1974, pp. 204–16.

Describes design and construction of an auditory substitute for the tactual cathode ray oscilloscope (CRO). Presents evaluative comments by a user.

3088. ———. Portable "seeing eye." *Science Digest,* May 1972, Vol. 71, No. 5, pp. 86–87.

Brief description of the latest version of the "Vision Substitution System" developed by Bach-y-Rita and Collins.

3089. Rand Corp. The Rand Corporation strikes again. *Hearing and Speech Action,* Jan.–Feb. 1975, Vol. 43. No. 1, p. 16.

Statements from Rand's report "Improving services to handicapped children" are summarized regarding visually and aurally handicapped children. Reviews report recommendations.

3090. Ritter, Charles G. Operations research. *New Outlook for the Blind,* June 1954, Vol. 48, No. 6, pp. 188–92.

Discusses purposes and usefulness of various appliances for the blind. Pictures of raised-line drawing kit, micrometer, and auditory circuit analyzer with braille dial.

3091. ———. *Technical research and blindness; Some recent trends and developments.* New York: AFB, 1956, 40 pp.

A description and evaluation of modern scientific achievements in aids for the blind.

3092. ———. Spending and research. *New Outlook for the Blind,* Feb. 1956, Vol. 50, No. 2, pp. 56–58.

Broad discussion of determining which inventors have good ideas for appliances for the blind and how to reward them since sales will rarely be in large enough quantity for profit.

3093. Scadden, Lawrence A. Recent advances in sensory technology for the blind. In George Attleweed, et al., Eds., *Sensory disabilities study group report.* Calif. Conference on Rehabilitation, Oct. 8–10, 1974. n.p., n.d., pp. 85–92.

Discusses optical-to-auditory translation devices, devices to translate visual images to vibrations, electronic mobility aids, and information storage and retrieval devices.

3094. ———. The Tactile Vision Substitution System: Applications in education and employment. *New Outlook for the Blind,* Nov. 1974, Vol. 68, No. 9, pp. 394–97.

The TVSS allows for the free use of the hands at the same time that the machine is in use thus widening applicability. It converts the visual image from a narrow-angle television camera to a tactual image on a display of vibrators placed against the abdomen of the blind person.

3095. Schneps, Jack A., Proj. Dir. What's new in electronic arts for the visually and auditorially handicapped. New York: Institute for Research and Development in Occupational Education, 1974, iv + 50 pp. Mimeo. Conference Material #74–7.

Detailed equipment description, including price, of products shown at the Electronics Aid Exhibit, New York, May 1974.

3096. Sensory Aids Evaluation and Development Center. *Evaluation and development of sensory aids and devices.* Cambridge, Mass.: Author, 1967, 86 pp., app., illus.

Achievements, administrative structure, and scope of activities of Sensory Aids Evaluation and Development Center, M.I.T., are described.

3097. Sterling, Theodor D. Report on progress in the development of visual prostheses. *New Outlook for the Blind*, Feb. 1970, Vol. 64, No. 2, pp. 41–45.

Discusses exploratory work based on the technique of electrical stimulation of visual cortex inducing phosphenes, experimental implantation done by Brindley & Donaldson, composition and construction of an electrode array, use of small computers, 4 components of a visual prosthesis system, and information exchange from conferences.

3098. Sterling, Theodor D., et al., Eds. *Visual prosthesis: The interdisciplinary dialogue.* New York: Academic Press, 1971, 382 pp.

Technical investigation of the potential of visual prosthesis and evaluation of available knowledge and techniques for construction of same by physiologists, neurologists, neurosurgeons, bioscientists, digital logicians, and specialists in miniaturized circuits.

3099. Topaz, Jeremy M. A photo stylus for mechanical sensing of images. *American Foundation for the Blind Research Bulletin 5*, July 1964, pp. 31–61, illus.

Preliminary study of a system to convert a 2-dimensional visual pattern into a pattern of forces which is sensed by a stylus moved about in the display. A television camera scans the image, and samples of the video signal are compared.

3100. Vaughan, Herbert G., Jr., & Schimmel, Herbert. Feasibility of electrocortical visual prosthesis. *American Foundation for the Blind Research Bulletin 21*, Aug. 1970, pp. 1–47.

The psychophysiological aspects of a useful prosthesis are examined and some of the biophysical factors in cortical stimulation are discussed.

3101. Webster, Frederic A. Active energy radiating systems: The bat and ultrasonic principles: Acoustical control of airborne interceptions by bats. *American Foundation for the Blind Research Bulletin 3*, Aug. 1963, pp. 134–99.

Unusually detailed report on the bat-moth encounter procedure with many pictures and diagrams. Ref.

3102. Welch, John R. A psychoacoustic study of factors affecting human echolocation. *American Foundation for the Blind Research Bulletin 4*, Jan. 1964, pp. 1–13.

Review of echolocation in lower animals and man is followed by an explanation of the use of a sound pulse generator and of the human ear to locate reflections of objects in the sound field. Four innovations needed in system before it can be effective in providing orientation and mobility assistance. Ref.

3103. Wexler, Abraham. A multipurpose sensory aid for the blind: Report on a field trial 1965-66. *American Foundation for the Blind Research Bulletin 15*, Jan. 1968, pp. 71–101.

Describes an audible conductance indicator for use in science classes. Diagrams and illustrations. Uses and evaluations by professionals given.

3104. White, Benjamin W. Perceptual findings with the vision-substitution system. *IEEE Transactions on Man-Machine Systems,* 1970, MMS-11, No. 1, pp. 54–58.

Reports the initial evaluation of a system for converting an optical image into a tactile display.

3105. ———. Psychological factors in the evaluation of sensory aids. In Proceedings of the Conference on New Approaches to the Evaluation of Blind Persons. New York: AFB, 1970, pp. 59–67. Mimeo.

An overall view and statement of opinion of the psychological factors involved in the evaluation of sensory aids for the blind. More than braille, the long cane, and the guide dog are discussed.

3106. White, Benjamin W., et al. Seeing with the skin. *Perception and Psychophysics,* 1970, Vol. 7, No. 1, pp. 23–27.

Evaluation of a system for converting an optical image into a tactile display to determine its value as a visual substitution system. Acquisition of skill with device was similar for blind and sighted *Ss.*

3107. Witcher, Clifford M. Physics without sight. *Physics Today,* Dec. 1954.

The problem in making physics data available to the blind is one of adapting measuring instruments into tactile and/or audible data. The author sees no limit to the adaptability of physical measuring devices for use of the blind.

3108. Witcher, Clifford M., & Washington, L. Echo-location for the blind. *Electronics,* Dec. 1954.

Describes 2 new types of sound projectors used as obstacle detection devices.

3109. Zimmerman, David R. Shall we have seeing aids for the blind? *Rehabilitation Teacher,* May 1970, Vol. 2, No. 5, pp. 3–19.

Reviews Brindley's work in the development of artificial sight for the blind using electrodes implanted in the brain. Also discusses vibrating tactile stimulators, the use of computers and light spot programs, an amauroscope, which uses facial nerves to carry signals to the brain, and reading machines.

29.   Deaf-Blind

3110. Alonso, Lou, Comp. *Directory of regional centers and educational programs providing services to deaf/blind children and youth in the United States (including Puerto Rico and the Virgin Islands).* East Lansing: Mich. State Univ., Feb. 1974, 30 pp.

Lists over 200 programs and services.

3111. American Assoc. of Workers for the Blind. *Contemporary papers, Volume II: The deaf/blind.* Washington, D.C.: Author, 1967, 40 pp.

Entirely about the deaf-blind, has 2 sections: (1) A portion of the Vocational Rehabilitation Amendments of 1967, with related testimony and House and Senate reports; (2) papers on rubella by Edward J. Waterhouse, Berthold Lowenfeld, & James F. Garrett.

3112. American Foundation for the Blind. *Training and employment of deaf-blind adults: Report on a workshop held in New York City, February 6–9, 1956.* New York: Author, 1956, 32 pp.

Committee studied specific vocational goals for "that group of blind individuals whose hearing loss is so severe that they cannot follow connected discourse through the ear, even with maximum amplification."

3113. ———. *Register of adult deaf-blind people in the United States, July 1, 1967.* New York: Author, 1967, 2 pp.

Listings by state and age group. State totals given.

3114. ———. *The preschool deaf-blind child.* New York: Author, 1969, 8 pp.

For parents of deaf-blind preschoolers.

3115. American Foundation for the Blind & National Study Committee on Education of Deaf-blind Children. *Workshop for teachers of deaf-blind children.* New York: AFB, 1956, 35 pp.

Report deals primarily with teaching methods, experience training, language development, and speech development.

3116. Bergman, Moe. Rehabilitating blind persons with impaired hearing. *New Outlook for the Blind,* Dec. 1959, Vol. 53, No. 10, pp. 351–56.

Describes the special program designed by Industrial Home for the Blind, Office of Vocational Rehabilitation, and AFB involving: A survey of hard-of-hearing blind persons served by IHB, assembling a staff to serve them, designing and constructing special physical facilities and electronic and mechanical equipment, establishing clinical services, and planning research.

3117. Berhow, Byron. Deaf-blind children—Their educational outlook. *New Outlook for the Blind,* Dec. 1963, Vol. 57, No. 10, pp. 399–401.

History of development of education of deaf-blind. General concepts and specific techniques useful in dealing with these handicaps.

3118. Berkan, Bill. Boarding homes for deaf/blind children. *Bureau Memorandum,* Summer 1973, Vol. 14, No. 4, pp. 27–30.

A 3-week pilot project involved 3 children, boarding house parents who were professionals in child development, and the natural parents, to provide support to the parents and exchange information about the child's behavior.

3119. Bernstein, Phyllis F., & Roeser, Ross J. *Audiological assessment of deaf-blind children.* Dallas: Callier Hearing & Speech Center, 1972, 15 pp.

Describes audiological assessment of 50 children, aged 16 months to 14 years, in an outpatient setting. Gives etiological factors, and testing procedures including play audiometry, conditioned orientation audiometry, behavior observation audiometry. Discusses results such as indication that 22% had normal-range hearing sensitivity with language and speech development precluded by other problems.

3120. Best, Anthony. Deaf-blind children and adolescents. *New Beacon,* Jan. 1974, Vol. 58, No. 681, pp. 2–6.

Discusses training program at British residential school for 10 deaf-blind children. Includes description of typical activities emphasizing self-care and communication, summary of admissions procedure.

3121. Bettica, L. J. Attitudes influencing the interaction between professional workers and deaf-blind clients. *New Outlook for the Blind,* Apr. 1966, Vol. 60, No. 4, pp. 120–22.

Summarizes 8 major findings of questionnaire survey of workers' attitudes. Makes 2 recommendations to remedy some attitudes which have unfortunate influence on positive interaction potential.

3122. Bettica, L. J., & Newton, David. Great expectations for deaf-blind people. *New Outlook for the Blind,* Jan. 1966, Vol. 60, No. 1, pp. 27–30.

Through discussion of IHB's Anne Sullivan Macy Service, stresses often overlooked undernurtured potentials of deaf-blind people.

3123. Bisno, Ann. An application of the Piaget model to a curriculum for deaf-blind children. In G. I. Lubin; J. F. Magary; & M. K. Poulsen, Eds., *Proceedings, Fourth Interdisciplinary Seminar: Piagetian theory and its implications for helping professions: February 15, 1974: University of Southern California.* Los Angeles: Univ. of S. Calif. 1975, 348 pp., $7.50.

3124. Blea, William A. *Proceedings of the national symposium for deaf-blind.* Sacramento: Southwestern Region Deaf-Blind Center, 1972, 114 pp.

Presents 9 conference papers. Topics include Piagetian theory, assessment and treatment, implications, etiology of hearing loss.

3125. ———, Ed. *Proceedings of the special study institute for teachers of deaf-blind multihandicapped.* Sacramento: Southwestern Region Deaf-Blind Center, 1972, 72 pp.

Three presentations describe the delivery of educational services, a curriculum of 359 tasks arranged in 22 progressive levels for profoundly retarded children, and a device and prototype system for screening hearing.

3126. Blea, William A., & Hobron, Robert. *Literature on the deaf-blind—An annotated bibliography.* Sacramento: Southwestern Region Deaf-Blind Center, 1970, 193 pp.

Covers a wide variety of sources and a lengthy period of time. Entries are listed by category, selected books and articles.

3127. Bowling, Wallace L. The introduction of signs and fingerspelling to a deaf-blind child. *Education of the Visually Handicapped,* Oct. 1970, Vol. 2, No. 3, pp. 89–90.

Report on treatment and progress of a 10-year-old deaf-blind girl. Instruction in manual signs and fingerspelling is briefly described.

3128. Brock, Margaret. There IS hope for these children. *Nursing Times,* Sept. 17, 1970, Vol. 66, No. 38, p. 1210.

Describes work in England with deaf-blind resulting from rubella. Parents are shown what can be done with children with these handicaps and reassured that other families have similar problems.

3129. ———. *Christopher—A silent life.* London: Macmillan, 1975, £2.95.

A mother's account of her severely handicapped rubella son.

3130. Bureau of Elementary and Secondary Education. *Policies and procedures: Centers and services for deaf-blind children.* Washington, D.C.: Office of Education, HEW, 1969, 43 pp.

Describes provisions for the establishment of centers and services for deaf-blind children under the Elementary and Secondary Education Act, Title VI, Part C. Explains criteria for agency eligibility, coordination among agencies, services provided by a comprehensive center, and activities authorized by the act.

3131. Burroughs, Judith R., & Powell, Frank W. Can we systematically meet the needs of all deaf children? *Peabody Journal of Education,* Apr. 1974, Vol. 51, No. 3, pp. 171–79.

Describes the systems approach to individualized instruction of the Callier Center for Communications Disorders (Tex.) for approximately 310 deaf, deaf-blind, and language-delayed children, 0–16 years of age.

3132. Burton, Derek. Deaf-blind children and adolescents—4. *New Beacon,* Feb. 1974, Vol. 58, No. 682, pp. 32–35. Last of series.

Discusses role and needs of social workers attempting to serve this population, present inadequate service, need for specialized training of workers, relevant legislation.

3133. Calif. State Dept. of Education, Div. of Special Education. *Directory of programs for deaf-blind children.* Sacramento: Author, 1971, 12 pp.

Lists programs by state for Calif., Nev., Hawaii, and Ariz.

3134. Calvert, Donald R.; Reddell, Rayford C.; Jacobs, Ursula; et al. Experiences with preschool deaf-blind children. *Exceptional Children,* Jan. 1972, Vol. 38, No. 5, pp. 415–21.

Discusses knowledge and insight gained during a pilot program for deaf-blind children adapted from prior experience with deaf preschool children. It is concluded that a preschool training program for deaf-blind Ss is beneficial when based on total child development with parental support and counseling.

3135. Carr, LaVernya K.; Zemalis, Charles; & Evans, William J. *Pre-career* *curriculum guide for deaf-blind: Parts I, II, & III.* [2 vols.] [n.p.]: Southwestern Region Center for Services to Deaf-Blind Children, 1975, 187 pp., app., illus.

Curriculum concentrated on expanding competencies of the deaf-blind so they may move from dependence to degrees of independence. I: Objectives, program synopsis; II: Precareer, daily living skills; III: Presheltered workshop manipulative activities for development of skills in simulated work experience.

3136. Cooper, Louis. The child with rubella syndrome. *New Outlook for the Blind,* Dec. 1969, Vol. 63, No. 10, pp. 290–98.

Relationship of rubella to visual handicaps is explored including: Rubella cataracts, cataract operations and prognosis, congenital glaucoma, ocular lesions, and myopia. Also discusses other defects and considers need for early identification in infants.

3137. Council for Exceptional Children. *Exceptional children conference papers: Deaf-blind, language, and behavior problems.* Reston, Va.: Author, 1971, 106 pp.

Includes 5 papers on aurally handicapped and deaf-blind, new trends in their education, area centers, parents, and evaluation.

3138. ———. *Exceptional Children Conference papers: Problems of auditory, visual, and speech impairments.* Washington, D.C.: Bureau of Education for the Handicapped, 1972, 91 pp.

Includes a paper on deaf-blind children and one on print reading for visually impaired children.

3139. Csapo, Marg, & Clarke, Bryan R. Deaf-blind children in Canada. *New Outlook for the Blind,* Sept. 1974, Vol. 68, No. 7, pp. 315–19.

Results of questionnaire survey, as well as description of educational facilities and recommendations for improving services.

3140. Csapo, Marg, & Wormeli, Ted. Functional diagnosis and educational treatment of a deaf-blind boy. *Canadian Teacher of the Deaf,* Oct.–Nov. 1973, Vol. 2, No. 4, pp. 16–23.

Discusses 8-week reinforcement program through which a 15-year-old profoundly deaf, partially sighted boy subject to highly inappropriate behavior was taught to communicate with others.

3141. Curtis, W. Scott, & Donlon, Edward T. *An analysis of evaluation procedures, disability types, and recommended treatments for 100 deaf-blind children.* Syracuse, N.Y.: Div. of Special Education and Rehab., 1969, 110 pp.

Descriptions of 70 deaf-blind children were examined for terminology used to describe child and his life situation. Suggests video tape for communication.

3142. ———. *Video tape recording evaluation protocol behavior rating form—part I: Communication.* Washington, D.C.: Office of Education, HEW, 1970, 9 pp.

Presents a behavior rating scale designed for use with a video-tape protocol for examination of multiply handicapped deaf-blind children.

3143. Curtis, W. Scott; Donlon, Edward T.; & Tweedie, David. Deaf-blind children: An examination procedure for behavior characteristics. *Educa-*

tion of the Visually Handicapped, Oct. 1974, Vol. 6, No. 3, pp. 67–72. 1st in 4-part series. (2nd, Dec. 1974; 3rd, Mar. 1975; last, May 1975.)

An examination of a procedure for studying deaf-blind children through the use of videotape. Included are behavior and summary rating forms, along with an analysis of variance for 37 behavioral judgments by 10 judges for 19 deaf-blind children.

3144. ———. Communicative behavior of deaf-blind children. *Education of the Visually Handicapped,* Dec. 1974, Vol. 6, No. 4, pp. 114–18. 2nd in 4-part series. (1st, Oct. 1974; 3rd, Mar. 1975; last, May 1975.)

Discussion of data on communication as obtained through a video-tape procedure.

3145. ———. Adjustment of deaf-blind children. *Education of the Visually Handicapped,* Mar. 1975, Vol. 7, No. 1, pp. 21–26. 3rd in 4-part series. (1st, Oct. 1974; 2nd, Dec. 1974; last, May 1975.)

Discussion of data on adjustment as obtained through a video-tape procedure described in the 1st part.

3146. ———. Learning behavior of deaf-blind children. *Education of the Visually Handicapped,* May 1975, Vol. 7, No. 2, pp. 40–48. Last in 4-part series. (1st, Oct. 1974; 2nd, Dec. 1974; 3rd, Mar. 1975.)

Discussion of data on learning as obtained through a video-tape procedure described in the 1st part.

3147. Curtis, W. Scott; Donlon, Edward T.; & Wagner, Elizabeth, Eds. *Deaf-blind children: A program for evaluating their multiple handicaps.* New York: AFB, 1970, 172 pp., $2.50.

A report of the deaf-blind children evaluation project conducted by the Syracuse Univ. Center of the Development of Blind Children.

3148. Dantona, Robert. Centers and services for deaf-blind children. *Hearing and Speech News,* July–Aug. 1970, Vol. 38, No. 4, pp. 12–13.

Discusses regional centers in terms of origin, services, administration, and current status.

3149. ———. Regional centers for deaf-blind children: A new hope. *Volta Review,* Oct. 1971, Vol. 73, No. 7, pp. 411–15.

Reviews concept and purposes of centers.

3150. Dantona, Robert, & Salmon, Peter J. The current status of services for deaf-blind persons. *New Outlook for the Blind,* Mar. 1972, Vol. 66, No. 3, pp. 65–70.

Identifies, in broad terms, the main functions of 2 programs—Regional Centers for Deaf-Blind Children and the National Center for Deaf-Blind Youths and Adults—and the eligibility requirements under each. Lists the centers and their directors.

3151. Dinsmore, Annette. National approach to the education of deaf-blind children. *American Annals of the Deaf,* 1953, Vol. 98, pp. 418–30.

A description of the establishment of the National Study Committee on Education of Deaf-Blind Children is given.

3152. ———. National approach to the education of deaf-blind children. *New Outlook for the Blind,* Jan. 1954, Vol. 48, No. 1, pp. 1–8.

Describes need for a national approach and efforts to stimulate such planning. The National Study Committee on Education of Deaf-Blind

Children has an ambitious and promising program but some possible problems are raised.

3153. ———. *Methods of communication with deaf-blind people*, rev. ed. New York: AFB, 1959, 48 pp., $2. (Braille also $2.)

Outlines the various methods of communication by hand and machine with the deaf-blind person. It is so written that a person does not need to see in order to understand the methods.

3154. ———. Services for deaf-blind adults and children: The role of the American Foundation for the Blind. *New Outlook for the Blind*, Apr. 1966, Vol. 60, No. 4, pp. 123–28.

Discussion includes the history of AFB's role and its various related services.

3155. ———. Field testing the Tactile Speech Indicator. *New Outlook for the Blind*, June 1967, Vol. 61, No. 6, pp. 192–93.

Reviews field testing by 7 deaf-blind persons of the Tactile Speech Indicator, a means of communication for deaf-blind persons.

3156. ———. Unmet needs of deaf-blind children. *New Outlook for the Blind*, Oct. 1967, Vol. 61, No. 8, pp. 262–66.

Describes characteristics and needs of deaf-blind children and 2 programs to meet these needs, the Syracuse Univ. and Perkins School programs.

3157. Dolan, William S. The first ten months of the Rubella Living-Unit. *New Outlook for the Blind*, Jan. 1972, Vol. 66, No. 1, pp. 9–14.

Gives daily schedule of unit and 6 case histories. Notes lack of adequate counseling services for families of these children.

3158. Donlon, Edward T., & Curtis, W. Scott. *The development and evaluation of a video-tape protocol for the examination of multihandicapped deaf-blind children*. Washington, D.C.: Office of Education, HEW, 1970, 79 pp.

Developed and evaluated a video-tape protocol for the examination of the communication skills of 20 multiply handicapped deaf-blind children. Project evaluation indicates the films are successful.

3159. English, Jack. Rehabilitation services for deaf-blind individuals: Need for planning. *Journal of Rehabilitation of the Deaf*, Jan. 1975, Vol. 8, No. 3, pp. 1–6.

Author feels that unless planning and coordination are begun immediately, vocational services will not be available to the number of deaf-blind adults needing these services.

3160. Esche, Jeanne, & Griffin, Carol. A handbook for parents of deaf-blind children. *Rehabilitation Teacher*, Aug. 1971, Vol. 3, No. 8, pp. 3–22.

Practical, nontechnical guide for parents.

3161. Forsythe, Patricia G., & Fein, Judith G. *A review of selected program activities in the education of the deaf*. Washington, D.C.: Dept. of Health, Education, and Welfare, 1967, 17 pp.

Reviews activities by HEW in education of the deaf. Summarizes centers and services for deaf-blind children, legislation for preparation of professional personnel, and research and demonstration programs. Gives addresses for further inquiries.

3162. Freeman, Peggy. *Understanding the deaf-blind child.* London: Hein-man Medical Book, 1975.

Mother of a rubella deaf-blind child relates her experiences.

3163. Friedlander, Bernard Z., & Knight, Marcia S. Brightness sensitivity and preference in deaf-blind retarded children. *American Journal of Mental Deficiency,* Nov. 1973, Vol. 78, No. 3, pp. 323–30.

Report on program to systematically evaluate light sensitivity in children for whom such evaluations are considered impossible. Results had implications for assessing boundary conditions of children's visual competence and disability prior to planning educational procedures. 16 *S*s, preschool, post-rubella.

3164. Friedlander, Bernard Z.; Silva, Dennis A.; & Knight, Marcia S. Selective responses to auditory and auditory-vibratory stimuli by severely retarded deaf-blind children. *Journal of Auditory Research,* Apr. 1973, Vol. 13, No. 2, pp. 105–11.

Evaluates response to sound in 15 retarded deaf-blind children (mean age 7.5 yrs.) by their choice between no sound and music at 80 db SPL. Numerical records document details.

3165. Gazely, D. J. Communication and mobility training with hearing-impaired blind clients. *New Beacon,* July 1973, Vol. 57, No. 675, pp. 170–73.

Presents tables designed to establish and standardize nonverbal correctional signals and command (e.g., "stop") signals, and rationale for such signals.

3166. Geltzer, Arthur I.; Guber, Donald; & Sears, Marvin L. Ocular manifestations of the 1964–65 rubella epidemic. *American Foundation for the Blind Research Bulletin 15,* Jan. 1968, pp. 35–48.

Study of 105 infants born during the epidemic, of whom 49 had post-rubella syndrome by viral culture and/or specific serologic response to the virus. Of proven rubella patients, 49% had ocular defects. Non-ocular defects are tabulated according to frequency and coexistence of eye lesions.

3167. Graham, Milton D. *The deaf-blind: Some studies and suggestions for a national program.* New York: AFB, July 1970, 25 pp.

Presents statistical data on the deaf-blind gathered in a national study of multiply handicapped children. Fourteen tables describe principal characteristics of the 1045 deaf-blind children such as degree of vision, sex, age distribution, degree of auditory impairment, age of onset of impairments, and lack of visual memory.

3168. Guldager, Lars. Progress in education for deaf-blind children. *Education of the Visually Handicapped,* Mar. 1971, Vol. 3, No. 1, pp. 18–21.

Discusses development of comprehensive regional centers to provide consultative and diagnostic services, training of personnel, and research and dissemination of information. Lists geographic areas served.

3169. ———. Using video tape in the education of deaf-blind children. *New Outlook for the Blind,* June 1972, Vol. 66, No. 6, pp. 178–83.

Is used in personnel training, as a teaching aid, and to record a student's progress; also to preserve samples of behavior, for language development, in learning speech-reading, and for programmed instruction.

3170. Halliday, Gordon W., & Evans, Joseph H. Somatosensory enrichment of a deaf, blind, retarded adolescent through vibration. *Perceptual and Motor Skills*, June 1974, Vol. 38, No. 3, pp. 880.

Brief report on a study investigating the effect of vibration on the smiling behavior of a deaf-blind, severely retarded, nonverbal, and nonambulatory adolescent girl.

3171. Hammer, Edwin K. *Deaf-blind children: A list of references.* Austin: Tex. Univ., Dept. of Special Education, 1969, 36 pp.

Lists references from journals, newspapers, and professional reports dealing with various aspects of the deaf-blind child.

3172. ————. *Area centers for services to deaf-blind children in Arkansas, Louisiana, Oklahoma, & Texas. Final report: Planning year.* Dallas: Callier Hearing & Speech Center, 1970, 33 pp.

Survey identified 454 deaf-blind children and adults in named states. Tables provide incidence and distribution data. Discusses services.

3173. ————. *Families of deaf-blind children: Case studies of stress.* Dallas: Callier Hearing & Speech Center, 1972, 17 pp.

Describes common needs and experiences of parents in critical times of stress.

3174. ————. *What is effective programming for deaf-blind children?* Dallas: Callier Hearing & Speech Center, 1973, 15 pp. Reprinted in *New Outlook for the Blind*, Jan. 1975, Vol. 69, No. 1, pp. 25–31.

Gives some suggestions on program effectiveness standards and how to meet them. This is a growing concern in view of increased educational programs for deaf-blind children.

3175. ————, Ed. *Behavior modification programs for deaf-blind children: Proceedings of a workshop held July 13 & 14, 1970, Pinecrest State School, Pineville, Louisiana.* Dallas: Callier Hearing & Speech Center, 1970, 85 pp.

Papers include Principles of behavior modification and the habilitation of deaf-blind children, Shaping behavior of deaf-blind crib patients, Medical aspects of deaf-blind children, and Administrative considerations for implementing programs for deaf-blind children.

3176. Hanaway, Thomas P., & Barlow, David H. Prolonged depressive behaviors in a recently blind deaf mute: A behavioral treatment. *Journal of Behavior Therapy & Experimental Psychiatry*, 1975, Vol. 6, No. 1, pp. 43–48.

Description of the behavior modification program used and its results.

3177. Harris, Gail A. The identification of deaf-blind school-age individuals in Michigan. *American Annals of the Deaf*, June 1972, Vol. 117, No. 3, pp. 386–88.

Survey yielded 52 deaf-blind individuals between ages 0–25 who would require special education designed for both impairments, an incidence of 12 deaf-blind per million persons under 24 years of age. Recommendations made re evaluation procedures as well as programs and services.

3178. Hatlen, Philip H. *Proceedings of a special study institute: Conference for teachers of deaf-blind children.* Sacramento: Calif. State Dept. of Education, Div. of Special Education, 1971, 84 pp.

Topics include early growth, diagnosis and evaluation, normal language development and stimulating hearing, vision, and motor development.

3179. ————, **Ed.** *Proceedings of the special study institute: Effects of pre-school service for deaf-blind children.* San Francisco: San Francisco State Col., 1969, 331 pp.

Topics include relationships with parents, descriptions of many preschool programs, regional centers, and implications for teacher preparation.

3180. Hayes, Gordon M. Teaching the deaf-blind to wrestle (a case study). *International Journal for the Education of the Blind,* Dec. 1953, Vol. 3, No. 2, pp. 224–29.

Study of 1 boy who attended school for the deaf until loss of vision, then attended school for blind. Covered in study: Difficulties, methods, results. Glossary. Ref.

3181. Henry, Virginia, & Lyall, Jerry H. Ability screening and program placement for deaf-blind children and adults. *Volta Review,* Apr. 1973, Vol. 75, No. 4, pp. 227–31.

Describes the Deaf-Blind Program and the Ability Screening Test and the need for such a test.

3182. Hill, Jessica. Deaf-blind children and adolescents. *New Beacon,* Dec. 1973, Vol. 57, No. 680, pp. 310–15.

Describes services of the National Association for Deaf-Blind and Rubella Children in England, teaching methods for parents to use with young deaf-blind children, and suggestions for social workers.

3183. Hill, Jessica, & Best, Tony. Survey of deaf/blind children in mental hospitals in England and Wales. *Teacher of the Blind,* Spring 1974, Vol. 62, No. 3, pp. 76–83.

Survey to find the probable number of deaf-blind children in mental hospitals and to gain some idea of their handicaps and needs. Results show that many classed as deaf-blind are functioning at a very low level. Where teaching has been provided to overcome their sensory handicaps, there has been a marked improvement in the level of attainment. Several ways of providing special educational facilities are suggested.

3184. Hoff, Joel R. Education and the deaf-blind child. *New Outlook for the Blind,* Apr. 1966, Vol. 60, No. 4, pp. 109–13.

Following brief history, states that medical advances are altering the characteristics of the handicapped population, offering new challenges. Discusses relevant school enrollment, evaluation, personalized curriculum, vocational activities, physical education, social experiences.

3185. Industrial Home for the Blind. *Rehabilitation of deaf-blind persons. Vol. V: Studies in the vocational adjustment of deaf-blind adults.* Brooklyn: Author, 1959, 324 pp.

Handbook for counselors and placement workers dealing with deaf-blind individuals. Provides a general review of vocational guidance, training and placement of deaf-blind adults.

3186. International Conference on the Education of Deaf-Blind Children. *Deaf-blind children and their education.* Rotterdam, Netherlands: Rotterdam Univ. Press, 1971, 150 pp.

From conference held at Sint Michielsgestel Aug. 1968.

3187. International Council of Educators of Blind Youth. *Fourth International Conference on Deaf-Blind Children, August 22–27, 1971, at Perkins School for the Blind, Watertown, Massachusetts.* Watertown, Mass: Perkins School for the Blind, 1972, 358 pp., $5.

Thirty-one papers are reprinted in the areas of early communication, learning difficulties, behavior modification, rubella children, social and sexual problems, training of personnel, and parent counseling. Several of the papers are descriptive of the programs and facilities in various countries.

3188. John Tracy Clinic. *Correspondence learning program for parents of preschool deaf-blind children.* Los Angeles: Author, 1973, illus., $9.50.

The program has been made available in book form as a professional resource. The lesson format covers all aspects of the development and education of the deaf-blind child.

3189. Jordan, Sidney. The deaf-blind: A clarification. *Perceptual and Motor Skills,* 1964, Vol. 18, No. 2, pp. 503–4.

Attention drawn to differences in behavior of the deaf person who later becomes blind and the blind person who later becomes deaf. Those with this double disability are usually characterized as a homogeneous group. It is contended that sufficient behavior differences indicate the need for separate classifications.

3190. Keane, George E. Historic conference on communications for the deaf-blind. *New Outlook for the Blind,* Oct. 1957, Vol. 51, No. 8, pp. 376–79.

Report of the 1st international conference on communications for the deaf-blind resulting in the hope for a single manual alphabet.

3191. Kennedy, Ann. Language awareness and the deaf-blind child. *TEACHING Exceptional Children,* Winter 1974, Vol. 6, No. 2, pp. 99–102.

Discusses the problems of the multiply handicapped child who has no concept of the function of language. Lists essentials of a language program and gives suggestions for teachers.

3192. Kiernan, Dennis W., & DuBose, Rebecca F. Assessing the cognitive development of pre-school deaf-blind children. *Education of the Visually Handicapped,* Dec. 1974, Vol. 6, No. 4, pp. 103–5.

The authors devised the Peabody Intellectual Performance Scale to fill an existing gap in the testing of deaf-blind children and evaluated the measure. Twenty-one children ranging in age from 10 to 102 months participated in this study. Seventeen were classified as Rubella Syndrome and the remaining 4 had multiple disabilities, including auditory and visual impairments.

3193. Kinney, Richard. How to make a friend of your deaf-blind client. *New Outlook for the Blind,* Oct. 1956, Vol. 50, No. 8, pp. 308–9.

Specific suggestions to the worker about identifying himself and communicating with deaf-blind persons.

3194. ———. *Independent living without sight and hearing.* Winnetka, Ill.: Hadley School for the Blind, 1972, 102 pp., $3.

Inkprint edition of the basic textbook used for the correspondence course offered by Hadley to deaf-blind persons throughout the world.

3195. Lawson, Lawrence J., & Myklebust, Helmer R. Ophthalmological deficiencies in deaf children. *Exceptional Children*, Sept. 1970, Vol. 37, No. 1, pp. 17–20.

Incidence of eye defects was twice that found in hearing children in a study of the ophthalmological status of school-aged deaf children. Precise association between visual deficiencies and deafness is not clear.

3196. Lowenfeld, Berthold. *Multihandicapped blind and deaf-blind children in California.* Sacramento: State Dept. of Education, 1968, 101 pp.

Data elicited by 2 questionnaires on the characteristics (number, nature, extent, location) of the multiply handicapped population under 21 years of age. Estimated to include 80–90% of the state's multiply handicapped blind children.

3197. ———. Multihandicapped blind and deaf-blind children in California. *American Foundation for the Blind Research Bulletin 19*, June 1969, pp. 1–72.

Detailed study of demography and characteristics of blind and deaf-blind children in the state. With ample statistical support, urges services for multiply handicapped. Bib.

3198. MacFarland, Douglas C. The rehabilitation service administration's role in the rehabilitation of deaf-blind persons. In George Attleweed, et al., Eds., *Sensory disabilities study group report*. Calif. Conference on Rehabilitation, Oct. 8–10, 1974, n.p., n.d., 49–54.

Reviews events which led up to the development of the proposal for the Center for Deaf-Blind Youths. The 3 major programs of the Center are reviewed and the implications the Center has for future planning are presented.

3199. Mescherjakov, A. I., & Apraushev, A. V. Services for the adult deaf-blind in the USSR. *New Beacon*, Apr. 1975, Vol. 59, No. 696, pp. 90–93.

Early education, vocational training, employment, and recreation described.

3200. Meshcheriakov, A. I. The main principles of the system for education and training of the blind and deaf and dumb. *International Journal for the Education of the Blind*, Dec. 1962, Vol. 12, No. 2, pp. 43–48.

Education, an absolute necessity to the development of the deaf-blind child, who can learn little from chance contacts with the environment, has 2 stages: (1) images of objects are accumulated and a system of habits of conduct created, (2) learning the structure of verbal speech.

3201. Mich. School for the Blind. *Environmental programming for the deaf-blind.* Lansing: Author, 1972, 126 pp.

Proceedings of a workshop at which principles, techniques of training, and examples of behavior modification for the deaf-blind were discussed and demonstrated. Training and maintenance procedures for skills of independent daily living stressed. Guidelines for instructing parents in home-based management techniques provided.

3202. Micropoulou, Evangelie. Grammagraphy system for the blind. *International Journal for the Education of the Blind*, June 1954, Vol. 3, No. 4, pp. 270–71.

Greek institutes for the blind use Braille system as well as Grammagraphy system. System explained as especially helpful to deaf-blind.

3203. Mira, Mary, & Hoffman, Sandra. Educational programming for multihandicapped deaf-blind children. *Exceptional Children*, Apr. 1974, Vol. 40, No. 7, pp. 513–14.

Briefly describes problems encountered in training 35 school-age deafblind children. Suggests that teachers of deaf-blind need preparation in multiple disabilities and that education of deaf-blind must begin in infancy.

3204. Mitchell, Paul C. The education of Jack Boyer. *International Journal for the Education of the Blind*, Oct. 1958, Vol. 8, No. 1, pp. 11–17.

Building around the story of 1 deaf-blind boy, describes education for deaf-blind children with a wide range of illustrations and somewhat philosophical discussion.

3205. Moriarty, Donald F., et al., Eds. *Diagnosis and evaluation.* Denver: Colo. State Dept. of Education, Mountain Plains Regional Center for Services to Deaf-Blind Children, 1972, 116 pp.

Eight papers focusing on the roles of various professionals working with deaf-blind children at the diagnostic stage.

3206. Myers, S. O. Deaf-blind children and adolescents. *New Beacon*, Jan. 1974, Vol. 58, No. 681, pp. 6–10.

Discusses results of a follow-up survey of 26 former pupils in a British special school. Includes excerpts of parents' letters regarding placement of their children.

3207. Myklebust, Helmer R. *The deaf-blind child.* Watertown, Mass.: Perkins School for the Blind, 1956, 24 pp.

Diagnostic procedures for investigating residual, sensory, neurological, and psychological capacities of the deaf-blind child are described, and general principles for education are suggested. Ref.

3208. National Academy of Sciences. *Communication and sensory aids for the deaf-blind.* Washington, D.C.: Author, 1975, v + 66 pp., illus.

Report of workshop held Nov. 1973 to stimulate technological innovation in communication and sensory aids. The principle needs cited were a telephone communication device and body-worn telephone bell, doorbell, and emergency alerting equipment.

3209. Nealey, Robert. A checkered career. *Nat-Cent News*, Jan. 1975, Vol. 5, No. 2, pp. 16–23.

Mr. N., who is totally deaf and has only light perception, has been playing checkers for over 55 years and is regarded as the greatest blind checkerist in the game.

3210. Nesbitt, John A., & Howard, Gordon K., Eds. *Program development in recreation service for the deaf-blind.* Iowa City: Univ. of Iowa (Recreation Education Program), 1974, 443 pp.

This comprehensive report is based on presentations, working papers, and proceedings of a National Institute on Program Development and Training in Recreation for Deaf-Blind Children, Youth, and Adults.

3211. Norris, Arthur G., Ed. *Deafness annual 1973, Volume III.* Silver Spring, Md.: Professional Rehabilitation Workers with the Adult Deaf, 1973, 389 pp.

Presents 21 papers on deafness and summaries of federal government programs. Includes information on the needs of deaf-blind.

3212. Nugent, Clare M. *The implications of play for the deaf-blind child in terms of growth and evaluation.* Watertown, Mass.: Research Library, Perkins School for the Blind, Apr. 1970, 37 pp.

Discusses play activity, its role in child development, teaching a deaf-blind child to play, and the use of play as a diagnostic tool for student placement.

3213. Office of Vocational Rehabilitation. *Rehabilitation of deaf-blind persons, Vols. I–VII.* Washington, D.C.: Author, 1958, 982 pp.

Reports on medical and psychological studies of the deaf-blind; useful as manual for professional workers.

3214. ———. *Report of Committee on Services for the Deaf-Blind to the World Assembly of the World Council for the Welfare of the Blind.* Washington, D.C.: U.S. Dept. of Health, Education & Welfare, 1959, 152 pp.

Reviews developed methods of communication and discusses the Basic Minimum Services Proposal for deaf-blind persons. Contains guidelines suggested for the helper of the deaf-blind and includes a bibliography of resource literature.

3215. Patton, William C. Services for deaf-blind persons in a small rural state. *New Outlook for the Blind,* Dec. 1968, Vol. 62, No. 10, pp. 309–12.

With 1 case report as an example, describes the coordination of public and private agencies in N.H. to serve deaf-blind clients.

3216. Perkins Research Library and the Evaluation Service of the Dept. for Deaf-Blind Children. *A selected bibliography relating to the education and training of deaf-blind children and communication-disordered children with sensory impairments: 1910–Spring 1972.* Watertown, Mass.: Perkins School for the Blind, 1972, 77 pp., $2.

This classified bibliography lists books, pamphlets, articles, and unpublished papers available in the Research Library. The table of contents gives the various categories and their subdivisions; there is also an index by author.

3217. Perkins School for the Blind. *Additions to bibliography: Education of deaf-blind, Fall 1972–June 1974.* Watertown, Mass.: Author, 1974, 12 pp.

Lists 134 sources of information including journal articles, workshop and conference proceedings, films, tapes.

3218. Prause, Robert J. Selective competitive placement of two deaf-blind persons in the New York Metropolitan area. *New Outlook for the Blind,* Feb. 1968, Vol. 62, No. 2, pp. 38–43.

Describes 2 deaf-blind clients, the jobs in which they were placed, and how the placements were made.

3219. Proscia, Vito A.; Silver, Sallie; & Zumalt, L. E. Joint enterprise undertaken between two centers for development and evaluation of a tactile communication aid for deaf-blind persons. *American Foundation for the Blind Research Bulletin 25,* Jan. 1973, pp. 205–10.

Describes the TAC-COM and some potential uses, such as use as a fire alarm system.

3220. Rees, Norma S., et al. The acquisition of a first language in a deaf-blind adult: A case study of a language development in an adult with a history of deaf-blindness. *Journal of Rehabilitation of the Deaf*, Oct. 1974, Vol. 8, No. 2, pp. 11–23.

Discusses 3-phase training program, procedures, response to auditory stimuli, reading, writing, used in the progress of a 19-year-old deaf-blind man over a 3-year rehabilitation period.

3221. Riley, Betty G. A new plan in Kansas—Its development and potentials. *New Outlook for the Blind*, May 1959, Vol. 53, No. 5, pp. 161–65.

Through the story of a particular deaf-blind child, services of the Univ. of Kansas Medical Center are described. Outlines additional services recommended by a conference and expresses need for research on diagnostic evaluation.

3222. Robbins, Nan. *Educational beginnings with deaf-blind children.* Watertown, Mass.: Perkins School for the Blind, 1960, 80 pp.

Presents a teacher's guide to activity with deaf-blind children including methods, principles, techniques, and goals. Discusses readiness and academic programs, development and growth of the child, and teacher-child/parent-child relationships in the context of Perkins.

3223. ———. *Speech beginnings for the deaf-blind child: A guide for parents.* Watertown, Mass.: Perkins School for the Blind, 1963, 57 pp.

Discusses processes by which deaf-blind children learn to speak and the relationships between communication and physical, mental, and social growth. Recommends activities for maintaining healthy, parent-child relationships.

3224. Robbins, Nan, & Stenquist, Gertrude. *The deaf-blind rubella child.* Watertown, Mass.: Perkins School for the Blind, 1967, 111 pp.

Twenty-eight children at Perkins School for the Blind with a prenatal history of maternal rubella were studied, and data were compiled on their characteristics. Preschool programs suggested in order to increase communicative abilities and foster language development.

3225. Root, Ferne K., & Riley, Betty G. Study of deaf-blind children: A developmental plan. *New Outlook for the Blind*, June 1960, Vol. 54, No. 6, pp. 206–10.

Describes dynamics of the diagnostic process at the Center for the Development of Blind Children at Syracuse Univ., where 2 children are studied each month for a 4-day period, on the basis of referrals from physicians, agencies or schools. Describes 1 case and gives sample findings in areas of ophthalmology, speech and hearing, etc.

3226. Rothschild, Jacob. Deaf-blindness. In James F. Garrett, & Edna S. Levine, Eds., *Psychological practices with the physically disabled.* New York: Columbia Univ. Press, 1962, pp. 376–407.

3227. Rusalem, Herbert. Development of the Anne Sullivan Macy Service for Deaf-Blind Persons. *New Outlook for the Blind*, Oct. 1962, Vol. 56, No. 8, pp. 278–82.

States that deaf-blind persons bentfit from rehabilitation services' specialized program. Notes barriers to such a program's implementation. Describes research project encompassing 15 states launched by OVR and IHB to provide for development of a regional rehabilitation service for the deaf-blind, incorporated into general agency programs.

3228. ———. The diffusion effect of an orientation program on deaf-blindness. *New Outlook for the Blind*, Feb. 1964, Vol. 58, No. 2, pp. 44–46.

Clerical workers were exposed to 6 formal sessions of information about and discussion of the deaf-blind. They attended a meeting with deaf-blind people. The diffusion of information that occurred from these workers to others they came in contact with caused the project planners to feel it was worthwhile.

3229. ———. Deprivation and opportunity: Major variables in the rehabilitation of deaf-blind adults. *New Outlook for the Blind*, Apr. 1966, Vol. 60, No. 4, pp. 114–20.

Describes IHB's service for deaf-blind. Despite neglect and deprivation, a regional rehabilitation service for deaf-blind can have positive results including at least partial social and vocational self-sufficiency. Case study.

3230. Rusalem, Herbert; Bettica, Louis J.; Haffly, John E.; et al. *New frontiers for research on deaf/blindness.* Brooklyn: Industrial Home for the Blind, 1966, 60 pp.

Proceedings of a seminar covering position papers, discussion, and research proposals on communication, learning, rehabilitation, and resettlement.

3231. Salmon, Peter J. Services for deaf-blind persons abroad: A personal view. *New Outlook for the Blind*, Apr. 1966, Vol. 60, No. 4, pp. 133–34.

Author notes British and European efforts for the deaf-blind which he feels merit emulation in the U.S.

3232. ———. Our responsibilities to the deaf-blind person. *Journal of Rehabilitation*, Jan.–Feb. 1967, Vol. 33, No. 1, pp. 25–26.

Reviews a demonstration project which discloses potential in deaf-blind despite years of neglect and extreme handicaps. Of 143 clients, majority became independent in self-care and mobility.

3233. ———. *Out of the shadows.* New Hyde Park, N.Y.: National Center for Deaf-Blind Youths and Adults, 1970, 103 pp., $1.

Describes Anne Sullivan Macy Service for Deaf-Blind Persons, a regional demonstration and research project. Describes the deaf-blind, dimensions of the problem, and rehabilitation program.

3234. ———. New directions for the deaf-blind. *Human Needs*, Jan. 1973, Vol. 1, No. 7, pp. 18–21.

Following discussion of history and present status of programs for deaf-blind, describes the projected National Center for Deaf Blind Youths and Adults, its planned staffing and services.

3235. Salmon, Peter J., & Rusalem, Herbert. Vocational rehabilitation of deaf-blind persons. *New Outlook for the Blind*, Feb. 1959, Vol. 43, No. 2, pp. 47–54.

With emphasis on how the program for the deaf-blind may differ from that of the blind person, describes vocational diagnosis, vocational counseling, prevocational training, vocational training, and placement for the deaf-blind.

3236. Salmon, Peter J., & Spar, Harry J. Some observations on services for deaf-blind persons. *New Outlook for the Blind*, Apr. 1975, Vol. 69, No. 4, pp. 172–81, 183.

Past, present, and future of services aimed at minimizing the limiting effects of the handicap through training and the use of sensory aids, with emphasis on functions of National Center for Deaf-Blind Youths and Adults.

3237. Schiff, William, et al. *A field evaluation of devices for maintaining contact with mobile deaf and deaf-blind children: Electronic communications with deaf and deaf-blind persons.* New York: New York Univ. Deafness Research and Training Center, May 1973, 35 pp.

Use of Vibralet, a vibrating portable signal system, with 24 deaf and hearing parents to maintain contact with their deaf children, showed that the majority liked and used the system. With deaf-blind adults comparison of Vibralet and another similar device (the M.I.T. TAC-COM), showed preference for Vibralet.

3238. Sculthorpe, Arthur. The deaf-blind. *New Beacon*, Aug. 1971, Vol. 55, No. 652, pp. 198–200.

3239. Search, David L. A special short-term evaluation/training program for deaf-blind adults. *New Outlook for the Blind*, Dec. 1974, Vol. 68, No. 10, pp. 444–46, 453.

A 3-week summer program to evaluate training potential as well as daily living and mobility skills of the client, to provide instruction in those skills, and to teach staff members to set up training programs for the deaf-blind.

3240. Shields, Joan. The Paget System at Pathways. *Special Education*, June 1971, Vol. 60, No. 2, pp. 11–14.

The Paget System, a systematic sign language, differs from other sign languages in that it is not based on finger spelling and can be used word-for-word as in spoken English. Many of the 2,500 words have signs which are pictorial representations. Most of the deaf-blind children in the training group had been handicapped from birth (maternal rubella) but none of them were totally blind.

3241. ———. Methods for teaching deaf children with visual difficulties. *Teacher of the Deaf*, Sept. 1972, Vol. 70, No. 415, pp. 370–73.

Describes teaching and communication methods, use of class trips, music, plays, and art activities to teach skills. Refers to social aspects of many of these learning situations.

3242. Silva, Dennis A.; Knight, Marcia S.; & Friedlander, Bernard Z. Visual tracking in deaf-blind retarded preschool children. *Exceptional Children*, Apr. 1973, Vol. 39, No. 7, pp. 574–75.

Brief report on research to study extent of functional connections between visual processing and body orientation in severely impaired deaf-blind children.

3243. Smith, Benjamin F. The social education of deaf-blind children at Perkins School for the Blind. *New Outlook for the Blind*, June 1966, Vol. 60, No. 6, pp. 183–86.

Describes the social training program: Roles and methods of attendants, housemother, liaison officer, principal, and orientation committee in working as a team.

3244. Spar, Harry J. What the future may hold for the deaf-blind child. *New Outlook for the Blind,* Dec. 1972, Vol. 66, No. 10, pp. 349–55, 360.

After reviewing the background of services for deaf-blind children and adults in this country, the author discusses future services, indicating that the development of special education and rehabilitation for deaf-blind persons is still many years behind that for other handicapped groups.

3245. Spein, Laszlo K., & Green, Mary B. Problems in managing the young deaf-blind child. *Exceptional Children,* Feb. 1972, Vol. 38, No. 6, pp. 481–84.

Defines general concepts regarding early management of deaf-blind children, including victims of maternal rubella, and the help that can be offered their parents.

3246. Starkovich, Paul. *Two-year study of Northwest Regional Center's summer sessions for preschool, rubella, deaf-blind children.* Vancouver, Wash.: Northwest Regional Center for Deaf-Blind Children, 1972, 122 pp.

Describes the short-term evaluative programs and how a coordinated program may be organized, administered, and evaluated.

3247. Stenquist, Gertrude. *The story of Leonard Dowdy: Deaf-blindness acquired in infancy.* Watertown, Mass.: Perkins School, 1974, viii + 64 pp., illus., $3.

The first section is a commentary by the author who taught *S*; the second contains information concerning norms of development, language learning, educational methods, etc., for those profoundly deaf-blind in early childhood.

3248. Stillman, Robert D. *Measuring progress in deaf-blind children: Use of the Azusa Scale.* Dallas: Callier Hearing & Speech Center, 1972, 46 pp.

Studies show scale is appropriate to evaluate behavioral change, instructional planning and programming.

3249. Stuckey, Ken, et al. *Education of deaf-blind: Bibliography.* Watertown, Mass.: Perkins School for the Blind, 1972, 84 pp.

Lists approximately 550 print materials and 26 film and videotapes relevant to education of deaf-blind children and adults. Also provides approximately 40 sources of information in Europe and the U.S.

3250. Torrie, Carolyn. *Affective reactions in some parents of deaf-blind children.* Dallas: Callier Hearing & Speech Center, 1972, 13 pp.

Parents' emotional problems and behavioral patterns are described clinically and in short case-studies. Includes consideration of childrens' isolation, parents' stress, the mourning period, anger, narcissistic insult, and possible role of agencies.

3251. Tweedie, David. Behavioral change in a deaf-blind multihandicapped child. *Volta Review,* Apr. 1974, Vol. 76, No. 4, pp. 213–18.

Reports project in which videotape programs documented behavioral change over a 4-year period.

3252. ———. Demonstrating behavioral change of deaf-blind children. *Exceptional Children*, Apr. 1974, Vol. 40, No. 7, pp. 510–12.

The behavior change of a deaf-blind girl, during 4 years at a residential school, was rated on communication, adjustment, and learning components by 10 observers on the basis of 8 video-tape recordings. Implications of video taping to show positive behavior changes and validity of special education programs.

3253. ———. Observing the communication behavior of deaf-blind children. *American Annals of the Deaf*, June 1974, Vol. 119, No. 3, pp. 342–47.

Reviews observational techniques for rating communication of deaf-blind multiply handicapped children. Reports initial study of diagnostic observational competency of 75 speech pathologists at 5 levels of training and experience. Discusses inadequacy of standardized tests for assessing speech and language of deaf-blind multiply handicapped children.

3254. ———. Videoaudiometry: A possible procedure for "difficult-to-test" populations. *Volta Review*, Feb. 1975, Vol. 77, No. 2, pp. 129–34.

Audiological information is obtained from behavioral responses of 21 deaf-blind children to stimuli. Video taping is used in measurement.

3255. ———. Identification and documentation of audio-behavioral responses in a deaf-blind multihandicapped population through the use of videotape. *Education of the Visually Handicapped*, Dec. 1975, Vol. 7, No. 4, pp. 108–11.

Through use of video tape, studied responses of 21 deaf-blind children. It was hoped that through identification of typical responses of each child, variations from the typical could be used in auditory testing.

3256. U.S. Dept. of Health, Education & Welfare & The Industrial Home for the Blind. *Rehabilitation of deaf-blind persons. Vol. 1: A manual for professional workers and summary report of a pilot study.* Brooklyn: Industrial Home for the Blind, 1958, xiv + 246 pp.

Provides information on: Communication, social casework services, health and medical aspects, psychological examination, vocational adjustment and a number of other services for the deaf-blind. 17-pp. bib.

3257. Van Dijk, Jan. The first steps of the deaf-blind child towards language. *International Journal for the Education of the Blind*, May 1966, Vol. 15, No. 4, pp. 112–14.

Suggestions for the presymbol or prelanguage stage with emphasis on use of gestures and whole-body involvement. Language growth depends upon the child's intelligence, emotional maturity, social awareness, and the experiences offered to him.

3258. Vernon, McCay. Usher's Syndrome—Deafness and progressive blindness: Clinical cases, prevention, theory, and literature survey. *Journal of Chronic Diseases*, Aug. 1969, Vol. 22, No. 10, pp. 133–51.

Presents a multidisciplinary survey and synthesis of the literature on Usher's Syndrome, a genetic condition resulting in a double handicap of congenital deafness and a progressive blindness.

3259. ———. Usher's Syndrome—Deafness and progressive blindness: An abstract. *New Outlook for the Blind*, Feb. 1970, Vol. 64, No. 2, pp. 51–52. Abstract of article of similar title in *Journal of Chronic Diseases*, 1969. Describes this cause of deafness, blindness, and central nervous system degeneration. Treatment is ineffective but prevention through high-risk diagnostic screening and genetic counseling is feasible.

3260. Verstrate, Donna. *Social group work with deaf-blind adults.* New York: AFB, 1959, 55 pp.

Author reports her experience as a social group worker with a club of deaf-blind adults, offering ideas and suggestions for similar workers.

3261. Walsh, Sara R. I'm me! *TEACHING Exceptional Children*, Winter 1974, Vol. 6, No. 2, pp. 78–83, illus.

A curriculum, primarily of language development, to establish self-identification. Used with 5 children at the Georgia Center for the Multihandicapped, all of which had some hearing loss but had some vision and knew a few colors.

3262. Waterhouse, Edward J. Helping the deaf-blind to face the future. *Journal of Rehabilitation*, 1957, Vol. 23, pp. 6–7.

Complexities of the dual handicap are discussed. Emphasis is placed on problems of education and the need for research in the areas of diagnosis and evaluation.

3263. ⸺⸺. Status of the deaf-blind in the world. *New Outlook for the Blind*, Apr. 1966, Vol. 60, No. 4, pp. 129–32.

Discusses programs for, availability of statistics on, definitions of, and prevalence of ignorance about deaf-blindness, internationally.

3264. ⸺⸺. Rubella: Implications for education. *New Outlook for the Blind*, Apr. 1967, Vol. 61, No. 4, pp. 106–12.

Describes 40 rubella children examined at Perkins School for the Blind, their characteristics, recommended educational programs, and staff needs. Reports plans of the National Committee for Deaf-Blind Children. Ref.

3265. ⸺⸺. *Why educate the deaf-blind. (Paper delivered at the 1974 Biennial Conference; Australian and New Zealand Association of Teachers of the Visually Handicapped. Brisbane, Queensland, January 1974).*

Stresses importance of educating the deaf-blind whichever of 5 levels of ability they belong in. Presents 3 cases illustrating this point.

3266. Watson, Marcia J., & Nicholas, Judith L. *A practical guide to the training of low-functioning deaf-blind children.* Hartford, Conn.: Oak Hill School, 1973, 49 pp., $2.

Outlines responsibilities that parents, teachers, aides, and houseparents should assume. Proposes behavioral objectives for training the child in discipline, body movement, toilet training, eating, dressing and undressing, washing, and social awareness.

3267. Weir, A. Charles, Ed. *Workshop in the education of deaf-blind children.* Lansing, Mich.: Midwest Regional Center for Services to Deaf-Blind Children, 1973, 63 pp.

The proceedings of a 1973 workshop provide 4 papers on aspects of diagnosis and remediation including such specific topics as vision and visual anomalies, implications of low-vision conditions, assessment and simulation role playing techniques, the nature of hearing disorders. Other material includes a list of tests appropriate for multiply handicapped children, a developmental inventory suitable for children aged 3 months to 9 years, a list of gross motor skills with achievement age.

3268. Wiedenmayer, Joseph. Look or listen. *Volta Review*, Feb. 1973, Vol. 75, No. 2, pp. 89–96.

Specific suggestions for legally blind hard of hearing persons such as development of listening ability, adjusting and seeking assistance, use of technical devices, includes suggestions on making verbal communication more intelligible and guidelines for relatives and friends.

3269. Wiehn, Virginia. An early childhood education program for deaf-blind children. *New Outlook for the Blind*, Dec. 1970, Vol. 64, No. 10, pp. 313–16.

Describes services to preschool deaf-blind children by a school for the blind. Institutes for parents and children, home visits by school staff to local families, and 1-week summer residential programs for entire families are discussed.

3270. Worchel, Philip, & Dallenbach, Karl M. "Facial vision": Perception of obstacles by the deaf-blind. *American Foundation for the Blind Research Bulletin 13*, July 1966, pp. 55–112. Reprinted from *American Journal of Psychology*, Oct. 1947.

Detailed account of experiments with 10 deaf-blind Ss. Although selected upon the basis of their ability to get about alone, these Ss did not possess the obstacle sense and were incapable of learning it. The pressure theory of the obstacle sense is untenable.

3271. Yu, Muriel. *The causes for stresses to families with deaf-blind children.* Dallas: Callier Hearing & Speech Center, 1972, 15 pp.

Described in 13 case studies of deaf-blind (as result of rubella) children are medical, economical, emotional, and professional factors that add to stresses of parents. Includes advice to professionals working with families.

3272. Zumalt, L. Eugene; Silver, Sallie; & Kramer, Lynne C. Evaluation of a communication device for deaf-blind persons. *New Outlook for the Blind*, Jan. 1972, Vol. 66, No. 1, pp. 20–25.

Description of study of an experimental instrument developed by the General Electric Company with 6 deaf-blind people. The aid divides words spoken into the microphone into various sound frequencies and, through 5 circuits, activates finger-sized vibrators mounted in a small box. Results suggest it may be a valuable adjunct to speech therapy.

30. Multiply Handicapped Blind Other Than Deaf-Blind

3273. Abel, Georgie Lee, et al. *The counseling process and the teacher of children with multiple handicaps.* San Francisco: San Francisco State Col., 1968, 93 pp.

Focus of this institute was on children with at least 1 sensory, emotional, or physical impairment in addtion to a visual handicap. Roles of specialist and teacher in counseling process and the determination of best educational placement for the child considered.

3274. Albrecht, Marcella. A curriculum for a class of mentally retarded blind children. *International Journal for the Education of the Blind*, Dec. 1957, Vol. 7, No. 2, pp. 33–42.

Describes an experimental class for the mentally retarded blind at the Wisconsin School for the Visually Handicapped. Provides daily schedules and the sequences for social studies, handwork, arithmetic, reading, phys. ed., writing, music, speech and phonics, and literature.

3275. Allen, Robert M., & Allen, Sue P. *Intellectual evaluation of the mentally retarded child: A handbook.* Beverly Hills, Calif.: Western Psychological Services, 1967, 69 pp., illus.

Designed for the psychologist, describes instruments commonly used for evaluation of children suspected of being mentally retarded, including section on visually handicapped.

3276. American Foundation for the Blind, Ed. *Proceedings of the regional institute on the blind child who functions on a retarded level.* New York: Editor, 1969, 107 pp., $2.

Institute dealt with growing concern about how the retarded blind child can best be served in an institutional setting.

3277. ———. *The blind child who functions on a retarded level: Selected papers.* New York: Editor, 1970, 73 pp., $1.

Papers dealing with the mentally handicapped blind child in the areas of: Effect on the family, rubella syndrome, teaching the child, the challenge for teacher preparation, psychological management, teaching techniques for institutionalized blind children, importance of motor development and motor skills, adapting school psychological evaluations, and behavior modification.

3278. Ashcroft, Samuel C. Delineating the possible for the multi-handicapped child with visual impairment. *International Journal for the Education of the Blind*, Dec. 1966, Vol. 16, No. 2, pp. 52–55.

After explaining why some clarification and hope seem to be coming out of the discouraging confusion about multiply handicapped children, describes program at Peabody Col. Therapeutic intervention must be drastic, and often emphasis on motor activity is the key.

3279. Ausman, James O., & Gaddy, Michael R. Reinforcement training for echolalia: Developing a repetoire of appropriate verbal responses in an echolalic girl. *Mental Retardation*, Feb. 1974, Vol. 12, No. 1, pp. 20–21.

Presents methods used successfully with 17-year-old severely retarded blind echolalic.

3280. Axline, Virginia. *To be a child among children.* New York: Institute of Physical Medicine & Rehabilitation, 1959.

Case histories of 3 multiply handicapped blind children and the attempt to solve their problems by play therapy.

3281. Bachelis, Leonard A. Symposium—Self-image: A guide to adjustment II. Some characteristics of sensory deprivation. *New Outlook for the Blind,* Nov. 1961, Vol. 55, No. 9, pp. 288–91.

Discusses ways of dealing with blind children who are also either mentally retarded, brain-injured, emotionally retarded, or deaf. Emphasis on communication problems.

3282. Bennett, Fay, & Oellerich, D. W. Institutional facilities for the visually handicapped mentally retarded: Results of a survey. *New Outlook for the Blind,* Oct. 1966, Vol. 60, No. 8, pp. 233–35.

Reports on survey of facilities for blind retarded outside state of Ga. Survey prompted by consideration of separate living units for this population at Georgia State School and Hospital. Questionnaire included.

3283. Benton, R. B.; Permenter, N. A.; Baylor, J.; et al. Evaluating the work potential of blind multiply handicapped persons for the manufacture of bath perfume. *New Outlook for the Blind,* Jan. 1974, Vol. 68, No. 1, pp. 20–24.

A model project in which 15 Ss attempted to master 1 or more of the 5 work-station tasks in the operation; 83% success rate. Severely mentally retarded were included.

3284. Bentzen, Billie L. Transfer of learning from school setting to life style in a habilitation program for multiply handicapped blind persons. *New Outlook for the Blind,* Sept. 1973, Vol. 67, No. 7, pp. 297–300.

Description of a program, in a residential setting, designed to provide full habilitation services for multiply handicapped blind adolescents and young adults. Program designed to help students achieve maximum level of self-sufficiency in personal care, care of immediate environment, social and community situations, independent travel and work.

3285. Best, John P., & Winn, Robert J. A place to go in Texas. *International Journal for the Education of the Blind,* Mar. 1968, Vol. 18, No. 1, pp. 2–10.

Describes the educational philosophy, procedures, curriculum and media of the Project for Multi-handicapped Children at the Texas School for the Blind. With aid of a chart, the subjects are described in detail. Key aspect of the program is its learning-problems approach.

3286. Bischoff, Robert W. Educating the retarded visually handicapped. *Utah Eagle,* Nov. 1973, Vol. 85, No. 2, pp. 1–4, 9.

Discusses various developmental areas such as speech, motor, cognitive, etc., and suggests methods and guidelines for teachers of retarded blind children.

3287. Blanchard, Irene, & Beard, Celeste. A program in basic communication development for retarded blind children. *Journal of Special Education*, 1968, Vol. 2, No. 3, pp. 337–40.

Description of program. Stresses: Whole-body contact, changes in body position, and touching common objects.

3288. Blanchard, Irene; Bowling, Don; & Roberts, R. Lincoln. Evaluation of an educational testing program for retarded blind children. *New Outlook for the Blind*, Apr. 1968, Vol. 62, No. 4, pp. 131–33.

Pre- and post-project assessment through systematic observation by several professionals made possible the evaluation of a summer program for 21 retarded blind children. Lists number of children improving in each of 14 areas of behavior.

3289. ——. Educational experience for the retarded blind. *Mental Retardation*, Dec. 1968, Vol. 6, No. 6, pp. 42–43.

A short report on an experimental program of concentrated educational activities with severely retarded blind children in Pomona, Calif.

3290. Blanchard, Irene, & Goodson, Frankie. Manipulation therapy for retarded blind children. *Education of the Visually Handicapped*, Oct. 1969, Vol. 1, No. 3, pp. 86–88.

Descriptions of behaviors of blind-retarded students in craft room. Advancements made by children.

3291. Bolkestein, G. Teaching blind retarded children in the Netherlands. *Phi Delta Kappan*, Apr. 1974, Vol. 55, No. 8, pp. 559–60.

Diagnosis stresses a multidisciplinary approach leading to a method of treatment identifying educational needs to increase independent functioning. Evaluation is followed by determination of educational objectives. School action plan stresses play at beginner level, crafts and skills at the middle level, work at the senior level.

3292. Boly, Louis F., & DeLeo, Gertrude M. A survey of educational provisions for the institutionalized mentally subnormal blind. *New Outlook for the Blind*, June 1956, Vol. 50, No. 6, pp. 232–36. Reprinted from *American Journal of Mental Deficiency*, Apr. 1956.

Results of a questionnaire to institutions concerning provision for mentally retarded blind. Responses from 52 institutions are presented through tables and discussion.

3293. Bongers, Kay H., & Doudlah, Anna M. Techniques for initiating visuomotor behavior in visually impaired retarded children. *Education of the Visually Handicapped*, Oct. 1972, Vol. 4, No. 3, pp. 80–82.

Reported observations, experiences as well as solutions. Recapitulation of sequence of perceptual motor development and control of sensory input were cited as major principles in developing remediation strategies.

3294. Boston Center for Blind Children. *Pamphlet Library.* Boston: Author, 1974, 17 pp.

An annotated bibliography of pamphlets intended to be useful to persons working with multiply handicapped, visually impaired individuals.

3295. Bucknam, Frank G. Multiple-handicapped blind children (an incidence suvery). *International Journal for the Education of the Blind*, Dec. 1965, Vol. 15, No. 2, pp. 46–49.

Records of 137 children, the entire student body of a residential school, were analyzed for presence of multiple handicaps, as determined by actual medical examinations. Tables report all findings, but significant is the data showing that 40 children had 1 handicap other than blindness, 35 had 2 other handicaps, and 21 had 3 or more.

3296. Budds, Frank C. Some initial experiences with mentally handicapped children who are attending schools for the blind. *International Journal for the Education of the Blind*, Oct. 1960, Vol. 10, No. 1, pp. 16–23.

Details the characteristics of children in a special class at the Michigan School for the Blind. Describes the curriculum, evaluation of growth, reporting to parents, and relevant administrative policies.

3297. Casabianca, Jamie. The case of Mr. K.: Rehabilitation vs. institutionalization. *New Outlook for the Blind*, Nov. 1975, Vol. 69, No. 9, pp. 416–17.

Case history of 65-year-old blind man illustrates problem of blind persons confined to mental institutions merely because they have not been taught the skills for living in a sighted world.

3298. Charney, Leon. Minority group within two minority groups. *International Journal for the Education of the Blind*, Dec. 1960, Vol. 10, No. 2, pp. 37–43.

After listing incidence of mental retardation in certain states and defining related terms, gives results of a questionnaire to units of National Assoc. for Retarded Children about their services to mentally retarded blind. Reviews relevant literature.

3299. Chiappone, Anthony D., & Libby, Bruce P. Visual problems of the educable mentally retarded. *Education and Training of the Mentally Retarded*, Dec. 1972, Vol. 7, No. 4, pp. 173–75.

Visual problems and implications for underachievement in the educable mentally retarded.

3300. Cicenia, Erbert F.; Belton, John A.; Myers, James J.; et al. The blind child with multiple handicaps: A challenge. *International Journal for the Education of the Blind*, Mar. 1965, Vol. 14, No. 3, pp. 65–71. Part 2, May 1965.

This, Part 1, gives philosophical background and organization of the unit for multiply handicapped blind at the Edward R. Johnstone Training and Research Center, Bordentown, N.J.

3301. ———. The blind child with multiple handicaps: A challenge. *International Journal for the Education of the Blind*, May 1965, Vol. 14, No. 4, pp. 105–12. Part 1, Mar. 1965.

This is Part 2 of a paper very fully describing the Blind Unit at Johnstone Training and Research Center. After several more academic programs failed, success resulted from providing emotional support and experiences to condition the child for training, especially in self-care.

3302. Cleland, Charles C., & Swartz, Jon D. Training activities for the mentally retarded blind. *Education of the Visually Handicapped*, Oct. 1970, Vol. 2, No. 3, pp. 73–75.

Describes the sport of fishing, games involving the sense of smell, and emotional experiences of simulation to evoke sensations of awe and grandeur.

3303. ———. The blind retardate—Three program suggestions. *Training School Bulletin*, Nov. 1970, Vol. 67, No. 3, pp. 172–77.

Adaptation of games, role of music in socialization, and ideas from the blind themselves are discussed.

3304. Cohen, Jerome. Development of a blind spastic child: A case study. *Exceptional Children*, 1966, Vol. 32, No. 5, pp. 291–94.

A case history is presented of a blind and spastic child who endured severe emotional deprivation and neglect as a baby. A rehabilitative program is described and discussed.

3305. Colligan, John C. *Opportunities for the additionally handicapped blind.* Washington, D.C.: Office of Vocational Rehabilitation, 1954.

Describes British program for multiply handicapped rehabilitation centers for newly blind with additional handicaps, and problems of deaf-blind.

3306. Council for Exceptional Children. *Multiply handicapped: A selected bibliography.* Exceptional Child Bibliography Series No. 614. Arlington, Va.: Author, 1972, 31 pp.

Contains approximately 100 abstracts with indexing information. Publication dates of included documents 1947–71.

3307. ———. *Multiply handicapped: A selective bibliography.* Reston, Va.: Author, 1973, 20 pp., Bibliography Series No. 614.

Lists references with descriptors and abstracts. Includes multiply handicapped blind and deaf-blind. Author and subject indexes.

3308. Cox, Lois V. The Maryland School for the Blind summer day school program for pre-school multi-handicapped blind children. *International Journal for the Education of the Blind*, Dec. 1968, Vol. 18, No. 4, pp. 97–99.

Lists program and services provided in a summer day school for 23 multiply handicapped blind youngsters. Lists objectives, visual status and other handicaps, and recommendations at close of the program.

3309. Cruickshank, William M. The multiple-handicapped child and courageous action. *International Journal for the Education of the Blind*, Mar. 1964, Vol. 13, No. 3, pp. 65–75.

Defines multiply handicapped children and role of residential centers, needed staff and research. Five major groups of blind children need service: Mentally retarded, emotionally disturbed, brain-injured, those with physical disabilities, and deaf-blind.

3310. Curren, Elizabeth A. Teaching water safety skills to blind multi-handicapped children. *Education of the Visually Handicapped*, Mar. 1971, Vol. 3, No. 1, pp. 29–32.

Details a swimming program for multiply handicapped blind children. Results of program positive, with 75% of the 13 children swimming without any support in deep water, and 100% of the transitional children swimming without support.

3311. Curtis, W. Scott. The evaluation of verbal performance in multiply handicapped blind children. *Exceptional Children*, Feb. 1966, Vol. 32, No. 6, pp. 367–74.

Team evaluations of communication skills has resulted in classification of children as apathetic or hyperactive. An outline of response categories provides cues to behavior patterns, and modality capacities are listed for receptive, expressive, and referential system. General recommendations included.

3312. Davidow, Mae E. A study of instructional techniques for the development of social skills of retarded blind children. *International Journal for the Education of the Blind*, Dec. 1962, Vol. 12, No. 2, pp. 61–62.

Studies need for social skill training in retarded blind children and offers a functional teaching procedure to meet the need.

3313. Dekaban, Anatole S. Mental retardation and neurologic involvement in patients with congenital retinal blindness. *Developmental Medicine and Child Neurology*, Aug. 1972, Vol. 14, No. 4, pp. 436–44.

Report on studies of 61 cases of congenital retinal blindness, a recessively inherited disorder occurring in about 10% of blind children.

3314. DeLeo, Gertrude M., & Boly, Louis F. Some considerations in establishing an educational program for the institutionalized blind and partially sighted mentally subnormal. *American Journal of Mental Deficiency*, 1956, Vol. 61, pp. 134–40.

Proposes a reorientation in teaching methodology and presents an experimental approach with a consideration of its compatibility with modern learning theory.

3315. Dept. of Institutions, Social and Rehabilitative Services. Visual Services. *Conference proceedings: Services to the visually impaired mental retardate.* Oklahoma City, Okla.: Author, 1972, 51 pp.

Report on conference held at Sand Springs, Okla., Sept. 11–13, 1972, designed to develop greater coordination between all units of the dept. serving the visually impaired mental retardate and to provide basic orientation for field staff involved with this group.

3316. Dolan, Cleo B. *Achieving rehabilitation potential with multiple disabled blind persons: Final demonstration report.* Cleveland, Ohio: Cleveland Society for the Blind, 1969, 35 pp., app., illus.

Results of project to demonstrate and report vocational rehabilitation services most essential to the return of the individual to employment potential and to evaluate patterns of joint service.

3317. Donlon, Edward T. An evaluation center for the blind child with multiple handicaps. *International Journal for the Education of the Blind*, Mar. 1964, Vol. 13, No. 3, pp. 75–78.

The Center for the Development of Blind Children, Syracuse Univ., evaluates multiply handicapped children through a dynamic process here described.

3318. Egland, George O. Teaching speech to blind children with cerebral palsy. *New Outlook for the Blind*, Oct. 1955, Vol. 49, No. 8, pp. 282–89. Reprinted from *Cerebral Palsy Review*, July–Aug. 1955.

Details the special approaches and attitudes needed to teach speech to a multiply handicapped child.

3319. Elonen, Anna S. & Zwarensteyn, Sarah B. Michigan's summer program for multiple-handicapped blind children. *New Outlook for the Blind*, Mar. 1963, Vol. 57, No. 3, pp. 77–82.

Pilot study to assemble an interdisciplinary team for diagnosis and evaluation of multiply handicapped blind children.

3320. Farrell, Malcolm J. A state facility for the blind retarded. *New Outlook for the Blind*, May 1955, Vol. 49, No. 5, pp. 166–68.

History, description, and services of the Ransom A. Greene building for the blind at the Walter E. Fernald State School, Mass.

3321. Fleming, Mary Jo. The partially sighted trainable mentally retarded child. *Journal for Special Education of the Mentally Retarded*, Winter 1973, Vol. 9, No. 2, pp. 118–23.

Considers instruction and the problem of identification, the need to avoid overprotection, and adapted techniques including Montessori tactual exercises.

3322. Fraenkel, William A. Blind retarded—or retarded blind? *New Outlook for the Blind*, June 1964, Vol. 58, No. 6, pp. 165–69.

Problems to be considered by those working with the blind retarded. Recommendations are made to these workers.

3323. Frampton, Merle E., et al. *Forgotten children: A program for the multihandicapped.* Boston: Porter Sargent, 1969, 287 pp.

Describes program in a cerebral palsy-blind experimental school unit for day and residential care, following developments as a staff of 13 serves 30 children in 6 years with 12–17 children yearly. Discusses the total program, group programs, individualized programs for each child, involvement with parents. Recommends total clinic and multifocal school. Case studies of 1 child through age 6, and 4 others.

3324. Freedman, Saul. Psychological implications of the multiply handicapped person. *New Outlook for the Blind*, June 1967, Vol. 61, No. 6, pp. 185–89.

Reviews factors which inhibit normal development, psychologically and socially, for the multiply handicapped. Suggests how agencies can meet these.

3325. Furst, R. Terry. An approach to multiply handicapped blind persons through physical recreation. *New Outlook for the Blind*, Sept. 1966, Vol. 60, No. 7, pp. 218–21.

Discusses program for young adults to arrest muscular deterioration, improve posture, develop common spirit, socialization, and participants' implementation, games, activities, interaction between staff and clients, positive results described.

3326. ———. Competitive team organization: A motivational technique for the multi-handicapped. *International Journal for the Education of the Blind*, May 1968, Vol. 18, No. 2, pp. 47–51.

A multiply handicapped group, aged 16–28, was quite uninterested in calisthenics or swimming for their health benefits, but simple team game activity gradually developed a sense of meaningful group goals which provided motivation.

3327. Gallagher, Patricia A., & Heim, Ruth E. The classroom application of behavior modification principles for multiply handicapped blind students. *New Outlook for the Blind*, Dec. 1974, Vol. 68, No. 10, pp. 447–53.

Three studies of multiply handicapped blind children in a special class in a residential school for visually handicapped children are reported.

3328. Goldblatt, Michael, & Steisel, Ira M. Behavior modification with multi-handicapped blind children. *Proceedings of the 81st Annual Convention of the American Psychological Association, Montreal, Canada,* 1973, Vol. 8, pp. 809–10.

The behavioral analysis, treatment plan, and results of programs designed to modify the behavior of 3 children who attend a day school for the blind are presented. The targeted, objectionable behaviors diminished, pro-social behavior was acquired, and the teachers were able to make more positive, educational approaches to the children.

3329. Graham, Milton D. *Multiply impaired blind children—A national problem.* New York: AFB, 1968, 82 pp., app., $2.50.

Mail questionnaire yielded a sample of 8,887 multiply impaired blind children, an estimated ⅔ of the total. Data implied the need for early detection, alternatives to institutionalization, planning of services, professional training, and educational innovation.

3330. ———. Multiply impaired children: An experimental severity rating scale. *New Outlook for the Blind,* Mar. 1968, Vol. 62, No. 3, pp. 73–81.

In detail, provides original and modified severity rating scales which can be used to describe individual children or calculate a teacher's potential class load.

3331. Greaves, Jessie R. Helping the retarded blind. *International Journal for the Education of the Blind,* Apr. 1953, Vol. 2, No. 3, pp. 163–64.

Problems: Eating, chewing, toilet training, hand development, speech difficulties, other handicaps such as deafness and spasticity. Suggestions and methods. Importance of music, conversation, much love, and home environment.

3332. Green, M. R., & Schecter, D. E. Autistic and symbiotic disorders in three blind children. *Psychiatric Quarterly,* 1957, Vol. 31, pp. 628–46.

A description of the 3 cases and of the therapeutic program which was followed.

3333. Greene, Frederick L. Resources for professionals involved with the education or treatment of multi-impaired, visually handicapped children. Greeley, Colo.: Rocky Mountain Special Education Instructional Materials Center, 1969, 62 pp. Mimeo.

References on the following: Deaf and hard of hearing, physically handicapped, mentally retarded, vocational rehabilitation, teacher resources, speech impaired, educationally handicapped, and emotionally disturbed, chiefly but not entirely in combination with blindness.

3334. Greene, Robert J., & Hoats, David L. Aversive tickling: A simple conditioning technique. *Behavior Therapy,* July 1971, Vol. 2, No. 3, pp. 389–93.

Aversive tickling reduced head-banging in 2 blind, retarded 13-year-old girls.

3335. Greene, Robert J.; Hoats, David L.; & Hornick, Adelbert J. Music distortion: A new technique for behavior modification. *Psychological Record,* Winter 1970, Vol. 20, No. 1, pp. 107–9.

Disruptive rocking behavior of a blind, retarded *S* was reconditioned through use of the aversive value of distorted music.

3336. Gruber, Kathern F., & Moor, Pauline M., Eds. *No place to go: A symposium.* New York: AFB, 1963, 89 pp., $2.

Text is addressed to teachers of blind retarded children. Discusses potentialities of family counseling, factors affecting development and appraisal, appraisal and evaluation, and the child in school. App. includes case studies, psychological measurements, and a suggested day's program.

3337. Guess, Doug. Mental retardation and blindness: A complex and relatively unexplored dyad. *Exceptional Children,* 1967, Vol. 33, No. 7, pp. 471–79.

Reviews aspects of multiple disability of mental retardation and blindness. Discussion includes: Assessment, prevalence estimates, behavior characteristics, treatment considerations, program development.

3338. Guess, Doug, & Rutherford, Gorin. Experimental attempts to reduce stereotyping among blind retardates. *American Journal of Mental Deficiency,* 1967, Vol. 71, No. 6, pp. 984–86.

Stereotyping rates among blind mental retardates observed under experimental, ward, and control conditions. Three experimental conditions included. Introduction of objects and sound-generating apparatuses significantly reduced stereotyping.

3339. Guess, Doug; Rutherford, Gorin; & Twichell, Alice. Speech acquisition in a mute, visually impaired adolescent. *New Outlook for the Blind,* Jan. 1969, Vol. 63, No. 1, pp. 8–14.

Describes an intensive speech development program with a severely retarded, mute adolescent blind boy. Theoretical as well as practical implications for severe language delay are suggested. Ref.

3340. Hall, Richard C. An experimental self-feeding program for a severely retarded male resident blind since birth. *Pennsylvania Psychiatric Quarterly,* 1969, Vol. 9, No. 3, pp. 41–43.

3341. Hallenbeck, Jane. Pseudo-retardation in retrolental fibroplasia. *New Outlook for the Blind,* Nov. 1954, Vol. 48, No. 9, pp. 301–7.

Study of 18 children (ages 3–6) representing the more severely disturbed and retarded of a larger group of RLF children. Study showed that a large part of their problems had emotional basis and could be altered by psychiatric treatment in all but 3 cases.

3342. Hamilton, Ross E. The research program of the National Association for Retarded Children. *International Journal for the Education of the Blind,* Oct. 1958, Vol. 8, No. 1, pp. 20–26.

Relates concerns of Association to many concerns in the field of blindness. NARC will benefit all mentally retarded, including those who are blind.

3343. Harley, Randall K.; Merbler, John B.; & Wood, Thomas A. The development of a scale in orientation and mobility for multiply impaired blind children. *Education of the Visually Handicapped,* Mar. 1975, Vol. 7, No. 1, pp. 1–5.

Describes need and development of a scale to measure orientation and mobility in multiply impaired blind children. Describes in detail the Peabody Mobility Scale. Conclusions reached as a result of the construction of the experimental scale are included.

3344. Harley, Randall K.; Wood, Thomas A.; & Merbler, John B., Jr. Programmed instruction in orientation and mobility for multiply impaired blind children. *New Outlook for the Blind*, Nov. 1975, Vol. 69, No. 9, pp. 418–421, 423.

In pilot study programmatic instruction was developed for each identified skill and field-tested by 5 teachers of multiply impaired blind children during 15-week period. Results showed significant gains. Need for further research indicated.

3345. Hart, Verna. The blind child who functions on a retarded level: The challenge for teacher preparation. *New Outlook for the Blind*, Dec. 1969, Vol. 63, No. 10, pp. 318–21.

The teacher program at Peabody Col. is described including techniques for programming learning situations, prescriptive teaching, establishing priorities and using other staff. Need for a structured program, the cooperation of parents, and student evaluation are emphasized.

3346. Hartlage, Lawrence C. Listening comprehension in the retarded blind. *Perceptual and Motor Skills*, 1965, Vol. 20, No. 3, pp. 763–64.

Listening comprehension has been found to be related to age, sex, and intelligence. With these variables controlled, no significant differences have been found in this area between the blind and sighted. Study aimed at assessing the generality of findings to an abnormal sample.

3347. ――――. Social maturity, listening comprehension, and intelligence in the retarded blind. *Psychology*, 1966, Vol. 3, No. 4, pp. 12–15.

Twelve blind retarded *S*s were matched with 12 sighted retarded *S*s on age, sex, intelligence, and length of institutionalization. There were no significant differences between blind and sighted *S*s on listening comprehension or social maturity. Correlation between intelligence and listening comprehension was high in both groups.

3348. Huffman, Mildred B. *Fun comes first for blind slow learners.* Springfield, Ill.: Charles C Thomas, 1957, 157 pp.

Written for classroom teachers, book illustrates how growth was promoted in slow-learning, blind elementary-age children in a residential school for the blind. Includes the application of educational goals, procedures used by the teacher, and practical teaching suggestions.

3349. ――――. Let's make life and words meaningful to them. *International Journal for the Education of the Blind*, Dec. 1958, Vol. 8, No. 2, pp. 65–67.

Argues against the verbalism imposed on many slow-learning blind children. Time, experiments in how to give words meaning, much patience and repetition, and faith on the part of the teacher are necessary to enable the slow child to learn.

3350. ――――. Teaching retarded, disturbed blind children. *New Outlook for the Blind*, Sept. 1960, Vol. 54, No. 7, pp. 237–39.

A primary teacher with 8 years' experience suggests that the teacher's attitude is the governing influence on the child's ability to progress. Presents 8 guidelines on the correct attitudes/address to the child. Cites some results which may be expected.

3351. Iverson, Lee A., & Hartong, Jack R. Expanded opportunities for multiply handicapped children. *New Outlook for the Blind*, Apr. 1971, Vol. 65, No. 4, pp. 117–19, 125.

Chiefly a description of Special Services Dept. of Illinois Braille and Sight Saving School, its staff, program, admission and termination policies.

3352. Johnson, Gil, & Tuttle, Dean. Education and habilitation of multiply handicapped blind youth. *New Outlook for the Blind*, Feb. 1971, Vol. 65, No. 2, pp. 56–61.

Based on project to meet needs of older students of a school for the blind, 3 basic groups are identified—high school group, transitional work experience group, and work evaluation group. Education, counseling, and services required for each group in the project presented and examined. Project was felt to point up need for adapted curriculum to the new experiences afforded, more available services, and on-going group counseling for parents.

3353. Johnston, Benjamin C. Total life rehabilitation for the mentally retarded blind person. *New Outlook for the Blind*, Dec. 1971, Vol. 65, No. 10, pp. 331–33, 336.

Describes a vocational rehabilitation program that attempts to duplicate real-life living and working situations. Placement of trainees in competitive employment and sheltered workshops suggests that the program is successful.

3354. Johnston, Benjamin C., & Corbett, Michael. Orientation and mobility instruction for blind individuals functioning on a retarded level. *New Outlook for the Blind*, Jan. 1973, Vol. 67, No. 1, pp. 27–31.

Reports method of training, beginning with very basic areas. Recommends follow-up.

3355. Jones, Lloyd. *Multihandicapped blind.* Garden Grove, Calif.: Garden Grove Unified School District, 1972, 134 pp.

Objectives of program included a self-contained classroom with low teacher-pupil ratio, individual programs, parental attitudinal change, and teacher training. Given for each of the 6 children are case histories, evaluation data, and parent attitude assessment. Also reports student volunteer activities and evaluations.

3356. Kass, Walter, et al. Treatment of selective mutism in a blind child: School and clinic collaboration. *American Journal of Orthopsychiatry*, 1967, Vol. 37, No. 2, pp. 215–16.

Case of a congenitally blind girl whose problems, psychiatric and educational, are proceeding towards satisfactory resolution in the collaborative context.

3357. Kass, Walter, & Gillman, Arthur E. *A mental health center for disturbed blind children.* New York: Jewish Guild for the Blind, 1965, 73 pp.

Describes a program offering diagnosis, treatment, special education, prevocational and socialization services to children and youth who are emotionally disturbed and visually handicapped. Program includes work with families.

3358. Klineman, Janet. Hidden abilities discovered among multiply handicapped blind children. *Education of the Visually Handicapped*, Oct. 1975, Vol. 7, No. 3, pp. 90–96.

Reasons for increase in multiply handicapped children and some problems they present, followed by suggested solutions to the problems. Discusses in detail a list of assessment instruments and the case study approach with 1 case study. Concludes that early assessment followed by individualized early education programs show positive results.

3359. Knight, John J. Building self-confidence in the multiply handicapped blind child. *New Outlook for the Blind,* May 1971, Vol. 65, No. 5, pp. 152–54.

How producing and recording a pseudo radio show enhances the self-image in multiply handicapped children.

3360. Lane, Harlan, & Curran, Charles. Gradients of auditory generalization for blind, retarded children. *Journal of the Experimental Analysis of Behavior,* 1963, Vol. 6, No. 4, pp. 585–88.

Severely retarded, blind children were conditioned to respond differentially to 2 intensities of a pure tone. Gradients of auditory generalization were obtained that were reliable and similar to those for normal adults, but often asymmetric and nonmonotonic.

3361. Larsen, Lawrence A. Behavior modification with the multi-handicapped. *New Outlook for the Blind,* Jan. 1970, Vol. 64, No. 1, pp. 6–15.

Very detailed description of teacher behaviors which can modify the behavior of severely handicapped children. Emphasizes that child cannot respond to a stimulus if the input has been inappropriate for him. Ref.

3362. Larsen, Lawrence A., & Bricker, William A. *A manual for parents and teachers of severely and moderately retarded children. IMRID papers and reports, Volume 5, Number 22.* Nashville: Institute on Mental Retardation & Intellectual Development, 1968, 146 pp.

Presents methods for educating the moderately and severely retarded child. App. includes materials needed for the activities, suggested reinforcers, sample forms for pre- and post-test, glossary, and applications to blind and deaf children.

3363. Leach, Fay. Multiply handicapped visually impaired children: Instructional materials needs. *Exceptional Children,* Oct. 1971, Vol. 38, No. 2, pp. 153–56.

Reports on a survey which included review of the literature, questionnaire to and interviews in educational organizations. Lists areas of identified need, proposals to meet need.

3364. Leverett, Jim, & Bergman, Allan I. Sunrise project for the blind. *New Outlook for the Blind,* Feb. 1970, Vol. 64, No. 2, pp. 38–40.

Great progress for 20 mentally retarded blind, ages 7–17, results from a generously staffed special project of individualized education.

3365. Lobenstein, John H., et al. *A curriculum for the residential visually handicapped child.* Union Grove, Wis.: S. Wis. Colony and Training School, 1964, 20 pp.

Curriculum used at Colony and Training School is described in outline form. Experiences offered are centered on situations of daily living. Includes self-care, self-help, body usage, social adjustment, basic knowledge, and self-expression.

3366. Long, Elinor H. *The challenge of the cerebral palsied blind child.* New York: AFB, 1952, 36 pp.

Attitudes of residential schools for the blind, of public schools with classes for the blind, and of agencies serving crippled children are reported as regards their willingness and ability to provide for the cerebral palsied blind child. Twelve-page bib. and listings of schools and agencies where help may be obtained.

3367. Long, Nancy T. Space exploration for young multi-handicapped blind. *California State Federation CEC Journal,* June 1971, Vol. 20, No. 3, pp. 31–34.

Activities to develop body image, explore topological space and the coordinates, and spatial relations between objects by manually and kinesthetically exploring.

3368. Loomis, Chester. *An introduction to development of curriculum for educable mentally retarded visually handicapped adolescents.* New York: AFB, 1968, 40 pp.

Covers academic and living areas with basic considerations in planning and developing curriculum set forth.

3369. McClennen, Sandra. Teaching techniques for institutionalized blind retarded children. *New Outlook for the Blind,* Dec. 1969, Vol. 63, No. 10, pp. 322–25.

Program described that emphasizes language and speech and use of the token system of motivation. Stresses the learning of socially acceptable behavior. Individual realistic goals are set.

3370. McDade, Paul R. The importance of motor development and mobility skills for the institutionalized blind mentally retarded. *New Outlook for the Blind,* Dec. 1969, Vol. 63, No. 10, pp. 312–17.

Assessment of 33 individuals showed that 20–40% of the mentally handicapped could profit from a mobility program. Level of presentation and time required for training are different for the retarded blind than for a nonretarded group.

3371. MacFarland, Douglas C. Serving multiply disabled blind persons. *New Outlook for the Blind,* Sept. 1964, Vol. 58, No. 7, pp. 206–8.

Details work with the multiply handicapped blind and sees positive signs in recent interest in working with this group.

3372. McGlinchey, Maureen A., & Mitala, Ronald F. Using environmental design to teach ward layout to severely and profoundly retarded blind persons: A proposal. *New Outlook for the Blind,* Apr. 1975, Vol. 69, No. 4, pp. 168–71.

A simple and inexpensive environmental design system utilizing wall and floor cues is proposed to decrease fear of the environment and to promote movement, independence and social interaction among the residents of a ward for severely and profoundly retarded blind men.

3373. McQuie, Bob. Severely disturbed blind children. *International Journal for the Education of the Blind,* Dec. 1960, Vol. 10, No. 2, pp. 34–37.

Provides rather specific suggestions and guidelines for either a day or residential school program to serve a small number of emotionally disturbed children. The key is coordinating community resources.

3374. Maron, Sheldon S. Training prospective teachers of multiply handicapped blind children. *New Outlook for the Blind,* June 1975, Vol. 69, No. 6, pp. 266–73.

Describes philosophy, course work, and practicum of new 5-year program to train teachers of multiply handicapped blind children.

3375. Maron, Sheldon S., & Scholl, Geraldine T. Use of dimension highlighting procedures with multiply impaired blind adolescents. *Exceptional Children*, Sept. 1974, Vol. 41, No. 1, pp. 50–51.

Two highlighting techniques, perceptual isolation and functional matching, as well as a combination of the 2, were used in tests designed to measure improvement in tactile discrimination ability.

3376. Mattis, Steven. An experimental approach to treatment of visually impaired multi-handicapped children. *New Outlook for the Blind*, Jan. 1967, Vol. 61, No. 1, pp. 1–5.

Describes 2 programs, Concept Formation and Day Treatment, developed in response to belief that in many emotionally/mentally disturbed children conceptual deficits of probable organic etiology result in inappropriate behavior and high anxiety.

3377. Michal-Smith, Harold. Rehabilitation of the mentally retarded blind. *Rehabilitation Literature*, July 1969, Vol. 30, No. 7, pp. 194–98.

Edited version of paper presented Nov. 1968 at Symposium on Rehabilitation of the Mentally Retarded Blind, Pottstown, Pa.

3378. Misbach, Dorothy L. Happy, gracious living for the mentally-retarded blind child. *New Outlook for the Blind*, Mar. 1953, Vol. 47, No. 3, pp. 61–66.

Examines the need for high quality and great flexibility in administrators, teachers, and the school program for mentally retarded blind. Includes many specific suggestions.

3379. *Modern approaches to the diagnosis and instruction of multi-handicapped children. Volume 2, Deaf-blind children and their education.* Rotterdam, Holland: Rotterdam Univ. Press, 1971, 150 pp.

Proceedings of international conference. Medical, behavioral, and educational aspects, teaching techniques, mental health, and relationships between motor and learning disorders.

3380. Moor, Pauline M. Who are the children and what are they like? *International Journal for the Education of the Blind*, Oct. 1965, Vol. 15, No. 1, pp. 20–22.

Largely demographic, with emphasis on large number of multiply handicapped blind children whose patterns of behavior are briefly described. Closes with challenging questions about further information needed.

3381. ――――. *No time to lose.* New York: AFB, 1968, 53 pp.

Discussions of educational methods and techniques to use with multiply handicapped blind children includes the variations among children, hints for teachers, 3 case studies, and needs for refinement in evaluation and parent and community involvement.

3382. Murphy, Thomas J. Teaching orientation and mobility to mentally retarded blind persons. *New Outlook for the Blind*, Nov. 1964, Vol. 58, No. 9, pp. 285–87.

Case study of teaching mobility to a partially sighted, mentally retarded male. Author feels techniques must be tailored to client.

3383. Myers, James J., & Deibert, Alvin N. Reduction of self-abusive behavior in a blind child by using a feeding response. *Journal of Behavior*

Therapy and Experimental Psychiatry, July 1971, Vol. 2, No. 2, pp. 141–44.

Reduced head beating in 11-year-old retarded blind male by creating a feeding response incompatible with it.

3384. Myers, S. O. *Where are they now?* London, England: Royal National Institute for the Blind, 1975, £2.

Follow-up study of more than 300 blind adults with additional handicaps. Reviews training, services, and life opportunities for multiply handicapped in Great Britain.

3385. N.Y. State Education Dept. *The challenge of educating the preschool blind child with multiple handicaps.* Washington, D.C.: Office of Education, HEW, 1970, 75 pp.

Proceedings from a Special Studies Institute. Includes discussion of the challenge of educating the multiply handicapped child with sensory defects; the physician's contribution in diagnosis, treatment, and consultation; adapting professional knowledge and skill to service; educational techniques; problems of multiply handicapped children in rural areas; and the impact of federal legislation.

3386. Office for the Blind and Visually Handicapped, Commonwealth of Pa. *Proceedings: In-service training conference on the rehabilitation of the multi-disabled industrially blind.* Harrisburg: Author, 1968, 134 pp.

Report on proceedings of 2 in-service training conferences designed to explore new approaches to providing more adequate services, particularly in the vocational area.

3387. O'Meara, Mary. An experimental program at the Illinois Braille and Sight Saving School for developmentally-delayed, visually-impaired children. *International Journal for the Education of the Blind,* Oct. 1966, Vol. 16, No. 1, pp. 18–20.

Three areas of instruction—living skills, sensory stimulation, and academic work—are offered on an individually planned basis. Various methods of communication are employed and ancillary services are available.

3388. Paraskeva, Peter C. A survey of the facilities for the mentally retarded-blind in the United States. *International Journal for the Education of the Blind,* May 1959, Vol. 8, No. 4, pp. 139–43.

Reports results of 29 responses to a questionnaire about residential school services for mentally retarded blind children. Lists number and percentage of such children in the responding schools and draws conclusions.

3389. Parker, Ann L. Reinforcement: One teacher's experiences and experiments with multiply handicapped blind children. *New Outlook for the Blind,* Mar. 1971, Vol. 65, No. 3, pp. 97–99.

Reviews some criticisms of operant conditioning. Reinforcement must be meaningful and appropriate. Two case studies illustrate this.

3390. Perry, Anna C. General music. *International Journal for the Education of the Blind,* Dec. 1958, Vol. 3, No. 2, pp. 220–22.

Discusses importance of music for retarded blind children: Appreciation, rhythm, manual ability, coordination, cooperation. Mentions types of songs, finger games, rhythm records, dances, folk tunes, toy orchestra.

3391. Pittsburgh Univ. School of Education. *Professional preparation of* *teachers of the multiply handicapped with special concern directed toward the child with both auditory and visual impairments. Proceedings of the Special Study Institute (Pittsburgh, Pennsylvania, June 28–August 6, 1971)* Harrisburg, Pa.: State Dept. of Education, 1971, 98 pp.

Reports selected examples of the preparation program for teachers. Appended is an extensive manual for development of self-help skills in multiply handicapped children.

3392. Rapaport, Irene. Symposium—Self-image: A guide to adjustment II. Mental handicap—diagnosis and placement. *New Outlook for the Blind*, Nov. 1961, Vol. 55, No. 9, pp. 291–93.

Discussion of the diagnostic process as an ongoing procedure divided into 3 phases: Initial evaluation, program and placement planning, and follow-up reevaluation.

3393. Regler, Jerry. An experimental program for slowly developing blind children. *International Journal for the Education of the Blind*, May 1960, Vol. 9, No. 4, pp. 89–92.

An experimental 4-week program at the Nebraska School for the Blind was set up (1) to evaluate the present preschool program, (2) to assist children to develop social skills, and (3) to recommend a permanent program for slow learners. Results and recommendations are reported.

3394. Rigby, Mary E. Some of the problems of the multiply handicapped. *International Journal for the Education of the Blind*, May 1963, Vol. 12, No. 4, pp. 97–102.

Problems in parent-child and educational areas are discussed. Lists special classes and ungraded rooms which have had considerable success in meeting the problems. Ref.

3395. Rigby, Mary E., & Woodcock, Charles C. *Development of a residential education program for emotionally deprived pseudo-retarded blind children, Volumes I, II, and III. Final report.* Salem: Oreg. State School for the Blind, 1969, 706 pp.

Vol. I describes a residential school program for multiply handicapped blind children and the identifying procedures for prospects for this type of program. Results indicated that 14 of the 15 children showed some improvement at end of the 12-month program. Vols. II and III are case studies of the 15 children.

3396. Rodden, Hannah. Teaching techniques for institutionalized blind retarded children. *New Outlook for the Blind*, Jan. 1970, Vol. 64, No. 1, pp. 25–28.

Suggested techniques include encouragement of self-care skills, counseling, remedial experience activities, and a nursery school to teach mobility and command responses.

3397. Rogow, Sally. The non-verbal blind child: Two paths to speech. *New Outlook for the Blind*, Jan. 1969, Vol. 63, No. 1, pp. 1–7.

Largely through the story of one 9-year-old blind girl who was so withdrawn as to be nonverbal, describes treatment which within 6 mos. led to speech and more rewarding relationships with the environment.

3398. ———. Retardation among blind children. *Education of the Visually Handicapped*, Dec. 1970, Vol. 2, No. 4, pp. 107–11.

Discusses the nature of retardation and ways in which blindness inter-feres with perceptual and cognitive learning. Sensory deprivation, percep-tual development, and limitations of environmental experience are also examined.

3399. ———. Blind retarded children in Canada. *Special Education in Canada*, Mar.–Apr. 1972, Vol. 46, No. 3, pp. 25–28.

Describes the blind mentally handicapped child's perception of the physical world and his language development.

3400. ———. Language acquisition and the blind retarded child. *Education of the Visually Handicapped*, May 1972, Vol. 4, No. 2, pp. 36–40.

Language development for the blind retarded child is impaired if the child does not receive educational training, stimulation, and social exper-ience. Includes personal experience with 9-year-old, nonverbal child.

3401. ———. Speech development and the blind multi-impaired child. *Education of the Visually Handicapped*, Dec. 1973, Vol. 5, No. 4, pp. 105–9.

Discusses types of oral/vocal sensory stimulation and activities. Ad-dresses need to assist transition from passive sensory experience to active experience and encourage integration of auditory and haptic systems in the multiply handicapped infant or child.

3402. ———. Beginning educational programmes for blind mentally re-tarded children. *Teacher of the Blind*, Winter 1973–4, Vol. 62, No. 2, pp. 40–46.

Based on an experimental programme in British Columbia with 7 chil-dren aged 2½–13. The main concern of the programming was the stimu-lation of play skills, self-initiated behavior, exploratory and manipulative skills.

3403. Root, Ferne K. Evaluation of services for multiple-handicapped blind children. *International Journal for the Education of the Blind*, Dec. 1963, Vol. 13, No. 2, pp. 33–38.

Discusses some of the ways in which needs of multiply handicapped blind children can be met and how to determine the best choice for a particular child. Counseling, diagnostic services, financial assistance, and information for future planning are needed. Describes services in N.Y.

3404. Royer-Greaves School, Staff Members. Academic subjects for retarded blind children. *International Journal for the Education of the Blind*, June 1952, Vol. 1, No. 4, pp. 84–88.

Discusses procedures used in presenting and teaching arithmetic, spell-ing, typing, and use of remaining vision.

3405. Rubin, Edmund J., & Monaghan, Sheila. Calendar calculation in a multiple-handicapped blind person. *American Journal of Mental Defi-ciency*, 1965, Vol. 70, No. 3, pp. 478–85.

Report of a 16-year-old, totally blind girl who functions at a retarded level. Her ability to give the day when different dates occurred was much above her general level of functioning. Different aspects of this talent are explored.

3406. Rubin, Judith. Through art to affect: Blind children express their feel-ings. *New Outlook for the Blind*, Nov. 1975, Vol. 69, No. 9, pp. 385–91, illus.

Describes feelings and fantasies, including those related to their blindness, expressed in and through art by multiply handicapped, visually impaired children.

3407. Rubin, Judith, & Klineman, Janet. They opened our eyes: Story of an exploratory program for visually-impaired multiply-handicapped children. *Education of the Visually Handicapped,* Dec. 1974, Vol. 6, No. 4, pp. 106–13.

Use of art programs with visually handicapped retarded children. Great growth seen both technically and emotionally in both students and teachers. Ref.

3408. Rusalem, Herbert, & Richterman, Harold. *Multi-handicapped blind persons can work.* New York: National Industries for the Blind, 1972, 85 pp.

Describes demonstration project with specially designed screening, product development, engineering, and rehabilitation techniques, with innovative approach to remunerative work—291 blind participants.

3409. Salmon, Peter J. Modern programs for blind persons with other disabilities. *New Outlook for the Blind,* Jan. 1965, Vol. 59, No. 1, pp. 15–17.

Illustrates recent changes in program by the new emphasis on public education to change attitudes about the multiply handicapped, use of diagnostic and service teams with specialists from other than the field of blindness, and cooperative agreements with other agencies.

3410. Schaeffer, M. Harris. Meeting the needs of the blind-mentally retarded at the Pennhurst State School and Hospital. *New Outlook for the Blind,* Oct. 1968, Vol. 62, No. 8, pp. 254–58.

Describes development of a special program for blind persons in a state institution for the mentally retarded.

3411. Schattner, Regina. *An early childhood curriculum for multiply handicapped children.* New York: John Day, 1971, 143 pp.

Chapters on the partially sighted child (pp. 100–105) and the blind child (pp. 106–13) concern special materials, especially those for teaching reading.

3412. Scott, Dwayne M. Blind retardates enter the job market. *Tennessee Public Welfare Record,* June 1972, Vol. 35, No. 3, pp. 46–50.

Brief report on a special training project at the Orange Grove Center for the Retarded. Although still in the experimental stage, the program has succeeded beyond expectations.

3413. Simon, G. B. The needs of the visually and mentally handicapped child—1. *New Beacon,* Feb. 1972, Vol. 56, No. 658, pp. 31–33. Part 2, Mar. 1972.

Author feels newly available education opportunities for these children have produced very positive results.

3414. ———. The needs of the visually and mentally handicapped child—2. *New Beacon,* Mar. 1972, Vol. 56, No. 659, pp. 63–65. Part 1, Feb. 1972.

Important steps of assessment, parental guidance, use of voluntary organizations, and research facilities are discussed. Residence unit is described, suggestions made to meet need in all of England.

3415. Sklar, Mark J., & Rampulla, Joanne. Decreasing inappropriate classroom behavior of a multiply handicapped blind student. *Education of the Visually Handicapped,* Oct. 1973, Vol. 5, No. 3, pp. 71–74.

A multiply handicapped 20-year-old student in a special, public school class was behaviorally reinforced with favorable results.

3416. Smeets, Paul M. The effects of various sounds and noise levels on stereotyped rocking of blind retardates. *Training School Bulletin,* Feb. 1972, Vol. 68, No. 4, pp. 221–26.

No clear relationship between rocking and noise level, type, or duration.

3417. Stephens, Roberta. Running free: The use of a "running cable" with blind adolescents who function on a retarded level. *New Outlook for the Blind,* Dec. 1973, Vol. 67, No. 10, pp. 454–56, illus.

Cables running between 2 telephone poles 38 yards apart provide opportunity for blind retarded adolescents to exercise, improve ambulation problems, and release excess energy in a constructive manner. By holding onto a strap connected to the cable by an inverted pulley, the adolescents are able to run independently with a minimum of supervision.

3418. Stolz, Stephanie B., & Wolf, Montrose M. Visually discriminated behavior in a "blind" adolescent retardate. *Journal of Applied Behavior Analysis,* 1969, Vol. 2, No. 1, pp. 65–77.

Description of the progress of the patient after training in discriminating visual stimuli.

3419. Stone, Alan A. Consciousness: Altered levels in blind retarded children. *American Foundation for the Blind Research Bulletin 19,* June 1969, pp. 235–41. Reprinted from *Psychosomatic Medicine,* 1964.

Observation suggested that there were 2 types of "blindisms" in 40 mentally retarded blind children. Electroencephalographic data shows relationship between the "blindisms" and altered levels of consciousness which may regulate the child's relation to reality.

3420. Strickland, Howard. Braille at Royer-Greaves School for the Blind. *International Journal for the Education of the Blind,* Feb. 1952, Vol. 1, No. 3, pp. 61–62.

Discusses methods of teaching students with more than 1 handicap who are also retarded, use of additional aids, individual instruction, nonexistant class graduation.

3421. ――――. Value of student organizations in our school. *International Journal for the Education of the Blind,* Sept. 1953, Vol. 3, No. 1, pp. 198–200.

Discussion of Royer-Greaves school for retarded (where children often have additional handicaps), student council, Girl Scouts, Victory Club, and projects, integration of rehabilitation.

3422. Sunland Training Center. *Outline of the program for trainable residents.* Gainesville, Fla.: Author, 1964, 17 pp.

Includes a program for the blind trainable retarded in discrimination skills, learning skills, music activities, self-expression, and social skills.

3423. Szuhay, J. A., Ed. *Report of proceedings of Institute on Continual Services for the Multi-Handicapped Blind.* Scranton, Pa.: Univ. of Scranton, 1968, 47 pp.

Description of conference discussions and copies of several papers on status of multiply handicapped blind.

3424. Talkington, Larry W. An exploratory program for blind-retarded. *Education of the Visually Handicapped*, May 1972, Vol. 4, No. 2, pp. 33–35.

Twelve blind retarded adolescents participated in a 12-week project that sought to develop and implement a program focusing on stimulus-behavior and motivation. Improvement noted between pre- and post-test.

3425. Tekawa, Toshi. Multi-handicapped blind children at the California School for the Blind. *Education of the Visually Handicapped*, May 1969, Vol. 1, No. 2, pp. 63–64.

Discussion of curriculum and problems in education of multiply handicapped.

3426. Terry, Grace F., & Schaffner, Fred G. Visually handicapped children who function on a retarded level: The Frances Blend School, Los Angeles. *New Outlook for the Blind*, May 1972, Vol. 66, No. 5, pp. 135–38.

Pictures with commentary supplement a description of goals of the school, individualized curriculum, prevocational training, and ultimate opportunities in a workshop.

3427. Thomas, E. J. Baylis. *Services and training methods in a day care center for severely retarded blind children.* New York: Jewish Guild for the Blind, 1969, 26 pp.

Discusses training methods used with 7 children, 3–14 years of age, during 1 year. Reviews program goals, staffing, research, demonstration. Analyzes 3 types of assessment used to determine effectiveness of training techniques.

3428. Thomas, John E. Mobility education for multiply handicapped blind children in day schools: What it encompasses. *New Outlook for the Blind*, Nov. 1972, Vol. 66, No. 9, pp. 307–14.

Description of a 6-part mobility program which includes coordination and postural exercises, sensory awareness, indoor orientation and travel skill building, outdoor mobility concept development and cane technique development, outdoor mobility in the school and home neighborhoods, and outdoor mobility in small business areas and on public transportation. Lists suggestions for a resource teacher that would assist a peripatologist.

3429. Tretakoff, M. I., & Farrell, M.J. Developing a curriculum for the blind retarded. *American Journal of Mental Deficiency*, 1958, Vol. 62, pp. 610–15.

Discussion of conclusions drawn as a result of study of the first 160 blind admissions to the Walter E. Fernald State School.

3430. Tupper, La Verne. The multiply handicapped blind child in New York State. *New Outlook for the Blind*, Sept. 1962, Vol. 56, No. 7, pp. 243–46.

After brief description of agency services, states that about ⅓ of blind population is multiply handicapped. Lists common combinations of handicaps and various helping services for children and parents.

3431. ———. *Suggestions for parents of a mentally retarded blind child.* Albany, N.Y.: Comm. for the Blind & Visually Handicapped, 1969?, 11 pp.

Includes such aspects of child rearing as good health practices, professional consultation, family attitudes, and provision of stimulating activities.

3432. Tuttle, Dean W. Shifting gears for multi-handicapped blind children. *Education of the Visually Handicapped*, Oct. 1970, Vol. 2, No. 3, pp. 76–79.

The development of personal relationships, awareness of individual differences, positive reinforcement of desired behavior, and utilization of community resources in the classroom are considered. Stressed are the totality of the child's experiences, realistic expectations, sharing and exchanging ideas, uniqueness of each child, activity learning, long-range commitments and goals, and research.

3433. Warburg, Mette. Prevention of blindness in mentally retarded children. *Sight-Saving Review*, Winter 1974–75, Vol. 44, No. 4, pp. 165–70.

Based on study of 201, discussion of causes of blindness found in MR population in Copenhagen.

3434. Wayne, Marvin R. *Report of proceedings: Institute on the Rehabilitation of the Multihandicapped Blind.* New York: Hunter Col., 1967, 74 pp.

Presents papers and discussions on various aspects of the multiply handicapped blind.

3435. Williams, Cyril E. Blind idiot who became normal blind adolescent. *Developmental Medicine and Child Neurology*, 1966, Vol. 8, No. 2, pp. 166–69.

A case report of a boy first seen at age 5 when he was considered an idiot with an MA of 9½ mos. on the Vineland Scale. At age 18, he had an IQ of 102 on the Williams Intelligence Test, had many interests and social skills, and was emotionally stable.

3436. Wilson, Diana A. Teaching multiply handicapped blind persons in a state hospital. *New Outlook for the Blind*, Oct. 1974, Vol. 68, No. 8, pp. 337–43, 362.

A compensatory education program for 14 blind retarded youths in a state institution is described. Teaching suggestions and guidelines are presented. Recreational skills are emphasized.

3437. Winn, Robert J., Jr. Two-year progress analysis of project for multi-handicapped visually-impaired children at the Texas School for the Blind. *International Journal for the Education of the Blind*, Dec. 1968, Vol. 18, No. 4, pp. 99–107.

Describes project subjects, discusses the philosophy and educational procedures, and provides detailed statistical analysis of the results, based on 24 children.

3438. Wolf, James M. Multiple disabilities—An old problem with a new challenge. *New Outlook for the Blind*, Oct. 1965, Vol. 59, No. 8, pp. 265–71.

Well-organized review of literature on multiple disabilities with special sections on deaf-blind and mentally retarded-blind. Ref.

3439. ———. *The blind child with concomitant disabilities.* New York: AFB, 1967, 112 pp.

Inquiry schedule sent to 48 residential schools and 53 classroom teachers conducting classes for mentally handicapped visually impaired children. Results indicate a trend for the schools to accept multiply handicapped children.

3440. Wolf, James M., & Anderson, Robert M., Eds. *The multiply handicapped child.* Springfield, Ill.: Charles C Thomas, 1969, 468 pp.

Articles presented in the area of the medical and educational challenge. Many types of handicaps are covered including those in children whose mothers had rubella. Also covered is psychological evaluation of the blind.

3441. Zwarensteyn, Sarah B., & Zerby, Margaret. A residential school program for multi-handicapped blind children. *New Outlook for the Blind,* June 1962, Vol. 56, No. 6, pp. 191–99.

Discusses, from points of view of administrators and teachers, the decisions, procedures, staff responsibilities, and housing of an experimental program for multiply handicapped blind.

31.   The Material Environment

3442. American Foundation for the Blind. *Travel concessions for blind persons: What every blind person should know,* rev. ed. New York: Author, 1965, 10 pp., free.

This large-print booklet provides information about travel concessions for blind persons and sighted companions.

3443. ————. *Nature trails, braille trails, foot paths, fragrance gardens. Touch museums for the blind: Policy statement.* New York: Author, July 1972, 2 pp.

3444. Arnold, Carolyn. Visually impaired persons in nursing homes. *New Outlook for the Blind,* Sept. 1972, Vol. 66, No. 7, pp. 227–29.

Through consultation with nursing home staff and direct contact with residents, the Lighthouse for the Blind of Houston helps older citizens adjust to changes in life style and provides direct services to the residents.

3445. Bankston, Alice. The Oral Hull story. *Braille Forum,* July–Aug. 1975, Vol. 14, No. 1, pp. 3–5.

History of a 22-acre recreational park, converted from a farm, in Oregon. Has 5 garden sections, 1 each for touch, taste, hearing, sight, and smell, with brailled as well as typed labels on plants, trees, and bushes.

3446. Bernardo, Jose R. Architecture for blind persons. *New Outlook for the Blind,* Oct. 1970, Vol. 64, No. 8, pp. 262–65.

Discusses ways an architect must alter his priorities and redefine architecture in nonvisual terms when designing buildings for blind persons. Suggests consultation with blind persons and recommends some possibilities for change while cautioning against a too protective and special environment.

3447. Braf, Per-Gunnar. *The physical environment and the visually impaired.* Bromma, Sweden: ICTA Information Center, 1974, 34 pp.

Reports results of project at the Swedish Institute for the Handicapped to determine needs of the visually impaired in the planning and adaptation of buildings and other forms of physical environment.

3448. Brett, James J. Pathways for the blind. *Conservationist,* June–July 1971, Vol. 25, pp. 13–16, illus.

Describes the design of the Oerwood Braille Trail in Pa.

3449. Brodey, Warren. Sound and space. *New Outlook for the Blind,* Jan. 1965, Vol. 59, No. 1, pp. 1–4.

A challenging discussion of how architecture and sound may interplay and how the sound of a room can be exciting, restful, etc. Also, a large room can be subdivided without visible walls by engineering different acoustical qualities in different parts of the room. Feels blind people are more sensitive to this than sighted people usually are.

3450. Campbell, Edward A. How safe are your shop facilities? *New Outlook for the Blind*, Apr. 1963, Vol. 57, No. 4, pp. 131–34.

Discusses accident prevention goals in a shop program including a clear outline of chief purposes of the shop, basic plan, adequate shop space, occupant safety, and shop environment.

3451. Chester Co. Board of School Directors. *Planning for a special education building for Chester County, Pennsylvania.* West Chester, Pa.: Author, 1966, 77 pp.

Discusses problems faced by Chester Co. in the construction of a special education building in the areas of facilities, equipment, staff and transportation. Suggestions of 10 consultants and graph and maps included. Program for the visually handicapped is described.

3452. Eisenberg, Arthur. Perspectives on living arrangements for blind people. *New Outlook for the Blind*, Oct. 1964, Vol. 58, No. 8, pp. 233–35.

Author thinks social agencies need to make community aware of need for adequate shelter for blind people.

3453. Fontaine, James. The one-fare travel concession. *New Outlook for the Blind*, June 1961, Vol. 55, No. 6, pp. 208–10.

Specific information as to eligibility and applicability of special travel rates for the blind.

3454. Froistad, Wilmer M. Housing: An aspect of services to blind persons. *New Outlook for the Blind*, Oct. 1964, Vol. 58, No. 8, pp. 239–43.

Social agencies must individualize housing advice to blind. Author feels that in general housing based on common factor of blindness is to be avoided unless there is an unusual reason for it.

3455. Governor's Committee on Employment of the Handicapped. *Proceeding of Architectural Barriers Conference (Ilikai Hotel, Honolulu, Hawaii, November 28, 29, 30, 1966).* Honolulu: Univ. of Hawaii, 1966, 58 pp.

Discussions are presented by handicapped and nonhandicapped speakers and focus on community attitudes, practical considerations (buildings and transportation), and economic considerations in eliminating architectural barriers.

3456. Johnson, Frank, & Smith, Byron M. The place of a home for the blind in a rehabilitation program. *New Outlook for the Blind*, Oct. 1954, Vol. 48, No. 8, pp. 271–72.

Describes a new residence for the blind in Minneapolis and how it fosters the personal independence and social integration of its residents.

3457. Kidwell, Ann M., & Greer, Peter S. The environmental perceptions of blind persons and their haptic representation. *New Outlook for the Blind*, Oct. 1972, Vol. 66, No. 8, pp. 256–76, illus.

Article is based on 2 chapters from authors' joint thesis written for masters of architecture degree at M.I.T. Compares physical-spatial maps and sequential maps. Limitations of the latter noted. Discusses 6 basic types of tactual map reproduction and indicates that polyvinyl chloride proved most promising. Success of 1st map encouraged planning of 2nd.

3458. ———. *Sites perception and the nonvisual experience: Designing and manufacturing mobility maps.* New York: AFB, 1973, 192 pp., app., illus.

Describes research and development of a tactual map of M.I.T. campus for blind students by M.I.T. architecture students. Includes discussion of spatial perception and concepts, adventitious and congenital blindness, aspects of mobility, student interviews, and the map itself.

3459. Library Assoc. *Clear print: Papers and proceedings of a conference sponsored by the Library Association and the National Association for the Education of the Partially Sighted.* London: Author, 1972, 65 pp.

Papers include factors in lighting, building design for providing correct quality and intensity of light, and library services.

3460. Lindsey, Robert. Travel for the handicapped eases as obstacles fall. *Rehabilitation Teacher,* Aug.–Sept. 1973, Vol. 5, No. 8–9, pp. 39–46.

Discusses attitudes of airlines that refuse to carry handicapped persons and improvements in architectural facilities such as in the Holiday Inn chains. Five agencies which arrange and conduct tours for the handicapped are listed with addresses.

3461. Mo. State Dept. of Education. *A master plan program of requirements for the Francis Jefferson Coates Country Campus of the Missouri School for the Blind.* St. Louis: Pearce & Pearce, Jan. 1966, 34 pp.

Facility requirements presented for indoor and outdoor living and learning facilities of proposed campus. Diagrammatic representations of proposed facilities included.

3462. Morris, Robert H. A play environment for blind children: Design and evaluation. *New Outlook for the Blind,* Nov. 1974, Vol. 68, No. 9, pp. 408–14, illus.

A play environment, comprised of 8 circular play courts arranged around a 9th court, was designed on basis of idea that play could be used to help blind children learn orientation skills that are essential for their development as individuals. The design was presented to a panel of experts, the majority of which judged it to be effective.

3463. Nugent, Timothy J. *Design of buildings to permit their use by the physically handicapped: A national attack on architectural barriers.* Chicago: National Society for Crippled Children & Adults, 1960, 15 pp.

Reviews research and implications for many handicaps, including making buildings more accessible for visually handicapped.

3464. N.Y. State Univ. *Making facilities accessible to the physically handicapped.* Washington, D.C.: Vocational Rehabilitation Admin., 1967, 40 pp.

Guidelines on performance criteria for N.Y. State Univ. considers the ambulant and semiambulant handicapped, including the visually and aurally handicapped. Includes detailed specifications for some aspects of exterior design including entrances, stairs, intersections, bus service. Interior design criteria are cited for general university facilities.

3465. Ontario Dept. of Education, School Planning and Building Research Section. *Soundstop: An experimental student housing study.* Bethesda: Leasco Information Products, 1969, 40 pp.

A detailed review of the design development of a housing facility for deaf and blind students. Each space in the final design is dealt with as to development, layout, and functional goals. Interiors for the various spaces are shown in several different schemes to meet the wide range of needs for the 6–20-year age range that will be served.

3466. "Please touch the flowers." *Seer*, Summer 1975, Vol. 46, No. 2, pp. 8–10.

Description of the Fragrance Garden at the Lancaster Co. Branch of the Pennsylvania Assoc. for the Blind. In the selection of plants great emphasis was placed on fragrance, texture, and size.

3467. Raskin, Nathaniel J. *A study of the living expenses of blind persons.* New York: AFB, 1955, 44 pp.

The living expenses of a sample of 65 blind single consumers and families including a blind member were compared with expenditures of a population of 143 sampled by Bureau of Labor Statistics in the same city to ascertain whether blind persons are confronted with special living expenses.

3468. Robinson, M. C., & Wood, H. A. Economic security in the twentieth century: Two views on philosophy and method of financial assistance to blind people. *New Outlook for the Blind*, Apr. 1955, Vol. 49, No. 4, pp. 124–31.

One paper favors a universal "expense of living" allowance to be given automatically to any person within the recognized definition of blindness regardless of financial circumstances. Mr. Wood's paper favors a means test but states that "the whole range of social needs . . . with an increasing standard of adequacy based upon valid needs rather than on arbitrary compensation for physical loss."

3469. Ruijter, C. W. *Architectural facilities for the disabled.* The Hague, Netherlands: Netherlands Society for Rehabilitation, 1973, 32 pp.

Presents 39 architectural engineering drawings to aid different classifications of disabled persons. Includes such things as telephone booths, pivoted doors, and ramps.

3470. Salmon, F. Cuthbert, & Salmon, Christine F. *The blind, space needs for rehabilitation.* Stillwater: Okla. State Univ., 1964, 82 pp., illus.

Based on analysis of 14 rehabilitation centers for the blind, presents recommendations for an ideal facility in terms of design and architecture. Ref.

3471. Shaw, John A. A blind man looks at color. *New Beacon*, Dec. 1973, Vol. 57, No. 680, pp. 15–17.

An adventitiously blind man discusses experiences with color deprivation, suggests a technique for teaching color concepts to congenitally blind people.

3472. ———. Stimulus appetite. *New Beacon*, June 1974, Vol. 58, No. 686, pp. 144–45.

Blind author discusses sensory stimulation and privation in general and in relation to blindness noting his own ways of satisfying his sensory appetite.

3473. Soyer, David. Living arrangements for blind adults. *New Outlook for the Blind,* Oct. 1964, Vol. 58, No. 8, pp. 246–51.

Discusses the social work philosophy of Jewish Guild for the Blind. History of Guild's residences, current work in field of living arrangements, and plans for future. Some case studies are given.

3474. Spinelli, Antonio J., & Earley, James E. Dual nature trails use both braille and printed markers for use of visually handicapped campers. *Camping Magazine,* Mar. 1972, Vol. 44, No. 3, p. 19.

Brief description of the construction of 2 natural trails at the Hale Camping Reservation, Westwood, Mass., designed for both visually handicapped and sighted persons.

3475. Stanford, Charles W., Jr. Knowing art in a museum through the perception of touch: The Mary Duke Biddle Gallery for the Blind. *North Carolina Museum of Art Bulletin,* Dec. 1968, Vol. 8, No. 2, pp. 4–11.

Story of the development of a special museum gallery based on sculpture and reliefs.

3476. Stephens, Alicia. "Seeing" by touch in a museum. *Rehabilitation Teacher,* Dec. 1972, Vol. 4, No. 12, pp. 7–10.

Describes a tour, for blind and partially sighted children, of Old Salem, restored.

3477. tenBroek, Jacobus. Proposal for a fixed grant to the blind and related constructive changes. *New Outlook for the Blind,* Nov. 1953, Vol. 47, No. 9, pp. 257–64.

Detailed statement of the need of blind people for an income security program, arguments against the means test, and a statement of valid welfare goals. Aid is a matter of right, and adequate exemption of earnings is necessary.

3478. Thornton, Walter. The typhlonaut in Scandinavia. *New Beacon,* Oct. 1975, Vol. 59, No. 702, pp. 253–257.

Semifictional account of travel by a blind person (typhlonautics = blind navigation).

3479. Toll, Dove. Should museums serve the visually handicapped? *New Outlook for the Blind,* Dec. 1975, Vol. 69, No. 10, pp. 461–64.

Describes research project and program at National Museum of Natural History of the Smithsonian Institution. Has cassette tours and braille guidebook. Lists other museums which have special exhibits and/or galleries. Bib.

3480. Tsunoda, Kazuichi, & Tanaka, Nobuo. An experimental study of the effects of environments on the seeing defectives: Summary report. *Tohoku Journal of Educational Psychology,* 1964, Vol. 1, No. 2, pp. 101–2.

Eighty blind children were divided into 2 equal groups with equal distribution in ages, IQs, physical conditions, etc. Experimental group was provided with an enriched diet, vitamins, and drugs of nutritious value to the brain. These children showed improvement in the constitutes of blood and urine, promotion of physical development and capacity, tendencies to stability of emotion and a few improvements in intelligence.

32.   The Human Environment

3481. American Foundation for the Blind. *National invitational symposium on attitudes about blindness: Special bibliography on attitudes affecting blindness.* New York: Author, 1971, 6 pp.

Developed especially for those attending the above symposium, lists selected references on attitudes related to blindness.

3482. Baker, Larry D., & Reitz, H. Joseph. Blindness, situational dependency, and helping behavior. *Proceedings of the 81st Annual Convention of the American Psychological Association, Montreal, Canada,* 1973, Vol. 8, pp. 807–8.

Conducted field research on whether blind persons would be helped more than sighted persons in situations in which sight was not essential to the person's plight. Results are related to the personality development of the blind.

3483. Barnett, Sara E. "Whatever Lola wants—" *New Outlook for the Blind,* Oct. 1955, Vol. 49, No. 8, pp. 293–94.

Criticizes the stereotypes of blindness presented by the media.

3484. Barraga, Natalie C. Utilisation of low vision in adults who are severely visually handicapped. *New Beacon,* Mar. 1975, Vol. 59, No. 695, pp. 57–63.

Advises concentrating on clients' use of residual vision, and treating low vision clients as "seeing" rather than "blind" individuals.

3485. Bateman, Barbara. The modifiability of sighted adults' perceptions of blind children's abilities. *New Outlook for the Blind,* May 1964, Vol. 58, No. 5, pp. 133–35.

Questionnaires to college students, followed by information-giving, disclose attitudes and the extent to which they can be improved.

3486. ———. Sighted children's perceptions of blind children's abilities. *American Foundation for the Blind Research Bulletin 8,* Jan. 1965, pp. 21–28. Reprinted from *Exceptional Children,* Sept. 1962.

Questionnaire listing 50 activities was administered to 115 sighted Ss who had not known a blind child and to 117 who had known 1 or more blind children, asking whether they believed a blind child their own age could perform the activities. Results are briefly reported.

3487. Beers, Nora. The preschool blind child in the hospital. *New Outlook for the Blind,* June 1958, Vol. 52, No. 6, pp. 216–21.

Discusses the premature blind child, the infant brought from the hospital, the hospital teacher, the blind toddler, the prekindergarten child.

3488. Bertin, Morton A. A comparison of attitudes toward blindness. *International Journal for the Education of the Blind*, Oct. 1959, Vol. 9, No. 1, pp. 1–4.

Following exploratory background discussion, reports results of a study of attitudes of 72 residential school blind students and 271 sighted public school students in similar grades.

3489. Bixby, Janet. A family the hard way. *Dialogue*, Winter 1974, Vol. 13, No. 4, pp. 2–5.

The difficulty experienced by blind persons who wish to adopt children is illustrated by the stories of 2 families.

3490. Carroll, Thomas J. The marriage of blind persons—A supplement. *New Outlook for the Blind*, Sept. 1963, Vol. 57, No. 7, pp. 267–68.

There are occasions when an individual blind parent is incapable of handling the situation, but it would be a gross error on the part of society to take blindness as prima facie evidence of the incompetence of the parent. Individual blind parents may show the highest competence in rearing children.

3491. Condl, Emma D. Ophthalmic nursing: The gentle touch. *Nursing Clinics of North America*, Sept. 1970, Vol. 5, No. 3, pp. 467–75.

Nursing techniques necessary in eye care including psychological adjustment of patient, admission and orientation procedures, pre- and postoperative care and home care.

3492. Differences between the congenital and the adventitious blind. *Lantern Light*, June 1974, Vol. 8, No. 2, pp. 30–31.

Brief description of differences in attitudes as they affect rehabilitation.

3493. Doherty, Jim. Jury duty in D.C. *Braille Monitor*, Jan. 1975, pp. 39–40.

Since blind persons are often excused from jury duty, the author relates his personal experiences in serving.

3494. English, R. William. Assessment, modification, and stability of attitudes toward blindness. *Psychological Aspects of Disability*, July 1971, Vol. 18, No. 2, pp. 79–85.

Use of tape recordings of simulated encounters shows that brief negative encounters between disabled and nondisabled persons have no measurable effect on attitudes.

3495. Ferguson, Linda T. Components of attitudes toward the deaf. *Proceedings of the Annual Convention of the American Psychological Association*, 1970, Vol. 5, Part 2, pp. 693–94.

Studied the reactions of hearing persons toward the deaf and relates the results to attitudes toward blindness, amputation, etc.

3496. Fleming, Juanita W. *Care and management of exceptional children.* New York: Appleton-Century-Crofts, 1973, 212 pp., $8.95.

Intended for nurses, offers a behavioral viewpoint of handicapped children and encourages nurses to help parents manage children for maximum development. Considers special needs, family dynamics, and behavior modification. Lists 29 agencies for nurses trying to help exceptional children and their families.

3497. Gioseffi, William V. Culture as an aspect of the total personality. *New Outlook for the Blind*, Mar. 1960, Vol. 54, No. 3, pp. 95–99.

Discusses culture (cultural patterns, cultural conditioning) as it helps form a total personality particularly with relationship to social work. Implications for consideration of workers with the blind: Different reactions to blindness among different ethnic groups, the blind as a subculture.

3498. Glister, Jim. "The gifties gien us." *New Outlook for the Blind*, Oct. 1963, Vol. 57, No. 8, pp. 316–18.

Discusses how ignorant sighted are about blind, yet fixed in their beliefs and disbeliefs. Author asks why loss of sight should make an otherwise ordinary person "different" and suggests it is a sort of superstition grown from a lack of understanding, an inability to explain away the apparently wonderful accomplishments of the blind.

3499. Goodman, William. When you meet a blind person. *New Outlook for the Blind*, June 1970, Vol. 64, No. 6, pp. 186–92.

Describes techniques for aiding the visually handicapped. Additional areas of concern are giving directions, mobility aids and devices, and dog guides.

3500. Gowman, Alan G. The role of companion. *New Outlook for the Blind*, Jan. 1957, Vol. 51, No. 1, pp. 17–24.

For the truly reciprocal role of companion to a blind person, the sighted individual must shed his stereotypes of blindness, the blind person must contribute equally to the relationship, and both must overcome the group pressures toward stereotyping.

3501. Haddle, Harold W., Jr. The modification of attitudes toward disabled persons: The case for using systematic desensitization as an attitude-change strategy. *American Foundation for the Blind Research Bulletin 28*, Oct. 1974, pp. 91–110.

Discusses relationship between anxiety theory and avoidance behavior. "There is evidence that attitudinal stimuli follow the context of a three-fold function: classical conditioning, reinforcement, and the discriminative controlling functions which such stimuli acquire." Ref.

3502. Haj, Fareed. On intermarriage among the blind. *New Outlook for the Blind*, May 1967, Vol. 61, No. 5, pp. 137–41.

Observations on whether blind people should marry, and especially whether they should marry other blind persons, and why they so often do marry blind partners. Suggests possible research.

3503. Handel, Alexander F. Community attitudes influencing psycho-social adjustment to blindness. *Journal of Rehabilitation*, 1960, Vol. 26, No. 6, pp. 23–25.

Discussion of the limitations placed upon the blind by a society acting in ignorance.

3504. ———. Community attitudes—A factor in the psycho-social adjustment to disability. *New Outlook for the Blind*, Dec. 1960, Vol. 54, No. 10, pp. 361–66.

Author suggests that remaining barriers to full integration are in the minds of the sighted and blind populations. Discusses stereotypes, vacillation between stifling sympathy and avoidance, progress made, and the role and responsibility of the social caseworker.

3505. Heeren, Ethel. Respectable and disrespectable diseases. *New Outlook for the Blind*, Jan. 1955, Vol. 49, No. 1, pp. 26–27.

Urges that the professional worker should not associate medical problems with morality or respectability or the lack thereof.

3506. Himes, Joseph S. Changing attitudes of the public toward the blind. *New Outlook for the Blind*, Nov. 1958, Vol. 52, No. 9, pp. 330–35.

Attempts to identify and characterize some forces and conditions influential on traditional American attitudes toward the blind. Includes discussion of the blind and the industrial labor market, the Social Security Act, wartime labor mobilization, agency programs, social consciousness, mass media.

3507. ———. The measurement of social distance in social relations with the blind. *New Outlook for the Blind*, Feb. 1960, Vol. 54, No. 2, pp. 54–58.

In a study carried out chiefly by means of questionnaires returned by undergraduate college students it was found that social distance increases directly with increase of the intimacy of social relationships and that in reciprocally committing relationships stereotypes become most decisive. Includes tables.

3508. Hingson, Michael. The disservice of service. In George Attleweed, et al., Eds., *Sensory disabilities study group report*. Calif. Conference on Rehabilitation, Oct. 8–10, 1974. n.p., n.d., pp. 45–48.

This paper is by a blind student whose message is that blind students should be provided with only those services that will enable them to compete with other students and will give them an opportunity for an equal education.

3509. Janicki, Matthew P. Attitudes of health professionals toward 12 disabilities. *Perceptual and Motor Skills*, Feb. 1970, Vol. 30, No. 1, pp. 77–78.

Presents a ranking of 12 disabilities in the order they were perceived as most disturbing. Blindness is 1st, with motor impairments following.

3510. Jastrzembska, Zofja S. Social and psychological aspects of blindness: A sampling of the literature. *American Foundation for the Blind Research Bulletin 25*, Jan. 1973, pp. 169–73.

Discusses lack of vision in the young child, adventitiously and aged blind, cross-cultural studies, and a 7-factor scale of attitudes toward blindness.

3511. Kim, Yoon Hough. *The community of the blind—Applying the theory of community formation.* New York: AFB, 1970, 151 pp., $3.50.

A monograph that studies the theory of community formation and how blind persons themselves form communities.

3512. Koch, Audrey S. Changing attitudes toward blindness: A role-playing demonstration for service clubs. *New Outlook for the Blind*, Nov. 1975, Vol. 69, No. 9, pp. 407–9.

Program designed and presented to 13 Lions and Rotary Clubs. Describes demonstration with blindfolded members of audience which was followed by discussion period. Pre- and post-questionnaires showed improvement in attitudes.

3513. Langdon, J. N. Some aspects of the employment and social life of young blind people in the midlands [England]. *New Beacon*, May 1970, Vol. 54, No. 637, pp. 114–22.

Young blind persons were interviewed concerning employment and social life. Results showed a well-established emphasis on the desirability of open employment when practicable. Most respondents were satisfied as to the suitability of vocational training received.

3514. Lowenfeld, Berthold. The social impact of blindness upon the individual. *New Outlook for the Blind*, Nov. 1964, Vol. 58, No. 9, pp. 273–77.

History of blind persons' relationship to society. Integration of blind persons into society. Role of vocational rehabilitation and social legislation in opportunities for the blind. Demise of homes for the blind. Advances in mobility training. Difficulties encountered with stereotyping. Goals still to be accomplished.

3515. Lukoff, Irving F., & Cohen, Oscar. *Attitudes toward blind persons.* New York: AFB, 1972, 74 pp., $2.

Two papers on social attitudes toward the blind and on discriminatory attitudes and the blind, along with 10 short papers designed as responses to the 2 initial papers.

3516. Lukoff, Irving F., & Whiteman, Martin. Attitudes toward blindness— Some preliminary findings. *New Outlook for the Blind*, Feb. 1961, Vol. 55, No. 2, pp. 39–44.

Findings relating to attitudes of sighted persons toward blindness and perceptions of blind persons of these attitudes. Through factor analysis several independent factors emerge leading to various implications for interaction between the two groups.

3517. ———. Intervening variables and adjustment: An empirical demonstration. *American Foundation for the Blind Research Bulletin 3*, Aug. 1963, pp. 55–65. Reprinted from *Social Work*, 1962.

Based on a sample survey of 500 legally blind persons in N.Y. State, evaluates "adjustment" in terms of: (1) employment, (2) travel independence, (3) independence in eating, and (4) independence in shopping. Related this to the attitudes of those around him as perceived by the blind person.

3518. ———. *The social sources of adjustment to blindness.* New York: AFB, 1970, 291 pp.

A study of the various aspects of the socialization process of blind persons and their implications. Ref.

3519. ———. Socialization and segregated education. *American Foundation for the Blind Research Bulletin 20*, Mar. 1970, pp. 91–107. Reprinted from #3518 above.

Studied a variety of factors which affected patterns of socialization. Found that attendance at a special school for the blind was most likely to result in the adult's saying most of his friends were blind. Ref.

3520. MacFarland, Douglas C. The public image of blindness. *New Outlook for the Blind*, May 1964, Vol. 58, No. 5, pp. 150–52.

Discusses public image of blindness and proposes to decide what image should be built by a study to ascertain: (1) what present public information is, (2) what agencies see as their role and what they do about public relations, and (3) what opinions of the blind clientele are.

3521. ———. Social isolation of the blind: An underrated aspect of disability and dependency. *New Outlook for the Blind*, Dec. 1966, Vol. 60, No. 10, pp. 318–19. Also in *Journal of Rehabilitation*, 1966.

Discusses isolation caused by inability to use the eye "as an instrument of social navigation," and inability to use many aids produced by and for the sighted majority. Mentions several ways helpful in breaking out of isolation, and types of training necessary to implement socialization.

3522. Marsh, Velma, & Friedman, Robert. Changing public attitudes toward blindness. *Exceptional Children*, Jan. 1972, Vol. 38, No. 5, pp. 426–28.

Reports an educational program with sighted high school freshmen to dispel mystery surrounding blindness and promote integration of blind students.

3523. Monbeck, Michael E. *The meaning of blindness: Attitudes toward blindness and blind people.* Bloomington: Ind. Univ. Press, 1973, 214 pp., $6.95.

Describes the various attitudes, investigates the cultural and historical sources of these attitudes, presents a broad outline of opinion and research dealing with the psychological origins of attitudes, interprets the meaning of blindness and discusses attitude changes and evaluates the various possibilities of improving attitudes.

3524. Moore, Virginia B. The white cane and I. *New Outlook for the Blind*, Apr. 1962, Vol. 56, No. 4, pp. 131–33.

Discusses her husband's early reluctance but gradual acceptance of cane.

3525. Morris, Harvey. The unhelped blind. *New Outlook for the Blind*, Sept. 1968, Vol. 62, No. 7, pp. 227–29. Reprinted from *New Society*, n.d.

Disabled people are not necessarily abnormal and should expect normal wages for their work. Society's attitude should be one of compassion.

3526. Muhlenkamp, A. F. Attitudes of nursing students toward eight major disabilities. *Psychological Reports*, Dec. 1971, Vol. 29, No. 3, pp. 973–74.

Nursing students ranked 8 disabilities according to degree of difficulty they felt they would experience were they to incur that disability. Results were compared with ranking by other professional groups.

3527. Murphy, Albert T. Attitudes of educators toward the visually handicapped. *International Journal for the Education of the Blind*, May 1961, Vol. 10, No. 4, pp. 103–07.

Results of a rating-scale study of attitudes toward various handicaps in 309 educators and education students.

3528. Okin, Tessie. Proceedings: Regional invitational symposium on attitudes toward blindness. New York: AFB, 1972, 85 pp. Mimeo.

This is a report of the symposium held by Region II. Includes the program with summaries of all areas of the symposium, presented in expanded outline form.

3529. Pascal, Joseph I. The changing attitude towards the blind and the partially sighted. *American Journal of Optometry*, 1954, Vol. 31, pp. 319–24.

Modern methods of rehabilitation of the visually handicapped are changing attitudes toward this group.

3530. Pa. Dept. of Public Welfare, Office for the Blind. *Attitudes and blind-*

ness: A workshop conducted for the staff of the Office for the Blind, Pennsylvania Department of Public Welfare. Harrisburg: Author, 1967, 73 pp. Papers resulting from a workshop on the formation and basic nature of attitudes.

3531. Rawls, Horace D. Cultural factors in disability. *New Outlook for the Blind*, Mar. 1957, Vol. 51, No. 3, pp. 87–92.

Traces the relationship of both material and behavioral aspects of a culture to the role of a disabled person in that culture. Changes in the culture are reflected in changes in that role.

3532. Ricketts, Peter. Always keep an open ear. *New Beacon*, May 1973, Vol. 57, No. 673, pp. 120–21.

Blind author decides idea is a myth that blind people, relying on other's voice for much information, assess others very accurately. Discusses what information voices may carry, "verbal prejudice."

3533. ———. Paying your way. *New Beacon*, July 1974, Vol. 58, No. 687, pp. 175–76.

Blind author discusses ways of sharing expenses for social activities though sighted participants dislike allowing blind man to pay his fair share.

3534. ———. Blind romance. *New Beacon*, Sept. 1975, Vol. 59, No. 701, pp. 228–30.

Author's personal attitudes toward marriage to another blind person.

3535. Rosenblum, Milton. The blind typhlophile. *New Outlook for the Blind*, Jan. 1965, Vol. 59, No. 1, pp. 18–20.

Describes 4 conflicting attitudes of the "blind typhlophile," all characterized by the blind person's claim to be normal and wish to be an accepted part of the community at the same time that he is claiming special privileges or speaking of "the blind." If blind people want respect rather than paternalism it is their responsibility to avoid the typhlophile image.

3536. Ross, Abraham S., & Braband, Janinne. Effect of increased responsibility on bystander intervention: II. The cue value of a blind person. *Journal of Personality and Social Psychology*, Feb. 1973, Vol. 25, No. 2, pp. 254–58.

Observed the reactions of 54 high school and 30 college males to an emergency which either threatened harm to themselves or to a person in another room. Results are explained in terms of the cue value of others present at the time of the emergency.

3537. Rossi, Peter, Jr., & Marotta, Michael. Breaking blind stereotypes through vocational placements. *New Outlook for the Blind*, Jan. 1974, Vol. 68, No. 1, pp. 29–32.

Discusses responsibility of relevant agencies to find unique, nonstereotyped placement for blind clients as one means of reducing stereotypical attitudes and concomitant limitations.

3538. Rotchford, Charlene. Helping sighted children develop realistic concepts of blindness. *New Outlook for the Blind*, Jan. 1961, Vol. 55, No. 1, pp. 16–18.

Fifth grade teacher of sighted children describes class projects designed to help students develop more understanding of blindness. "Children's Pledge to the Blind" was developed as a result.

3539. Rottman, Robert R. Attitude toward the blind and the "integrated" school. *New Outlook for the Blind*, Mar. 1958, Vol. 52, No. 3, pp. 78–82.

Discusses the implications of matter-of-factness for the blind child as well as resource room benefits in creating confidence in the blind child.

3540. Royster, Preston M. Proper hospital techniques can help sightless patients. *New Outlook for the Blind*, May 1965, Vol. 59, No. 5, pp. 184–85.

Rather detailed and specific suggestions for staff handling a hospitalized blind person to provide greater emotional security and comfort for the patient.

3541. Rusalem, Herbert. A study of college students' belief about deaf-blindness. *New Outlook for the Blind*, Mar. 1965, Vol. 59, No. 3, pp. 90–93.

With 132 college freshmen as Ss, attitude questionnaires show perception of deaf-blind persons as dependent, ingratiating, inhibited, socially conforming, and unsuccessful. Public education is needed.

3542. Rusalem, Herbert, & Rusalem, Roslyn. Students' reactions to deaf-blindness. *New Outlook for the Blind*, Oct. 1964, Vol. 58, No. 8, pp. 260–63.

Report of a study exposing high school students to a very successful deaf-blind person and studying their reactions via a questionnaire. Interest and learning momentum was aroused among the students; however, author thinks without follow-up these feelings may be shortlived.

3543. Schmidt, Leo J., & Nelson, Calvin C. Special class teacher attitudes toward affective and cognitive goals for visually handicapped students. *New Outlook for the Blind*, Dec. 1968, Vol. 62, No. 10, pp. 297–300.

Attitudinal study of 14 teachers of the visually handicapped indicates they do not perceive visual disability as necessarily associated with intellectual or achievement retardation, and they view the cognitive structure of the child as normal.

3544. Schulz, Paul J. The sight of blindness and the phenomenon of avoidance. *New Outlook for the Blind*, June 1975, Vol. 69, No. 6, pp. 261–65.

The sighted population's avoidance of blind people can be countered by more personal contact between blind and sighted persons and by agencies showing the abilities of blind persons in their programs.

3545. Sewell, Ray, & Sewell, Gloria, as told to Renate Wilson. *House without windows*. Toronto, Canada: Peter Martin Assoc., 1974, $8.95.

Through their own very personal story, the Sewells show how blind people go about their daily lives: Working, learning, housekeeping, socializing. A church group discussion on blindness led by them provides a summary of sighted people's attitudes toward the blind and how blind people would like the sighted to treat them.

3546. Shaw, John A. Sighted children and the blind. *New Beacon*, May 1974, Vol. 58, No. 685, pp. 117–19.

Blind author considers factors in sighted children's attitudes towards blind people/blindness: Spontaneous untutored reactions, openness, obviously learned reaction, supernatural associations, fear, etc.

3547. Siller, Jerome. Personality determinants of reaction to the physically disabled. *American Foundation for the Blind Research Bulletin 7*, Dec. 1964, pp. 37–52.

Reports initial findings for a 574-item self-report personality questionnaire which was administered to junior high school, high school, and college students. Suggests that accepting feelings toward the disabled exist only when the individual has a positive self-image and stable object relationships.

3548. ———. Reactions to physical disability by the disabled and the nondisabled. *American Foundation for the Blind Research Bulletin 7*, Dec. 1964, pp. 27–36.

A clinical and theoretical analysis of dynamics underlying (1) reaction to personal physical disability, and (2) negative attitudes of the nondisabled toward the disabled, using the concept of narcissism.

3549. Siller, Jerome, et al. *Studies in reaction to disability, XI: Attitudes of the nondisabled toward the physically disabled.* Washington, D.C.: Rehabilitation Services Admin., HEW, 1967, 105 pp.

One study used college, high school, and junior high school Ss to examine the relationships among measures of attitude toward the disabled. Demographic variables and indexes of personality traits described. Another study dealt with the relationship between personality structure and attitude toward the disabled.

3550. ———. *Studies in reaction to disability. XII: Structure of attitudes toward the physically disabled; disability factor scales—amputation, blindness, cosmetic conditions.* Washington, D.C.: Rehabilitation Services Admin., HEW, 1967, 106 pp.

Seven identical factors emerged from the amputation and blindness analysis: Interaction strain, rejection of intimacy, generalized rejection, authoritarian virtuousness, inferred emotional consequences, distressed identification, imputed functional limitations.

3551. Siller, Jerome; Ferguson, Linda T.; Vann, Donald H., et al. Structure of attitudes toward the physically disabled: The disability factor scales—Amputation, blindness, cosmetic conditions. *Proceedings of the 76th Annual Convention of the American Psychological Association*, 1968, Vol. 3, pp. 651–52.

3552. Spence, Ruth. Blank faces. *New Beacon*, May 1972, Vol. 56, No. 661, pp. 115–18.

Personal narrative by a blind woman concerning difficulties experienced in communicating with the sighted public.

3553. Steinzor, Luciana V. School peers of visually handicapped children. *New Outlook for the Blind*, Dec. 1966, Vol. 60, No. 10, pp. 312–14.

Presents summary of study to find out if sighted childrens' attitudes toward blindness related to contact with visually handicapped children in school settings. Implications include unreserved recommendation of full participation of visually handicapped adolescents in schools for the sighted.

3554. ———. Visually handicapped children: Their attitudes toward blindness. *New Outlook for the Blind*, Dec. 1966, Vol. 60, No. 10, pp. 307–11.

Do visually handicapped elementary and junior high students think of the blind and sighted as opposite and irreconcilable groups; how do they define sightedness and blindness; do they perceive some behavior patterns as more proper for each group? Conclusions given.

3555. Sterne, Richard S. Whose external reality? *Social Work*, 1963, Vol. 8, No. 1, pp. 127–28.

A critique of a report on role determinants for the blind. Questions the statistics presented.

3556. Swieringa, Marilyn. Robin A. Jensen, Illus. *See it my way.* Grand Rapids, Mich.: Institute for the Development of Creative Child Care, 1972, 48 pp., $1.50.

Based on author's experiences as a newly blinded person. She describes the types of people who both helped and hindered her in adjusting to new circumstances, new roles, and new demands. A down-to-earth guide, enlivened by stick figure illustrations.

3557. Thomas, Elizabeth C., & Yamamoto, Kaoru. School-related perceptions in handicapped children. *Journal of Psychology*, Jan. 1971, Vol. 77, No. 1, pp. 101–17.

Examines perceptions of specific curriculum areas and of school personnel by 500 handicapped children, including blind.

3558. ———. A note on the semantic structures of the school-related attitudes in exceptional children. *Journal of Psychology*, July 1972, Vol. 81, No. 2, pp. 225–34.

Administered a semantic differential form to 620 retarded, disturbed, blind, and deaf students. Classmates, teachers, parents, self, and 4 curriculum areas were rated.

3559. Whiteman, Martin, & Lukoff, Irving F. Public attitudes toward blindness. *New Outlook for the Blind*, May 1962, Vol. 56, No. 5, pp. 153–58.

Discusses attitude structure, development, change, and function. Considers effects of introjected attitudes upon the blind person, his self-concept, and his attitudes toward the sighted.

3560. ———. A factorial study of sighted people's attitudes toward blindness. *Journal of Social Psychology*, 1964, Vol. 64, No. 2, pp. 339–53.

Questionnaires on attitudes toward blindness were administered to 2 college groups. Factors identified were: (1) degree to which respondents have negative view of general adequacy of the blind, (2) degree to which they see blind as socially competent, (3) degree to which blindness is perceived as potentially threatening or uniquely frustrating, (4) tendencies to be protective of blind, (5) readiness for personal interaction with blind people.

3561. Wolman, Marianne J. Preschool and kindergarten child attitudes toward the blind in an integrated program. *New Outlook for the Blind*, Apr. 1958, Vol. 52, No. 4, pp. 128–33.

Discusses purpose, procedures, reactions of sighted children to partially sighted peers and attitudes of adults toward integrated classes.

3562. Wright, Beatrice A. An analysis of attitudes—Dynamics and effects. *New Outlook for the Blind*, Mar. 1974, Vol. 68, No. 3, pp. 108–18.

Factors influencing attitudes toward blind people and their abilities as well as guidelines for the improvement of attitudes and environmental opportunities are discussed.

33. Art, Music, Literature

3563. Allen, Alfred. Current developments in progress toward international uniformity in the field of braille music. *New Outlook for the Blind*, May 1953, Vol. 47, No. 5, pp. 121–25.

History of the problems and progress in developing, over about 100 years, uniform braille music notation.

3564. Alvin, Juliette. *Music for the handicapped child.* New York: Oxford Univ. Press, 1965, 150 pp.

Musical sensibility in the handicapped child and the contribution of music to a child's general emotional, intellectual, and social maturation are assessed.

3565. Anderson, Muriel. Art for visually handicapped. *School Arts*, June 1956.

Describes an experimental class at Milwaukee Art Institute.

3566. Andrews, F. M. Art experiences for blind children. *International Journal for the Education of the Blind*, May 1956, Vol. 5, No. 4, pp. 86–87.

Report on panel discussion of tactual art experience and interest in making art available for blind. Discusses the relationship between ability of appreciation and degree of blindness and age when became blind. Suggestions for improvements in ideas, art forms, use of tapes, etc.

3567. Beddoes, M. P. Toward an improved Optophone—Experiments with a musical code. *American Foundation for the Blind Research Bulletin 16*, May 1968, pp. 41–64, illus.

Notes that the Optophone is little used because difficult to learn. Proposes a "musical" code, less complex and easier to identify. Reports on 40–50 hours of training with blind and sighted Ss.

3568. Coon, Nelson. Blindness in the ceramic art of ancient Peru. *New Outlook for the Blind*, Dec. 1959, Vol. 53, No. 10, pp. 374–75, illus.

Archeological finds show that potters of ancient Peru clearly depicted blind persons, often as beggars or musicians.

3569. Dauterman, William L. Aesthetic considerations in the rehabilitation of the blind. *New Outlook for the Blind*, Feb. 1959, Vol. 53, No. 2, pp. 61–65.

Describes the effects of introducing music therapy and a variety of 3-dimensional art forms into the experience of blind persons at the Kansas Rehabilitation Center for the Blind. Suggests that the experience facilitated emotional acceptance of blindness.

3570. DeWyngaert, Laura. Art for the blind. . . . *Arts and Activities*, Feb. 1973, pp. 30–32, illus.

A junior high school art teacher writes concerning the efforts of her sighted class in developing art forms that would appeal to blind and partially sighted people.

3571. Ditzler, Harry J. To sound accord on braille music. *International Journal for the Education of the Blind*, Dec. 1955, Vol. 5, No. 2, pp. 37–39.

Presents the history of the Conference of Braille Music assisted by UNESCO, with list of representatives. Discusses research, projects, new note-for-note system, and changes from present system.

3572. Eaton, Allen H. Beauty for the sighted and the blind. New York: St. Martin's Press, 1959, 191 pp., illus. (Forward by Helen Keller.)

A description of aesthetic response to beauty of both seeing and blind persons with the object of encouraging communication between sighted and blind on aesthetic experience. Introduces objects which are beautiful to both sight and touch.

3573. Fukurai, Shiro. *How can I make what I cannot see?* Margaret Haas & Fusako Kobayashi, Trans. New York: Van Nostrand Reinhold, 1974, 127 pp., illus., $5.95.

Author relates his experiences in teaching art at a school for the blind and his understandings of blind children's thoughts and perceptions gained there.

3574. Goodenough, Forrest, & Goodenough, Dorothy. The importance of music in the life of a visually handicapped child. *Education of the Visually Handicapped*, Mar. 1970, Vol. 2, No. 1, pp. 28–32.

Discusses influences of music on blind child in following areas: Physical development in auditory discrimination and motor development, emotional development, opportunity for emotional outlet, creativity, increased attention span, ability to memorize, interaction with groups. Also discusses music in relation to gifted and multiply handicapped blind children.

3575. Gorson, Albert G. A comprehensive music service. *New Outlook for the Blind*, Mar. 1954, Vol. 48, No. 3, pp. 71–72.

Describes bimonthly publication, the record club, and the music information service of the Louis Braille Music Institute of America.

3576. Haupt, Charlotte. Self realization—But not through painting. *New Outlook for the Blind*, Feb. 1966, Vol. 60, No. 2, pp. 43–46.

Discusses need of blind persons for first-hand experience, for self-realization, and various media appropriate as vehicles of self-expression, artistic and other.

3577. Lisenco, Yasha. *Art not by eye: The previously sighted visually impaired adult in fine arts programs.* New York: AFB, 1972, 114 pp., $3.75, illus.

Designed to assist teachers and administrators of art programs to understand problems of the previously sighted visually impaired adult and guide him towards media and techniques giving the greatest aesthetic satisfaction. Discusses teacher attitudes and methods.

3578. Maynard, Merrill A. Painting by blind artists. *New Outlook for the Blind*, Nov. 1965, Vol. 59, No. 9, pp. 318–21.

A blind painter explains some of the satisfaction he finds in art, his methods, and why painting should be taught to blind children.

3579. Pitman, Derek J. The musical ability of blind children. *American Foundation for the Blind Research Bulletin 11*, Oct. 1965, pp. 68–80. Also in *Review of Psychology in Music*, 1965, No. 2.

Musical ability and general ability of 90 blind children and a matched group of 130 sighted children was measured. Results showed that the sighted group excelled significantly in English attainment and that the blind group was significantly superior in music.

3580. Revesz, G. *Psychology and art of the blind.* H. A. Wolff, Trans. New York: Longmans, Green, 1950, 338 pp.

The 1st part of the book centers on the haptics of form, particularly on establishment of principles of haptic perception, and attempts to provide a theoretical foundation for haptics and for psychology of the blind. The 2nd part is devoted to the aesthetic experience and to the sculptural activity of the blind.

3581. Ricketts, Peter. Learning to write. *New Beacon*, Sept. 1973, Vol. 57, No. 677, pp. 236–37.

The author, a blind adult, describes his experience in integrated creative writing class, and benefits, social as well as literary, it provided him.

3582. Rowland, William. An experiment in art appreciation by touch. *New Beacon*, May 1974, Vol. 58, No. 685, pp. 115–17.

Blind author and adviser to South African National Gallery discusses tactile values in art, sculpture exhibitions for the blind, opportunities for creative self-expression, establishment of a touch gallery.

3583. Sherman, Robert M. Why popular music for the blind? *New Outlook for the Blind*, Mar. 1958, Vol. 53, No. 3, pp. 89–92.

Discusses the term "popular music" in its various meanings. Lists suggestions for training and discusses opportunities for employment.

3584. Slatoff, Howard A. Integrated art experiences for blind children. *International Journal for the Education of the Blind*, Oct. 1962, Vol. 12, No. 1, pp. 17–18.

Rather general dicussion of art as an integrative experience; the child may identify with the whole object or the relationship of its parts. Art experiences should not be denied the child because he cannot experience them visually.

3585. Stoesz, Gilbert. *A suggested guide to piano literature for the partially seeing.* New York: National Society for the Prevention of Blindness, 1966.

The 262 selections are identified by degree of difficulty, size of notehead, name of publisher, and type of composition—collection, ensemble, solo, instructional. A selective listing.

3586. Swerdlow, David. Audio Drama: A mobile theater by the blind. *Rehabilitation Record*, May–June 1972, Vol. 13, No. 3, pp. 11–14.

Describes activities of a troupe of blind adults who travel around the New York City area bringing dramatic reading productions of major plays to numerous communities.

3587. Trevor-Roper, Patrick. *The world through blunted sight.* New York: Bobbs-Merrill, 1970, 191 pp., illus.

Considers influence of altered (other than normal) vision on art and literature. Writers and painters whose sight was impaired are used as examples. Text demonstrates how the nature of the impediment affected or is evident in the pattern of their artistry.

3588. Twersky, Jacob. *Blindness in literature: Examples of depictions and attitudes.* New York: AFB, 1955, 57 pp.

Reviews the ways in which blindness and blind people have been represented in the literature for the past 200 years.

3589. Wintle, Mary J. An answer to the blind musician's plight. *New Outlook for the Blind,* Apr. 1964, Vol. 58, No. 4, pp. 120–21.

Description of collection of music scores in braille available from Library of Congress.

34.   Recreation and Leisure Activities

3590. American Foundation for the Blind. *Integrating blind and visually handicapped youths into community social and recreational programs.* New York: Author, 197–, free.

An informative pamphlet giving many valuable pointers on "how to."

3591. Baird, Beatrix; Monsky, Millie; & Kratz, Laura E. A program of dance for visually handicapped young people: A symposium. *International Journal for the Education of the Blind,* Mar. 1958, Vol. 7, No. 3, pp. 85–89.

Combines 3 brief articles on values of a social dancing program, a program based on modern dance, and folk dancing. Describes the programs as developed in 3 different schools.

3592. Barnett, Marion W. Blind girl in the troop. *New Outlook for the Blind,* Nov. 1966, Vol. 60, No. 9, pp. 277–78.

Stating that there are about 1,000 visually handicapped girls in Scouting, author then gives general guidelines and assurances useful to troop leaders about to welcome blind members into their troops.

3593. Bean, Margaret A. Camp Lighthouse. *American Journal of Nursing,* May 1972, Vol. 72, No. 5, pp. 950–53.

Description of recreational and learning activities at summer camp for legally blind.

3594. Belenky, Robert. *A swimming program for blind children.* New York: AFB, 1955, 44 pp.

3595. Bisbee, Margaret K. Adapted horseshoes for the blind. *Rehabilitation Teacher,* Feb. 1970, Vol. 2, No. 2, pp. 33–36.

Horseshoes adapted for the blind described in terms of equipment, court, playing, and scoring.

3596. Bischoff, Robert W. Recreational activities for the visually handicapped. *Utah Eagle,* Jan. 1973, Vol. 84, No. 4, pp. 1–4, 7, 9.

Discusses a wide variety of recreational activities including dance, tumbling, swimming, wrestling, team sports, camping, fashion shows, and the keeping of pets.

3597. Boninger, Walter B. The small planning committee: A tool for meeting human needs. *New Outlook for the Blind,* June 1973, Vol. 67, No. 6, pp. 258–65, 271.

By dividing a social club of blind adults into small committees, psychogenic needs are met. Explains mechanics of setting up groups and suggestions for conducting meetings. Benefits noted for volunteer and professional staff as well as club members.

3598. ———, **Ed.** *Proceedings of the Special Demonstration Workshop for Integrating Blind Children with Sighted Children into Ongoing Physical Education and Recreation Programs* (Cleveland, Ohio, Oct. 9–10, 1969.) New York: AFB, 1970, 38 pp.

Social and psychological aspects of blindness as they relate to participation in physical activities.

3599. Boy Scouts of America. *Involving Handicapped Scouts: Scoutmaster's Guide.* North Brunswick, N.J.: Author, 1974.

3600. Brandt, L. C. Scouting at the Maryland School. *International Journal for the Education of the Blind,* Mar. 1956, Vol. 5, No. 3, p. 63.

Description of a blind Boy Scout troop and its similarity to other Scout troops. Information on activities and accomplishments (merit badges, etc.).

3601. Briller, Stanley, & Morrisson, Becky. Teaching rock and roll dancing to totally blind teenagers. *New Outlook for the Blind,* Apr. 1971, Vol. 65, No. 4, pp. 129–31.

Describes need for high school students to participate in the dancing of their sighted peers and how rock and roll dancing was taught to a group of blind teenagers in a community agency.

3602. Brownson, George. Visually-handicapped persons play baseball. *CCB Outlook,* Apr. 1972, Vol. 25, No. 2, pp. 20–22.

Detailed description of equipment and rules in baseball as adapted for the blind at the Canadian National Institute.

3603. Buell, Charles. Ten active games for blind children. *International Journal for the Education of the Blind,* Mar. 1955, Vol. 4, No. 3, pp. 62–64.

List and description of games which can be played by the blind. Mainly ball games.

3604. ———. Recreational and leisure-time activities of blind children. *International Journal for the Education of the Blind,* Mar. 1962, Vol. 11, No. 3, pp. 65–69.

With emphasis on integration and having the blind child do, as nearly as possible, what sighted children do, author discusses activities under 6 classes: Community, organizational, commercial entertainment, neighborhood, family, and individual activities.

3605. ———. Hiking aids physical, mental growth of blind children. *New Outlook for the Blind,* May 1965, Vol. 59, No. 5, pp. 175–76.

Describes values of hiking and how hikes can be organized for blind children.

3606. Carter, V. R. Bowling into the spotlight. *International Journal for the Education of the Blind,* Mar. 1959, Vol. 8, No. 3, pp. 100–101.

Explains how the National Bowling League of Schools for the Blind functions and invites participation of schools which are not already in the league. Bowling is done at the school, scores are exchanged by mail, and certain rules must be followed.

3607. Case, Maurice. The specialized recreation center for blind adults. *New Outlook for the Blind,* May 1959, Vol. 53, No. 5, pp. 176–78.

Reasons for a specialized recreation center, describes benefits with several brief case histores, and generally defends the specialized center.

3608. ———. *Recreation for blind adults.* Springfield, Ill.: Charles C Thomas, 1966, 208 pp.

Many adult activities can be used for youth groups. Includes discussion of arts and crafts, study and participation in dance and drama, literary and language activities, nature outings, sporting events. Qualifications of paid and volunteer staff are considered, as is their training.

3609. Castleton, David. True sportsmanship in Vienna. *St. Dunstan's Review,* Aug. 1973, No. 644, pp. 14–18.

Report on the 1st Austrian International Games for the Blind held in Vienna during June 1973. The 5 events were 50 meter sprint, shot put, long jump, medicine ball, and sling ball.

3610. Cohill, Audrey. Hobbies and the handicapped. *Top of the News,* Apr. 1969, Vol. 25, No. 3, pp. 282–85.

Description of a club to interest handicapped children in hobbies. Guest speakers used, sample hobbies shown, talking books and records available.

3611. Cohn, H. H. Skiing for the blind. *New Beacon,* Mar. 1974, Vol. 58, No. 683, pp. 68–70.

A blind individual describes skiing courses for the visually handicapped in France, Switzerland, Germany, Austria, and Norway.

3612. Coleman, Philip W. Photography for the partially blind. *New Beacon,* Jan. 1973, Vol. 57, No. 669, pp. 6–8.

Justification of photography as a hobby for the partially sighted, and of various camera equipment, its functions, pros and cons.

3613. Cornacchia, Theresa, & Spenciner, Loraine. Camp program for pre-school children with auditory and visual handicaps. *Education of the Visually Handicapped,* Oct. 1969, Vol. 1, No. 3, pp. 88–89.

Program used by, and adjustment problems of, camp. Positive and negative effects on children and their families.

3614. Dept. of the Interior, Bureau of Outdoor Recreation. *Outdoor recreation planning for the handicapped.* Washington, D.C.: National Recreation & Park Assoc., 1967, 43 pp.

Discusses planning and modification of play grounds, facilities, equipment to accommodate the handicapped, including the visually handicapped. Notes that such special consideration is prerequisite to state participation in the Land and Water Conservation Program. Gives addresses of some potentially helpful agencies, histories of some extant projects.

3615. Derganc, Mildred. Arts and crafts as related to vocational opportunities. *New Outlook for the Blind,* Feb. 1959, Vol. 53, No. 2, pp. 66–68.

Argues for the skill, creativity, and real beauty to be found in crafts. Describes use of crafts in rehabilitation and prevocational experiences.

3616. de Silva, Anthony. Back to the Ben. *New Beacon,* Sept. 1973, Vol. 57, No. 677, pp. 234–236.

One of 20 blind members of the Milton Mountaineers (7 sighted "companion" members) describes their 5th annual gathering and an ascent of Lochnagar Mt. (3,768 ft.).

3617. ———. Milton Mountaineers on the Glyders. *New Beacon,* July 1975, Vol. 59, No. 699, pp. 172–74.

How a group of blind mountain climbers functions with the aid of guides who are phys. ed. students.

3618. Dickman, Irving R. *I'm blind, let me help you.* New York: AFB, 1974, 20 pp.

Discussion of the merits of integrating the blind into volunteer service programs.

3619. DiMattia, Ralph. Sailing—A new experience. *New Outlook for the Blind*, May 1970, Vol. 64, No. 5, pp. 139–41.

Describes a summer sailing program for the blind including discussion of the benefits of increased confidence, independence, and socialization.

3620. Duggar, Margaret P. What can dance be to someone who cannot see? *Journal of Health, Physical Education, and Recreation*, May 1968, Vol. 39, No. 5, pp. 28–30.

Suggests methods of teaching blind children to dance, of developing spatial awareness, body awareness, rhythmic perception.

3621. Eastman, E. Elaine, & Blix, Sue. The importance of community recreation programs for visually handicapped people. *New Outlook for the Blind*, May 1971, Vol. 65, No. 5, pp. 144–48.

Recreation not only provides diversion and physical activity, but can be an excellent means of integration with sighted. Details a program, chiefly in camping.

3622. Felleman, Carroll. Integration of blind children in a recreational setting. *New Outlook for the Blind*, Sept. 1960, Vol. 54, No. 7, pp. 252–55.

Presents arguments for and against integration, and concludes in favor of integration. Discusses integration process at Jamaica Jewish Center Day Camp, and gives examples of several blind children involved.

3623. Fender, Linda. *Aquatic/swimming orientation manual.* Bethany, Okla.: Children's Convalescent Hospital, 1975.

This manual for volunteers discusses aims and values of aquatic swimming programs for special populations, including the deaf-blind. Also included are a glossary of hospital terminology and discussion of teaching hints for specific swimming skills.

3624. Fischer, Ernst. "I ski, though blind." *Ski*, Jan. 1954, Vol. 18, No. 4.

Describes methods of learning and continuing technique for blind skier, also skiing by groups in formation.

3625. Fisher, David. Blind students learn karate. *Journal of Rehabilitation*, July–Aug. 1972, Vol. 38, No. 4, pp. 26–27.

Karate training exercises aid in the development of kinesthetic awareness and could be of special value to the blind, who often have problems related to balance, posture, and coordination.

3626. Fullard, Bob. Merioneth mountaineers. *St. Dunstan's Review*, Aug. 1974, No. 655, pp. 14–16.

Four St. Dunstaners, including the author, made the climb of Cader Idris (2,927 ft.) in North Wales.

3627. Glass, Robert. Report of an integrated day-camp program. *New Outlook for the Blind*, Feb. 1959, Vol. 53, No. 2, pp. 55–57.

How 10 blind children were integrated in 2 day-camp programs and the favorable effects reported.

3628. Graeff, James W. School camping at the Michigan School. *International Journal for the Education of the Blind*, Mar. 1956, Vol. 5, No. 3, pp. 60–62.

Explanation in detail of 1st camping experience including planning (choice of site, group of children, materials, foods, utensils, etc.). Details of how all was accomplished, including activities.

3629. Graham, Milton D., & Clark, Leslie L. A model for contemporary society. *New Outlook for the Blind*, Dec. 1966, Vol. 60, No. 10, pp. 303–4.

Study of war-blinded veterans shows their use of leisure is personally rewarding and socially useful; may have much to teach a sighted society.

3630. Gravitz, Leonard. A study: Social participation of blind adults. *New Outlook for the Blind*, May 1954, Vol. 48, No. 5, pp. 149–51.

Results of interviewing 100 blind adults concerning their participation in social groups and less formal social contacts. Summary of a master's degree thesis.

3631. Gunston, David. Personal tapes. *New Beacon*, Oct. 1972, Vol. 56, No. 666, pp. 257–59.

Experience allows author to give "tips" on tape recording and listening, correspondence, purchase and use of equipment, subjects to tape for entertainment, and sense of involvement.

3632. Hack, Walter A. Marksmanship for the blind. *International Journal for the Education of the Blind*, Oct. 1965, Vol. 15, No. 1, pp. 24–25.

How sound coming through a target makes possible shooting practice and the values of a rifle club.

3633. Halliday, Carol. School camping—A meaningful experience. *New Outlook for the Blind*, Mar. 1964, Vol. 58, No. 3, pp. 81–82.

Benefits of school camping (moving classroom outdoors) are detailed, and it is emphasized that the positive aspects of the experience would be even more important to those with visual handicaps.

3634. Hanneman, Ralph. Bicycles provide recreation opportunities for the blind. *New Outlook for the Blind*, Feb. 1968, Vol. 62, No. 2, pp. 57–59.

Describes various ways in which cycling has been used by the blind, including the tandem, riding in parallel with a sighted companion, and unicycling.

3635. Hartman, R. Eugene. The perilous game of football. *International Journal for the Education of the Blind*, Feb. 1952, Vol. 1, No. 3, pp. 64–66.

Author believes football should neither be encouraged nor permitted among students of schools for the blind. Reasons given.

3636. ———. A game for totally blind boys. *International Journal for the Education of the Blind*, May 1958, Vol. 7, No. 4, pp. 138–39.

Exact description and instructions for "Floor Ball." This is a game for the totally blind.

3637. ———. Ball games for visually handicapped children. *New Outlook for the Blind*, Oct. 1974, Vol. 68, No. 8, pp. 348–55.

In addition to allowing students to interact actively with their classmates, a series of progressively more difficult games can help in the improvement of visual-physical efficiency. Full descriptions of a number of games are given.

3638. Held, Marian. Day camp as a step toward integration. *New Outlook for the Blind*, Dec. 1955, Vol. 49, No. 10, pp. 372–77.

General discussion of the values of camping and description of a day camp run by the Lighthouse, New York City.

3639. Hordines, John. Competitive rowing for blind boys. *International Journal for the Education of the Blind*, Mar. 1955, Vol. 4, No. 3, pp. 58–62.

Describes rowing in competition with sighted. Advantages of sport, general information: Size of boats, terminology, techniques and enjoyment of boys, special equipment, problems, coaching procedure.

3640. Huckins, Ross L. Camping for children who are blind. *New Outlook for the Blind*, Mar. 1963, Vol. 57, No. 3, pp. 91–94.

Discusses the chief goals of camping, preparing firewood, preparing the fireplace and lighting the fire, cooking over the campfire, sleeping quarters.

3641. Ireland, Ralph R. Recreation's role in rehabilitating blind people. *New Outlook for the Blind*, Apr. 1958, Vol. 52, No. 4, pp. 134–38.

Discusses factors in assessing importance of recreation, recreation opportunities, recreation in rehabilitation, recreation goals in rehabilitation of blind people, how to help and understand blind people.

3642. Jackson, Claire L. Recreation and the blind child. *New Outlook for the Blind*, Nov. 1957, Vol. 51, No. 9, pp. 402–6.

How to help the younger blind child integrate in the social and recreational activities of his community.

3643. Jones, Peter. Woodwork for the visually handicapped. *New Beacon*, Sept. 1974, Vol. 58, No. 689, pp. 229–32. 1st of series.

The author, a blind woodworker, discusses some problems, giving advice and information on ways to overcome them. Measurement, cutting, assembly, and finishing considered. Lists recommended tools.

3644. ———. Woodwork for the visually handicapped. *New Beacon*, Oct. 1974, Vol. 58, No. 690, pp. 256–58. 2nd of series.

Blind author discusses techniques for drilling holes and using woodscrews. Reviews somewhat sophisticated equipment and aids available to sighted, and also useful to the visually handicapped.

3645. ———. Woodwork for the visually handicapped. *New Beacon*, Nov. 1974, Vol. 58, No. 691, pp. 286–89. 3rd of series.

Discusses tools and aid useful to the visually handicapped person wishing to improve his woodworking results: Measuring/marking tools, screws, drills, cutting aids, power tools and attachments, integral tools, new products.

3646. ———. Woodwork for the visually handicapped. *New Beacon*, Dec. 1974, Vol. 58, No. 692, pp. 318–19. 4th of series.

Blind author gives detailed instructions on use of woodscrews for fixing hinges (which he says is difficult for blind worker), and general discussion of types of woodscrews and their uses.

3647. ———. Woodwork for the visually handicapped. *New Beacon*, Jan. 1975, Vol. 59, No. 693, pp. 5–6. 5th of series.

Tells how to "wall-plug," an operation which may be necessary when hanging something heavy on a wall; i.e., replace brick or concrete with material which can accept a screw or nail.

3648. ———. Woodwork for the visually handicapped. *New Beacon*, Feb. 1975, Vol. 59, No. 694, pp. 33–35. 6th of series.

Description of how to build a bookcase to hold standard braille books. Included are the materials and tools needed, and how to assemble it. Terms and prices are British.

3649. ———. Woodwork for the visually handicapped. *New Beacon*, Mar. 1975, Vol. 59, No. 695, pp. 65–67. 7th of series.

Reviews various kinds of joints employable in construction of furniture and evaluates them in terms of difficulty for a visually handicapped woodworker.

3650. ———. Woodwork for the visually handicapped. *New Beacon*, Apr. 1975, Vol. 59, No. 696, pp. 95–96. 8th of series.

Detailed instructions for making a bedroom stool.

3651. ———. Woodwork for the visually handicapped. *New Beacon*, May 1975, Vol. 59, No. 697, pp. 122–23. 9th of series.

How to finish a piece of woodwork, especially how to sand prior to staining or polishing.

3652. ———. Woodwork for the visually handicapped. *New Beacon*, June 1975, Vol. 59, No. 698, pp. 150–51. 10th of series.

General overview of some of the materials available in Great Britain to the woodworker and how he can tailor them to his needs.

3653. ———. Woodwork for the visually handicapped. *New Beacon*, July 1975, Vol. 59, No. 699, pp. 174–75. 11th of series.

Specific instructions for using a kit to make a tea wagon.

3654. ———. Woodwork for the visually handicapped. *New Beacon*, Aug. 1975, Vol. 59, No. 700, pp. 200–203. 12th of series.

Specific instructions for building a bedside cabinet.

3655. ———. Woodwork for the visually handicapped. *New Beacon*, Sept. 1975, Vol. 59, No. 701, pp. 230–32. 13th of series.

Specific instructions for construction of a storage cupboard.

3656. ———. Woodwork for the visually handicapped. *New Beacon*, Oct. 1975, Vol. 59, No. 702, pp. 257–59. 14th of series.

Specific instructions for building a bedhead as a link between 2 wardrobes.

3657. ———. Woodwork for the visually handicapped. *New Beacon*, Nov. 1975, Vol. 59, No. 703, pp. 285–88. 15th of series.

Review and evaluation of some specific materials and tools available to the woodworker in Great Britain.

3658. ———. Woodwork for the visually handicapped. *New Beacon*, Dec. 1975, Vol. 59, No. 704, pp. 311–13. 16th and last of series.

Specific instructions for building a cupboard.

3659. Josephson, Eric. *The social life of blind people.* New York: AFB, 1968, 150 pp., $2.25.

Article discusses leisure in relation to free time, age, impairment, and poverty. Also discussed are leisure time preferences, radio and television, social life, cultural activity, reading habits and methods, and the need for integration into the sighted world. Ref.

3660. Kempter, Richard R., Jr. Recreation concepts for the adult blind. *New Outlook for the Blind*, Nov. 1968, Vol. 62, No. 9, pp. 282–85.

Therapeutic recreation should meet the educational and development needs of the individual as well as providing happiness and fun. Acceptance and the development of independence are keys.

3661. Kirkland, Jack A. Integrated group work and recreation. *New Outlook for the Blind*, May 1962, Vol. 56, No. 5, pp. 166–68.

Discusses how we can make better use of recreation and group work in an integrated setting. Lists factors of integration with suggestions on coping with them.

3662. Koch, Audrey. Blind people as volunteers. *Rehabilitation Teacher*, June 1974, Vol. 6, No. 6, pp. 3–7.

The author, who is the rehabilitation teacher for the Aging Project of the Columbia Lighthouse for the Blind, reports on her success in finding satisfying service projects for some of her clients.

3663. Kraus, Richard. *Therapeutic recreation service: Principles and practices.* Philadelphia: W. B. Saunders, 1973, 234 pp., $9.

Various handicaps are satisfactorily described, but discussions on practical programming are limited.

3664. Laufman, Marjorie. Blind children in integrated recreation. *New Outlook for the Blind*, Mar. 1962, Vol. 56, No. 3, pp. 81–84.

Discusses ways of helping blind children become participants in recreational facilities available to other children in their own communities. Pamphlets such as "What to do when not in school," and "When you meet a blind child," proved helpful to leaders and camp directors.

3665. Laughlin, Sheila. A walking-jogging program for blind persons. *New Outlook for the Blind*, Sept. 1975, Vol. 69, No. 7, pp. 312–13.

Description of program at Tucson Assoc. for the Blind begun because blind individuals tend to be inactive physically. Walkers have stated that they feel 50–100% better since beginning the program.

3666. Leonard, Charles E. Sailing blind. *Yachting*, Aug. 1971, Vol. 130, No. 2, pp. 62–63, 90, 92.

The author, an engineer by profession, who had many years of sailing experience before he became blind, describes how he has adapted his sailing techniques and gives details of the audio compass he devised.

3667. Lions International. Idleness isn't on the agenda. *Lion*, Jan. 1972, Vol. 54, No. 7, pp. 10–13.

Picture story of the Colorado Lion's Foundation Center on the edge of Pike National Forest, a summer camp for blind and partially sighted children.

3668. Lloyds, A. D. The blind in an age of science: sports and hobbies for the blind. *New Beacon*, Nov. 1969, Vol. 53, No. 631, pp. 287–90.

Includes discussion of rowing, football, road walking, swimming, braille car rally, horseback riding, and golf. Discusses adaptations for the blind in darts, bowling, shooting, fishing, gymnastics. Hobbies discussed.

3669. McMullen, A. Robert, Ed. *Scouting for the visually handicapped.* North Brunswick, N.J.: Boy Scouts of America, 1974, 48 pp., app., $1.50.

Intended for parents of visually handicapped boys. Describes advantages, opportunities of Scouting, practical ways to compensate for lack of sight, possible modifications in various advancement areas.

3670. Matheson, Arnold E. Delivering recreation services to blind youth. *New Outlook for the Blind*, May 1969, Vol. 63, No. 5, pp. 153–56.

Staff, functions, and guidelines for an agency seeking to integrate blind youth into community recreation.

3671. Miller, Irving. Camping with the handicapped. *New Outlook for the Blind*, Nov. 1957, Vol. 51, No. 9, pp. 411–15.

Camping services for everybody meet an important social need. Integration in camping fights the isolation so likely to result from a handicap.

3672. Miller, Oral O. Cross-country skiing by the blind—A reality and a success. *Braille Forum*, May–June 1975, Vol. 13, No. 6, pp. 15–19.

Brief report on "Race For Light"—a cross-country ski race for the blind in Colo., Feb. 1975. Includes brief description of cross-country vs. downhill skiing.

3673. Moore, Dennis. To Westminster by canoe. *New Beacon*, July 1975, Vol. 59, No. 699, pp. 176–78.

Training for and participating in a canoe race.

3674. Paske, Valdemar, & Weiss, Walter. A study of leisure time activities of school students. *American Foundation for the Blind Research Bulletin 25*, Jan. 1973, pp. 233–40.

Results of a questionnaire of leisure time activities of 34 normal, 30 visually handicapped, and 14 deaf 8th and 9th graders in Denmark.

3675. Peterson, Carol A. Sharing your knowledge of folk guitar with a blind friend. *New Outlook for the Blind*, May 1969, Vol. 63, No. 5, pp. 142–46, illus.

Step-by-step instruction in how a sighted person can teach a blind friend folk guitar.

3676. Pitzer, John R. Nordic ski touring for the visually handicapped. *Education of the Visually Handicapped*, May 1974, Vol. 6, No. 2, pp. 63–64.

Cross-country skiing can be mastered quickly by the visually handicapped and is an excellent inexpensive activity for physical education, recreation and physical fitness.

3677. Pomeroy, Janet. *Recreation for the physically handicapped.* New York: Macmillan, 1964, 382 pp.

Modifications for a handicap are mentioned only when they are necessary.

3678. ———. Recreation for severely handicapped persons in a community setting. *New Outlook for the Blind*, Feb. 1972, Vol. 66, No. 2, pp. 50–55, 58.

Describes activities, benefits of program, enrollment policy, staff, etc.

3679. Pringle, Dough, & Winthers, Jim. *Ya see what we mean: Teaching the blind to ski.* Carmichael, Calif.: National Inconvenienced Sportsman's Assoc., 1974, 14 pp.

Illustrated manual contains instructions for teaching blind and partially sighted students to ski.

3680. Pruger, Robert. Standards for a comprehensive camping program with blind adults—A point of view. *New Outlook for the Blind*, Apr. 1963, Vol. 57, No. 4, pp. 121–26.

Discusses intake procedures, staff training, program, auxiliary services and philosophy.

3681. Resnick, Rose. Recreation: A gateway to the seeing world. *New Outlook for the Blind*, Nov. 1971, Vol. 65, No. 9, pp. 291–96.

Role of recreation in the process of personal and social adjustment for the blind child is discussed. Includes discussion of various categories of recreational activities and the therapeutic effects of each: Hiking, nature study, swimming, rowing, sports and games, folk and social dancing, dramatics, and music.

3682. ————. The specialized camp as preparation for integration. *New Outlook for the Blind*, Dec. 1972, Vol. 66, No. 10, pp. 374–76.

Describes camp in which handicapped are integrated with nonhandicapped peers with suggestions to make this experience a success.

3683. Richie, S. J. 48 Years of Scouting in the Kentucky School. *New Outlook for the Blind*, June 1959, Vol. 53, No. 6, pp. 221–22.

History, activities, and current status of Scouting at this school.

3684. Ritter, Charles. *Hobbies for the blind.* New York: AFB, 1953, 52 pp.

Covers hobbies for blind adults and youth.

3685. Scott, Eileen. Integrating blind children into community recreation. *New Outlook for the Blind*, June 1960, Vol. 54, No. 6, pp. 221–23.

Explains, with 3 examples, how blind children join in social activities of sighted, explaining counseling to parents and findings of parent groups.

3686. Stewart, Ian. Blind cricket. *New Beacon*, Aug. 1972, Vol. 56, No. 664, pp. 201–3.

Description of the game as it is played on an organized basis in Australia.

3687. Swerdlow, David. The beginning. *Rehabilitation Teacher*, Sept. 1974, Vol. 6, No. 9, pp. 3–14.

Sighted author recounts his experiences at a camp for the blind, resulting in new attitudes. Describes the camp's features, activities, programs.

3688. Teager, D. P. Technical aspects of coaching blind sportsmen. *New Beacon*, Mar. 1974, Vol. 58, No. 683, pp. 66–68.

Guidelines are given for the athletic coach.

3689. Tillinghast, Edward W. Hiking across the Grand Canyon. *International Journal for the Education of the Blind*, May 1957, Vol. 6, No. 4, pp. 94–95.

Describes the hike as done by 6 blind youths, how the boys prepared for this arduous outing, the challenges, and the feeling of success.

3690. Turner, Robert, & Biblarz, Arturo. Blind people can do more than tread water. *Braille Monitor*, Nov. 1971, pp. 920–22.

Report on techniques involved in adapting scuba diving as an activity for the blind.

3691. Wall, John A. On equal terms. *New Beacon*, Dec. 1972, Vol. 56, No. 668, pp. 316–17.

Discusses chess as game in which blind and sighted can meet on equal terms, and the *Braille Chess Magazine*.

3692. Watney, John. Sailing blind. *New Beacon*, Dec. 1970, Vol. 54, No. 644, pp. 311–15.

Sailing techniques practiced by blind headmaster of Rushton Hall, Kettering, England.

3693. Webster, Richard W. Jogging and the blind veteran. *New Outlook for the Blind*, Mar. 1973, Vol. 67, No. 3, pp. 116–18.

A discussion of the introduction of jogging as a recreational activity at a VA rehabilitation center. The specific, easy-to-learn techniques to be used by a sighted person acting as guide for a blind jogger are explained. Jogging is shown to be a practical, inexpensive activity that should be available to those blind persons who are interested in it.

3694. Williams, Chester T. A community drama project. *New Outlook for the Blind*, Feb. 1968, Vol. 62, No. 2, pp. 44–48. Also in *Therapeutic Recreation Journal*, 4th Quarter 1969.

How an agency for the blind developed a community drama group half of whose members were blind, the other half sighted. To the recreational values of drama were added public education and an integration experience.

3695. Williams, Chester T., & Coltoff, Kay. Sharing responsibility for an integrated day camp. *New Outlook for the Blind*, Mar. 1965, Vol. 59, No. 3, pp. 100–103.

Tells just how an agency for the blind related to other community agencies in developing and running integrated day camp experiences for blind children.

3696. Williams, Chester T., & Whitney, Polly. An experiment in day camping. *New Outlook for the Blind*, Mar. 1964, Vol. 58, No. 3, pp. 83–84.

Positive and negative aspects of a trial day camp program for visually handicapped children.

3697. Wolfe, Herbert J. The Key Club. *International Journal for the Education of the Blind*, May 1957, Vol. 6, No. 4, pp. 73-78.

The Key Club is a service group sponsored by Kiwanis. Tells how the club serves school and community and the benefits for the students involved.

3698. Wood, Tom, Ed. Highbrook: Vacation camp for blind persons. *Rehabilitation Teacher*, Mar. 1970, Vol. 2, No. 3, pp. 3–14.

Describes a camp for blind children and adults providing information on activities. App. presents information in learning skills of orientation, using a white cane, eating, clothing care, personal care, money handling, and general housekeeping.

3699. Woodcock, Charles C. School camping in Oregon. *New Outlook for the Blind*, June 1956, Vol. 50, No. 6, pp. 205-9.

Describes the interest and educational values of camping.

3700. Worden, Phyllis, Comp. *National Invitational Training Conference on Working with Youth With Special Needs through 4-H.* St. Paul: Univ. of Minn., 1971, 51 pp., $2.

Papers concern the mentally retarded, physically and visually handicapped.

3701. Young, Charles R. Scouting in residential schools for the blind. *International Journal for the Education of the Blind*, Oct. 1957, Vol. 7, No. 1, pp. 22–25.

Following background on Scouting in residential schools, describes a questionnaire study of the nature of Scouting programs in these schools, progress, weaknesses and strengths, and recommendations. Results from 29 participating schools are analyzed and 10 recommendations are made.

3702. Zok, Joseph E. *Instructional manual for blind bowlers.* Washington, D.C.: American Univ. & American Blind Bowling Assoc., 1970, 46 pp., illus.

Guide for sighted persons working with blind.

35.   Blind Persons and Other Biographies

3703. Barnett, M. Robert. Helen Keller and the American Foundation for the Blind. *New Outlook for the Blind*, Sept. 1968, Vol. 62, No. 7, pp. 201–5.

Recounts the story of Miss Keller's relationship with AFB with some personal reminiscences.

3704. Barnett, M. Robert; Henney, Nella B.; Migel, M. C.; et al. Saluting Helen Keller. *New Outlook for the Blind*, June 1955, Vol. 49, No. 6, unnumbered.

A special insert with pictures and tributes from many of Miss Keller's friends in honor of her 75th birthday.

3705. Brooks, Richard S. Blind, he leads the blind. *Rotarian*, May 1974, Vol. 124, No. 5, pp. 32–33, 51.

The story of Bryon Eguiguren, chairman of the Dept. of Romance Languages at Hadley School.

3706. Brooks, Van Wyck. *Helen Keller: Sketch for a portrait.* New York: Dutton, 1956, 166 pp.

A biography of Helen Keller.

3707. ———. For the blind. *New Outlook for the Blind*, Sept. 1968, Vol. 62, No. 7, pp. 209–13.

The story of Helen Keller's life beginning with 1917 and especially recording her services to the blind.

3708. Castleton, David. Don't shut me in—Charles Cummings. *St. Dunstans Review*, July 1974, No. 654, pp. 10–14.

Interview with Cummings, a blinded English veteran of World War II who has successfully continued farming in England, specializing in livestock.

3709. Coon, Nelson. New light on Louis Braille. *International Journal for the Education of the Blind*, Dec. 1954, Vol. 4, No. 2, pp. 41–42.

Recounts some of the lesser known accomplishments of Louis Braille.

3710. ———. Prospero Fagnani. *New Outlook for the Blind*, Feb. 1955, Vol. 49, No. 2, pp. 62–64.

The history of an eminent teacher of canon law who was blind, and some of his views about blindness.

3711. ———. Luigi Groto: His life and work. *New Outlook for the Blind*, Apr. 1955, Vol. 49, No. 4, pp. 137–38.

The story of a mid-16th-century Italian scientific commentator, political ambassador, and author.

3712. ———. Gottlieb Conrad Pfeffel 1736–1809. *New Outlook for the Blind*, Jan. 1958, Vol. 52, No. 1, pp. 33–34.

In addition to his many books of poetry and prose and his success as a schoolmaster, he was a prominent Protestant religious leader being in his last years president of the Evangelical Consistory of his city. He was totally blind by age 22.

3713. ———. Sir John Fielding. *New Outlook for the Blind*, Mar. 1958, Vol. 52, No. 3, pp. 95–96.

After receiving a "gentleman's education" Fielding lost his sight at the age of 19 and thereafter established what is now rated as the predecessor of the travel agency and general service organization.

3714. ———. George Eberhard Rumph. *New Outlook for the Blind*, Apr. 1958, Vol. 52, No. 4, pp. 147–48.

Biography of the blind author of a book which, for 3 centuries, was the main source of knowledge of plants in the East Indies.

3715. ———. William Hickling Prescott. *New Outlook for the Blind*, Jan. 1959, Vol. 53, No. 1, pp. 33–34.

One of a series of sketches of notable blind persons. Prescott was a historian and one of the founders of Perkins School for the Blind.

3716. ———. Morrison Heady (1829–1915). *New Outlook for the Blind*, Feb. 1959, Vol. 53, No. 2, pp. 73–74.

Brief account of a deaf-blind poet.

3717. ———. John Metcalf (1717–1810). *New Outlook for the Blind*, Mar. 1959, Vol. 53, No. 3, pp. 108–9.

Describes the varied talents of a blind man who, despite lack of formal education, engineered and managed difficult road construction.

3718. Fisher, Harold S. No greater light. *Nursing Mirror*, Oct. 9, 1970, Vol. 130, No. 15, pp. 39–40.

First-person report of secretary-accountant who went blind. Negative outlook finally turned positive. Now working as free-lance writer.

3719. Frank, Morris, & Clark, Blake. *First lady of the Seeing Eye.* New York: Henry Holt, 1957, 156 pp.

Essentially the story of Seeing Eye, told through the history and anecdotes of the people who developed it.

3720. Fraser, Ian. *Conquest of disability.* New York: St. Martin's Press, 1956, 224 pp.

A compilation of accounts, in 1st or 3rd person, of the processes involved in living with a disability. Five chapters have to do with blindness, 2 with multiple handicaps.

3721. ———. Understanding blindness. *Nursing Mirror*, Dec. 12, 1969, Vol. 129, No. 24, p. 44.

First person account of secretary who became blind in her middle 50s. Mentions problems and positive aspects of her life.

3722. Freund, Elisabeth D. *Crusader for light: Julius R. Friedlander, Founder of the Overbrook School for the Blind 1832.* Philadelphia: Dorrance & Co., 1959, 153 pp.

Biography. Tells much of condition of the blind and beginnings of education for them.

3723. Harper, Grace S. Major Migel: The early years. *New Outlook for the Blind*, Dec. 1958, Vol. 52, No. 10, pp. 365–67.

Reviews the history of Migel's work for the blind from before World War I until his death in 1958.

3724. Henney, Nella B. Annie Sullivan—A teacher's preparation. *New Outlook for the Blind*, Apr. 1966, Vol. 60, No. 4, pp. 102–5.

Brief history of Sullivan's early years.

3725. Hickok, Lorena. *Story of Helen Keller.* New York: Grosset & Dunlap, 1958, 181 pp.

3726. ———. *The touch of magic: The story of Helen Keller's great teacher, Anne Sullivan Macy.* New York: Dodd Mead, 1961.

3727. Irvine, Paul. Pioneers in special education: Robert Benjamin Irwin (1883–1951): A biographical sketch. *Journal of Special Education*, Winter 1970, Vol. 4, No. 1, pp. 1–2.

Describes major events in Irwin's life.

3728. Irwin, Robert B. *As I saw it.* New York: AFB, 1955, 205 pp.

Essentially a history of work with the blind over the 50 years of the author's experience, including changes in braille, libraries, the Talking Book, periodicals, education, and occupations.

3729. Keller, Helen. *Teacher: Anne Sullivan Macy.* New York: Doubleday, 1955, 247 pp.

Biography and tribute to Anne Sullivan Macy by her famous student.

3730. ———. The heaviest burden on the blind. *New Outlook for the Blind*, Sept. 1968, Vol. 62, No. 7, pp. 214–16.

Adaptation of an address by Helen Keller first printed in *Outlook*, April 1907. Urges intelligent help toward independence for blind people rather than disorganized charity.

3731. ———. On her deprivations. *New Outlook for the Blind*, Sept. 1968, Vol. 62, No. 7, p. 220.

Quoted from *The Open Door* by Miss Keller. Brief reflections on her feelings, or lack of feelings, of deprivation due to blindness and deafness.

3732. ———. Why men need woman suffrage. *New Outlook for the Blind*, Sept. 1968, Vol. 62, No. 7, pp. 217–19.

Article originally appeared in the Oct. 17, 1915, edition of the *New York Call*. Urges suffrage for women.

3733. Krents, Harold. *To race the wind: An autobiography.* New York: G. P. Putnam, 1972, 282 pp., $6.95.

The story of a very capable young man and the dramatic events of his growing up without vision. Basis for the play and motion picture *Butterflies Are Free.*

3734. Kugelmass, J. Alvin. *Louis Braille: Windows for the blind.* New York: Julian Messner, 1951, 160 pp.

Recounts life of Louis Braille. Includes his development of a 43-symbol code of punched dots used by the blind for reading, writing, and musical notation.

3735. Lende, Helga. Major Migel: His broad contribution. *New Outlook for the Blind*, Dec. 1958, Vol. 52, No. 10, pp. 363–65.

Presents overview of Migel's contributions to the good of blind persons, relating chiefly those activities involving him as head of AFB. Eulogy.

3736. Mulholland, Mary E. Helen Keller: 1880–1968. *New Outlook for the Blind*, Sept. 1968, Vol. 62, No. 7, pp. 201–5.

Upon the death of Miss Keller, this brief biography and tribute were published with illustrations and a quotation from her.

3737. Parsons, Patricia. Charles Cadwell. *New Beacon*, July 1973, Vol. 57, No. 675, pp. 173–75.

Profile/success story of blind man who started the Tape Recording Service for the Blind.

3738. Potts, P. C. The Migel Medal. *New Outlook for the Blind*, Jan. 1959, Vol. 53, No. 1, pp. 28–32.

Lists recipients of the Migel Medal from 1937 through 1958, with brief statements of the achievements of the recipients.

3739. Roblin, Jean. *The reading fingers: Life of Louis Braille.* Ruth G. Mandalian, Trans. New York: AFB, 1955, 66 pp.

Originally published in French in 1952.

3740. Ross, Ishbel. *Journey into light.* New York: Appleton, Century, Crofts, 1951, 213 pp.

The life stories of many blind people over the centuries.

3741. Rusalem, Herbert. Anne Sullivan: An analysis of her teaching techniques. *New Outlook for the Blind*, Apr. 1966, Vol. 60, No. 4, pp. 106–8.

Through excerpts from Helen Keller's writings and Sullivan's letters to a former Perkins employee, article compares Sullivan's techniques and methods favorably with those currently in use and declares her an innovative precursor of 20th-century techniques.

3742. Russell, Robert. *To catch an angel: Adventures in the world I cannot see.* New York: Vanguard Press, 1962, 317 pp.

Blind author recounts and reflects upon his life and the experiences which led him to a career of college teaching.

3743. ———. *The island.* New York: Vanguard Press, 1973, 274 pp., $6.95.

The author, accidentally blinded at age 5, recounts experiences at a summer cottage on a Canadian island in the St. Lawrence River over a 15-year period, describing such activities as cabin repair, camping, independent fishing experiences. Describes influences of others in the environment and the effects of his summer experiences.

3744. Simpson, Dorothea. Edward Rushton. *New Outlook for the Blind*, Nov. 1953, Vol. 47, No. 9, pp. 275–77.

History and accomplishments of a pioneer in work with the blind in Great Britain.

3745. ———. Stetson K. Ryan: An appreciation. *New Outlook for the Blind*, Sept. 1954, Vol. 48, No. 7, pp. 230–34.

Fairly detailed description of the life and accomplishments of Ryan and the Connecticut Board of Education of the Blind which he served as executive for 36 years.

3746. Smith, Geoffrey. A frank speaker. *New Beacon*, Oct. 1972, Vol. 56, No. 666, pp. 254–56.

Profile of Michael A. Killoran, liaison officer of the British N.F.B., relates his position on agencies, employment, etc., and gives relevant biographical information.

3747. ————. The fighter. *New Beacon*, Mar. 1974, Vol. 58, No. 683, pp. 62–65.

Profile of Bob Noon, a blind man who feels integration is the responsibility of the blind, and whose many activities, especially winning admission to judo classes and gaining the black belt, show positive results for his philosophy.

3748. ————. Henry and Chris. *New Beacon*, Sept. 1974, Vol. 58, No. 689, pp. 232–35.

Profile of blind couple who produce a talking newspaper and live very independently.

3749. ————. Profile: The sight saver. *New Beacon*, May 1975, Vol. 59, No. 697, pp. 113–16.

Biography of John Wilson, leader in work with the blind in United Kingdom.

3750. ————. The singer. *New Beacon*, Sept. 1975, Vol. 59, No. 701, pp. 225–28.

Biography of Margaret Townshend, a successful lyrical soprano.

3751. tenBroek, Jacobus. Newell Perry: Teacher and humanitarian. *New Outlook for the Blind*, Nov. 1954, Vol. 48, No. 9, pp. 328–31.

A short review of his life, activities, and achievements.

3752. A tribute to Murray B. Allen. *New Outlook for the Blind*, Feb. 1954, Vol. 48, No. 2, pp. 49–51.

Story of Allen's life and many services to blind people.

3753. Waterhouse, Edward J. The emergence of Anne Sullivan. *International Journal for the Education of the Blind*, Mar. 1966, Vol. 15, No. 3, pp. 82–83.

A tribute to Anne Sullivan 100 years after her birth.

3754. Weiner, Margery. *Helen Keller.* London: Heron Books, 1970, x + 327 pp., illus.

3755. Yates, Elizabeth. *The lighted heart.* Dublin, N.H.: William L. Bauhan, 1974, 251 pp., $3.95.

Soft-cover edition of a book originally published in 1960. The personal story of the author and her husband during the difficult period of adjusting to his blindness.

3756. Zook, Deborah. *Debby.* Scottdale, Pa.: Herald Press, 1974, 128 pp., $3.95.

Personal experience of losing sight, going to college, obtaining special training, securing employment, and finding fulfillment in life.

3757. Zwang, David. How I waged war against blindness. *Science Digest*, Mar. 1974, Vol. 75, No. 3, pp. 52–56.

Author's experiences in undergoing treatment for diabetic retinopathy by means of laser beam photocoagulation.

Associations and Agencies

American Association of Workers for the Blind, Inc.
1511 K Street, NW—Suite 637
Washington, D.C. 20005

American Council of the Blind, Inc.
106 Northeast Second Street
Oklahoma City, Okla. 73104

American Foundation for the Blind, Inc.
15 West Sixteenth Street
New York, N.Y. 10011

American Foundation for Overseas Blind, Inc.
22 West 17th Street
New York, N.Y. 10011

American Printing House for the Blind, Inc.
1839 Frankfort Avenue
Louisville, Ky. 40206

Association for Education of the Visually Handicapped, Inc.
    [formerly American Association of Instructors of the Blind, Inc.]
919 Walnut Street—4th floor
Philadelphia, Pa. 19107

Blinded Veterans Association
1735 DeSales Street, NW
Washington, D.C. 20036

Braille Institute of America, Inc.
741 North Vermont Avenue
Los Angeles, Calif. 90029

Bureau of Education for the Handicapped
2100 Regional Office Bldg. #3
Washington, D.C. 20202

Canadian Council of the Blind
96 Ridout Street (P.O. Box 2640)
London, Ontario, Canada

Canadian National Institute for the Blind
1929 Bayview Avenue
Toronto 17, Ontario, Canada

Christian Record Braille Foundation, Inc.
4444 South Fifty-second Street
Lincoln, Nebr. 68506

Clovernook Printing House for the Blind
7000 Hamilton Avenue
Cincinnati, Ohio 45231

The College for Teachers of the Blind
Royal School for the Blind
Church Road North
Wavertree
Liverpool L15 6TQ, England

The Council for Exceptional Children
1920 Association Drive
Reston, Va. 22091

Delta Gamma Foundation
6940 West Floyd Avenue
Lakewood, Colo. 80227

Dialogue Publications, Inc.
3100 Oak Park Avenue
Berwyn, Ill. 60402

Episcopal Guild for the Blind
157 Montague Street
Brooklyn, N.Y. 11201

Guide Dogs for the Blind, Inc.
P.O. Box 1200
San Rafael, Calif. 94902

Guiding Eyes for the Blind, Inc.
106 East Forty-first Street
New York, N.Y. 10017

Hadley School for the Blind
700 Elm Street
Winnetka, Ill. 60093

Howe Press of Perkins School for the Blind
175 North Beacon Street
Watertown, Mass. 02172

Jewish Braille Institute of America, Inc.
110 East Thirtieth Street
New York, N.Y. 10016

John Milton Society for the Blind
366 Fifth Avenue
New York, N.Y. 10001

Library of Congress
Division for the Blind and Physically Handicapped
1291 Taylor Street, NW
Washington, D.C. 20542

Lions International
York and Cermak Roads
Oak Brook, Ill. 60521

Louis Braille Foundation for Blind Musicians, Inc.
112 East Nineteenth Street
New York, N.Y. 10003

Matilda Ziegler Magazine for the Blind
20 West Seventeenth Street
New York, N.Y. 10011

National Accreditation Council for Agencies Serving the Blind
    and Visually Handicapped
79 Madison Avenue
New York, N.Y. 10016

National Association for Visually Handicapped, Inc.
3201 Balboa Street
San Francisco, Calif. 94121

National Braille Association
85 Godwin Avenue
Midland Park, N.J. 07432

National Braille Press, Inc.
88 Saint Stephen Street
Boston, Mass. 02115

National Center for Deaf-Blind Youths and Adults
105 Fifth Avenue
New Hyde Park, N.Y. 11040

National Committee for Research in Ophthalmology and Blindness
Wills Eye Hospital
1601 Spring Garden Street
Philadelphia, Pa. 19130

National Federation of the Blind
Randolph Hotel Building
DesMoines, Iowa 50309

National Industries for the Blind
1455 Broad Street
Bloomfield, N.J. 07003

National Institutes of Health, National Eye Institute
Bethesda, Md. 20014

National Retinitis Pigmentosa Foundation
8331 Mindale Circle
Baltimore, Md. 21207

National Society for the Prevention of Blindness, Inc.
79 Madison Avenue
New York, N.Y. 10016

Office of Education
400 Maryland Avenue, SW
Washington, D.C. 20201

Office of Education, Bureau of Education for the Handicapped
7th and D Streets, SW
Washington, D.C. 20202

The President's Committee on Employment of the Handicapped
1111 20th Street, NW
Washington, D.C. 20210

Recording for the Blind, Inc.
215 East Fifty-eighth Street
New York, N.Y. 10022

Rehabilitation Services Administration, Office for the Blind
    and Visually Handicapped
330 C Street, SW
Washington, D.C. 20201

Royal Commonwealth Society for the Blind
Commonwealth House
Heath Road
Hayward's Heath
Sussex RH16 3AZ, England

Royal National Institute for the Blind
224 Great Portland Street
London W1N 6AA, England

The Seeing Eye, Inc.
P.O. Box 375
Morristown, N.J. 07960

Social Security Administration
6401 Security Boulevard
Baltimore, Md. 21235

U.S. Civil Service Commission, Office of Selective Placement Programs
1900 E Street, NW
Washington, D.C. 20415

Veterans Administration
Office of the Administrator
810 Vermont Avenue, NW
Washington, D.C. 20420

Volunteer Services for the Blind, Inc.
919 Walnut Street
Philadelphia, Pa. 19107

Xavier Society for the Blind
154 East Twenty-third Street
New York, N.Y. 10010

Author Index

Aamoth, Lillie, 854
Abel, Georgie Lee, 4, 686, 687, 713, 714, 1262, 1263, 1264, 1265, 2756, 2912, 2913, 3273
Abels, H. Leola, 1585
Adair, Elly, 1226
Adams, George L., 2136
Adams, Sherrill, 1831
Adamshick, Donald R., 2685
Adaptive Physical Education Task Force, 855
Adelson, Edna, 478, 2248
Ahmad, Shahab, 2273
Ahr, Paul, 2414
AIM for the Handicapped, Inc., 856
Airasian, Peter W., 2543
Akau, Lindo Jo, 857
Alabama State Dept. of Education, 715
Alameda County Public Schools
  See Alameda County School Dept.
Alameda County School Dept., 2544, 2545
Alaska State Dept. of Education, 716
Alavi, S. Hassan, 370
Albrecht, Marcella, 3274
Albright, Tacy B., 858
Alekseev, O. L., 2938
Alexander Graham Bell Association for the Deaf, 279
Alfano, Joseph E., 519
Alford, Albert L., 280
Alford, Milton M., 1586
Allan, Dennis, 2458
Allegheny County Schools, 479
Allegheny Intermediate Unit No. 3, Exceptional Children's Program, Pittsburgh, Pa., 480
Allen, Alfred, 154, 3563
Allen, Edward E., 6
Allen, Gordon W., 1587
Allen, Robert M., 3275

Allen, Sue P., 3275
Allison, Louise, 697
Allwein, Herman, 1456
Alonso, Lou, 859, 860, 1755, 2546, 3110
Altman, Anne, 1588
Altmann, John, 2547
Altshuler, Kenneth Z., 13, 2137
Alvin, Juliette, 3564
Amadeo, Marco, 2274
American Academy of Ophthalmology and Otolaryngology, 3017
American Association for Health, Physical Education and Recreation, 861, 862
American Association of Instructors of the Blind
  See Association for Education of the Visually Handicapped
American Association of Workers for the Blind, 1, 2, 3, 4, 5, 6, 7, 8, 9, 10, 11, 12, 13, 1589, 1913, 2138, 3111
American Foundation for Overseas Blind, 371
American Foundation for the Blind, 14, 15, 16, 17, 155, 156, 157, 482, 483, 863, 864, 865, 866, 1268, 1328, 1412, 1457, 1458, 1459, 1590, 1591, 1592, 1593, 1756, 1914, 1915, 1974, 1975, 2479, 2480, 2481, 2482, 2483, 2548, 2549, 2757, 2758, 2759, 3112, 3113, 3114, 3115, 3276, 3277, 3442, 3443, 3481, 3590
American Library Association, 1757
American Optometric Association, 325
American Printing House for the Blind, 158, 1758, 2760, 2761, 2762
Ames, A. C., 326
Ammons, Carol H., 2550
Amster, Clarence H., 2830
Andermann, K., 1919

Grannis, Florence, 2856
Gravitz, Leonard, 3630
Gray, P. G., 405
Greater Detroit Society for the Blind, 1650
Greaves, Jessie R., 3331
Green, M. R., 3332
Green, Mary B., 3245
Greenberg, Herbert M., 697, 2196
Greene, Frederick L., 3333
Greene, Robert J., 3334, 3335
Greenhalgh, Robert, 199
Greenwood, E., 2857
Greenwood, Ernest, 1439
Greer, Peter S., 3457, 3458
Gregg, Nancy J., 1580
Grier, Timothy L., 341
Griffin, Carol, 3160
Griffis, Gretta, 2506
Griffith, Carolynn, 550
Griggs, Norman J., 1289
Grim, Rosemary A., 1933
Gross, Joseph, 2334
Grossberg, Sidney H., 1651
Grossman, Rose T., 549
Grosvenor, Theodore, 406
Grosz, Hanus J., 2197, 2198, 2271
Groth, Hilde, 407
Grover, Edward C., 768
Grover, Wayne, 985
Groves, Doris, 550
Groves, Paul A., 1204, 1224, 1225
Gruber, Kathern F., 70, 290, 1390, 1545, 3336
Grumpelt, Howard R., 2858
Grunwald, Arnold P., 2859
Grupp, James W., 986
Guarniero, G., 3071
Guber, Donald, 3166
Guess, Doug, 2335, 3337, 3338, 3339
Guldager, Lars, 769, 3168, 3169
Gulkus, Steven P., 2126
Gumm, Mrs. Harvey, 770
Gunderson, Robert, 1652
Gunston, David, 3631
Gust, Tim, 1236
Gwaltney, John L., 408

Haase, Kenneth W., 342
Habel, Adelaide, 1820, 1902
Hack, Walter A., 2860, 3632
Hadary, Doris, 1137
Haddle, Harold W., 3501

Hadley School for the Blind, 1653
Haffly, John E., 3230
Hagberg, Carolyn L., 1862
Haj, Fareed, 3502
Haliczer, S. L., 988
Hall, George C., 551
Hall, Margaret M., 989
Hall, Richard C., 3340
Hall, William, 771
Hallam, Kris, 552
Hallenbeck, Charles E., 7, 1654
Hallenbeck, Jane, 553, 3341
Hallenbeck, Phyllis N., 2031, 2199, 2200
Halliday, Carol, 554, 3633
Halliday, Gordon W., 3170
Hallman, Heinz E., 2634
Halpin, Gerald, 2336, 2337, 2338
Halpin, Glennelle, 2336, 2337, 2338
Hambrecht, F. T., 3072
Hamilton, Ross E., 3342
Hamilton-Wilkes, Monty, 2610
Hammer, Edwin K., 3171, 3172, 3173, 3174, 3175
Hammill, Donald D., 2032, 2033, 2034, 2299, 2342
Hampshire, Barry E., 2861, 2862, 2863
Hanaway, Thomas P., 3176
Handel, Alexander F., 71, 72, 190, 291, 1440, 1655, 3503, 3504
Haney, R. R., 2399
Hanley, Leo F., 2864
Hanneman, Ralph, 3634
Hanninen, Kenneth A., 772, 2339, 2340
Hans, Michael A., 2341
Hansen, Carl E., 1383
Hanson, Howard H., 343
Hapeman, Lawrence, 2611, 2612
Harding, G. F. A., 2363
Hardy, Richard E., 73, 74, 1385, 1475, 1493, 1656, 1657, 2035, 2201, 2202, 2300
Hare, Betty A., 2342
Harford, Earl, 2704
Hargrove, Eugene A., 2138
Harkness, Charles A., 1658
Harley, Randall K., 344, 345, 346, 347, 409, 1272, 2343, 2865, 2866, 2867, 3018, 3343, 3344
Harley, Robison D., 1952
Harlow, Steven D., 2203, 2955
Harper, Florine W., 990
Harper, Grace S., 3723

Analytical Subject Index

Abbreviations

sa   *See also*. Indicates a reference to a related or subordinate topic

xx   *See also from*. Indicates a related topic from which a *sa* reference is made

ABACUS, 882, 897, 932, 981, 982, 983, 994, 1010, 1042, 1045, 1056, 1086, 1089, 1992
    sa APPLIANCES
Ability Tests
    See TESTS AND TESTING
Accidents, Prevention of
    See SAFETY
ACCREDITATION, 124, 190, 191, 194, 196, 207, 232, 237, 260, 272, 788, 831, 836, 837, 838, 839, 1264, 1688
    sa EDUCATION
    xx AGENCIES—Standards
Achievement Tests
    See TESTS AND TESTING— Achievement
Adjustment Centers
    See REHABILITATION CENTERS
ADJUSTMENT TO BLINDNESS, 49, 125, 587, 632, 646, 655, 693, 711, 1104, 1115, 1421, 1470, 1486, 1495, 1527, 1581, 1931, 2016, 2045, 2051, 2136, 2137, 2141, 2144, 2145, 2152, 2153, 2154, 2165, 2173, 2175, 2177, 2184, 2189, 2210, 2218, 2222, 2224, 2225, 2231, 2241, 2242, 2243, 2244, 2246, 2254, 2256, 2258, 2266, 2270, 2291, 2382, 2458, 2473, 2515, 2531, 2604, 2732, 3145, 3517, 3518, 3545, 3569, 3718, 3720, 3721, 3755, 3756
    sa BLINDNESS
    xx NEWLY BLINDED; PSYCHOLOGY OF THE BLIND

ADOLESCENT BLIND, 228, 686, 687, 690, 692, 693, 695, 697, 698, 699, 703, 704, 705, 706, 707, 708, 710, 711, 739, 959, 1088, 1331, 1350, 2139, 2156, 2192, 2259, 2427, 2602, 2607, 2671, 2755, 3375, 3601
ADVENTITIOUS BLINDNESS, 1490, 2102, 2172, 2294, 2304, 2695, 3492, 3510
    xx AGE AT ONSET OF BLINDNESS; WAR-BLINDED
AFRICA, 406, 417, 451, 469
AGE AT ONSET OF BLINDNESS, 553, 2184, 2275, 2313, 2354, 2375, 2399, 2400, 2415, 2420, 2426, 2428, 2449
    sa ADVENTITIOUS BLINDNESS
    xx NEWLY BLINDED
AGENCIES, 23, 39, 88, 112, 115, 118, 125, 130, 135, 141, 152, 155, 156, 157, 159, 161, 170, 171, 172, 177, 182, 183, 187, 192, 193, 194, 197, 200, 201, 202, 204, 208, 210, 214, 219, 223, 227, 228, 246, 249, 251, 252, 253, 256, 258, 259, 262, 264, 265, 285, 381, 440, 459, 466, 574, 611, 675, 729, 756, 790, 1382, 1386, 1407, 1433, 1442, 1481, 1712, 1742, 2480, 2497, 3030, 3096, 3130, 3148, 3149, 3150, 3172, 3300, 3320, 3506, 3520
    sa RADIO NETWORKS FOR BLIND; STATE COMMISSIONS;